Geriatric Medicine

Geriatric Medicine

SECOND EDITION

John W. Rowe, M.D.
Professor of Medicine and Director, Division
on Aging, Harvard Medical School; Chief,
Gerontology Division, Beth Israel and
Brigham and Women's Hospitals, Boston,
Massachusetts

Richard W. Besdine, M.D.
Associate Professor of Community Medicine
and Internal Medicine and Travelers Professor
of Geriatrics and Gerontology, University of
Connecticut School of Medicine; Director,
Travelers Center on Aging, University of
Connecticut Health Center, Farmington,
Connecticut

Little, Brown and Company
Boston   Toronto

Contents

Contributing Authors

BURT ADELMAN, M.D.
Assistant Professor of Medicine, Medical College of Virginia; Member, Division of Hematology/Oncology and Staff Physician, Hunter Holmes McGuire Medical Center, Richmond, Virginia

JERRY AVORN, M.D.
Associate Professor of Social Medicine, Harvard Medical School; Attending Physician, Gerontology Division, Department of Medicine, Beth Israel and Brigham and Women's Hospitals, Boston, Massachusetts

RICHARD W. BESDINE, M.D.
Associate Professor of Community Medicine and Internal Medicine and Travelers Professor of Geriatrics and Gerontology, University of Connecticut School of Medicine; Director, Travelers Center on Aging, University of Connecticut Health Center, Farmington, Connecticut

BRUCE J. BAUM, D.M.D., PH.D.
Clinical Director and Chief, Clinical Investigations and Patient Care Branch, National Institute of Dental Research, National Institutes of Health, Bethesda, Maryland

PETER BONIS, B.S.
Student, New York University School of Medicine, New York, New York

HARVEY J. COHEN, M.D.
Professor of Medicine and Director, Center for the Study of Aging and Human Development, Duke University; Director, Geriatric Research Education and Clinical Center, Veterans Administration Hospital, Durham, North Carolina

NAOMI K. FUKAGAWA, M.D., PH.D.
Instructor, Division on Aging and Department of Pediatrics, Harvard Medical School, Boston, Massachusetts; Assistant Director, The Clinical Research Center and Instructor, Whitaker College, Massachusetts Institute of Technology, Cambridge, Massachusetts

TERRY T. FULMER, PH.D., R.N.
Associate Professor of Nursing, Columbia University, New York, New York

RICHARD A. GARIBALDI, M.D.
Professor of Medicine, University of Connecticut School of Medicine; Vice-Chairman, Department of Medicine, University of Connecticut Health Center, Farmington, Connecticut

TOBIN N. GERHART, M.D.
Instructor in Orthopaedic Surgery, Harvard Medical School; Attending, Department of Orthopaedic Surgery, Beth Israel Hospital, Boston, Massachusetts

DAVID F. GIANSIRACUSA, M.D.
Associate Professor of Medicine, University of Massachusetts Medical School; Director, Division of Rheumatology/Immunology, Department of Medicine, University of Massachusetts Medical Center, Worcester, Massachusetts

BARBARA A. GILCHREST, M.D.
Professor and Chairman, Department of Dermatology, Boston University School of Medicine; Senior Scientist, U.S.D.A. Human Nutrition Research Center on Aging, Tufts University, Boston, Massachusetts

SUSAN L. GREENSPAN, M.D.
Instructor in Medicine, Harvard Medical School; Associate in Medicine, Gerontology Division and Department of Endocrinology, Beth Israel and Brigham and Women's Hospitals, Boston, Massachusetts

DONALD A. JURIVICH, D.O.
Fellow, Division of Geriatrics, Department of Medicine, Duke University Medical Center, Durham, North Carolina

FRED G. KANTROWITZ, M.D.
Assistant Professor of Medicine, Harvard Medical School; Associate in Medicine, Rheumatology Unit, Beth Israel Hospital, Boston, Massachusetts

JONATHAN KAY, M.D.
Clinical and Research Fellow in Medicine, Harvard Medical School and Department of Rheumatology/ Immunology, Brigham and Women's Hospital, Boston, Massachusetts

LEWIS A. LIPSITZ, M.D.
Director, Geriatric Fellowship Program, Harvard Medical School; Director of Education and Clinical Research, Hebrew Rehabilitation Center for the Aged, Boston, Massachusetts

BENJAMIN LIPTZIN, M.D.
Assistant Professor of Psychiatry, Harvard Medical School, Boston, Massachusetts; Director of Geriatric Psychiatry, McLean Hospital, Belmont, Massachusetts

KENNETH G. MANTON, PH.D.
Research Professor, Demographic Studies, Duke University; Medical Research Professor, Community and Family Medicine, Duke University Medical Center, Durham, North Carolina

GRAYDON S. MENEILLY, M.D., F.R.C.P. (C)
Instructor in Medicine, Division on Aging, Harvard Medical School; Physician, Department of Medicine, Beth Israel and Brigham and Women's Hospitals, Boston, Massachusetts; Physician, Geriatric Research Education and Clinical Center, Brockton/ West Roxbury Veterans Administration Medical Center, West Roxbury, Massachusetts

KENNETH L. MINAKER, M.D., F.R.C.P. (C)
Assistant Professor of Medicine, Harvard Medical School; Associate Physician, Department of Medicine, Beth Israel and Brigham and Women's Hospitals, Boston, Massachusetts; Deputy Director, Geriatric Research Education and Clinical Center, Department of Medicine, Brockton/West Roxbury Veterans Administration Medical Center, West Roxbury, Massachusetts

ELLEN G. NEUHAUS, M.D.
Assistant Professor of Medicine, University of Connecticut School of Medicine, Farmington, Connecticut; Chief of Infectious Diseases and Hospital Epidemiologist, Rockville General Hospital, Rockville, Connecticut

BRENDA A. NURSE, M.D.
Assistant Professor of Medicine, University of Connecticut School of Medicine, Farmington, Connecticut; Chief, Infectious Diseases and Epidemiology, The New Britain Memorial Hospital, New Britain, Connecticut

TERRENCE A. O'MALLEY, M.D.
Instructor in Medicine, Harvard Medical School; Associate Physician, Department of Medicine, Massachusetts General Hospital, Boston, Massachusetts

TANIA J. PHILLIPS, B.SC., M.B.B.S., M.R.C.P.
Fellow in Geriatric Dermatology, Boston University School of Medicine, Boston, Massachusetts

CAROL C. PILBEAM, M.D., PH.D.
Assistant Professor of Internal Medicine, University of Connecticut School of Medicine; Assistant Director, Travelers Center on Aging, University of Connecticut Health Center, Farmington, Connecticut

MICHAEL S. RABIN, M.D.
Research Fellow in Medicine, Harvard Medical School; Research Fellow, Hematology/Oncology Division, Beth Israel Hospital, Boston, Massachusetts

NEIL M. RESNICK, M.D.
Assistant Professor of Medicine, Harvard Medical School; Chief, Geriatrics Unit and Director, Continence Center, Brigham and Women's Hospital, Boston, Massachusetts

JOHN W. ROWE, M.D.
Professor of Medicine and Director, Division on Aging, Harvard Medical School; Chief, Gerontology Division, Beth Israel and Brigham and Women's Hospitals, Boston, Massachusetts

CARL SALZMAN, M.D.
Associate Professor of Psychiatry, Harvard Medical School; Director of Psychopharmacology, Massachusetts Mental Health Center, Boston, Massachusetts

LOWELL E. SCHNIPPER, M.D.
Theodore W. and Evelyn G. Berenson Associate Professor of Medicine, Harvard Medical School; Chief, Division of Oncology, Beth Israel Hospital, Boston, Massachusetts

BETH J. SOLDO, PH.D.
Chair, Department of Demography, Georgetown University, Washington, D.C.

DAVID SPARROW, D.SC.
Assistant Professor of Public Health, Boston University School of Medicine; Epidemiologist, Normative Aging Study, Veterans Administration Outpatient Clinic, Boston, Massachusetts

THOMAS M. WALSHE, M.D.
Assistant Professor of Neurology, Harvard Medical
School; Associate Chief of Neurology, Brockton/
West Roxbury Veterans Administration Medical
Center, Brockton, Massachusetts

SAN WANG, M.D., PH.D.
Instructor in Medicine, Harvard Medical School;
Associate Attending Staff, Beth Israel Hospital,
Boston, Massachusetts

JEANNE Y. WEI, M.D., PH.D.
Associate Professor of Medicine, Harvard Medical
School; Director, Gerontology Research Lab-
oratory, Gerontology and Cardiovascular Divisions,
Beth Israel Hospital, Boston, Massachusetts

SCOTT T. WEISS, M.D.
Associate Professor of Medicine, Harvard Medical
School; Associate Physician, Beth Israel Hospital,
Boston, Massachusetts

TERRIE WETLE, PH.D.
Assistant Professor of Medicine, Harvard Medical
School, Boston, Massachusetts; Director for
Research, Braceland Center for Mental Health and
Aging, Institute of Living, Hartford, Connecticut

T. FRANKLIN WILLIAMS, M.D.
Director, National Institute on Aging, National
Institutes of Health, Bethesda, Maryland

VERNON R. YOUNG, PH.D., D.SC.
Professor of Nutritional Biochemistry, Department
of Applied Biological Sciences, Massachusetts
Institute of Technology, Cambridge, Massachusetts

Preface to the Second Edition

This volume represents the second edition of *Health and Disease in Old Age,* which was first published in 1982. The substantial growth of information in the field of geriatrics over the past six years is reflected both in the expansion of all the chapters that appeared in the first edition and in the addition of several new chapters. The subjects of the new chapters include functional assessment, which is rapidly becoming the new technology of geriatrics; abuse, neglect, and inadequate care; rehabilitation; the oral cavity; cancer; and Paget's disease of bone.

In this edition we have maintained our emphasis on providing substantial information on the physiologic and psychosocial changes that occur with age, both in introductory chapters and in the initial portions of the organ-specific chapters.

American geriatrics has taken major strides in the 1980s. In 1988, the first examination leading to certification of added competence in internal medicine and family practice was given, and the first cohort of geriatric medicine fellowship programs was reviewed for certification by the Accrediting Council for Graduate Medical Education. By the 1990s admission to the examination in geriatrics will require satisfactory completion of a two-year fellowship in an accredited program. Despite this progress, recent reports from the National Institute on Aging and the Institute of Medicine document the urgent need for many more clinical and academic geriatricians. Federal, foundation, and state initiatives are developing support for establishment of robust academic programs in geriatrics. These centers will produce a cadre of clinicians/teachers and investigators who will establish academic activities in most or all medical schools and ensure that the next generation of physicians will have been taught the principles and practice of geriatric medicine.

We are pleased to contribute to the rapid development of the data base for geriatric medicine and its ongoing maturation to its proper place in academic medicine. We hope this text is useful for the growing number of students, practitioners, fellows, and faculty concerned with geriatric medicine.

J.W.R.
R.W.B.

Preface to the First Edition

The past 10 years have seen American geriatrics advance from obscurity to visibility through numerous programs in medical schools and teaching hospitals. This increasing interest has been accompanied by an increased demand for educational materials and curriculum offerings in geriatric medicine at the undergraduate levels. We offer this textbook in the hope that it will be of value to medical students, physicians-in-training, and practitioners. In its development, we have attempted to strike a balance between the desire for completeness and the recognition that much of what is generally considered to be geriatric medicine is discussed very adequately in textbooks of primary care or general internal medicine.

This book has several characteristics that we hope will make it useful. We have included substantial information about the normal physiologic and psychosocial changes that occur with age, both in introductory chapters and in the initial portions of each individual chapter. This reflects our belief that much of the influence of age on disease presentation, response to treatment, and ensuing complications results from the interaction of a disease process with an age-altered physiologic substrate. The juxtaposition of normal age-related changes and disease characteristics should help the physician to identify the separate clinical consequences of aging and disease. This book generally contains information only on diseases that occur late in life or that present special characteristics in the elderly as compared to younger individuals. Since our aim was to write a book that could appropriately serve as a supplement to a more general text rather than to reproduce a textbook of internal medicine, we have chosen not to include information regarding many diseases and, in the case of hematology, an entire organ system. We have included subjects not usually found in general texts, such as the biology and physiology of aging, the social context of geriatric medicine, long-term care, nutrition, ethical issues in geriatrics, and a consideration of the research methodologies appropriate for clinical gerontologic investigations.

We hope that this book will provide physicians with a gerontologic data base and with principles of geriatric medical practice so that they can better arm themselves to care for the disproportionate burden of illness borne by our increasingly large elderly population.

J.W.R.
R.W.B.

Geriatric Medicine

1

The Biology and Physiology of Aging

JOHN W. ROWE
SAN WANG

ALTHOUGH AGING IS a universal phenomenon that affects every one of us in profound ways, the study of aging has not been a part of mainstream biologic research. Indeed, most textbooks of biology make no mention of the subject. Yet aging is intrinsic to all higher animals, and its inevitability and universality beg for biologic explanations. This chapter reviews some commonly held theories of aging, the biologic and physiologic changes associated with aging and their clinical impact, and some recent promising approaches to the study of human aging.

What Is Aging?

For most people, the term *aging* evokes an array of changes based on their own experiences and their observations of others. Generally, aging may be considered an irreversible process that begins or accelerates at maturity and results either in an increasing number or range of deviations from the ideal state or in a decreasing rate of return to the ideal state, or both. Kohn [1] defines aging in several contexts: (1) chemical aging, manifested by changes in the structure of crystals or in macromolecular aggregations; (2) extracellular aging, manifested by progressive cross-linkage of collagen and elastin fibers or by amyloid deposition; (3) intracellular aging, manifested by changes in normal cellular components or by accumulation of substances such as lipofuscin in cells; and (4) aging of entire organisms.

Aging is inevitable, and every living organism has a finite life span. Moreover, each species has a characteristic maximum attainable life span. Improved nutrition and health care have increased the average human life span from less than 20 years in ancient Greece to well over 70 years in the United States today, but they have not altered the approximately 110-year maximum life span of our species.

It is interesting that the maximum life span, which is so constant within a species, may vary tremendously even among closely related animals such as mammals—50-fold between mice and men, for example. Relations have been determined between species life span and body weight or brain weight, basal metabolic rate, reproductive rate, and ability to repair DNA damage [2].

Biologic Theories of Aging
THEORIES RELATING TO ALTERATIONS IN MACROMOLECULES
Errors in Protein Synthesis
The theory of protein synthesis errors holds that age-associated impairments in cellular function result from an accumulation of errors in protein synthesis [3]. It is reasoned that random mutations in DNA, or errors in transcription or

translation, accumulate with aging to a level that markedly impairs cell function. A "catastrophe" resulting in loss of function would be particularly likely if the error were present in factors responsible for DNA synthesis. Substantial basic research in aging during the past two decades has shown that both transcription and translation maintain their fidelity with advancing age and that aging is characterized by a remarkable constancy of the amino acid sequence of a variety of physiologically important proteins. Specific findings inconsistent with the error catastrophe theory include (1) aged fibroblast cultures infected with viruses do not have a decreased virus yield; (2) newly synthesized enzymes from tissues in the aged are found to contain no synthetic errors; (3) experimentally induced errors fail to produce an error catastrophe; (4) there is no increase in the infidelity of codon recognition by transfer RNA molecules with age; and (5) there are no age-related differences in the accuracy of poly(U)-directed protein synthesis. Thus, the error theory is considered by many to be disproven.

Posttranslational Modifications
(Cross-Linkage Theory)
The cross-linkage theory is based on the finding that, although transcription and translation remain intact with age, *altered* proteins accumulate with advancing age. Thus, posttranslational modifications may be important in mediating age-related losses in cell and organ function. A number of physiologically critical enzymes have been shown to undergo posttranslational modifications with age, though these changes are by no means universal. One important posttranslational modification—glycosylation—appears to be important in age-related development of increasing opacification in crystalline lens protein and eventual development of cataracts [4]. Another modification, increased cross linking, is central to the major aging changes that occur in collagen and might have direct clinical consequences for arteriosclerosis and other diseases. Cross links should not be considered important only in extracellular tissues because an age-related increase in cross links has also been shown to occur in DNA. There are a number of important criticisms of this theory,

including the lack of evidence for varied rates of posttranslational change in the same class of molecules in different species despite the remarkable diversity in species specificity of life span [5]. Although it is unlikely that posttranslational modifications are central to all age-related biologic decrements, there is general agreement that they may play an important role in the emergence of some clinical consequences of aging.

Altered Protein Turnover
Another aspect of protein chemistry that has attracted substantial gerontologic attention is the alterations in the *rate* of protein biosynthesis that occur with age. Although, as previously stated, there appears to be no mis-synthesis of proteins with age, many proteins are *produced more slowly* in aged cells than in their younger counterparts. Delays have been identified in all of the four major stages of protein synthesis, including aminoacylation of tRNA, initiation, elongation, and termination [6].

In addition, it has been shown that lysosomal pathways for elimination of proteins are substantially altered with age. Some proteins are degraded more quickly than in younger cells, whereas others are turned over much more slowly. Future experiments in recombinant DNA techniques to correct modifications in these lysosomal pathways will permit evaluation of the impact of these changes on cell aging.

DNA Damage, Repair, and Somatic Mutation
The intact fidelity of protein synthesis with age does not exclude major age-related alterations in DNA, since a substantial portion of DNA is responsible for regulatory rather than synthetic activities. The DNA damage and repair theory focuses on the fact that DNA is constantly damaged throughout life and that age-related impairment in the repair mechanisms might be expected to be associated with progressive declines in cellular function [7]. Although modifications in DNA repair capacity with age have been identified, these have generally not been well correlated with life span, suggesting either that DNA repair defects are not important in

aging or that, to date, investigations have not focused on the critical repair mechanisms.

The somatic mutation theory of aging also falls under this rubric. There is evidence from karyotype banding studies that chromosomal aberrations increase in somatic cells with aging. Schimke et al. [8] postulated that this increase is due to disruptions in the timing and number of the multiple initiations of DNA replication on single chromosomes, leading to overreplication of certain segments of DNA and subsequently to the generation of a wide variety of rearrangements and aberrations. Shmookler Reis et al., studying senescence of normal somatic human cells in vitro, found substantial interclonal and intraclonal variations in genotype and phenotype. They postulate that stochastic influences or random environmental events, accumulating over the life span of the organism, generate cellular heterogeneity, which may in turn explain the age-related increase in diseases that are of clonal origin, such as cancer and atherosclerosis [9].

FREE RADICAL THEORY

Free radicals are highly reactive atoms or molecules bearing an unpaired electron that can cause random damage to structural proteins, enzymes, lipids, informational macromolecules, and DNA. In mammals the most important source of free radicals is the reduction of oxygen, with subsequent generation of hydrogen peroxide. The free radical theory holds that advancing age is associated with an accumulation of low-level free radical damage, which leads to the physiologic and clinical consequences associated with aging [10]. Normal defense mechanisms against free radical damage include a number of endogenous antioxidants, including selenium-containing glutathione peroxidase, superoxide dismutase, bilirubin, and tocopherol, as well as DNA repair mechanisms. Preliminary support for this theory rests on studies indicating that animals whose oxygen consumption is high in proportion to their size have shorter life spans and that administration of antioxidants results in modest increases in life expectancy. In primates, the levels of the cellular antioxidant superoxide dismutase correlate well with life span. Additionally, in lower forms of life mutations leading to defects in

production of free radical quenching enzymes are associated with shorter life spans [5].

ORGAN SYSTEM THEORY (PACEMAKER THEORY)

The organ system (or pacemaker) theory holds that certain organs or organ systems decline with advancing age, and their loss of function drives the systemic aging process. The organs that have attracted the most attention as the "pacemakers" of aging are the immune system and the neuroendocrine system, particularly the hypothalamus.

Immunosenescence is well documented in humans and experimental animals. Aging is associated with declines of over 75 percent in T-lymphocyte function as well as a progressive development of autoantibodies. Although clinical consequences of immunosenescence have not been experimentally demonstrated, there are obvious potential clinical ramifications such as increased morbidity from infections, increased risk of cancer, and perhaps autoimmune damage as well [11]. Support for the importance of these changes in the aging process is found in studies of mice that are identical except for the major histocompatibility complex (MHC); these studies show a close relation between MHC and life span [12].

The neuroendocrine system is another central control complex in which marked age-related changes have been identified and that has been proposed as a possible aging pacemaker. Sympathetic nervous system responsiveness is increased with age, and it has been postulated that this increase may be responsible for a number of age-related changes such as hypertension, impaired carbohydrate tolerance, and altered sleep architecture [13]. Investigators have also sought to identify the presence of a "death hormone," a substance that is produced in increasing amounts with advanced age. To date, no firm data are available to support the presence of such substances.

These theories focusing on individual organ systems as major regulators of systemic aging suffer from the weakness that not all organisms known to age have well-developed immune or neuroendocrine systems and that such theories fail to explain the origin of the changes in the pacemaker system itself.

GENETIC THEORIES OF AGING

Despite the apparent lack of evolutionary value of increases in life span beyond the reproductive years, gerontologists have long been attracted to the notion that just as growth and development are clearly regulated by a systematic turning on and off of various genes, so aging might represent a process in which systematic modifications in gene expression result in age-related and pathologic changes. Several of the theories of aging discussed above are linked by the likelihood that the basic mechanisms of aging, whether they be decreases in the production of antioxidants, impairments in DNA structure or repair, age-related modifications of protein disposal systems, or modifications of T-cell function, may all have a genetic basis.

Substantial information exists that supports the view that genetic factors are important to the aging process. There is a remarkable species specificity to life span. Within a particular species, the life expectancy of identical twins is more similar than that of nonidentical twins, and this in turn is more similar than that of siblings. On a more basic level, recent studies in *Caenorhabditis elegans,* a nematode, have identified mutant varieties with life spans that exceed the normal life spans of this species by 50 percent [14]. In some of these strains, the life span extension appears to be due to a single gene change. These findings suggest that more intensive genetic approaches are promising avenues for future research in aging, as will be discussed later.

Prominent among the genetic theories of aging is the program theory. This theory holds that cells have an intrinsic biologic clock, a sequence of events programmed into the genome that generates the aging process, an extension of the program of growth and development from the fertilized egg [5]. The finding by Hayflick and Moorhead [15] that normal human diploid cells have a finite proliferative capacity when cultured in vitro and that cells from old adults divide fewer times than cells from young adults before becoming senescent [16, 17] is the strongest support for this theory (Fig. 1-1). There is also a correlation between the maximum life span of a species and the number of doublings that fibroblast-like cells isolated from it can undergo in tissue culture before reaching

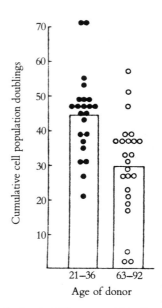

FIGURE 1-1. *In vitro life spans of skin fibroblast cultures from young and old men in cumulative number of cell population doublings. (From E. L. Schneider and Y. Mitsui. The relationship between in vitro cellular aging and in vivo human age. Proc. Natl. Acad. Sci. U.S.A. 73:3584, 1976.)*

a growth crisis or senescence [18] (Fig. 1-2). It is not generally thought that organisms age because their cells have used up their replicative capacity but rather that their finite replicative capacity is an expression of their aging program. Hayflick and Moorhead's discovery gave an enormous stimulus to modern research on the cell biology of aging; some of these findings are reviewed below.

Cellular Aging

The study of aging at the cellular level has largely focused on aging in the readily obtainable, fibroblast-like cell cultures, particularly on the mechanisms of their loss of replicative capacity with an increasing number of passages in culture. With in vitro senescence, Gl, the initial phase of the cell replication cycle, becomes extended, and eventually the cycle at the interface of Gl with the S or synthesis phase is arrested, preventing initiation of a new round of DNA synthesis and replication. Cell fusions between normal diploid cells that senesce and virally or spontaneously transformed immortal

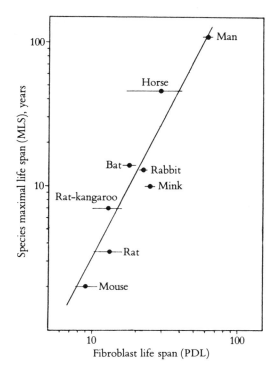

FIGURE 1-2. *Linear correlation (log/log) between species maximal life span (MLS) and their fibroblast life spans in vitro (PDL). (From D. Rohme. Evidence for a relationship between longevity of mammalian species and life spans of normal fibroblasts in vitro and erythrocytes in vivo. Proc. Natl. Acad. Sci. U.S.A. 78:5009, 1981.)*

cells have shown that the phenotype of limited proliferation is dominant over the phenotype of immortality [17]. Senescent cells produce a membrane-associated protein that inhibits initiation of DNA synthesis [19]. Microinjection of poly(A) messenger RNA from senescent cells inhibits DNA synthesis in proliferation-competent cells [20]; presumably, these RNA molecules code for factors that suppress initiation of DNA synthesis. Cell proliferation also requires external growth factors, and as cells become senescent, they lose their response to mitogenic growth factors. Epidermal growth factor (EGF) is one of the best characterized peptide mitogenic factors, and Carlin and her colleagues [21] have shown that in senescent cells, although EGF receptor density does not change, its kinase activity, measured by autophosphorylation of tyrosine residues on stimulation by EGF, is strikingly decreased.

Human cells, unlike rodent cells, almost never escape senescence when grown in vitro, and O'Brien et al. [22] have postulated that cellular senescence, or resistance to immortalization, plays a key role in protection against cancer in humans. In summary, cells have a range of proliferative behavior: regulated proliferation during growth and development, inhibited proliferation with aging, and uncontrolled proliferation in cancer. Understanding the control of cell replication is an active arena of research of crucial importance to all three of these areas.

Modifiers of Aging

In any discussion of the biology of aging, the question naturally arises whether any environmental, dietary, or pharmacologic interventions can be made to diminish the negative impact of aging and perhaps to extend life. This subject has recently been thoughtfully reviewed by Schneider and Reed [23]. Among the more plausible interventions are (1) regular exercise, which may decrease plasma lipid and insulin levels, retard bone mineral loss, and enhance cardiovascular performance; (2) dietary antioxidants [24], particularly vitamins C and E, which are postulated to inhibit free radical interactions with cell macromolecules and membrane lipids; (3) trace minerals, notably selenium, whose deficiency may be a risk factor for coronary heart disease and cancer; (4) aspirin, which affects platelet aggregation and inhibits thromboembolic events; and (5) the omega-3 fatty acids, found in especially high concentrations in fish oils, which may have beneficial effects on platelet and vascular endothelial functions, plasma lipids, cell membrane fluidity, and neutrophil functions [25]. Controlled clinical trials to test objectively the efficacy of some of these interventions in preventing human diseases are being planned or carried out, but the huge public interest in favorable interventions, especially by simple dietary means, and the workings of the free market system do not favor waiting for hard data.

One specific intervention to extend life span in laboratory rats and mice, namely caloric restriction, has been known for 50 years and has reattracted considerable attention. For instance, Yu and his colleagues [26] have shown that food restriction to 60 percent of ad libitum intake in barrier-reared Fischer-344 male rats increased mean length of life and life span by 40 percent. Food restriction delayed the appearance of pathologic lesions associated with aging in this strain. The reasons for this effect remain to be elucidated. Also, the effect may not apply to humans. Andres has analyzed insurance data from over 4 million policies taken out between 1954 and 1972 and has found that the body mass index (a measure of obesity) associated with the lowest mortality increases with age [27]. Andres' analysis of the available literature suggests that individuals who are initially lean and gain 20 to 25 pounds between young adulthood and age 60 have lower overall mortality risk than lean individuals who do not gain weight.

New Approaches to the Study of the Biology of Aging

Recent developments in cell biology, molecular biology, and recombinant DNA technology have opened new vistas for aging research that promise to increase our understanding of the biology and physiology of aging. Among these developing areas for study are the following.

1. *Cell growth and trophic factors.* The great majority of the cells in adult animals are nondividing cells. Many of these cells have been found to require trophic factors to maintain their differentiated functions. Furthermore, it has become clear that even cells generally thought to be terminally differentiated, such as neurons in the central nervous system, can exhibit plasticity in response to injury. Cells that do divide throughout life, such as hematopoietic cells, require growth factors to stimulate division and other factors to differentiate. Some of the cellular protooncogenes expressed in all cells code for growth factors or their receptors. On a simplistic level, one could postulate that many aging changes may be due to decreased production, decreased action, or altered expression of growth and trophic factors and normal products of cellular protooncogenes and that correction of these deficiencies could alleviate some of aging's effects on the cells involved.

2. *Detailed mechanistic studies of physiologic changes with aging.* Many physiologic changes with aging in humans are well characterized, and

the contributory effects of disease and environmental factors have been largely identified. Among these are impaired glucose tolerance, decreased baroreceptor responses, increased sympathetic nervous system activity, and defective diuretic responses to salt and water loads. In many of these systems, both the effector organs and the receptor tissues can be isolated (e.g., for glucose homeostasis, the islets of Langerhans and the fat cells), and detailed biochemical studies are possible. Such studies may allow one to pinpoint specific steps that are impaired with aging at the cellular and subcellular levels and then to generalize to the steps in other physiologic systems that are likely to be affected by aging, eventually targeting interventions to these steps when they lead to important clinical dysfunction.

3. *Longevity genes.* Modern techniques in molecular biology, particularly recombinant DNA technology, have markedly facilitated comparisons of gene expression by cells under differing conditions. These techniques are being applied to detection of proteins and messenger RNA molecules present in cells near the limit of their in vitro proliferative capacity and comparison of them with molecules present in cells at early doubling levels. Once a partial protein sequence is known or a specific messenger RNA molecule isolated, a nucleic acid probe can be produced, and the gene responsible for the protein or message can be isolated and sequenced. It may be possible using this approach to identify "longevity" genes that are preferentially expressed in long-lived animals or humans versus their short-lived counterparts. Identification of the genes should eventually lead to identification of the function of these genes and thus to understanding how the aging process is controlled. It is assumed that the number of genes that affect longevity or aging is a small subset of the 100,000 or so genes in the human genome. Indeed, this approach has recently been used in the study of the most clinically important geriatric disorder, Alzheimer's disease, generating exciting new leads in understanding the genetic components of its pathogenesis.

With the increased longevity of our population, the aging process has a large and ever increasing impact on health and disease. Application of modern biomedical research techniques will bring the study of the biology and physiology of aging into the mainstream of biomedical research, hasten our understanding of aging, and facilitate development of interventions to lessen the functional disability and disease that aging engenders.

Clinical Impact of the Aging Process
PHYSIOLOGY OF NORMAL AGING
A thorough understanding of the age-related physiologic changes that occur in humans in the absence of disease is critical to the diagnosis and the mangement of disease in old age. These physiologic changes influence the presentation of disease, its response to treatment, and the complications that ensue. Cross-sectional and longitudinal studies in carefully screened community-dwelling groups across the adult age range indicate that increasing age is accompanied by inevitable physiologic changes that are separate from the effects of disease. Growth and development, characterized by rapid increases in many physiologic functions, generally continue into early adulthood, peaking in the late twenties or early thirties. In those variables that change with age after adulthood (and not all do), a linear decline begins at the end of the growth and development phase and continues into old age. There is generally no pleasant plateau during the middle years during which physiologic function is stable, but rather a progressive age-related reduction in the function of many organs.

The loss of function of most variables that do change with age is linear into the eighth and ninth decades and does not increase as we become older. Thus, the rate of aging does not change in most cases—an 80-year-old man is aging just as fast as a 30-year-old man. The 80-year-old is more aged than his younger counterpart, having accumulated more of the changes secondary to age, but he is not losing function at a more rapid rate.

An important characteristic of age-related changes is their *variability*. There are several sources of variability, including changes within individuals from organ to organ and changes

from individual to individual in a given population. Such functions as glomerular filtration rate and carbohydrate tolerance change rather dramatically, whereas others, such as nerve conduction velocity and hematocrit, undergo little significant change into the eighth or ninth decade.

Changes in one organ are not necessarily predictive of changes with age in other organs. If an apparently healthy 60-year-old is found on serial prospective measurements to have a cardiac output that is falling at a certain rate, perhaps at the rate average for his age group, this information is of no value in predicting the rate at which his kidneys, lungs, sympathetic nervous system, or any other organ is changing with time. This apparent failure of the various organs to be synchronized in regard to age-related changes is thought by some to rule against the presence of a basic biologic clock. The within-person variability and unpredictability has stymied investigators seeking to construct a variable termed *functional age* that predicts performance on a physiologic or psychologic test better than an individual's chronologic age.

The variability in human aging from individual to individual is also substantial. In studies of variables that undergo major changes with age the variance is often large, and one can easily identify apparently healthy 40-year-olds who perform at the same level as the average 80-year-old. Likewise, many 80-year-olds can be found who perform like the average 40-year-old.

NORMAL AGING—DISTINCTION BETWEEN USUAL AND SUCCESSFUL SUBTYPES
As noted above, the elderly population is characterized by substantial variability in the severity of age-related physiologic changes. Physiologically, it seems that the older individuals become, the less like each other they become, not more like each other. This may be due in part to life-style differences that confound the effects of aging. For instance, although maximal oxygen consumption has repeatedly been shown to decline with age, studies also indicate that oxygen consumption increases in response to exercise training in older persons, with older master athletes achieving levels higher than those seen in average young adults but not as high as those observed in young, equally condi-

tioned athletes. In addition to their variability, evidence is accumulating that many of the physiologic changes that have been considered normal with aging are not, as previously believed, harmless but actually carry risk. Thus, age-related increases in systolic blood pressure and blood glucose that are not large enough to qualify as diseases may be harmful. This concept becomes increasingly important because studies indicate that many of these changes, formerly considered to be due to the intrinsic aging process per se, are actually related to extrinsic factors such as diet, exercise, and body composition and can be modified. As increasing attention is paid to the potential beneficial effects of exercise, diet, smoking cessation, moderation in alcohol intake, and so on, we may encounter increasing numbers of robust elders who demonstrate successful aging—i.e., not only lack of disease but also physiologic performance that is only moderately below that of healthy young adults. However, the fact remains that most older adults exhibit another syndrome, that of *usual aging* [28], in which the effects of aging per se are mixed with the adverse effects of confounding environmental, dietary, or life-style factors. Most studies in the literature on the physiology of aging, although they exclude diseased subjects, describe usual rather than successful aging.

DISTINCTION BETWEEN AGING AND DISEASE

Increasing age after adulthood is associated with an exponential increase in the mortality rate, and this mortality is preceded by a similar exponential increase in the presence of pathologic changes. This association has stimulated controversy about whether aging should be considered a disease state, and if not, what is the relation of normal aging to disease-related changes. There is now general agreement that increasing age is accompanied by inevitable physiologic changes that represent normal aging and are separable from the effects of disease states that become increasingly prevalent with age.

One superficial and simple way of separating disease effects from the influence of normal aging is the inevitability of the changes. Although a change may vary from individual to

individual in its time of onset or the rate of loss of function, some loss of function should be demonstrable in all old subjects if the change is due to aging. Aging is a universal phenomenon, whereas many disease states, which occur with increasing prevalence as age advances, affect only a small portion of the elderly population. Evaluation of the presence of a change secondary to a disease state or some other factor not age-related in an elderly cohort often shows two populations: one with the effect and one with no evidence of the effect. The utility of this approach in determining whether or not a change is likely to be related to age can be seen in, for example, mental failure or dementia. This loss of mental function with advancing age is thought by some individuals to be characteristic of aging itself. When populations are studied in detail, however, it is shown that the presence of an intact intellect and the absence of mental failure is consistent with normal aging and is in fact the rule rather than the exception. Thus, mental failure cannot be considered a normal consequence of aging but more properly represents the impact of diseases that have increasing prevalence in advanced years. This condition can be contrasted with the menopause, which, although variable in time of onset, is universally present in aged women and thus is more likely to be a result of normal aging.

Since age has an important influence on numerous physiologic variables, and since detection of disease depends on the determination that an individual is different from what would be expected by virtue of his or her age, it is important to establish age-adjusted criteria for clinically relevant variables to facilitate differentiation of the physiologic consequences of usual aging from those of concomitant diseases. Such criteria have been in wide clinical use for many years for several clinically important functions. For example, spirometric measures of pulmonary function are commonly expressed as "percent expected" for age and body size. Similarly, the validity of an exercise tolerance test as a suitable stress test for detection of ischemic heart disease is judged on the basis of age-adjusted maximum heart rate achieved. Standardized criteria are also available for age-related changes in glomerular filtration rate

(GFR) and oral glucose tolerance, although it must be reemphasized that variability is great among the elderly for these functions, and individual determinations are required to guide diagnosis or therapy. If an individual measurement of GFR is not available, application of age-related standards is facilitated by the fact that the marked decline in creatinine clearance with advancing age (approximately 10 ml/min/decade) is balanced by similar reductions in endogenous creatinine production as serum creatinine levels remain unchanged [29]. Thus, similar criteria for levels of serum creatinine can be applied in older individuals and their younger counterparts as evidence of renal disease, while recognizing that a given level of serum creatinine reflects a substantially lower GFR in the older patient. Familiarity with age changes in renal function and the hepatic oxidizing system are of particular importance in guiding drug therapy in the elderly (see later discussion).

INTERACTION OF AGING AND DISEASE

Physicians treating elderly patients should be aware that the differences between these patients' clinical status and that of healthy younger individuals are a mixture of age-related and disease-related effects and that these factors interact with one another. There is a wide spectrum of interaction between aging processes and diseases, ranging from a lack of interaction at one extreme to age changes that have direct adverse clinical sequelae. Two of the clinically relevant points along this continuum include those variables that do not change with age and those whose declines limit the homeostatic capacity of older persons.

Physiologic Variables that Do Not Change with Age

Perhaps the most important phenomenon seen in the aged, from a clinical standpoint, is no age-related change at all. Too frequently, clinicians attribute a disability or abnormal physical or laboratory finding to "old age" when the actual cause may be a specific disease process. Often there is no influence of age on the specific variable being evaluated [30]. For example, old patients with low hematocrit values may be incorrectly characterized as having "anemia of old age" and be assured that no diagnostic evaluation or treatment is warranted. Data from several sources clearly indicate that in healthy community-dwelling elders no age-related change in hematocrit occurs. Thus, a low hematocrit level in an elderly individual cannot be ascribed to normal aging and requires prompt investigation and treatment. Other common clinical measures not strongly influenced by age include fasting blood glucose level, serum electrolyte concentrations, blood pH and carbon dioxide content, and numerous hormone levels, including insulin, cortisol, thyroxine, and parathyroid hormone.

Impaired Homeostasis in the Elderly

The category of impaired homeostasis encompasses age-related reductions in the function of numerous organs that place the elderly person at special risk of increased morbidity from coincident pathologic changes in those organs. Although normal age-related declines in physiologic function are not severe enough to result in impairments in function under basal circumstances, these declines are of sufficient magnitude to reduce physiologic reserve significantly, placing old individuals close to the clinical threshold for the emergence of symptoms. Thus, declines in basal immune, renal, and pulmonary function and declines in glucose tolerance and cardiac function during physiologic stress all place the elderly at risk for earlier emergence or greater severity of clinical disease. This statement can be illustrated with several clinically relevant examples:

1. Aging is associated with significant progressive reductions in the *dopamine content* of the substantia nigra [30]. These decreases may interact with pathophysiologic changes to account for the increasing prevalence of Parkinson's disease in late life, and they are also consistent with the well-recognized enhanced susceptibility of older individuals to extrapyramidal side effects of neuroleptic agents.

2. Age-related reductions in *pulmonary function* are so substantial that healthy individuals in the ninth decade of life frequently have pulmonary function equal to only half of their 30-year-old counterparts. Thus, acute bacterial pneumonias of equal initial severity are much more likely to induce serious clinical

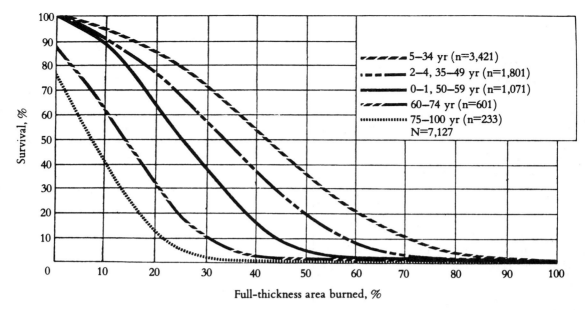

FIGURE 1-3. *Survival of patients as a function of the total percentage of body surface burned and age. From I. Feller, et al. Baseline results of therapy for burn patients. J.A.M.A. 236:1943, 1976. Copyright 1976 American Medical Association.*

Graph legend:
- 5–34 yr (n=3,421)
- 2–4, 35–49 yr (n=1,801)
- 0–1, 50–59 yr (n=1,071)
- 60–74 yr (n=601)
- 75–100 yr (n=233)
- N=7,127

Y-axis: Survival, %
X-axis: Full-thickness area burned, %

manifestations in the elderly because of their markedly lessened pulmonary function reserve. Additionally, the marked decline in *immune function* with age may also be expressed as an impaired capacity of the older individual to respond to the infecting agent and a subsequent worsening of the clinical picture.

3. Since normal *renal function* in older persons may be as much as 40 percent less than that in healthy younger adults [29], the loss of one kidney due to ureteral obstruction, vascular occlusion, or trauma is more likely to result in a clinically significant reduction in overall renal function in an old patient than a similar loss of function of one kidney in a healthy younger individual.

4. The mortality associated with *severe burns* increases dramatically with advancing age throughout adulthood (Fig. 1-3). This effect, which reflects the multiple parallel reductions in physiologic function during middle age and early senescence, is apparent well before diseases become highly prevalent and exemplifies the impaired homeostasis associated with the physiologic changes with age.

Age-related alterations in disease presentation due to physiologic changes characteristic of aging have long been recognized as being of major importance to the practice of geriatric medicine. As detailed in Chap. 3, many diseases that occur in both young and old adults have manifestly different clinical presentations and natural histories depending on the age of the individual. These disorders should be regarded as being neither more nor less severe in the elderly, just different.

References

1. Kohn, R. R. *Principles of Mammalian Aging* (2nd ed.). Englewood Cliffs, N.J.: Prentice-Hall, 1978. P. 240.
2. Sacher, G. A. Relation of Lifespan to Brain Weight and Body Weight in Mammals. In G. E. W. Wolstenholme and M. O'Connor (eds.), *The Lifespan of Animals* (Ciba Foundation Colloquy on Aging, Vol. 5). Boston: Little, Brown, 1959.
3. Orgel, L. E. The maintenance of the accuracy of protein synthesis in its relevance to aging. *Proc. Natl. Acad. Sci. U.S.A.* 49:517, 1963.
4. Garlick, R. L., et al. Nonenzymatic glycation of human lens crystallin: Effect of aging and diabetes mellitus. *J. Clin. Invest.* 74:1742, 1984.
5. Hayflick, L. Theories of Biological Aging. In R. Andres, E. L. Bierman and W. R. Hazzard (eds.), *Principles of Geriatric Medicine.* New York: McGraw-Hill, 1985. Pp. 9–22.

6. Reff, M. E. RNA and Protein Metabolism. In C. E. Finch and E. L. Schneider (eds.), *Handbook of the Biology of Aging* (2nd ed.). New York: Van Nostrand Reinhold, 1985. Pp. 225–254.

7. Hart, R. W., and Setlow, R. B. Correlation between deoxyribonucleic acid excision-repair and lifespan in a number of mammalian species. *Proc. Natl. Acad. Sci. U.S.A.* 71:2169, 1974.

8. Schimke, R. T., et al. Overreplication and recombination of DNA in higher eukaryotes: Potential consequences and biological implications. *Proc. Natl. Acad. Sci. U.S.A.* 83:2157, 1986.

9. Shmookler Reis, R. J., et al. Clonal Diversification of DNA Structure and Transcription During Cellular Senescence. In R. S. Sohal (ed.), *Molecular Biology of Aging: Gene Stability and Gene Expression.* New York: Raven, 1985. Pp. 37–48.

10. Harman, D. The aging process. *Proc. Natl. Acad. Sci. U.S.A.* 78:7124, 1981.

11. Hausman, P. B., and Weksler, M. E. Changes in the Immune Response with Age. In C. E. Finch and E. L. Schneider (eds.), *Handbook of the Biology of Aging* (2nd ed.). New York: Van Nostrand Reinhold, 1985. Pp. 414–432.

12. Smith, G. S., and Walford, R. L. Influence of the main histocompatibility complex on aging in mice. *Nature* 270:727, 1977.

13. Rowe, J. W., and Troen, B. R. Sympathetic nervous system activity and aging in man. *Endocr. Rev* 1:167, 1980.

14. Russell, R. L., and Jackson, L. A. Some Aspects of Aging Can Be Studied Easily in Nematodes. In C. E. Finch and E. L. Schneider (eds.), *Handbook of the Biology of Aging* (2nd ed.). New York: Van Nostrand Reinhold, 1985. Pp. 128–145.

15. Hayflick, L., and Moorhead, P. S. The serial cultivation of human diploid cell strains. *Exp. Cell. Res.* 37:614, 1961.

16. Martin, G. I., Sprague, C. S., and Epstein, C. J. Replicative lifespan of cultivated human cells. Effects of donor's age, tissue, and genotype. *Lab. Invest.* 23:66, 1970.

17. Norwood, T. H., and Smith, J. R. The Cultured Fibroblast-like Cell as a Model for the Study of Aging. C. E. Finch and E. L. Schneider (eds.), *Handbook of the Biology of Aging* (2nd ed.). New York: Van Nostrand Reinhold, 1985. Pp. 291–321.

18. Rohme, D. Evidence for a relationship between longevity of mammalian species and life spans of normal fibroblasts *in vitro* and erythrocytes *in vivo. Proc. Natl. Acad. Sci. U.S.A.* 78:5009, 1981.

19. Stein, G. H., and Atkins, L. Membrane-associated inhibitor of DNA synthesis in senescent human diploid fibroblasts. *Proc. Natl. Acad. Sci. U.S.A.* 83:9030, 1986.

20. Lumpkin, C. K., et al. Existence of high abundance antiproliferative mRNA's in senescent human diploid fibroblasts. *Science* 232:393, 1986.

21. Carlin, C. R., et al. Diminished *in vitro* tyrosine kinase activity of the EGF receptor of senescent human fibroblasts. *Nature* 306:607, 1983.

22. O'Brien, W., Stenman, G., and Sager, R. Suppression of tumor growth by senescence in virally transformed human fibroblasts. *Proc. Natl. Acad. Sci. U.S.A.* 83:9030, 1986.

23. Schneider, E. L., and Reed, J. D. Life extension. *N. Engl. J. Med.* 312:1159, 1985.

24. Ames, B. N. Dietary carcinogens and anticarcinogens. Oxygen radicals and degenerative diseases. *Science* 221:1256, 1982.

25. Glomset, J. A. Fish, fatty acids and human health. *N. Engl. J. Med.* 312:1253, 1985.

26. Yu, B. P., et al. Life span study of SPF Fischer 344 male rats fed *ad libitum. J. Gerontol.* 37:130, 1982.

27. Andres, R. Effect of obesity on total mortality. *Int. J. Obesity* 4:381, 1980.

28. Rowe, J. W., and Kahn, R. L. Human aging: Usual versus successful. *Science* 237:143, 1987.

29. Rowe, J. W., et al. The effect of age on creatinine clearance in man: A cross-sectional and longitudinal study. *J. Gerontol.* 31:155, 1976.

30. Rowe, J. W. Clinical research in aging: Strategies and directions. *N. Engl. J. Med.* 297:1332, 1977.

31. Feller, I., et al. Baseline results of therapy for burn patients. *J.A.M.A.* 236:1943, 1976.

Suggested Reading

Finch, C. E., and Schneider, E. L. (eds.). *Handbook of the Biology of Aging* (2nd ed.). New York: Van Nostrand Reinhold, 1985.

2

Demography: Characteristics and Implications of an Aging Population

BETH J. SOLDO
KENNETH G. MANTON

IT IS IRONIC that one of the greatest achievements of this modern world—extending life expectancy well into the seventies—is more commonly lamented for its implications than celebrated as a victory over early death. One does not need to look very far for examples of this mentality: A banner on the cover of a weekly news magazine a few years ago asked, "Can we afford our older population?" and the crisis in financing the social security and Medicare systems regularly make front page news.

Yet the aging of populations, like that of individuals, is inevitable [1]. Since at least the turn of the century, increases in both relative and absolute numbers of elderly have been carefully documented [2]. The origins of aging populations in declining fertility and mortality at younger ages also are well known and have been extensively documented [3]. Chapters like this often present the demographic parameters of population aging as static "facts." Although appealing in its simplicity, this approach ignores the dynamics of an aging population. Demographers have a poor track record in anticipating the rapid growth in the size of the older population and its key compositional changes [4]. Furthermore, the effects of population "metabolism" seldom play out in a linear fashion because they interact with evolving societal factors, some of which are susceptible to planned intervention. For example, changes in the health status of the elderly cause major shifts in the age structure of the entire U.S. population and in the needs of future cohorts of older persons. But the health needs of the elderly also respond to the amount of resources allocated to disease prevention, treatment, and palliation. Ultimately, resource allocation decisions affect the future course of old age mortality and life expectancy and the status of tomorrow's elderly.

Demographic "Aging"

The three basic demographic features of population "aging" include (1) growth in the absolute size of the elderly population, (2) changes in the relative number of older persons, that is, structural aging, and (3) increases in life expectancy.

INCREASES IN THE SIZE OF THE ELDERLY POPULATION

The simple increase in the absolute number of older persons is a basic indicator of population aging. This growth is tracked from 1960 to 2040 in Table 2-1. Since 1960, the older population has grown at a rate twice that of the total U.S. population, recording an average annual net gain of nearly 452,000 elderly. Over the next 30 years, this growth will decelerate as the small, depression-era cohorts reach age 65. For several decades thereafter (2010–2030), how-

TABLE 2-1. *Total number of persons 65 years of age and over: Estimates, 1960–1980; Projections, 1990–2040[a] (numbers in thousands)*

YEAR	NUMBER	65 YEARS OF AGE AND OVER % INCREASE IN PRECEDING DECADE
Estimates		
1960	16,675	—
1970	20,087	20.5
1980	25,708	28.0
Projections[b]		
1990	31,799	23.7
2000	35,036	10.2
2010	39,269	12.1
2020	51,386	30.9
2030	64,344	25.2
2040	66,642	3.6

Key:— = not applicable.
[a] Estimates and projections as of July 1, for each year; base date of projections is July 1, 1982. Data pertain to the total population of the 50 states and the District of Columbia.
[b] Projections assume "middle level" mortality (ultimate life expectancy of 81.0 years in 2080), fertility (ultimate number of births per woman of 1.9) and net immigration (450,000 per annum).
SOURCE: U.S. Bureau of the Census. *Current Population Report.* Series P-23, No. 138. Washington, D.C.: U.S. Government Printing Office, 1984.

FIGURE 2-1. *Total number of elderly in the United States by broad age groups and sex. Data for 1960–1980 are estimates. Data for 1990–2040 are projections. (From U.S. Bureau of Census.* Current Population Report. *Series 25, no. 952.)*

ever, the post–World War II "baby boom" will swell the ranks of the elderly, with average annual net increases of 1.3 million older persons. After this dramatic growth, the rate of increase will slow as the so-called "baby-bust" cohorts of the mid-1960s and 1970s cross the threshold into old age. Hence, an uneven pace of growth will be a hallmark of population aging in the late twentieth and early twenty-first centuries as the number of elderly increases from 26 million in 1980 to 51.4 million in 2020 and to 66.6 million in 2040.

It is tempting to equate increases in the total number of elderly with changes in the volume of demand for a variety of goods and services. The data presented in Figure 2-1 display three major facets of population aging that will strongly influence demand: the predominantly female character of the older population, especially at the oldest ages; the rapid growth in the oldest old; and the impact of the baby boom.

Female Preponderance
Although the number of females per 100 males will change little from its current base of 148, the relative gap in the number of very old (85+) women per 100 comparably aged men will widen, peaking in 2010 at 266. These anticipated changes, like all projection-based estimates, are a direct function of the underlying

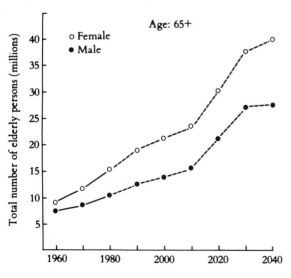

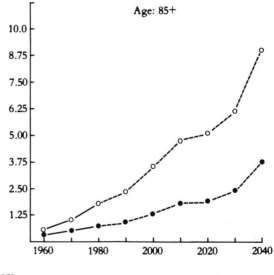

Years

assumptions. Since 1970 the male-female gap in life expectancy has risen to 7.8 years [6], but the future course of this differential is subject to much debate. Fries [7], for example, argues that the male-female difference will converge as female life expectancy first approaches the upper limit of natural "life span." Others anticipate a divergency of as much as 10 to 12 years by the turn of the century [8]. The projections discussed above and shown in Figure 2-1 are based on more moderate assumptions of a gradual widening to an 8.5-year difference in male-female life expectancy in 2080 [9].

Sex differentials in survivorship are important planning considerations because, as discussed below, older men and women have quite different resources available for coping with a variety of age-related changes. In general, older women have fewer financial assets, and, because they typically outlive their spouses, are most dependent on adult children and formal services (including the nursing home) for meeting their personal care needs [10].

Rapid Growth of the Oldest Old
Those 85 years of age and over are already the fastest growing age group within our entire population and will pose special challenges, since per capita hospital and nursing home costs peak at these ages [11, 12]. Indeed, the current influx of the oldest old has already saturated existing nursing home facilities, and the 85+ population is projected to nearly triple by the year 2020 and nearly double again by 2040. Particularly dramatic, though speculative, is the expected increase in the number of centenarians from 32,000 in 1982 to 597,000 in 2040.

Impact of the Baby-Boom Cohorts
The baby-boom cohorts will rapidly swell the 65+ population between the years 2000 and 2020, and a comparable increase will occur in the over-85 population 20 years later. Because of the staggered impact of the aging of the baby boom, pressures for societal adaptation will shift quickly from one aspect of planning and policy making to another. As these large cohorts reach 54, for example, they will have an immediate effect on income transfer programs, such as social security, and private pension funds. Within a few decades concerns with fi-

nancing retirement income programs will give way to a new focus on the ability of various health care programs and institutions to absorb an unprecedented number of very old and probably frail elderly.

STRUCTURAL ASPECTS OF POPULATION AGING
Strictly speaking, the age of a population is defined by its proportion of elderly. A convenient way to track the aging of a population is to compare the relative numbers of elderly over time. These estimates are shown in Table 2-2.

At the turn of this century the United States was a demographically youthful country with an elderly population of only about 4 percent. By 1950 the United States reached what is currently considered to be a "mature" age structure, with 8.2 percent of the population concentrated in the older ages. In 1980, when one in nine Americans was elderly (11.2 percent), the U.S. age structure was already considered to be "aged." The United States, however, is far from being the "oldest" of the developed countries. In both Sweden and the German Democratic Republic over 13 percent of the population was age 65 or over in 1980 [13].

TABLE 2-2. *Percentage of total population 65 years of age and over, 1960–1980; and projections under varying assumptions, 1990–2040*

YEAR	% OF TOTAL POPULATION AGED 65 AND OVER
Estimates	
1960	9.3
1970	9.9
1980	11.3
Projections*	
1990	12.7 (12.4–13.0)
2000	13.1 (12.2–13.9)
2010	13.9 (12.3–15.5)
2020	17.3 (14.7–20.1)
2030	21.1 (17.2–25.5)
2040	21.6 (16.5–27.6)

*Base date of projections is July 1, 1982. Main projection is from series 14 (middle fertility, mortality and immigration). Ranges in parentheses are from series 27 (high fertility, mortality, migration) and from series 1 (low fertility, mortality, and immigration). Range was chosen to illustrate largest possible spread and not to indicate uncertainty intervals around the main projections.
SOURCE: U.S. Bureau of the Census. *Current Population Report.* Series P-23, No. 138. Washington, D.C.: U.S. Government Printing Office, 1984.

Future increases in the relative number of elderly depend primarily on the course of fertility. If the United States were to witness another baby boom, the base of the population pyramid would widen and the proportion of elderly could actually decline. The projections shown in Table 2-2 of the relative number of elderly result from projections of the U.S. Bureau of the Census [9] chosen to illustrate the largest possible range of changes in the relative number of elderly.

Dependency Ratios

If increasing numbers of elderly suggest major changes in the volume of demand, increasing proportions of elderly suggest difficulties in absorbing the costs of meeting this escalating demand, since many programs directly benefiting the elderly are structured as intergenerational transfers. Recent depressed fertility levels and increased numbers of elderly are combining to result in fewer persons of working age relative to the number of older people.

Aged-support (-dependency) ratios are a crude way of plotting the future of the various transfer programs that figure so predominantly in both the total federal budget and the quality of life of older persons. In 1980 there were almost 19 retirement-age persons benefiting from the hypothetical contributions of every 100 working-age persons (Table 2-3). By the year 2000 this ratio is projected to increase to 21:100, and by 2040 the aged-dependency ratio will more than double from its 1980 level to 38:100. This increase implies an increasing financial burden on workers if the current system of intergenerational transfers continues into the next century.

These ratios probably err on the optimistic side, since delayed entry into the labor force and earlier retirement characterize recent patterns of labor force participation. Nor do the ratios shown in Table 2-3 reflect the disproportionate claim that the very old—those 85 and over—make on our collective resources.

LIFE EXPECTANCY CHANGES

The 1950s and 1960s were a time of relative stability in life expectancies in the United States. Since the early 1970s, however, this country has once again witnessed major increases in life ex-

TABLE 2-3. *Aged-dependency ratios: Estimates, 1960–1980, and projections, 1990–2040—United States*

YEAR	AGED DEPENDENCY RATIO[a]	INDEX OF RELATIVE CHANGE[b]
Estimates		
1960	16.8	90
1970	17.6	94
1980	18.6	100
Projections[c]		
1990	20.7	111
2000	21.2	114
2010	21.9	118
2020	28.7	154
2040	37.7	203

[a] Number of persons aged 65 and over per 100 persons aged 18–64.
[b] Base year is 1980.
[c] Projections from series 14, or "middle-level" series.
SOURCE: U.S. Bureau of the Census. *Current Population Report*. Series P-23, No. 138. Washington, D.C.: U.S. Government Printing Office, 1984.

pectancy. These improvements may be seen by examining the data shown in Figure 2-2. Even at ages 65 and 85, and particularly for older women, the improvements made in the last 20 years have been substantial. Unlike earlier improvements, which were due to reductions in acute and infectious disease death rates, more recent improvements reflect declines in chronic disease mortality risks.

Nearly three-quarters of all elderly deaths are attributable to three chronic diseases: heart disease, cerebrovascular disease, and malignant neoplasms [14]. Because diseases of the heart account for nearly half of all deaths among those 65 and over, changes in the structure of mortality among the elderly have largely been dictated by recent substantive declines in the rates of heart disease.

Prolongation of Morbidity

Mortality reductions have increased the survival time for individuals affected by the major life-threatening chronic diseases. Manton [15] estimates (Table 2-4) that true mortality reductions have been accomplished by delaying the mortal impact of chronic disease. The average age at death has increased by 2.75 years during the last three decades for males dying from either heart disease or cancer. The mean age at death for women with heart disease increased by 5.44

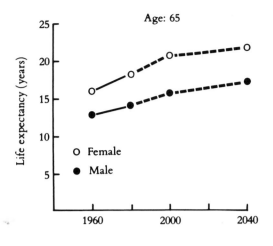
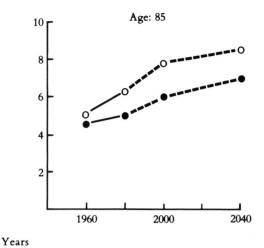

Years

FIGURE 2-2. *Life expectancy by sex for the U.S. population at ages 65 and 85. (From Social Security Administration, Office of the Actuary.* Life Tables for the United States, 1900–2050. Actuarial Study No. 87, SSA Publication No. 11-11534. *Washington, D.C.: U.S. Government Printing Office, 1982.)*

TABLE 2-4. *Changes, 1950–1980, in life-table estimated proportions affected by heart disease and cancer and the mean age at death for each disease, by sex*

SEX AND TIME OF OBSERVATION	LIFE TABLE ESTIMATES	
	PROPORTION AFFECTED BY DISEASE	MEAN AGE AT DEATH
HEART DISEASE		
Males		
1950	40.0	71.14
1960	41.3	71.49
1970	39.2	72.11
1980	36.9	73.89
Females		
1950	38.9	76.87
1960	40.4	78.41
1970	39.5	79.90
1980	38.1	82.31
CANCER		
Males		
1950	13.4	67.13
1960	15.1	67.23
1970	17.1	67.88
1980	20.8	69.88
Females		
1950	15.2	67.39
1960	15.3	68.35
1970	16.0	69.26
1980	18.4	71.38

SOURCE: Adapted from K. G. Manton. Mortality patterns in developed countries. Paper presented at the 1983 Annual Meeting of the Population Association of America, Pittsburgh, PA, 1983.

years (to 82.3 in 1980) and for women with cancer by nearly 4 years. At the same time, however, the proportion of the population affected by cancer increased for both males and females, while the proportion affected by heart disease declined moderately for males and negligibly for females. In combination, these two sets of estimates raise the specter of a population living longer but in a diseased condition—that is, a population in which life extension has been accomplished at the expense of increased morbidity.

Although increases in the mean age at death and survival time since disease onset coupled with gains in life expectancy at the older ages are likely to be interpreted by most individuals as "good news" for their own survival prospects, from a societal perspective these same data portend a future characterized by increasing numbers of disabled with high per capita health care costs. If gains in later life expectancy are independent of age-specific risks of morbidity and disability, the recent advances will extend the period of functional dependence prior to death. On the other hand, if age at onset of disability is postponed proportionate to survivorship improvements, increases in life expectancy imply additional years of active life expectancy (see Chap. 4).

Morbidity of the Elderly in the Community
Chronic degenerative diseases increase in prevalence with age. In part this is because many chronic illnesses become evident clinically only after a long period of latency. Thus, those who survive into old age are increasingly likely to manifest the symptoms on which detection and diagnosis of disease are based.

Cross-sectional data, such as those shown in Table 2-5, indicate that the risk of chronic disease accelerates rapidly with age. Four of every five community-based elderly have at least one chronic condition, most commonly arthritis, hypertension, auditory impairments, and heart disease. Together, these conditions account for nearly 60 percent of all chronic conditions reported by the noninstitutionalized elderly. In each case, the disease prevalence among those aged 65 and over is five times that observed in younger individuals. The fact that the etiologies of many of the common chronic diseases of old age are associated with a middle-aged life-style (e.g., cigarette smoking, excessive sodium and cholesterol intake) and subclinical risk factors

(e.g., elevated blood pressure) gives direction to public health initiatives designed to reduce chronic disease incidence in future elderly cohorts. If successful, such efforts would tend to reduce the impact of selective survivorship on future cohorts, thereby increasing the heterogeneity of tomorrow's elderly, particularly at the extremes of old age [16].

Patterns of risk and disease prevalence vary substantially by sex. Some diseases, such as polymyalgia rheumatica and osteoporosis, are much more common in older women, whereas others, such as coronary heart disease, disproportionately affect older men. In general, older women have higher rates of most chronic diseases and consequently higher rates of disability. However, diseases common to older men tend to be more life threatening than those prevalent among older women.

Not all major chronic conditions threaten quality of life or compromise functional capacity. Nonetheless, the risk of functional disability consequent to chronic disease increases rapidly after age 65. Although only 6.7 percent of persons aged 65 to 74 require personal care assistance, the prevalence of such need more than doubles (to 15.7 percent) for those 75 to 84 years of age and surges to 44 percent at age 85 or older. This translates into some 2.8 million elderly with various kinds of functional dependencies. Approximately 69 percent of these elderly dependent persons, or 1.9 million in 1979, were women [17].

Prevalence rates of personal care dependencies are shown for individuals aged 75 to 84 and 85+ years in Figure 2-3. For each type of dependency, the rate for those 85+ years is more than double that for persons 75 to 84 years of age, although in terms of absolute numbers there are more 75 to 84-year-old dependent persons in the community than comparably impaired individuals 85 years of age and over. These same age differences in both relative and absolute numbers are evidenced in recent data from the 1982 Long-Term Care Community Survey [10].

It is, of course, hazardous to attempt to infer aging dynamics from cross-sectional data. The estimates of functional transition probabilities prepared by Branch et al. [18] suggest the tra-

TABLE 2-5. *Prevalence by age of top 15 chronic conditions affecting persons 65 years of age and over, 1981 (numbers in thousands)*

CHRONIC CONDITION	PREVALENCE		
	<45	45–65	65+
Arthritis	47.7	246.5	464.7
Hypertension	54.2	243.7	378.6
Hearing impairments	43.8	142.9	283.8
Heart conditions	37.9	122.7	277.0
Chronic sinusitis	58.4	177.5	183.6
Visual impairments	27.4	55.2	136.6
Orthopedic impairments	90.5	117.5	128.2
Arteriosclerosis	.5	21.3	97.0
Diabetes	8.6	56.9	83.47
Varicose veins	19.0	50.1	83.2
Hemorrhoids	43.7	66.6	65.9
Frequent constipation	9.2	22.4	59.2
Diseases of urinary system	25.8	31.7	56.1
Hay fever	100.2	77.5	51.9
Corns and callosities	14.0	35.8	51.9
Hernia of abdominal cavity	8.9	33.1	49.1

SOURCE: National Center for Health Statistics. Unpublished data reported in U.S. Senate, Select Committee on Aging. *Aging America: Trends and Projections.* Washington, D.C. 1984.

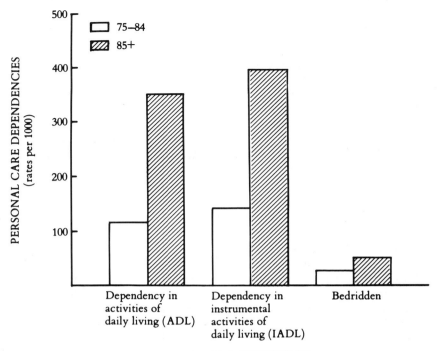

PERSONAL CARE DEPENDENCIES (rates per 1000)

500

400

300

200

100

☐ 75–84

▨ 85+

Dependency in activities of daily living (ADL)

Dependency in instrumental activities of daily living (IADL)

Bedridden

TYPE OF DEPENDENCY

jectory of disability at advanced ages. Compared with those 65 to 74 years old and functionally independent at year 1.25 of the study, those 85 years or over had a threefold greater risk of losing their independence, seven times the chance of entering a nursing home, and two-and-a-half times the risk of dying during the observation interval. These same general age differences remain for those who were functionally dependent at the baseline, but in this group those 85 and over had but 3 chances in 100 of regaining their independence—a probability 11 times lower than that estimated for the youngest age group.

In sum, the health of the elderly in the community shows a considerable prevalence of both morbidity and disability but no inevitable linkage between the two at any specific age or point in time. Although very few elderly in the community are disease .free, a majority manifest little if any functional incapacity consequent to chronic disease.

Morbidity of the Institutionalized Elderly
To this point we have been concerned only with the health of older persons in the community,

FIGURE 2-3. *Rates of personal care dependencies, by type, among noninstitutionalized persons, by age, 1979. Activities of daily living (ADL) dependency describes those who require assistance in walking, going outside, bathing, dressing, toileting, getting out of bed or chair, and eating. Instrumental activities of daily living (IADL) dependency describes those who require assistance managing money, making telephone calls, grocery shopping, or doing routine chores. (From National Center for Health Statistics. Americans needing help to function at home. In* Vital and Health Statistics. *Advanced Data Report No. 92. Washington, D.C.: U.S. Government Printing Office, 1983.)*

but approximately 1.1 million of the aged are nursing home residents. The relative number of nursing home residents increases rapidly after age 75. Although only 1.5 percent of those aged 65 to 74 are nursing home residents, this figure increases to 6.8 percent for those aged 75 to 84 and to 21.6 percent among the oldest old.

Nursing home residents differ substantially from their peers in the community. Nursing home residents are disproportionately very old, female, white, and currently unmarried. Table 2-6 examines the health of older nursing home residents using three different indicators. Panel A of this table displays cross-sectional age dif-

TABLE 2-6. *Rate per 1,000 nursing home residents of selected health status indicators of older nursing home residents, by age: United States, 1977*

HEALTH STATUS INDICATOR	AGE			
	65+	65–74	75–84	85+
A. PRIMARY DIAGNOSIS AT LAST EXAMINATION[a]				
Circulatory diseases	437.7	333.3	427.4	497.3
Arteriosclerosis	231.2	106.4	227.8	293.3
Stroke	82.4	131.0	90.2	51.4
Mental disorders	164.1	247.2	163.1	126.1
Chronic brain syndrome	75.3	73.0	80.0	71.6
Other diagnoses	330.9	357.5	335.3	313.8
Arthritis	46.6	30.3	46.9	53.8
Cancer	23.5	31.1	23.0	20.3
B. CHRONIC CONDITIONS OR IMPAIRMENTS				
Arteriosclerosis	496.6	354.2	508.7	604.9
Hypertension	177.0	189.1	192.9	145.4
Stroke	199.2	237.0	222.9	134.7
Heart trouble	382.4	289.6	372.8	476.3
Chronic brain syndrome	247.2	221.3	286.4	217.6
Senility[b]	306.0	182.1	319.9	395.7
Arthritis and rheumatism	189.4	132.2	195.8	230.9
Diseases of nervous system and sense organs	57.5	36.5	47.8	88.8
Cancer	73.7	57.4	70.8	91.8
C. FUNCTIONAL STATUS INDICATORS				
Incontinence problems[c]	526.0	624.0	529.0	478.0
Mobility restrictions[d]	692.0	568.0	668.0	775.0
Dependent in all ADL activities[e]	245.0	176.0	243.0	279.0

[a]Primary diagnosis is condition that currently affects the resident most seriously.
[b]Includes senility without psychosis.
[c]Includes those who have difficulty with control of bowel and/or bladder and those with either a bowel or bladder ostomy.
[d]Includes those who are chairfast and bedfast as well as those who need assistance walking.
[e]Dependent in bathing, dressing, toileting, mobility, eating, and incontinent.

SOURCE: National Center for Health Statistics. Characteristics of nursing home residents, health status and care reviewed. *Vital and Health Statistics,* Series 13. Data from the National Health Survey, No. 51. DHHS Pub. No. (PHS) 81-1712. Washington, D.C.: U.S. Government Printing Office, 1981.

ferences in the primary or most serious diagnostic condition recorded at the resident's last medical examination. Circulatory diseases in general and arteriosclerosis in particular are the causes of most of the serious health problems in elderly nursing home residents. The rate at which circulatory diseases are reported as the primary diagnosis increases with age (as does the rate for arthritis), whereas the prevalence of most other diagnoses generally drops with age. These age differentials reflect in part the increasing complexity of chronic disease symptomatology and differential diagnosis at the extremes of old age.

Total prevalence estimates of chronic disease and impairment (Table 2-6, panel B) provide a more comprehensive profile of the health of older nursing home residents. Most residents aged 75 and over show the symptoms of arteriosclerosis, although it is a primary problem for only about 30 percent. Nearly 40 percent of all older residents have some type of heart disease, and approximately one-third are reported to be "senile." The prevalence of most chronic diseases and impairments increases with age.

The functional status indicators shown in panel C of Table 2-6 demonstrate the substantial prevalence of disability in the older nursing home population. More than half are incontinent, nearly three-quarters are restricted in their mobility, and one-fourth are dependent in all activities of daily living (ADL). Of the three general indicators shown in Table 2-6, the elderly in nursing homes are most clearly differentiated from their community counterparts in terms of functional dependencies.

Numerous investigators have attempted to predict nursing home placements at advanced ages reliably. Need, per se, whether measured in terms of functional incapacity or medical condition, has proved to be an imperfect predictor, and no one set of factors consistently differentiates institutionalized from community elderly [19]. Nonetheless, a majority of previous studies have found that advanced old age is a significant risk factor for other predictor variables. Most studies also point to the importance of a supportive family network and factors that are likely to undermine the caregiver's capacity or commitment to noninstitutional care. Among these latter factors are incontinence, need for nearly constant supervision, and the presence of cognitive impairments or behavioral problems.

Planning for the Future

As recently as the mid-1970s, the aging of our population was described as the "quiet demographic revolution." In light of the recent media attention accorded the crises in financing Medicare and social security, the description *quiet* may no longer be apt. Likening population aging to a force as powerful as a revolution in the social order is not inappropriate. Upward shifts in our age structure will ultimately require profound and far-reaching adaptations in all social structures and institutions. Long-range comprehensive planning can ease the transition to a future in which as many as one in five individuals will be elderly.

Last, the ultimate worth of any planning schema will be tested against its ability to isolate the impact of alternative policies and the trade-offs among them. In anticipating the needs of future elderly and alternative policies responsive to those needs, it is important to recognize that few outcomes of interest are discrete. There is an inherent linkage among numerous policy areas affecting the elderly. It is inadequate, for example, to assess the relative merits of competing housing proposals without also examining their effects on the volume, timing, mix, and duration of health care needs within the population. Even within one broad policy area such as health, there are a multitude of trade-offs. Initiatives aimed at extending life expectancy imply a very different future for health care financing than those that seek to postpone the onset of chronic disability.

One model with potential value for planning purposes is the life table, which can be used to dis-

play changes in individual risk. The population implications of age-variable risk is illustrated in Figure 2-4. This figure represents life-course changes in health for a hypothetical cohort. The outermost line is the survival curve from a standard life table—that is, the probability of surviving to age X. The innermost line represents the probability of surviving to age X free of disease, and the middle curve is the probability of surviving to a given age with disease but free of disability. The relationship of the three curves during age and time portrays the linkages of various health outcomes.

The area between the disability and mortality curves represents the number of expected person-years to be lived in the disabled state; this is a summary measure of the requirements for long-term care services in a population. The area between the morbidity and disability curves represents the number of person-years to be lived in a morbid but nondisabled state. Individuals in this state, for example, might be socially and economically autonomous but nonetheless dependent on some types of medical services.

Kramer [21] and Gruenberg [22] suggest that the time spent in both the morbid and disabled states is increasing because most of our biomedical resources are being expended on pro-

FIGURE 2-4. *Mortality (observed), morbidity (hypothetical), and disability (hypothetical) survival curves for U.S. females in 1980. Sx = percentage of individuals who have not yet developed the characteristics described (i.e., morbidity, disability, or mortality).*

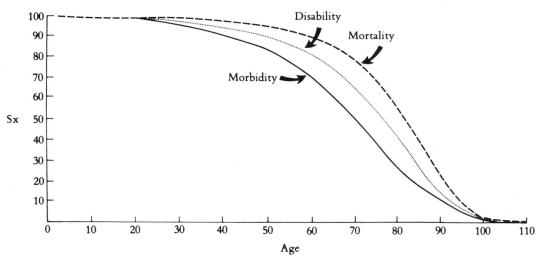

longing survival rather than on enhancing the quality of life. Strehler [23] suggests that the survival curve could be greatly modified as a byproduct of aging research and that with increases in life span, the proportion of the life span spent free of disease and disability would increase. In terms of Figure 2-4, the morbidity and disability curves would move parallel to the survival curve, since the basic parameters of aging would be unchanged. Fries [24], on the other hand, argues that the morbid period could be "compressed." He posits (1) that we have nearly reached the point at which further life expectancy increases will be bounded by biologic limits, and (2) that at very advanced ages death is due to biologic senescence. In other words, the morbidity curve could be shifted to the right to meet the survival curve.

Fries's model modifies the model originally proposed by Riley [25, 26], in which compression of morbidity is possible, but, in recognition of recent scientific evidence, efforts to improve health can also modify the rate of basic aging changes. We propose a model of "dynamic equilibrium" to understand the relationship of morbidity and mortality in the wake of increased life expectancy. This concept draws attention to the basic mathematical relationship between disease incidence, prevalence, and duration. If, as the data indicate, disease incidence is constant, then recent mortality reductions can only be accomplished by increasing the duration of disease. Rather than emphasizing increased duration consequent to the management of lethal sequelae, we focus on the duration-extending effects achieved by reducing disease severity. The concept of equilibrium, therefore, implies that both the severity and the rate of disease progression are correlated with mortality reductions in such a way that increases in life expectancy at the older ages are accompanied by a "corresponding reduction in the rate of progression of the 'aging' of the vital organ systems of the body" [27].

References

1. Coale, A. J. How a Population Ages or Grows Younger. In R. Freedman (ed.), *Population: The Vital Revolution*. Garden City, NY: Doubleday, 1964.
2. Soldo, B. J. America's elderly in the 1980s. *Population Bull.* 35 (4), 1980.
3. U.S. Bureau of the Census. Demographic and socioeconomic aspects of aging in the United States. *Current Population Reports.* Series P-23, No. 138. Washington, D.C.: U.S. Government Printing Office, 1984.
4. Myers, G. C. Future Age Projections and Society. In A. J. J. Gilmore (ed.), *Aging: A Challenge to Science and Social Policy.* Vol. 2. Oxford: Oxford University Press, 1981.
5. Manton, K. G., and Soldo, B. J. *A Dynamic Model of Population Aging and Health Status Change: Implications for Development and Implementation of National Health Policy.* Durham, NC: Center for Demographic Studies, Duke University, 1983.
6. Myers, G. C., and Manton, K. G. Recent changes in the U.S. age at death distribution: Future observations. *Gerontologist* 24:572, 1984.
7. Fries, J. F. The compression of morbidity: Miscellaneous comments about a theme. *Gerontologist* 24:354, 1984.
8. Crimmins, E. Implications of recent mortality trends for the size and composition of the population over 65. *Rev. Public Data Use* 11:37, 1983.
9. U.S. Bureau of the Census. Projection of the population of the United States, by age, sex, and race: 1983 to 2080. *Current Population Reports,* Series P-25, No. 952. Washington, D.C.: U.S. Government Printing Office, 1984.
10. Manton, K. G., and Liu, K. Future growth of the long-term care population: Projections based on the 1977 National Nursing Home Survey and the 1982 Long-Term Care Survey. Paper prepared for presentation at the Third Leadership Conference on Long-Term Care Issues: The Future World of Long-Term Care, Washington, D.C., 1984.
11. Fisher, C. R. Differences by age groups in health care spending. *Health Care Financing Rev.* 1:65, 1980.
12. National Center for Health Statistics. Characteristics of nursing home residents, health status, and care received: National nursing home survey, United States 1977. *Vital & Health Statistics,* Series 13, No. 51. Washington, D.C.: U.S. Government Printing Office, 1981.
13. U.S. Senate. *Aging America: Trends and Projections.* Washington, D.C.: U.S. Government Printing Office, 1984.
14. National Center for Health Statistics. Changes on the mortality among the elderly: United States, 1940–1978. *Vital & Health Statistics,* Series 3, No. 22. Washington, D.C.: U.S. Government Printing Office, 1982.

15. Manton, K. G. Mortality Patterns in Developed Countries. In R. F. Tomassen (ed.), *Comparative Social Research* Vol. 7. Greenwich, CT: JAI Press, 1983.

16. Manton, K. G., and Soldo, B. J. Dynamics of health changes in the extreme elderly: New perspectives and evidence. *Milbank Memorial Fund Q, Health and Society* 53(2):206, Spring 1985.

17. Verbrugge, L. M. Women and Men: Mortality and Health of Older People. In M. W. Riley, B. B. Hess, and K. Bond (eds.), *Aging in Society: Selected Reviews of Recent Research*. Hillsdale, NJ: Lawrence Erlbaum Associates, 1983.

18. Branch, L. G., et al. A prospective study of functional status among community elders. *Am. J. Public Health* 74:266 , 1984.

19. Branch, L. G., and Jette, A. M. A prospective study of long-term care institutionalization among the elderly. *Am. J. Public Health* 72:1373, 1982.

20. Weissert, W., and Scanlon, W. *Determinants of Institutionalization of the Aged*. Working Paper No. 1466-21 (Rev.). Washington, D.C.: Urban Institute, 1983.

21. Kramer, M. N. The rising pandemic of mental disorders and associated chronic diseases and disabilities. *Acta Psychiatr. Scandi.* 62 [Suppl. 285]: 382, 1980.

22. Gruenberg, E. M. The failures of success. *Milbank Memorial Fund Q, Health and Society* 55:3, 1977.

23. Strehler, B. L. Implications of aging research for society. Proceedings of the 58th Annual Meeting of the Federation of American Societies for Experimental Biology 34:5, 1975.

24. Fries, J. F. Aging, natural death and the compression of morbidity. *N. Engl. J. Med.* 303:130, 1980.

25. Riley, M. W. Health Behavior of Older People: Toward a New Paradigm. In D. L. Parron, F. Soloman, and J. Rodin (eds.), *Health, Behavior, and Aging*. Institute of Medicine Interim Rep. No. 5. Washington, D.C.: National Academy Press, 1981.

26. Riley, M. W., and Bond, K. Beyond Ageism: Postponing the Onset of Disability. In M. W. Riley, B. B. Hess, and K. Bond (eds.), *Aging in Society: Selected Reviews of Recent Research*. Hillsdale, NJ: Lawrence Erlbaum Associates, 1983.

27. Manton, K. G. Changing concepts of morbidity and mortality in the elderly population. *Milbank Memorial Fund Q, Health and Society* 60:183, 1982.

3

Clinical Approach to the Elderly Patient

RICHARD W. BESDINE

BEYOND THE DEMOGRAPHIC, FISCAL, AND MORAL IMPERATIVES driving our health care system toward increasing attention to and involvement with older persons, there are emotional and intellectual attractions to geriatric care for the physician and other health professionals. The aged survivors who are our geriatric patients are the shape of things to come for us, their clinicians. They link the past with the present and aim us toward our own futures, stimulating our learning and experience in geriatrics. More objectively pertinent, orchestrating salubrious clinical outcomes in older persons is more challenging intellectually and thus more gratifying for caregivers when successful. The thoughtfulness and scope of approach demanded of the clinician require that the best the health professions can provide be brought to bear on the decompensated, functionally disabled, sick old patient. In response to these multiple imperatives, there has been an extraordinary growth of knowledge in all areas of aging during the past two decades, and centers of excellence in clinical geriatric care, solidly based on robust research and education programs, have developed in a dozen or more universities nationwide. The proliferation of new information from the broad spectrum of current investigation related to aging has taken advantage of methodologies initially developed in other areas, including gene probes, computer modeling, imaging techniques, and large population-based studies.

Although there is certainly need for more good human aging research, a body of gerontologic data does now exist and new knowledge is accumulating rapidly. These relevant data are the intellectual frontier of geriatric care and must be assimilated into the specifics of diagnosis and treatment for the elderly. Most physicians have not been taught fundamental data about normal human aging and thus may not know what to expect of cardiac output, kidney function, blood pressure, ventilatory capacity, immune function, or glucose metabolism in a healthy old person. When illness is superimposed on age-related changes, the classic parallel lines of normal human biology and disease converge at the elderly patient, causing a dilemma for the clinician unschooled in gerontology and geriatric medicine. Here also, there has appeared a substantial new knowledge base concerning differences in clinical phenomena in the elderly, largely attributable to the altered substrate produced by the impact of normal aging.

The need for detailed elucidation of normal biologic aging and its influence on disease is obvious when we consider the potential for confusion of the practitioner encountering a sick old person. This patient has biobehavioral and functional abnormalities not found in younger healthy individuals, but whether the observed differences are attributable to normal aging or to disease cannot be ascertained without a detailed understanding of the multiple changes resulting from normal human aging. Only with a clear view of normative age-related changes can the physician properly evaluate and treat a sick old person. Ignorance of these data has two equally dangerous consequences. First, normal age-related changes may be attributed to disease, provoking treatment that will certainly be ineffective and will likely do harm. Alternatively, disease effects are mistakenly attributed to normal aging and neglected, allowing unchecked progression of a potentially treatable underlying disease. A third outcome, and perhaps the most destructive, is the avoidance of elderly patients altogether by clinicians who are frustrated and discouraged by unsuccessful interactions with aged individuals whose multiple problems have disease- and age-related components. Accordingly, we systematically review here the interplay between normal aging and disease to inform or remind clinicians of the unusual or unique aspects of providing health care to older persons.

Illness Behavior in the Elderly

Under this heading we discuss both the ways in which older persons behave differently from younger ones when ill and the special aspects or behavior of diseases themselves when they occur in old patients.

BEHAVIOR OF SICK OLDER PERSONS

There is now substantial information documenting that human behavior in health and illness is influenced by a variety of social, ethnic, psychologic, and clinical phenomena, including subjective assessment of illness severity, degree of interference with daily life, degree of denial, alternatives to explain symptoms, and the availability of care [1, 2]. It has become apparent that aging exerts a powerful modulating effect on the phenomena already known to influence health and illness behavior, and thus it is crucial to examine the impact of aging on behavior.

Subjective Health Assessment
Although the assessment of one's personal health is most obviously related to the objective reality of health status and illness burden, we are also powerfully influenced by the peer group

in which we function and its reference standards concerning health [3]. For example, an older person living in the community, whose reference group consists of relatively healthy elders, would tend to evaluate more severely the same condition that an institutionalized elder would consider less serious. It seems that as people age, their health expectations diminish, regardless of objective health status; for example, 75-year-olds reported more physical conditions and disability than 65- to 74-year-olds but tended to be more positive in their self-ratings of health [4].

Overestimating healthiness is obviously potentially dangerous to older people because it produces denial or neglect of disease. Sometimes called "normalization," this process leads the patient to attribute problems to some common phenomenon rather than disease; for example, a fall is caused by the fatigue, diminished vision, or just unsteadiness that "all old people get." But equally dangerous is the tendency to underestimate the severity or seriousness of a disease when the older person finally does acknowledge illness. Ischemic chest pain becomes muscle strain from innocent activity. Getting lost in once-familiar places is protectively attributed to failing vision. Past experiences with the health care system also influence the elder's evaluation of health. Health professionals previously may have minimized the seriousness of legitimate complaints, and thus an older person may delay seeking care from a physician on subsequent occasions when serious problems surface. If older people expect disability and functional decline in late life, they are likely to minimize the seriousness of symptoms and delay treatment for improvable conditions. These behavioral phenomena exert a powerful clinical influence on older people and on the outcomes of their health care encounters.

Reporting of Symptoms
Another crucial psychobehavioral phenomenon seen in older people is the underreporting of signs of illness. Legitimate symptoms heralding serious but often treatable disease are concealed, or at least not reported, by elderly patients. The first suggestion that older persons did not seek medical attention when suffering health-related functional decline came from Scotland. In the

1950s and 1960s, several pioneer geriatricians screened elderly individuals, seeking information about health status in older persons residing in the community [5, 6]. The findings in these and subsequent corroborating studies were landmarks. An iceberg of concealed disease was discovered among Scottish elderly enrolled in the British National Health Service, which appeared to have the necessary features to provide adequate service to the elderly: doctors responsible for each older person's outpatient care, free care, and numerous, accessible doctors' offices. Yet startling numbers of problems hitherto unknown to and untreated by the patients' responsible physicians were discovered. Nor were the problems esoteric, requiring sophisticated diagnostic methodology. Frequently encountered disorders included congestive heart failure, correctable hearing and vision deficits, tuberculosis, urinary dysfunction, anemia, chronic bronchitis, claudication, cancers, nutritional deficiencies, uncontrolled diabetes, foot disease hampering mobility, dental disease impeding nutrition, dementia, and depression.

American investigations have corroborated and extended the British data. In an early survey of older persons, nearly 90 percent had experienced symptoms of illness in the month prior to interview, but less than one-third had notified or visited a physician about the problem [7]. More than four-fifths of subjects surveyed, when asked whom they would consult in the event of a health crisis, named a family member; less than 10 percent said they would consult a physician, clergyman, or social worker. When the family members of the surveyed group were questioned, one-third thought that their elderly relatives were not getting as much medical care as they needed and that they viewed their symptoms as normal and expected in old age. Another community-based study of symptoms and reporting in older persons revealed that although a slight majority told someone about symptoms, a large proportion told no one at all [8]. More than half of all symptoms were not reported to a health professional. The usual confidant for the symptomatic older person was a family member, and when symptoms were unreported, explanations included "no big deal," "nobody cares," "nothing can be done about it," or "don't want to bother people."

One study examined in detail the health beliefs and practices of adults across the age span through a series of questionnaires concerning attitudes toward health and illness, as well as responses to hypothetical personal clinical situations [9]. The oldest subjects had the highest levels of health-promoting baseline behavior but were least responsive to symptoms consistent with serious systemic illness. Mild symptoms were most likely to be attributed to age alone by subjects of all ages, but all symptoms (brief, severe, brief mild, and chronic mild) were increasingly likely to be attributed to aging by subjects of increasing age. Subjects who thought symptoms were due to aging also were more likely to react passively to the perception of symptoms by doing one of the following: (1) waiting and watching, (2) accepting the symptoms, (3) denying or minimizing the threat, or (4) postponing or avoiding medical attention. Thus we see continued documentation of risk to older persons by underreporting of symptoms and their misidentification as only age-related.

It appears that older people perceive pain, malaise, and disability adequately but choose to conceal their distress or at least not seek treatment. The most common explanation for symptom tolerance and nonreporting seems to be the pervasive belief that old age is inextricably associated with illness, functional decline, and feeling sick. Old and young, lay and professional, men and women, all believe that to be old is to be ill. Obviously this "ageist" view of health and disease guarantees that older individuals, even when afflicted with the same symptoms that impel the middle-aged sick into the mainstream of the health care system, will not seek care, will suffer in silence the progression of many diseases, and will endure the functional losses engendered by untreated illness. That old age in the absence of disease is a time of good health and persisting function has been documented by numerous studies of normal aging (see Chap. 1), but while our society continues in ignorance of gerontologic information, elders will continue to expect decline and dysfunction. A useful geriatric maxim to be remembered is that sick old people are sick because they are sick, not because they are old. Although certainly decline in numerous physiologic functions characterizes normal human aging, these declines are gradual, and their functional impact is ameliorated by the decades over which they occur and by the remaining, if diminishing, reserve capacities of the individual. Thus, major functional decline, especially if abrupt in an individual already old, is usually attributable to disease, not age.

Other possible explanations for old people not reporting illness include depression and intellectual loss. Though never normal, the increasing prevalence of cognitive loss with age is doubly dangerous to the detection of disease. Cognitively impaired individuals have a diminished ability to complain and are also evaluated less enthusiastically for associated medical disease or even reversible disease that produces the intellectual losses itself.

The abundant documentation that disease is not being reported by the elderly appears to contradict a clinical rule of thumb that identifies hypochondriasis as common among aged patients. Many clinicians caring for elderly patients cite one or two individuals who try their patience and good-will with endless complaints rooted in trivial or nonexistent illness. Yet when studied, the hypochondriacal, doctor-shopping, old person appears to be one more unverifiable mythical figure in people's ideas about aging [10]. Not only is hypochondriasis less common among older people, but when elders do complain, important disease is found underlying their complaints substantially more often than in younger, nonhypochondriacal individuals [11].

Nonreporting of symptoms of underlying disease in elderly persons is an especially dangerous phenomenon when coupled with the American organizational structure of health care delivery. Our health care system is passive, especially for elderly people, and lacks prevention-oriented or early detection efforts. American medical care of the critically ill, elderly hospitalized patient is the best in the world. Science and technology are most expertly blended to help the sick. But American hospital beds, health maintenance organizations (HMOs), physicians' offices, emergency rooms, and neighborhood health centers all wait passively for the symptomatic patient to activate the system. For the most part, this passive system of health care provision is adequate for children,

who have parental advocates, and for young and middle-aged adults who have the need to work and earn impelling them to seek medical relief of function-impairing symptoms. But aged persons, without advocates and usually without jobs, burdened by society's and their own ageist views of functional loss in the elderly, cannot be relied upon to initiate appropriate health care for themselves, especially early in the course of an illness when intervention is most likely to have a favorable outcome. In summary, our health care system relies on the patient to enter the system and initiate care, and that is precisely the one illness behavior most often missing in aged individuals. These factors make undetected decline especially likely and suggest that adding a more active case-finding facet to the system for the elderly would be beneficial (see Chap. 5).

Behavior of Disease in Older Persons
"PREDEATH" AMONG HOSPITALIZED ELDERLY

A year-long Scottish study of 4,000 hospital deaths in individuals over 65 years of age revealed a recurring pattern of preadmission debility and surprisingly long stays for those patients destined to die [12]. The older the patients were, the longer they survived before dying in the hospital. A high proportion—nearly three-quarters—of the deaths were preceded by a period of increasing dependency prior to hospitalization. A high correlation of dependency with advancing age and death following hospitalization led to naming the dependent period "predeath." The most common causes of predeath dependency were immobility, incontinence, and mental impairment, often in combination. The durations of predeath and attendant hospitalization were strikingly age-related, as was the likelihood of hospital death. Although deaths of the very old occurred more often in beds allotted to geriatric or psychiatric patients (in which average hospital stays were substantially longer than for patients in American beds used for acute or short-term care) than in those used for patients undergoing medical or surgical care, it was astonishing to find that the average hospital stay before death was three months for patients 65 to 74 years of age, six months for those 75 to 84 years of age, seven months for men 85 years and older, and 13 months for women more than 85 years old! Retrospective analysis of a small subject sample revealed that a high proportion had potentially reversible or at least improvable causes of the predeath dependency if appropriate evaluation and treatment had been undertaken early. Immobility, incontinence, and dementia are clarions of serious underlying disease in old people and demand prompt evaluation. Long, costly, discouraging dependency among old people may be avoided by prompt evaluation and intervention on detection of decline.

MULTIPLE PATHOLOGY

Another characteristic of illness in old age that is important in planning geriatric health care and predisposes elderly individuals to functional decline based on late detection of potentially treatable disease is the common occurrence of illness clustering in aged patients. Usually called multiple pathology, the existence of several concurrent diseases in an old person who either is not obviously ill or is under treatment for a different problem has a profound negative influence on health and functional independence in old age. A random sample of community-dwelling subjects over 65 years of age found nearly 3.5 important disabilities per person [6]. An earlier study of elderly patients being admitted to hospitals documented six pathologic conditions per person [13]. An American clinical experience tabulated common problems often coexisting in elderly individuals (Table 3-1) [14]. Isaacs (1972) has coined the phrase "survival of the unfittest" to describe the most vulnerable disease-burdened group of elders.

Multiple pathologic conditions can exert a detrimental influence on elderly individuals in at least two important ways. In treatment-disease interaction, the diagnostic evaluation or treat-

TABLE 3-1. *Common coexisting conditions in the elderly*

Congestive heart failure	Urinary incontinence
Depression	Vascular insufficiency
Dementia	Constipation
Chronic renal failure	Diabetes
Angina pectoris	Sensory deficits
Osteoarthritis	Sleep disturbance
Osteoporosis	Adverse drug reactions
Gait disorder	Anemia

ment of one identified illness interacts adversely with one or several undiagnosed conditions, producing iatrogenic harm. For example, an old man with ankle edema and pulmonary congestion of mild heart failure is given a potent diuretic, which rapidly clears a liter of excess fluid from his circulation and improves the identified problem of heart failure. The rippling secondary effects are not beneficial. The abrupt diuresis overwhelms the emptying capacity of his bladder, previously compromised by prostatic enlargement, and produces acute urinary retention. The secondary kidney damage and pain of retention produces acute confusion, worsened by early memory loss of Alzheimer's disease. The diuretic raises already high but previously asymptomatic levels of blood sugar and uric acid due to undiagnosed diabetes and gout, respectively. Each of these now becomes symptomatic, with impaired consciousness and dehydration of hyperosmolar diabetes and the exquisitely painful foot of gout.

An example of disease-disease interaction is the old woman with unreported urinary tract infection that produces frequent urgent urination that exceeds the mobility limit of her degenerative osteoarthritis and makes her incontinent. Uncorrected poor vision and urine on the floor cause a fall, with fracture of her osteoporotic hip and secondary decompensation of heart failure. The retrospective identification of functional losses in a once independent elder is a truly depressing but improvable aspect of geriatric medical care.

The number of pathologic conditions in an individual is strongly related to age, often rising to more than a dozen in the very old. If the entire spectrum of multiple pathologic conditions is not identified and carefully considered, virtually any diagnostic or therapeutic initiative is as likely to produce harm as benefit through a treatment-disease adverse interaction. In the absence of an obvious flare-up of one problem, major danger still exists for the patient with multiple pathologies. Korenchevsky [16] first pointed out the destructive, insidious virulence of unattended multiple pathologies in the uncomplaining elderly patient through disease-disease adverse interaction. Undetected, untreated diseases create ricocheting stress in several organ systems or tissues, producing deterioration of a previously diseased but compensated physiologic function. As each overburdened organ fails, a concatenation of deteriorations is created that rapidly becomes irreversible, passing multiple points of no return and leading to infirmity, dependence, and, if uninterrupted, death.

CHRONICITY OF DISEASE

Disease in old age is characterized by a high prevalence of chronic conditions. Chronic disease is defined as any condition lasting more than three months [17]. Among the population aged 65 years and older, 80 percent have at least one such chronic disease [18], and it is estimated that a large number also experience multiple chronic conditions. Although some elderly advance to old age with chronic illnesses that were acquired during their earlier years, for many, chronic disease is first experienced in late life, and this interacts with many age-related changes, resulting in accelerated loss of organ reserve.

Given the lack of population-based epidemiologic studies, it is difficult to estimate the true prevalence of chronic disease among the aged. However, mortality statistics do provide information on the link between chronic disease and eventual mortality, and chronic diseases do account for most deaths in persons over age 65.

Diseases of the heart account for nearly half of all deaths at these ages, and diseases of the heart, malignant neoplasms, and cerebrovascular diseases account for nearly 80 percent of deaths among the aged (Table 3-2).

The prevalence of chronic disease among the aged has several implications. It is currently estimated that over 80 percent of all health care resources in the United States are devoted to chronic diseases [19]. As the population continues to age, chronic disease will become more prevalent and disability a more common occurrence. In addition, the management of chronic diseases poses challenges for health care providers. Success requires a sensitive and accurate ability to assess functional status initially and over time (see Chap. 4). Moreover, health care providers working with the chronically ill elderly must shift their traditional treatment emphasis from cure to efforts aimed at managing the existing condition, improving function, postponing further deterioration and disability, and preventing secondary complications.

ATYPICAL PRESENTATION OF DISEASE

A fundamental principle of geriatric medicine is that many diseases may present with signs and symptoms in the elderly that differ from those seen characteristically or classically in younger persons. Although it has been suggested that

TABLE 3-2. *Death rates for the 10 leading causes of death for ages 65 and over, by age: 1976*

CAUSE OF DEATH BY RANK	65 YEARS AND OVER	65–74 YEARS	75–84 YEARS	85 YEARS AND OVER
	DEATHS PER 100,000			
All causes	5,428.9	3,127.6	7,331.6	15,486.9
1. Diseases of the heart	2,393.5	1,286.9	3,263.7	7,384.3
2. Malignant neoplasms	979.0	786.3	1,248.6	1,441.5
3. Cerebrovascular diseases	694.6	280.1	1,014.0	2,586.8
4. Influenza and pneumonia	211.1	70.1	289.3	959.2
5. Arteriosclerosis	122.2	25.8	152.5	714.3
6. Diabetes mellitus	108.1	70.0	155.8	219.2
7. Accidents	104.5	62.2	134.5	306.7
Motor Vehicle	25.2	21.7	32.3	26.0
All other	79.3	40.4	102.2	280.7
8. Bronchitis, emphysema and asthma	76.8	60.7	101.4	108.5
9. Cirrhosis of the liver	36.5	42.6	29.3	18.0
10. Nephritis and nephrosis	25.0	15.2	34.1	64.6
All other causes	677.5	427.8	908.6	1,683.8

SOURCE: National Center for Health Statistics, U.S. Public Health Service. Advance report—Final mortality statistics, 1976. *Monthly Vital Statistics Report* 26 (12), Suppl. 2, March 1978; and unpublished data provided by the National Center for Health Statistics.

atypical presentation may have been overemphasized during early efforts to establish and validate a unique data base for geriatric medicine, and it is certainly true that diseases often present typically in older persons, there is also abundant documentation of atypical presentation. One way in which disease presentation can be atypical is that manifestations of illness may be nonspecific, meaning that general or functionally related problems become the first or major or sole indicator of disease (see Chap. 4). The new appearance of confusion, incontinence, falls, appetite loss, or other unfocused problem usually announces systemic illness with no clue as to the origin of the pathology. Pneumonia [20, 21] and myocardial infarction [22, 23] are prime examples of diseases frequently presenting nonspecifically, without their usual features, in older persons (Table 3-3).

A second variety of atypical presentation consists of diseases that have specific and characteristic manifestations in the older person that differ from their appearance in the young (Table 3-4). For example, young diabetics out of control present with modest blood sugar elevations and profound acid-base and electrolyte disorders of ketoacidosis, provoked by insulin insufficiency and consequent free fatty acid metabolism. Elderly decompensated diabetics present with

TABLE 3-3. *Diseases likely to present nonspecifically in the elderly*

Pneumonia
Meningitis
Tuberculosis
Myocardial infarction
Pulmonary embolism
Digitalis toxicity
Myxedema
Alcoholism
Accidental hypothermia

TABLE 3-4. *Altered presentation of disease in the elderly*

DISEASE	GERIATRIC PRESENTATION
Diabetes, out of control	Hyperosmolar state, without ketoacidosis
Thyrotoxicosis	Apathetic—psychomotor retardation, dementia Masked—single organ system without usual hyperthyroid features
Depression	Cognitive impairment

striking elevations of blood sugar, often in the range of 1,000 to 2,000 gm/dl, and dehydration due to the obligate diuresis of severe hyperglycemia. Obtundation proceeding to coma, without important acid-base abnormalities, accompany the syndrome (see Chap. 28).

DISEASES MORE COMMON OR SEVERE

More common or severe diseases derive from age-related reductions in the function of numerous organs and tissues, which put the older person at special risk for increased frequency of and morbidity from disorders in those organs. Losses of function in the renal, immune, pulmonary, and musculoskeletal systems, combined with restricted homeostatic capacity in most organ systems, reduce dramatically the ability of older persons to compensate for otherwise modest perturbations of organ functions produced by illness. Problems that thus are more common and probably severe in older persons are particularly important to keep in mind when approaching elderly patients (Table 3-5).

Examination of the Older Person

Adequate and successful evaluation of the older person requires modification and supplementation of the usual doctor-patient interaction used for the young and middle-aged person. Different components of the history and physical examination need to be emphasized for older individuals, and the physical environment and interpretation of laboratory data require attention as well. Perhaps most important, comprehensive functional assessment must be coupled with the usual medical evaluation strategies (Chap. 4).

ENVIRONMENT AND INTERACTION

The physical environment in which the older person is assessed should be modified in consideration of common difficulties in old age. Frail older persons are more easily intimidated and frightened by the advanced technology presented by the ordinary accoutrements of the doctor's office. Sensory impairments, physical discomfort, and communication disorders demand a considerate and individualized approach to each older person, but some general prin-

TABLE 3-5. *Problems more common or severe in the elderly*

Falls
Syncope
Hip fracture
Urinary incontinence
Fecal incontinence
Fecal impaction
Pressure sores
Hearing and vision impairment
Stroke
Dementia syndrome
Parkinsonism
Normal pressure hydrocephalus
Polymyalgia rheumatica/giant cell arteritis
Osteoporosis
Osteoarthritis
Paget's disease
Carpal tunnel syndrome
Spinal stenosis
Diabetic hyperosmolar nonketotic coma
Inappropriate antidiuretic hormone secretion
Accidental hypothermia
Chronic lymphatic leukemia
Basal cell carcinoma
Angioimmunoblastic lymphadenopathy with
  dysproteinemia
Solid tumors
Tuberculosis
Herpes zoster
Arteriosclerosis
Amyloidosis
Colonic angiodysplasia
Isolated systolic hypertension
Postural hypotension

ciples are useful for the physician dealing with substantial numbers of elders. Time spent at the beginning of the interaction to reassure and comfort an older person and establish a friendly relationship is usually worthwhile and productive, and most older persons are reassured rather than put off by a gentle touch on the hand or arm during conversational interaction. The interview and examining rooms should be quiet to allow communication and prevent distraction for those with impaired hearing. Speech should be uttered with an emphasis on clarity and diction while directly facing the patient to allow lip reading and other visual clues. Increasing the volume of speech is often helpful and may be necessary in communicating with a hearing-impaired older person because the prevalence of clinically relevant hearing impairment exceeds 50 percent in the elderly population. Yet not all older persons are hearing disabled, and thus it is most sensible to begin the interview by inquiring about hearing and the adequacy of the doc-

tor's speech for the patient. Given the fatigue provoked by constant shouting for the physician and the discomfort for the individual with normal hearing who has to listen to it, it only makes sense to be direct and unembarrassed in discussing hearing loss. If hearing is impaired and an increase in voice volume is necessary for adequate audition, the voice should be raised in the lower frequency range rather than the high range in which most of us tend to raise our voices, since high-tone loss is most common in the elderly. Also, the physician should be sure to inquire about both the presence and the adequacy of a hearing aid. Discovering at the conclusion of a shouted interview that the patient had a hearing aid in her purse, or worse, in her ear but not turned on, is frustrating for all concerned.

Since visual impairment is nearly as common as hearing loss in the older person, lighting should be carefully considered for safety, comfort, and accurate perception by the patient. Deep shadows in the environment can make walking about the room dangerous for the visually impaired older person, and intensely bright light, especially from above, can be painful for those who have had cataract surgery without lens implantation. Back-lighting of the interviewer is intensely unpleasant because aging eyes accommodate less well. As with hearing aids, glasses should be available and worn during the visit to the physician.

Physical safety and comfort demand that furniture, if not specifically designed for use by older and disabled persons, at least not be unusable or unsafe. Chairs of adequate height to allow easy arising are essential. The examining table should be of a height and size that will not imperil an unsteady older person in the process of mounting, dismounting, and being examined. Examining gowns should be manageable with arthritic joints of diminished mobility and should be short enough not to produce tripping or falling by an elderly woman under five feet in height. Allowing the patient sufficient time to undress and dress again after examination is essential to provide the relaxation and attentiveness required for retaining information and advice communicated by the physician at the conclusion of the evaluation. Finally, since geriatric patients tend to be years, if not decades, older than their physicians and nurses, it is only seemly and polite for the health professional to initiate a relationship with an older person by using formal address such as Mr., Miss, Mrs., or Ms., at least until invited to use first names. At no time should the impersonal and generic term "dear" be used.

HISTORY-TAKING

Gathering adequate historic information from the older person concerning illness and health care in the present, recent past, and remote past is more complex and time-consuming than it is in younger individuals. In addition to the patient interview, previous medical records, friends and family members, and other physicians and health professionals generally must be included in data collection. Although family members are an important source of information in history-gathering, total reliance on the family or allowing them to dominate an interview with the patient can interfere with a sensitive assessment of the patient's perceptions as well as with cognitive and emotional evaluation. The presence of cognitive impairment, mild or severe, should not automatically abort the history. It is common for demented patients to be able to report adequately useful information about their symptoms. In most instances, the patient should be seen alone first to the limit of the interaction's utility, and only then should the family join the interview or be seen separately. It should be emphasized that much of the preliminary data gathering can be accomplished by someone other than the physician; only after there is a base of information to target the history-taking need the physician personally interview the patient.

One of the early lessons learned by physicians who deliver primary care to older patients is that the chief complaint is not the key to unlocking the puzzle of disease in the elderly. Rarely is there a single chief complaint from a sick old person. The multiple pathology of accumulated chronic disease generally burdens the older person with numerous chronic and fluctuating complaints. When clinical decompensation is driven by a single illness, either flare of a chronic disease or acquisition of a new acute problem, it usually provokes ripples of symptoms in a variety of tissues and organ systems as well as tipping the psychosocial and economic status of the old person, guaranteeing multiple presenting complaints. Each complaint may originate in a different problem on the problem list, and the law of parsimony, or Occam's razor, does not usually apply in geriatric care. Even in those uncommon instances when there is a single presenting complaint by a decompensated older person, the complaint is far less reliable in narrowing the differential diagnosis in the older patient compared with a younger one.

The family history is usually less relevant to a thorough elucidation of pathology in older persons, although the strong familial trend in Alzheimer's disease and its relationship to Down's syndrome is a notable exception. But if time can be saved in truncating the family history, the social history must be greatly expanded to include and highlight items usually of secondary importance in younger individuals. The social interaction of friends and family plays a major role in the overall well-being and mental health of older retired persons compared with younger individuals, who derive so much of their sense of self and social interaction in the workplace. In addition, resources in the community, including friends, family, and clergy, are critical to identify the kind and intensity of disability that can be managed at home subsequently. Given the escalation of percentage of income and assets allocated to health care by older persons, a detailed listing of resources and insurance coverage should also be documented. An accurate diet history is relevant for individuals in whom disease management includes food restriction or alteration—for example, diabetes, hypertension, acid peptic disease, or congestive heart failure. Although the status of polio, pertussis, and smallpox immunization is not useful in older persons, pneumococcus, influenza, and tetanus vaccination histories are important.

Although enumeration of medications accompanies virtually every written medical record for an older person, reliance on these written lists can lead to iatrogenic harm through either duplication of medication not reported to the current physician or neglect of treatment by assuming that a medication previously listed is still being taken. Regardless of abundant historical information from written or verbal reports, the only reliable medication list is generated by physically inspecting and inquiring about all medications currently in the possession of the patient. Instructing patient, friends, and family members to bring all medications to the doctor's office or to the hospital at the time of admission is essential; and when all medications are in hand, including prescription and over-the-counter drugs, the patient should be asked which ones are taken, for what symptoms, and at what intervals ("brown bag evaluation"). Major discrepancies between instructions on the label and patient practice are common at any age but are especially frequent and dangerous in the elderly (see Chap. 9).

PHYSICAL EXAMINATION

Patients of any age deserve a careful and thorough physical examination, and given the increase in pathology in the elderly, it is usually more time-consuming to conduct an examination in an older person. Thus it is of particular concern to note the diminished time allocated to older patients in physician encounters [24]. Given this peculiar phenomenon, it is incumbent on us as geriatricians to recommend as little extra in the physical examination of the elderly person as we can. Nevertheless, there are certain points and measurements in the physical examination that do require special attention in older patients.

Vital signs deserve emphasis. Because of the high prevalence of orthostatic hypotension in older persons (see Chap. 16), blood pressure should be measured with the patient recumbent and then standing for at least three minutes to exclude postural hypotension. Whether the patient becomes symptomatic or not, objective recording of any blood pressure or pulse change is essential. Because orthostatic drop appears to be greater in some older individuals with higher systolic blood pressure, the presence of hypertension, with or without hypotensive drug treatment, should not exclude postural recordings. The vulnerability of older persons to accidental hypothermia requires that recording of low normal temperatures in the winter be verified with appropriate low-reading thermometers, especially when clinical abnormalities are consistent with the multisystem declines in function typical of hypothermia (see Chap. 28). Pulse recordings should be done routinely, but

awareness of baroreflex blunting in older persons demands that absence of cardioacceleration when blood pressure falls on standing be noted prominently in the record (see Chap. 16). Although height measurement is generally of little relevance, weight should be recorded under similar conditions at all encounters. In addition to the value of weight in following nutritional status and degree of fluid loss or retention in patients on chronic diuretic therapy for congestive heart failure, it has been documented that involuntary weight loss in older patients is generally ominous [25]. Among 90 Veterans Administration patients over 60 years of age with involuntary weight loss, 25 percent died in one year, and another 15 percent deteriorated in a major way. A comprehensive history and physical examination were usually adequate to identify etiology, and evaluation was undertaken if either weight loss was documented in the medical record or convincing evidence thereof could be found (change in clothing size, corroborating information from a close friend or family member, ability to give exact weight loss by home scale measurement). Aged skin usually reveals numerous abnormalities (see Chap. 12). Turgor is notoriously difficult to assess due to loss of supporting subcutaneous tissue and wrinkling, but the lateral aspect of the cheek is often a reliable site for evaluation.

Although many abnormalities appear in the head and neck examination of older persons, a majority are not of major clinical importance. The arcus senilis, long emphasized as a marker of premature cardiovascular disease, has been identified simply as depigmentation within the iris and is associated with healthy aging [26]. Although glaucoma is the second leading cause of blindness in America and is increasingly common with age, measurement of intraocular pressure by Schiotz tonometry may not be reliable because there is considerable diurnal variation of pressure. Thus, funduscopic examination and testing for visual field loss are at least as important [27]. The temporal arteries should be palpated for thickening or tenderness routinely, regardless of complaints related to possible temporal arteritis, in view of the vague nature of presentation of polymyalgia rheumatica and its spectrum of associated disorders. Recording of carotid bruits is worthwhile to document change over time, but their presence does not have relevance to cerebrovascular insufficiency symptoms and is only a marker of generalized atherosclerosis. The oral cavity should be examined carefully with dentures in place to check for comfort and adequacy of mastication and with dentures removed to look for sores or possibly cancerous lesions.

Deferring breast or pelvic examination in an elderly woman is indefensible in view of the increased incidence of malignancy and of other problems whose elucidation is greatly enhanced by careful examination. Genital and rectal examination in men and women provides an excellent opportunity to assess bowel and bladder function as well as the presence of impaction or more ominous rectal lesions. Atrophic vaginitis, urethritis, cystocele/rectocele, uterine prolapse, and evidence of incontinence all can easily be noted and addressed. In addition, this is the time at which an adequate sexual history should be taken. A pelvic examination and Papanicolaou (Pap) smear should be done at least every two years in elderly women [28].

Adequate neurologic examination is crucial given the high prevalence and incidence of neurologic disorders in the elderly and the common expression of other illnesses through secondary dysfunction in the nervous system. A mental status evaluation is central and primary in assessing elderly individuals presenting for medical evaluation, both for establishment of baseline norms and for detection of subtle or severe abnormalities that are to be followed and worked up (see Chaps. 4 and 27). In addition, the diminution or disappearance of both gag and ankle jerk reflexes must be kept clearly in mind, lest these isolated age-related changes be misinterpreted as disease related. Furthermore, frontal release signs, often touted as indicative of dementing disease, have been shown to occur with normal aging and do not predict cognitive impairment [29].

LABORATORY DATA

The great majority of laboratory values do not have an age adjustment, although within the wide limits of normal ranges, some individual tests do reveal, on average, statistically significant but clinically unimportant deviations up or down in healthy old people compared with younger ones [30, 31]. Some tests in healthy older persons deviate beyond the upper or lower normal limits [30, 31, 32], and these few are important and must be learned by clinicians. Finally, in rare instances, values that do not change with age belie or overestimate the "normality" of the underlying organ function being evaluated.

Among the values that do not change with age are clinical measures of red cell concentration in the blood. Although it is commonly held that there is an "anemia of old age," it has been shown that hematocrit does not decline during the adult life span in the absence of disease [33]. Likewise, hemoglobin concentration, red cell and platelet counts, and red blood cell indices do not change in old age. Yet there is a decline in red cell mass, which is indicated by normal, but not elevated, hematocrit levels in the presence of diminution in intravascular volume and total body water [34]. Likewise, there is no change in total leukocyte count, nor do polymorphonuclear or lymphocytic elements decline, although there is apparently a decline in total lymphocyte count during the three years preceding death in previously healthy elderly men [35].

The erythrocyte sedimentation rate (ESR) rises slightly with age, but values above 19 mm in men and 22 mm in women suggest disease, not aging, and deserve investigation [36]. More important in approaching overall patient management in the elderly is the finding that half of the older patients with diseases predicted to cause elevation of ESR (autoimmune disorders, malignancy, pyelonephritis, obstructed airways disease) have values within the normal range. Accordingly, the ESR should be regarded as relevant in elderly patients if elevated, but normal values should be of no comfort to the clinician. Although serum proteins do not change with age, albumin diminishes substantially in the healthy elderly [37], and reductions of 0.5 to 0.9 gm/dl are reported, but values remain within the limits of normal. The decline in albumin has direct relevance to the ratio of free to bound drug in the older person and may be one of many factors contributing to increased adverse drug reaction rates in the elderly (see Chap. 9). Fasting blood sugar rises with age but remains within normal limits as opposed to postprandial blood sugar, which rises in reflection of increasing age-related carbohydrate intolerance (see Chap. 28).

Although electrolyte composition of the blood does not change, blood urea nitrogen (BUN) and serum creatinine both show statistically significant but clinically trivial increases with increasing age [31]. Far more important, BUN and creatinine levels remain well within normal ranges for healthy older persons in spite of a major decline in creatinine clearance because of concurrent changes in body composition, and thus these parameters seriously overestimate renal function in the elderly (see Chap. 18).

There is no age adjustment in normal ranges for any clinical liver function tests, although alkaline phosphatase rises within the normal range [31]. In addition, many older persons show frank elevation above the upper limits of normal for alkaline phosphatase in the presence of clinical stability and apparent good health. In most cases, modest degrees of Paget's disease or osteomalacia, rheumatoid arthritis, or fracture underly the abnormality, and measurement of the bone and liver fractions is helpful in working up the elevation. When the liver fraction is elevated, chronic gallbladder disease is the most common cause in the elderly.

Physician Decisions in Evaluation of the Elderly Patient

The physician caring for sizable numbers of older persons has two decisions to make in the allocation of time and choice of assessments for individuals receiving that care. The first decision concerns the evaluation of the elderly patient who is palpably ill, the person with symptoms or signs of illness, no matter how nonspecific, altered, atypical, or functional the presentation may be. We would argue, and good data support the argument [5, 6, 38, 39, 40], that decline of any sort requires a comprehensive evaluation, including history, physical examination, laboratory screening, and functional assessment, because symptom specificity "breaks the rules" in older persons who are ill. Furthermore, the above studies amply document the benefit to patients of early and comprehensive

medical evaluation prompted by nonspecific or peculiar functional deterioration. The unique details of geriatric patient evaluation are considered in this and the next chapter and are defensible in these fiscally austere times by continued documentation of patient benefit.

The second decision is more difficult because of fewer data to inform it, larger numbers of persons to be considered, and thus greater costs. What is appropriate "screening" for the truly asymptomatic, at least once-evaluated, clinically stable older person? Should the venerable annual physical examination, now regarded as both expensive and useless in young and middle-aged persons, also be abandoned in the elderly [41]? Or are there reasons to continue this otherwise archaic practice for our more ancient citizens? For persons seeking the "complete physical examination" the physician may be best advised to undertake the assessment, since motivation may well include the perception of unreported symptoms, recognition of deleterious health habits, or psychosocial stress highly relevant to health. Recommendations for screening the asymptomatic elderly have been summarized and compiled [42, 43, 44]. Although these differ, a majority advise annual contact after age 60 for blood pressure measurement, breast, rectal and pelvic examinations, influenza vaccination and one-time-only pneumococcal vaccination, stool examination for occult blood, and mammography, and a Pap smear every other year. A complete history and physical examination have been recommended as a part of screening only once [45]—annually after 74 years of age and every other year from age 60 to 74.

In most discussions, laboratory screening of asymptomatic persons has been thought to be unrewarding, but only recently has the common practice of periodic laboratory testing in the nursing home been scrutinized. This special population, with its impressive burden of disease, disability, and health care costs, appears to be fertile ground for early detection of imminent health status decline by periodic laboratory assessment. When scrutinized, routinely performed laboratory tests, although yielding abnormal results nearly 10 percent of the time, resulted in further diagnostic tests in only 0.7 percent of patients, and only 0.1 percent of tests "led to changes in patient management, none of which benefited the patient in an important way" [46]. Lest we take this and a corroborating study [47] as evidence against laboratory tests for nursing home residents, Domoto and the accompanying editorial [48] pointed out that the Boston study examined the most functionally independent residents in an institution providing atypically exemplary medical care, which provided prompt clinical assessment at the first sign of decline. In such an environment, annual screening would actually detect only laboratory changes that occurred entirely covertly in a carefully medically scrutinized group of functionally independent and thus easily monitored people.

References

1. Mechanic, D. *Medical Sociology* (2nd ed.). New York: Free Press, 1978.
2. Besdine, R. W., Levkoff, S. E., and Wetle, T. Health and illness behaviors in elder veterans. In T. Wetle and J. W. Rowe (eds.), *Older Veterans: Linking VA and Community Resources.* Cambridge: Harvard University Press, 1984.
3. Neugarten, G. L., Moore, I. W., and Lowe, J. C. Age Norms, Age Constraints, and Adult Socialization. In B. L. Neugarten (ed.), *Middle Age and Aging.* Chicago: University of Chicago Press, 1968.
4. Ferraro, K. Self-ratings of health among the old and the old-old. *J. Health Soc. Behav.* 21:377, 1980.
5. Anderson, W. F. *The Prevention of Illness in the Elderly: The Rutherglen Experiment in Medicine in Old Age.* Proceedings of a conference held at the Royal College of Physicians of London. London: Pitman, 1966.
6. Williamson, J., et al. Old people at home: Their unreported needs. *Lancet* 1:1117, 1964.
7. Shanas, E. *The Health of Older People.* Cambridge: Harvard University Press, 1962.
8. Brody, E. M., and Kleban, M. H. Physical and mental health symptoms of older people: Who do they tell? *J. Am. Geriatr. Soc.* 29:442, 1981.
9. Leventhal, E. A., and Prohaska, T. R. Age, symptom interpretation and health behavior. *J. Am. Geriatr. Soc.* 34:185, 1986.
10. Costa, P. T., Jr., and McCrae, R. R. Somatic complaints in males as a function of age and neuroticism: A longitudinal analysis. *J. Behav. Med.* 3:245, 1980.
11. Stenback, A., Kumpulainen, M., and Vauhkonen, M. L. Illness and health behavior in septuagenarians. *Gerontologist* 33:57, 1978.
12. Isaacs, B. The concept of pre-death. *Lancet* 1:115, 1971.
13. Wilson, L. A., Lawson, I. R., and Brass, W. Multiple disorders in the elderly. *Lancet* 2:841, 1962.
14. Besdine, R. W. Geriatric medicine: An overview. *Ann. Rev. Geront. Geriatr.* 1:135, 1980.
15. Isaacs, B. *Survival of the Unfittest.* London: Routledge & Kegan Paul, 1972.
16. Korenchevsky, V. *Physiology and Pathological Aging.* New York: Basel/Karger, 1961.
17. National Center for Health Statistics, Public Health Service. Current estimates from the National Health Interview Survey, United States, 1979. S. Jack, and P. Ries (eds.), *Vital and Health Statistics* Series 10, No. 136, DHHS Pub. No. (PHS) 81-1564. Washington, D.C.: U.S. Government Printing Office, April, 1981.
18. Kovar, M. G. Health of the elderly and use of health services. *Pub. Hlth. Rep.* 92:9, 1977.
19. Cluff, L. F. Chronic disease, function and quality of care. *J. Chronic Dis.* 34:299, 1981.
20. Osler, W. *Principle and Practice of Medicine.* New York: D. Appleton & Co., 1892.
21. Gleckman, R. A. Community-acquired Pneumonia. In R. A. Gleckman and N. M. Gantz (eds.), *Infections in the Elderly.* Boston: Little, Brown, 1983.
22. Bayer, A. J., et al. Changing presentation of myocardial infarction with increasing old age. *J. Am. Geriatr. Soc.* 34:263, 1986.
23. Kannel, W. B., and Abbott, R. D. Incidence and prognosis of unrecognized myocardial infarction. *N. Engl. J. Med.* 311:1144, 1984.
24. Keeler, E. B., et al. Effect of patient age on duration of medical encounters with physicians. *Med. Care* 20:1101, 1982.
25. Marton, K. I., Sox, H. C., and Krupp, J. R. Involuntary weight loss: Diagnostic and prognostic significance. *Ann. Intern. Med.* 95:568, 1981.
26. Editorial. *Lancet* Feb. 18, 1984. P. 376.
27. Eddy, D. M. The value of screening for glaucoma with tonometry. *Surv. Ophthalmol.* 28(3):194, 1983.
28. Gunby, P. Compromise reached on suggested intervals between Pap tests. *J.A.M.A.* 244 (13):1411, 1980.
29. Basavaraju, N. G., Silverstone, F. A., and Libow, L. S. Primative reflexes and perceptual sensory tests in the elderly—their usefulness in dementia. *J. Chronic Dis.* 34(8):367, 1981.
30. Hodkinson, H. M. *Biochemical Diagnosis of the Elderly.* London: Wiley, 1977.
31. Kelly, A., et al. Patterns of change in selected serum chemical parameters of middle and later years. *J. Gerontol.* 34:37, 1979.

32. Dybkaer, R., Lauritzen, M., and Krakauer, R. Relative reference values for clinical chemical and hematological quantities in "healthy" elderly people. *Acta Med. Scand.* 209:1, 1981.

33. Garry, P. J. Iron status and anemia in the elderly: New findings and a review of previous studies. *J. Am. Geriatr. Soc.* 31:389, 1983.

34. Vestal, R. E., et al. Aging and ethanol metabolism. *Clin. Pharmacol. Ther.* 21:343, 1977.

35. Bender, B. S., et al. Absolute peripheral blood lymphocyte count and subsequent mortality of elderly men. *J. Am. Geriatr. Soc.* 34:649, 1986.

36. Griffiths, R. A. Normal erythrocyte sedimentation rate in the elderly. *Br. Med. J.* 289:724, 1984.

37. Greenblatt, D. J. Reduced serum albumin concentrations in the elderly: A report from the Boston Collaborative Drug Surveillance Program. *J. Am. Geriatr. Soc.* 27:20, 1979.

38. Hodkinson, H. M. Non-specific presentation of illness. *Br. Med. J.* 4:94, 1973.

39. Larson, E. B., et al. Dementia in elderly outpatients: A prospective study. *Ann. Intern. Med.* 100:417, 1984.

40. Lowther, C. P., MacLeod, R. D. M., and Williamson, J. Evaluation of early diagnostic services for the elderly. *Br. Med. J.* 3:275, 1970.

41. Canadian Task Force on the Periodic Health Examination. The periodic health examination. *Can. Med. Assoc. J.* 121:1193, 1979.

42. Canadian Task Force on the Periodic Health Examination. The periodic health examination: 1984 update. *Can. Med. Assoc. J.* 130:1278, 1984.

43. Fletcher, S. W. The periodic health examination and internal medicine: 1984. *Ann. Intern. Med.* 101:866, 1984.

44. American College of Physicians Medical Practice Committee. Periodic health examination: A guide for designing individual preventive health care in the asymptomatic patient. *Ann. Intern. Med.* 95:729, 1981.

45. Breslow, L., and Somers, A. R. The lifetime health-monitoring program: A practical approach to preventive medicine. *N. Engl. J. Med.* 296:601, 1977.

46. Domoto, K., et al. Yield of routine annual laboratory screening in the institutionalized elderly. *Am. J. Public Health* 75:243, 1985.

47. Wolf-Klein, G. P., et al. Efficacy of routine annual studies in the care of elderly patients. *J. Am. Geriatr. Soc.* 33:325, 1985.

48. Golodetz, A. Good medical care in nursing homes. *Am. J. Publ. Health* 75:227, 1985.

4
Functional Assessment in the Elderly

RICHARD W. BESDINE

Definition and Scope

FUNCTIONAL ASSESSMENT may be defined as the systematic, multidimensional, detailed evaluation of an individual's ability to perform various tasks associated with independent daily living. Functional assessment typically measures disabilities in the physical, mental, social, psychological, and economic domains and usually is coupled with appropriate medical evaluation as well. Functional assessment is most useful when standard instruments are used to measure and record impairment. It is especially valuable and important in evaluating older persons, for whom independent capabilities are easily perturbed by the broad array of illnesses and problems common in old age. Although interdisciplinary teams are properly regarded as the "gold standard" for the performance of functional assessment, individual physicians, nurses, social workers, and other health professionals certainly *can* satisfactorily assess patients. Who actually performs the assessment in a given clinical setting is less important than getting it done objectively and routinely and using the results appropriately. Functional assessment can and should be used clinically as a clue to the presence and severity of illness, to determine service needs and eligibility, and to follow change over time.

Understanding and using instruments to assess the functional capabilities of impaired older persons is intimately associated with the successful planning and delivery of health and social care required by dependent elders. This chapter focuses on the usefulness of geriatric functional assessment (GFA), both in the education of health professionals responsible for the care of older persons and in the delivery of that care. The uses of GFA are discussed under five headings. First, the intrinsic worth and necessity of GFA are considered, particularly in relation to the special features of geriatric medicine and of educational programs for geriatric health care providers. The next three components of the chapter consider GFA in the nursing home, in the acute hospital, and in the community, major sites in which functionally disabled elders receive care [7]. The final section discusses principles and specifics of instrument selection.

Need for GFA
FUNCTIONAL LOSS IN THE ELDERLY

Restriction of independent functional ability is the final common pathway for many disorders in the elderly. Functional impairment means decreased ability to meet one's own needs and is measured by assessing activities of daily living (ADL), including mobility, eating, toileting, dressing, and grooming, and by assessing instrumental activities of daily living (IADL), including housekeeping, cooking, shopping,

TABLE 4-1. *Functional presentations of illness*

Stopping eating or drinking
Falling
Urinary incontinence
Dizziness
Acute confusion
New onset, or worsening of, previously mild dementia
Weight loss
Failure to thrive

banking, and driving or using public transportation. In addition, objective assessments of cognition and behavior and of the elder's social, economic, and emotional state are required to document health-related function of older persons. Unlike the situation in young persons, when elderly individuals get sick, the first sign of new illness or reactivated chronic disease is rarely a single specific complaint that helps to localize the organ system or tissue in which the disease occurs. Instead, elderly persons usually present when ill with one or more nonspecific problems, which themselves are manifestations of impaired function (Table 4-1) [6]. These problems quickly impair independence in the previously self-sufficient elder without necessarily producing obvious, typical signs of illness by most lay and even general professional standards. Why disease presents first with functional loss in old patients, usually in organ systems unrelated to the locus of illness, is not well understood. It appears that disruption of homeostasis by any disease is likely to be expressed in the most vulnerable, most delicately balanced systems in previously independent, functional elderly persons. And these most vulnerable systems, or weakest links, are likely to fail and produce problems of ADL or IADL function rather than the usual classic signs and symptoms of disease. Thus, difficulties in mobility, cognition, continence, and nutrition are frequently the first manifestations of disease in an old person, regardless of the organ system or tissue in which the disease resides. Progressive restriction of the ability to maintain homeostasis, or the occurrence of "homeostenosis," is a physiologic principle that capsulizes much phenomenology of biologic aging [8].

The lesson for health care providers, family members, and elders themselves is that deterioration of functional independence in active, previously unimpaired elders is an early and subtle sign of untreated illness, and life quality can only be maintained by rapid and thorough clinical evaluation when such functional impairments develop. These disease-generated functional impairments in old people are usually treatable and improvable, but detection and evaluation are essential before treatment can be applied [52]. Since disease is likely to present with abrupt impairment of function in elderly individuals, GFA is critically important to allow early detection and thus intervention during the beginning phases of active illness. Early therapeutic intervention has been repeatedly emphasized as essential for successful health care of elderly persons. Often called "prevention" or "preventive geriatrics" [1,51], early response to functional loss and treatment of disease is tertiary prevention at best but is still crucial to restoring independence. Success of these health maintenance or early intervention strategies in geriatrics requires a sensitive and accurate ability to assess functional status initially and at subsequent evaluations in vulnerable elders in all settings. Accordingly, GFA emerges as a vital capability for front-line health care providers dealing with the elderly. GFA is available as an objective and rapid surveillance instrument to be used by all health providers for elderly persons. Periodic formal assessment, coupled with rapid response to any detected declines in independence, is a central requirement for satisfactory geriatric care and must be included in the basic, postgraduate, and continuing education of health care professionals working with the elderly.

DISABILITY IN THE ELDERLY
Chronic functional impairment increases with increasing age, and thus individuals over 65 years of age carry a disproportionate burden of disability compared with younger persons. Fifty percent of community-dwelling elders have ADL limitations, and more than three-quarters have at least one chronic illness. More than a third cannot perform their major activity independently, and 5 percent are confined to home [19,45]. Beyond the age of 75, 15 percent are confined to their homes, and over the age of 80 nearly one-quarter cannot go outdoors independently [44]. The disability figure should also have added into it the 5 percent of the over 65

population dwelling in nursing homes at any one time. In view of this impressive level of functional disability in the geriatric population, it seems only sensible that objective, reproducible, quantifiable assessment of functional impairment should be used in designing and distributing supportive services for disabled elders. Those chronic functional losses that are not a result of treatable or reversible pathology still should be evaluated by GFA so that the type and intensity of compensatory care needed to buttress function in those elders can be estimated accurately. Although functional disability may often be due to stable but disabling chronic illness, insufficient supportive services and unappreciated, unmet functional dependency needs themselves are likely to produce cascading further functional loss and deteriorating independence. Accordingly, another important value of GFA is its usefulness in determining and then providing supportive care to prevent further accumulation of disability.

ACTIVE LIFE EXPECTANCY

Another purpose for which GFA has substantial applicability is in the prediction of functional decline. Using a modification of the Katz ADL index [29] and life-table techniques, calculations were made of remaining years of independent or active life expectancy (ALE) for noninstitutionalized older persons in Massachusetts [28]. The onset of dependency was defined by accumulation of ADL assistance need. Years of ALE remaining declined with increasing age, shrinking from 10 years for persons 65 to 70 years of age, to less than 3 years for those 85 and above. ALE was less at all ages for the poor elderly. Although ALE was similar for men and women at most ages, because of the greater longevity of women the percentage of life spent without dependency was greater for men at each 5-year interval. Besides its obvious value in predicting the need for supportive services and in further research on the condition of older persons, the concept of ALE has a major impact on our thinking about the future of older persons. For the first time, we have predictive data to frame the discussion of the burden of disability and its onset associated with the increasing life expectancy of Americans. The opportunity to quantify objectively the duration of dependency that comes with longer life should be seized by support of further study in this arena.

RELATIONSHIP OF FUNCTION AND DISEASE

A major task in the education of health professionals, especially physicians, is the systematic and detailed identification of the clinical signs and symptoms associated with specific pathologic conditions. We have already discussed the frequent functional presentation of disease in old age, characterized by absence of classic or typical clinical findings of illness. GFA illustrates and clarifies another phenomenon common in geriatric medicine, in which there is poor correlation between type and severity of functional disability and the disease problem list. Since the burden of illness and functional loss both increase with increasing age, it is often assumed that the number of diseases or conditions enumerated on the problem list of an old person correlates with and identifies the kind and intensity of functional disability. But the accumulation of many problems or illnesses by an old person does not necessarily result in serious loss of function. Instead, it is common to find independent and vigorous elderly persons with shockingly long and serious lists of problems [53]. Another common but erroneous assumption is that the specific functional impairment in an old person is determined by the organ or tissue with disease—mobility problems are due to musculoskeletal or neurologic disorders, confusion arises from brain disease, incontinence from the bladder, and so on. This causality principle, usually valid for disease in the young and middle-aged, does not hold in geriatric medicine. Instead, certain particularly vulnerable tissues and organ systems, which are responsible for functional integrity in the elderly, are especially likely to decompensate owing to the systemic influence of disease anywhere in the body.

Furthermore, the severity of illness, as measured by objective data, does not necessarily determine the presence or severity of dependency. For example, cardiac arrhythmias may be discovered on routine electrocardiagram or Holter monitor, or chronic elevation of the alkaline phosphatase level may be discovered on multiphasic screening in an independently functional old person. When there is impressive laboratory abnormality with minimal or no obvious functional disability, objective GFA can support withholding treatment for a symptomless problem, particularly if the treatment carries with it considerable cost, discomfort, or health risk. Accordingly, the use and the sensitivity of GFA will allow health professionals maximum capacity to enhance independence among elders and detect declines driven by potentially treatable illnesses. Special features of history-taking, physical examination, and interpretation of laboratory data for older persons and their linkage to GFA have been well described [5].

The lessons taught by these noncorrelations between function and diagnoses are crucial for good geriatric care. First, functional impairment must be assessed and quantified independently of the medical problem list. Second, although functional deterioration is specific and can involve capacities served by a single organ system, the loss of function in a single organ system does not in any way mean that primary pathology exists in that particular organ system, nor does it allow us to attribute causality for functional loss to disease found in that organ system. For example, evaluation of an old man with urinary incontinence may show that he has a normal urinary tract and is incontinent because his diuretic works faster than his feet. Even if prostatitis were documented, treatment of the infection may well not alleviate the incontinence. Only the restoration of normal organ function by successful treatment of the disease in that organ system allows us to identify a causal relationship with certainty.

The crucial importance of lost function to the elderly person emphasizes the value and need for GFA. Although health care providers may focus concern and attention on objective measurements of disease such as physical findings and abnormal laboratory values, for the elderly person these parameters are unimportant compared with the impact of lost function on their daily lives. Therapeutic interventions for the patient must be measured by restoration of lost function and the resulting improvement of life quality. The value of GFA is again clear in that it allows gratification for the health care profes-

sional and satisfaction for the patient by targeting and relieving the most troubling problems.

The educational objective for health professionals caring for vulnerable elders is to acquire an awareness of and skill in using GFA in parallel with classic disease-oriented evaluation techniques [34]. Enumerating functional impairments side-by-side with the problem list can facilitate matching diagnosis with lost function. A list of functional impairments and their severity will allow identification of those medical problems that are probably causing the most troublesome functional losses in the elderly individual. Using a functionally oriented priority system is most likely to satisfy the patient and the clinician by producing important gains in independence. Finally, if interventions are not beneficial, they can be confidently abandoned and replaced by functionally relevant new treatment.

INTERDISCIPLINARY TEAMS AND GFA
Successful geriatric health care requires a wide array of collaborating professionals, posing both an opportunity and a challenge [13,27]. When clinicians from multiple disciplines sequentially evaluate an elderly patient, leave their recommendations, and depart having made no communication with any of the other professionals involved, the likely outcome is uncoordinated and possibly conflicting therapeutic initiatives. In contrast, the hallmark of good geriatric health care is interdisciplinary, coordinated team function, in which primary care provider teams, usually including but not limited to a physician, nurse, and social worker, evaluate, plan treatment for, and follow elderly patients using each profession's perspective on functional assessment. Communication and coordination are crucial to success. Additional professionals from medical subspecialties such as psychiatry, physiatry, and neurology as well as from the professions of podiatry, dentistry, restorative therapies, nutrition, pharmacy, law, and other potentially useful disciplines are consulted for evaluation and therapeutic recommendations from their respective bodies of knowledge or can be recruited to the team but always in the context of interdisciplinary team function [11].

One report concerning GFA and interdisciplinary geriatric team care is reassuring about the value and efficiency of formal GFA using one particular instrument [36]. The consensus evaluation of a group of experienced members of a well-functioning team, based on prolonged clinical contact with a group of elderly veterans receiving care from a hospital–based home care program, correlated very highly with the scores generated for that population (by one observer, who did not have prior knowledge of the patients assessed) using the Functional Assessment Inventory [10]. The suggestion that formal assessment with a standardized instrument can generate data about frail dependent elders that correlate with expert interdisciplinary team evaluation identifies a potential for saving time and money in developing accurate and useful functional profiles of older persons.

For maximum effectiveness, GFA and health care should be administered by professionals using a common language of functional assessment [24]. Discipline-specific jargon interferes with communication and coordination of care. Functional assessment provides a common language that can be used to facilitate interdisciplinary evaluation and management of disease across disciplines. Agreement on nomenclature and instruments is long overdue. When each discipline uses its own nonintegratable methodology, communication is impeded and frustration grows. GFA provides interdisciplinary teams with functional data that enable each discipline to see and discuss the problems of the old person as they affect life and independence. Using the language and methods of GFA, practitioners in several disciplines can be taught simultaneously. GFA makes evaluation, treatment planning, therapeutic interventions, and follow-up easier and measurable. Teaching geriatric care in any discipline and at any level of training is simplified and enchanced by GFA.

Geriatric Assessment Units

In light of the substantial flurry of exhortation and reasoning about functional assessment as a useful component of geriatric care, it is not surprising that there has been a proliferation of care units reporting integration of functional assessment into the routine evaluation and management of elderly patients. The best of these clinical programs have recruited teams of health professionals who cooperate in an integrated and interdisciplinary structure of care aimed at the especially vulnerable, functionally impaired, and medically complex older patient. These units have developed in acute care hospitals, chronic disease hospitals, nursing homes, and health maintenance organizations (HMOs), and they are particularly prevalent in Veterans Administration medical centers. Geriatric assessment or evaluation units (GA-EUs) ideally address the social, medical, rehabilitative, and emotional problems of older persons, using the "technology of geriatrics" [18]. This technology consists of a coordinated, interdisciplinary, functional and clinical assessment coupled with a team care planning approach.

Advantages of GA-EUs for older patients have been reported in many domains of patient care. Most units have made larger numbers of important medical diagnoses and with increased accuracy and have identified treatable, improvable problems [12,38]. Accuracy and durability of discharge site is another benefit claimed by such units [40,50]. One study demonstrated a major reduction in drug use while also augmenting the number of diagnoses made [38]. Improved overall social, cognitive, and ADL function is commonly recorded [3,38,40,41]. One prospective study examined the impact of a home health care team on service utilization, functional status, and patient and informal caregiver satisfaction [55]. Experimental patients showed reductions in hospitalization time, nursing home admissions, and ambulatory visits as well as in overall cost of care compared with controls. Caregiver satisfaction was especially high. Although most information points to the benefits of GA-EUs, a majority of data come from uncontrolled studies [3,12,38,40,41,50], which describe clinical care outcomes for the patients within the particular unit reported on. Additionally, some studies have shown little or no advantage of a GA-EU [31,43,47], although these studies are also cited to emphasize the need for targeting of services by GA-EUs for special high-need, high-risk elderly subpopulations. The strongest evidence in support of GA-EU care comes from a prospective randomized study of inpatient care in a VA hospital with continued outpatient follow-up [39], which showed, in addition to most of the previously mentioned advantages, a decrease in nursing home admissions, in cost of care, and in mortality. The atypical nature of the population and site, as well as the continued control of care matched only against routine follow-up, make additional studies mandatory. Further questions about GA-EU care include: (1) What is the optimal site for such a unit? (2) What personnel are essential for successful outcomes? (3) Is continuing input from the team required, or is one consultative evaluation sufficient for benefit? (4) What are the real costs of development and operation of GA-EUs? One comprehensive review of studies examining the impact of GA-EUs discusses in detail the findings of all published studies in the English language literature [37].

A survey of existing GA-EUs at medical schools and Veterans Administration medical centers documents many aspects of their structure and function [18]. More than 90 percent of the 114 such units identified responded to a questionnaire, and a majority (80 percent) were hospital-based, although 60 percent served ambulatory as well as inpatients. Half had not existed before 1983, and of those that had, two-thirds have grown substantially since that time (Fig. 4-1). Half the physicians involved lacked

training in geriatric medicine. Though variability was great, the average time spent in evaluating new referrals in outpatient sites exceeded two and one-half hours. Conclusions argue powerfully for more and better policy-informing studies about the design and operation of GA-EUs, but data are increasingly persuasive that some form of this addition to the clinical care collage in geriatrics is advisable.

GFA in Long-Term Care Institutions

Although only a small minority of Americans over 65 years of age live in nursing homes (less than 5 percent at any one time), and although nursing home admission is even rarer under age 75, the nursing home experience is not uncommon or irrelevant for elderly persons. Among individuals reaching age 65, one-quarter will spend time in a nursing home during the remainder of their lives, and individuals over the age of 80 are most likely to die in a nursing home bed. Additionally, because nursing home residents are among the most functionally impaired and sick elderly persons in our society, the nursing home provides concentrated management and health care challenges [42].

HISTORICAL CONSIDERATIONS

Organization of care in the nursing home has evolved from acute hospital models and from constraints of regulatory bodies. Although informal level-of-care systems have existed in nursing homes for 50 years, titles XVIII and XIX of the Social Security Act created the first formal system more than 20 years ago by establishing what is now called the skilled nursing facility (SNF). Soon afterward the less costly, less intense type of care, called the intermediate care facility (ICF), came into existence. These institutions and the stratification-of-care systems generated by their development and growth violate a principle of long-term geriatric care based on attention to functional disability. Eligibility for SNF or ICF care and placement within one stratum of any similarly designed system of care are based on the need for specific nursing treatments related to diseases identified through the usual medical as-

FIGURE 4-1. *Proliferation of geriatric assessment units, based on information provided by 101 units for the initial year of operation. Data given for all units (circles), outpatient units (triangles), and inpatient units (squares); values for 1985 were computed for only those units developed in the first two months of the year. (From A. M. Epstein, et al. The emergence of geriatric assessment units: the "new technology of geriatrics." Ann. Intern. Med. 106:299, 1987.)*

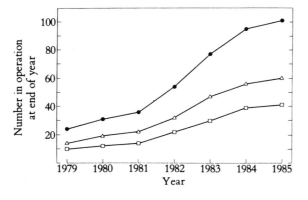

sessment procedures. These systems of care, using need for procedure-oriented nursing intervention as the sole criterion for placement of nursing home residents, are all vulnerable to the same criticism and fail on the same flaw. Cumulative functional disability, which is the dominant determinant of the need for nursing home care, is ignored in favor of diagnosis-related treatments that usually account for a very small proportion of the total care and dependency burden in the institutionalized elder. As a result, elderly nursing home candidates with sizable total care burdens spanning the disciplines of nursing, medicine, social work therapies, and others may not be eligible for care in the very setting that can provide an adequate volume of service because they lack a demonstrable need for specific technical therapeutic nursing interventions. Education of the regulators and providers of nursing home care in the theory and practice of GFA is a crucial first step in improving the match of need in nursing home residents with available services [17].

A second problem in the organization of nursing home care arose from two confluent phenomena. First, deinstitutionalization from state mental hospitals suddenly confronted nursing homes with demented and behavior-disordered elderly individuals who had been previously treated in the mental health system, usually long-stay geriatric wards. Second, although this occurred more gradually, the continuing survival of severely impaired nursing home residents aggravated the deinstitutionalization problem by generating an internal population of residents with cognitive impairment, behavior disorders, double incontinence, and severe physical dependency. The accumulation of substantial numbers of these multiply and seriously impaired individuals in nursing homes adversely influenced life quality for the majority of nursing home residents who were less impaired and confounded any diagnosis-based stratification system that attempted to provide sensible placement. GFA can offer help in addressing the problem produced by the adverse interactions of nursing home residents with dramatically different degrees and types of deficits. Quantitative and qualitative assessment of functional impairments allows the creation of nursing home resident groupings that will in-

sulate the more functional residents from the more mentally and behaviorally disordered.

BENEFITS

Using GFA in the nursing home to group residents with similar types and intensities of impairments has many benefits. First, scarce personnel can be used most efficiently by assignment to groups of residents with similar needs, ensuring that staff time is used wisely. Second, residents with diverse nursing care needs are guaranteed adequate attention, since those with different quantities and types of care needs are unlikely to be grouped together, a circumstance in which those with less urgent or obvious needs would be at risk for neglect in favor of the most impaired. Third, new admissions can be appropriately coordinated with the existing mix of residents and the staffing pattern within each group. Fourth, more pleasant living environments can be created by providing peer groups of residents who will be able to socialize with one another based on similar strengths and weaknesses. Fifth, cognitively normal residents can be insulated from severely demented, incontinent, or behavior-disordered residents. Sixth, residents with grossly disruptive behavior can be isolated. Seventh, residents with severe behavior disorders that would likely provoke physical or verbal abuse from other residents can be protected. Eighth, specialization and refinement of care, particularly among nurses, is facilitated, and nursing preferences as to type of resident problems to be dealt with can be considered. The opportunity to specialize enhances job stability and satisfaction for nursing staff. Last, maximum independence among residents is fostered by not placing those with less care needs in environments where large amounts of care are provided and are likely to be applied to all residents in the group regardless of specific need.

Interdisciplinary care team discussions of resident problems and needs in the nursing home are facilitated by the language of GFA. Information sharing is simplified, and it is common for professionals at different levels in different disciplines, such as nursing aides, physicians, and social workers, to communicate concisely and clearly, aided by the language of functional assessment [39].

GFA in Acute Care Hospitals

The acute hospital appears to be a poor site in which to emphasize GFA. Certainly it is one in which functional assessment does not appear prominently in the array of clinical activities. Because elderly patients, particularly under the impact of diagnosis-related groups (DRGs), have brief stays in the hospital and are being treated for life-threatening and rapidly evolving illnesses, GFA appears to be irrelevant to the situation of these patients. By the time assessment could be undertaken and quantified, it would seem that the patient might change, and the results would quickly become obsolete. These assumptions about GFA in the acute care hospital do not stand up under rigorous scrutiny. GFA is both useful and manageable in the acute hospital setting; it not only is helpful to professionals sorting out the disabilities of sick, old patients but also brings clinical benefits to the patients themselves by identifying and treating functional disabilities [46]. The acute hospital is a locus of intense geriatric care. Elderly patients now dominate acute hospital beds on an annual basis, and national data reveal that among 1,000 Americans over the age of 65, more than 400 admissions to a hospital occur annually. These elderly patients, in spite of DRG-driven early discharge, have a longer average length of stay than younger patients and a much higher rate of recidivism. Thus, the acute hospital is a hotbed of geriatric activity, and it would be erroneous and neglectful to emphasize only the long-term care institution and the community in a discussion of functional assessment in relation to geriatric care. Although nursing home days outnumber acute hospital days for elderly patients each year, acute care hospitals consume a much larger share of the public and private health care dollars spent annually for care of the elderly. While in the hospital, most elderly patients are seriously functionally disabled by the admitting disease and its complications. This functional decline usually requires continuing treatment, supportive care, or both following discharge from the hospital, and it is typical for elderly patients to receive formal services well beyond the day of hospital discharge. Planning for that care and identifying its need and scope are made far easier through the use of GFA. It is not unusual for hospital administrators to emphasize the need to consider discharge planning literally at the point of hospital admission. Identifying functional disability and the type and intensity of additional services needed following hospital care cannot be done in the absence of careful and accurate quantification of functional impairment. It is not the diagnosis or hospital-generated problem list that will determine the need for care after hospitalization but rather the functional disability regardless of etiologic disease.

It is well understood by most practitioners that elderly patients respond differently to disease compared with younger ones. Prolonged rehabilitation and late recovery of independent function as well as unexpected improvement or decline characterize the responses of elderly patients to serious systemic illness. GFA can thus define the need for care as well as provide the most accurate estimates of the specific type, intensity, and duration of care required. By performing GFA during hospitalization, the double-edged sword of erroneous estimation of after-care need can most likely be avoided. On the one hand, underestimation of need for care with resulting neglect of patient need and increase in likelihood of rehospitalization because of neglect can be avoided. Equally important to the patient and the system, overestimation of need and unnecessary provision of costly services or even nursing home admission also can be avoided. The values of GFA for providers of hospital service as they consider discharge planning are substantial. Use of GFA enhances caregivers' appreciation that functional capability can change dramatically over time in elderly patients. Understanding that elderly patients will continue to show functional change with time after hospitalization, especially given shorter hospital stays under DRGs, will enhance realistic planning for care after discharge. GFA, performed repeatedly during hospitalization, will allow prediction and formulation of an accurate discharge plan, particularly if functional capability before admission is documented and used as a standard against which to measure hospital progress in functional independence and as a goal for restorative efforts.

GFA is useful in another way as elderly hospitalized patients are followed during the course of an illness. Given that diseases and their complications often present in the elderly first and most dramatically with impairment in functional capacity, frequent GFA in the hospital setting allows documentation of response to treatment and thus early detection of decline due to disease progression or complications of the admitting illness. For example, the elderly man admitted with urosepsis and confusion who, during the course of apparently successful antibiotic treatment, loses the ability to stand at the bedside to assist in his transfers, may be re-evaluated more quickly, and the development of thrombophlebitis in one leg may be detected earlier as a result of investigation prompted by detecting loss of the ability to stand. The quantification of function resulting from GFA provides a major additional resource for clinicians and planners by yielding tangible parameters to follow over time that are as valid and objective as serum sodium or glucose determinations.

GFA in the Community

The community, or home environment, in which 95 percent of older Americans live at any one time, is the site in which functional impairment first appears most often. One cross-sectional study of more than 1,200 patients receiving primary care in New England quantified physical and mental function and compared the results with the impressions of the physicians delivering care [35]. For both physical and mental impairment, physician opinions underestimated major disability by more than 50 percent in each domain. Functional losses were greatest and most underestimated in the elderly. Many of the principles articulated above for elderly in nursing homes and acute hospitals apply equally to older persons at home. If GFA is to become a successful and commonly employed clinical technique, useful in the numerous domains for which it has been suggested (diagnosis, placement, treatment and rehabilitation planning, outcome measurement, cost savings, teaching, and research), then assessment must be easily performed in the communities where older people live and receive care. The relationship of a GA-EU to an acute hospital or nursing home may facilitate access to space, equipment, and personnel, but the routine availability of GFA must be targeted to the older person at home in the mainstream of ambulatory care.

An important review identifies three ways in which GFA can be integrated into the process of care in the community [49]. The first model is designated the "recognized specialty" and is found primarily among British systems of health care. Soon after the founding of the National Health Service in 1948, geriatrics became identified as a bona fide clinical specialty with responsibility for organization and delivery of care to older persons in each of the countries embracing the model (United Kingdom, Australia, and New Zealand). Teams composed of professionals specifically trained in their discipline's geriatric component accept referrals and perform evaluation of the most challenging and functionally impaired older persons to plan treatment. Allocation of scarce resources, especially long-term care institutional beds, is under their control. Although attractive to many Americans in their discovery of geriatrics, this model travels poorly and probably has little relevance to the planning of care for older Americans.

The second model has been called "consolidated" [54] and comprises a comprehensive system of care including an assessment component for a geographically defined population. The social health maintenance organization (SHMO) is the most common form of the consolidated model use of GFA in the United States. Allocation of organizational resources is made only after assessment, using the data obtained. Although available to any patient enrolled in the particular system, it is the older group who receives this special geriatric assessment service on a regular basis.

The third alternative for bringing functional assessment to the community is the "brokerage" model [49]. Here, the primary focus is evaluation by an organization that has been authorized to control and allocate funds for services, usually Medicare, Medicaid, or both. The services being funded are virtually always long-term, whether in or out of an institution. The emphasis is on comprehensive assessment, which includes community resources, so that home dwelling can be preserved and enhanced and premature and more costly nursing home admission delayed. One of the earliest projects of this type was the Triage program in Connecticut, which showed client benefit and economy but was discontinued [25].

Although much evidence has been marshalled arguing strongly for strengthening the front line of primary care for older persons in the community by building in a routine functional assessment component to that care, there has been little systematic or quantitatively important response. Numerous demonstration projects have shown patient benefit and conservation of scarce resources by coupling GFA to delivery of care, and perhaps some states are beginning to respond rationally by requiring assessment prior to Medicaid-funded nursing home admission. Yet we must acknowledge that, despite a decade of successful demonstration projects, integration of GFA into an overall system of care serving large numbers of older Americans in the community is distinctly uncommon. It may be that further demonstration of a fourth or "consultative" model of community-based GA-EUs providing GFA will succeed where others have not in making assessment a routine component of geriatric care.

Choosing Instruments

The measurement of functional capacity in older persons is of vast importance in the early detection of illness and evaluation of response to therapeutic intervention. Numerous other uses and values for GFA have been discussed. If the reasoning is persuasive and an individual practitioner or organization decides to integrate GFA into the process of care, a second decision concerning instruments or tools for measurement must also be made. Frequently, even in contemporary geriatric care, informal clinical impressions are used to assess function in older persons instead of the numerous formal instruments currently available [48]. The decision to assess "by the seat of the pants" is usually made under the pressure to accomplish a clinical or administrative goal, which may make this method seem more convenient and time-saving than choosing and learning to use standard tools for assessment. There are several reasons for using standardized protocols for GFA. First, standard instruments ensure that assess-

ment will be complete. Informal evaluation may omit key observations under the time pressure of clinical care. In addition, use of formal tools ensures comprehensive functional assessment, including domains not immediately obvious or important at that moment to individual assessors. Second, standard instruments guarantee that the same observations are quantified from one assessment to another, allowing accurate comparisons over time. Third, objective assessment permits valid research observations to be made in the process of managing older patients. Fourth, and closely related, standard instruments allow comparison across populations of individuals in different places. Fifth, formal assessment leaves a record of function that is easily transferrable from one clinician or institution to another. Sixth, use of formal instruments makes the detection of small differences in function more likely, which has substantial implications for the assessment of disease progression or therapeutic impact for clinical or research purposes. A comprehensive text is available that reviews the strengths and weaknesses of most assessment measures and reproduces many useful instruments, and it should be consulted for further discussion [27].

One important and useful caveat concerning adoption of formal instruments by clinicians has been noted recently [2]. The validity and reliability of tools developed for specific research purposes may make them inappropriate for other, usually clinical, applications. A persuasive argument has been made for carefully identifying goals before using functional assessment, and then selecting instruments based on their relevance to and utility in achieving these goals.

Physical functioning is best assessed using ADL and IADL measures. Many ADL scales have been reported in the literature, but the Katz index [29] is very widely used and has been extensively validated. Like most scales, the Katz rates bathing, dressing, toileting, transferring, continence, and feeding. It has been shown that these capacities are lost and regained in a hierarchy (as ordered above) during disability progression and subsequent recovery. A disadvantage of the Katz and many pure ADL scales is sensitivity. The Katz index does not begin to register impaired function until substantial disability has accumulated, and it is best suited for use with moderately severely dependent individuals. Thus, the Katz index is most useful for working with institutionally placed persons, and more sensitive instruments for detecting early decline are helpful in the community.

To increase sensitivity to detect only modest functional loss in older persons living in the community and needing assistance, IADL measurements are useful [33]. Although IADL functions are more sensitive to less severe physical decline than ADL losses, they are also more complex and thus vulnerable to emotional and motivational factors, especially in the frail, potentially discouraged older person. Another liability in using IADL scales is that in most institutional settings, particularly nursing homes, the exercise of IADL skills is preempted by the staff, even in those elders entirely competent before and after institutionalization. In spite of the difficulties inherent in IADL measurements, they are important and useful in assessing elders in the community, particularly those who are currently receiving few or no supportive services. Two generally useful geriatrically oriented IADL scales are a subsection of the Older Americans Research and Service Center Instrument (OARS) [16] and the Philadelphia Geriatric Center IADL scale [32]. A detailed description of specific instruments and the many factors influencing their choice and utility is available and should be consulted [9].

Cognitive functioning is a major determinant of functional capacity in virtually all other domains, and thus impairment must be documented and quantified as a starting point for any other aspect of GFA. Having asserted the primacy of the intellect and the impact of its loss, it must be acknowledged that the severity and extent of impaired cognition are poor predictors of functional capacity in other domains. The inability to predict physical, behavioral, and social functioning by measurement of cognitive impairment apparently relates more to the state of instrument development than to mystery about the interrelationship of these capacities. At present, cognitive assessment is primarily useful in documenting loss and initiating comprehensive medical evaluation designed to detect underlying curable or treatable conditions producing the loss. In addition, detection

of intellectual impairment alerts both professionals and family to a possible need for remedial or protective services. Repeated assessment also is essential to monitor and document change over time, both decline due to disease progression and improvement from treatment [23]. Because tests in clinical use only screen for deficits, neuropsychological consultation should be sought in uncertain cases.

Numerous tests of cognition are currently in use for mental status evaluation. None is perfect, but some have definite advantages. The mental status questionnaire (MSQ) is a ten-question test that has had wide use during more than two decades [26] and has been validated extensively. Low scores correlate well with impaired cognition. The test is short and requires little training to administer. Although convenient, the MSQ has several drawbacks. Sensitivity is lacking, and severe impairment must be present for scores to be low. Up to moderate intellectual losses are not usually detected, and erroneous determinations of "normal" mental function can be generated by exclusive use of this test. The brevity of the test results in omission of several domains of cognitive function from assessment, domains that are crucial and may be early or sole deficits during the progressive stages of diseases impairing intellect. Functions not tested include reasoning, many aspects of language, and visual-spatial relationships.

The short portable MSQ is a subtest from the OARS [16] and is more sensitive than the MSQ in asking somewhat more difficult questions. In addition, it tests domains of mental function, such as arithmetic skills, which are not included on the MSQ. Overall, it adds only modestly to the MSQ but is probably preferable if a very brief ten-question test is to be used. The English Dementia Rating Scale [30] is unusual in that it rates cognitive impairment by questioning someone else who knows the patient well rather than by direct examination. It is also one of the few instruments used in several research protocols whose questions probe practical ADL and IADL functions and impairments *due solely to cognitive losses*. This scale has the potential to relate impaired cognition to self-care capacity and the need for remedial services based solely on intellectual impairment. This scale is also a brief instrument.

The mini-mental state examination [20] is a more elaborate test of cognitive function than the others mentioned. The designation "mini" refers to the measurement only of cognition to the exclusion of other mental functions such as affect, behavior, paranoia, hallucinations, and so forth. The assessment of cognitive ability includes memory, orientation, attention, calculation, recall, language, and visual-spatial relations. Since administration and scoring take five to ten minutes depending on subject abilities and cooperation, it obviously does not test any domain in depth. The maximum score of 30 points corresponds roughly to 30 questions, and the mini-mental is the most sensitive and informative of commonly employed clinical mental status tests. Scores below 23 correlate well with moderate or worse cognitive impairment, and this test is recommended for routine clinical use. When any of the clinical mental status tests are equivocal, or if the patient or family insists that results of assessment are erroneous, either positively or negatively, more elaborate neuropsychologic testing should be done, and complicating psychiatric disease should be considered.

Affective functioning measurement in the elderly is equivalent to the assessment of and search for depression [21]. Unfortunately for nonpsychiatrists, psychiatric assessment by a skilled clinician remains by far the best instrument for detecting depression, and most scales or tests have been extensively criticized [22,27]. Nevertheless, two widely used instruments are the Zung Self-Rating Depression Scale [56] and the Beck Depression Inventory [4]. Both are clinically oriented and probe for standard psychic or organic accompaniments of depression. A major difference between them is that, as its name states, the Zung is self-administered and the Beck is not. If the correlation between poor scores on commonly used mental status tests and impaired overall function is not robust, the relationship of high scores for depression on the Zung or Beck scale to functional disability is even more frail. The recently developed geriatric depression scale (GDS) is designed for use with the elderly, comes in a brief version, and has been validated [53a]. Despite certain valid criticisms, one of these or some other scale should be used routinely to identify older persons at risk for the negative consequences of untreated depressive symptoms or depressive illness. Once identified, they should be referred for evaluation and possible treatment by an experienced clinician.

Behavioral functioning is rarely considered part of formal GFA unless major behavioral abnormalities are reported by family or other observers. Recently, agitated behavior, including wandering, repetitive verbal or physical acts, physical or verbal abuse toward self or others, and inappropriate sounds or actions including disrobing, have begun to be studied systematically. Agitation, defined as "inappropriate verbal, vocal or motor activities that are not explained by needs or confusion per se" [14], was studied among cognitively impaired nursing home residents using a frequency rating scale [15]. Major findings were that agitated behaviors were interrelated, were most often not aggressive, and usually provoked the use of medication. It is fair to say that for now no formal assessment instrument for behavior is sufficiently developed or validated to be useful in routine clinical assessment of older persons and that the best advice to care providers and planners is to be alert to the clinical detection and quantification of behavioral abnormalities, especially in the setting of cognitive impairment.

Social function measurement is a crucial aspect of assessment of older persons. Though often relegated to "soft" or tangential status by biologically oriented clinicians, social functional assessment illuminates critical aspects of life quality and health status that we cannot afford to overlook. First, social functional integrity makes it more likely that the older person will be able to manage in the face of adversity. Personal and family/friend social resources are often the key determinant of successful community coping with an illness and disability burden that threatens independence and produces institutionalization for the less socially robust. Second, social function in part both predicts and is determined by physical and cognitive capacities or limitations. Social withdrawal or breakdown in previously strong relationships may be the first manifestation of physical, emotional, or dementing illness. Deteriorating interpersonal contacts or loss of friends or family can produce illness in each sphere. Third, deep and elaborate social activities are an independent marker of good life quality and thus are important in a wide array of secondary impact measurements in caring for older persons. In addition, a rich social life should be an independent goal in the overall approach to managing health care of older citizens.

Specific aspects of social function to be measured include the persons who can help in meeting dependency needs as well as the type, frequency, importance, and quality of social interactions. Measurement of ability to cope, self-assessed well-being or life quality, and suitability of the individual's living arrangement have also been identified as useful [27]. Instrument selection for the clinical setting is challenging, since research is a major focus of most validated tools, and they are long and cumbersome. The OARS social resource scale is more manageable and is widely used [16].

Economic assessment should be mentioned for completeness, and its importance appears self-evident. If money for health care, including medications, care and life-style alterations, and basic necessities, is insufficient, the entire array of sensible and potentially successful health care interventions will fail. Open and detailed discussion of the older person's resources, as well as current choices concerning expenditures, must be part of assessment.

Conclusions

The intimate relationship between disease and functional loss in old age demands that clinicians and health planners who have responsibility for geriatric care learn to use standard instruments for the detection and quantification of functional disability in the domains of ADL, IADL, cognition, social function, and affect. Behavioral scales require further development and validation for routine use. GFA is important for understanding and measuring the burden and impact of disease in elderly patients, whether they are ambulatory in the community or receiving care in nursing homes or acute hospitals. Teaching and using GFA in planning and organization of health services for the elderly ensures coordination of care and rapid response of the system of care to subtle fluctuations of need. GFA is a useful strategy for teaching

across the health professions and makes communication and team care feasible within the time constraints of practical clinical care. In the nursing home, GFA permits classifying of residents in efficient and humane groupings. Teaching GFA to hospital discharge planners will likely increase accuracy in predicting discharge needs and rehabilitation potential. In the community, GFA allows early detection of decline and rational allocation of services. Finally, GFA offers predictive information and a substantial opportunity for generating useful research data to inform and improve the increasing utilization of health services by older persons in America.

References

1. Anderson, W. F. Preventive aspects of geriatric medicine. *Postgrad. Med.* 52:157, 1972.
2. Applegate, W. B. Use of assessment instruments in clinical settings. *J. Am. Geriatr. Soc.* 35:45, 1987.
3. Applegate, W. B., et al. A geriatric rehabilitation and assessment unit in a community hospital. *J. Am. Geriatr. Soc.* 31:206, 1983.
4. Beck, A. T., et al. An inventory for measuring depression. *Arch. Gen. Psychiatry* 4:53, 1961.
5. Beers, M. and Besdine, R. Medical assessment of the elderly patient. *Clin. Geriatr. Med.* 3:17, 1987.
6. Besdine, R. W. The Data Base of Geriatric Medicine. In J. W. Rowe and R. W. Besdine (eds.), *Health and Disease in Old Age.* Boston: Little, Brown, 1982, Pp. 1–14.
7. Besdine, R. W. The educational utility of comprehensive functional assessment in the elderly. *J. Am. Geriatr. Soc.* 31:651, 1983.
8. Besdine, R. W., Levkoff, S. E., and Wetle, T. Health and Illness Behaviors in Elder Veterans. In T. Wetle and J. W. Rowe (eds.), *Older Veterans: Linking VA and Community Resources.* Cambridge, MA: Harvard University Press, 1984. Pp. 1–33.
9. Branch, L. G., and Meyers, A. R. Assessing physical function in the elderly. *Clin. Geriatr. Med.* 3:29, 1987.
10. Cairl, R. E., Pfeiffer, E., and Keller, D. An evaluation of the reliability and validity of the functional assessment inventory. *J. Am. Geriatr. Soc.* 31:607, 1983.
11. Campbell, L. J., and Cole, K. D. Geriatric assessment teams. *Clin. Geriatr. Med.* 3:99, 1987.
12. Cheah, K. C., and Beard, O. W. Psychiatric findings in the population of a geriatric evalua-

tion unit: Implications. *J. Am. Geriatr. Soc.* 28: 153, 1980.

13. Coe, R. M. Comprehensive Care of the Elderly. In R. D. T. Cape, R. M. Coe, and I. Rossman (eds.), *Fundamentals of Geriatric Medicine.* New York: Raven, 1983. Pp. 5–6.

14. Cohen-Mansfield, J., and Billig, N. Agitated behaviors in the elderly. I. A conceptual framework. *J. Am. Geriatr. Soc.* 34:711, 1986.

15. Cohen-Mansfield, J. Agitated behaviors in the elderly. II. Preliminary results in the cognitively deteriorated. *J. Am. Geriatr. Soc.* 34:722, 1986.

16. Duke University Center for the Study of Aging and Human Development. *Multi-dimensional Functional Assessment: The OARS Methodology.* Durham, NC: Duke University, 1978.

17. Falcone, A. R. Comprehensive functional assessment as an administrative tool. *J. Am. Geriatr. Soc.* 31:642, 1983.

18. Epstein, A. M., et al. The emergence of geriatric assessment units: The "new technology of geriatrics." *Ann. Intern. Med.* 106:299, 1987.

19. Filner, B., and Williams, T. F. Health Promotion for the Elderly: Reducing Functional Dependency. In A. R. Somers and D. R. Fabian (eds.), *The Geriatric Imperative: An Introduction to Gerontology and Clinical Geriatrics.* New York: Appleton-Century-Crofts, 1981. Pp. 187–204.

20. Folstein, M. F., Folstein, S., and McHugh, P. R. Mini-mental state: A practical method for grading the cognitive state of patients for the clinician. *J. Psychiatr. Res.* 12:189, 1975.

21. Gallagher, D. Assessing affect in the elderly. *Clin. Geriatr. Med.* 3:65, 1987.

22. Gallagher, D., Thompson, L. W., and Levy, S. M. Clinical Psychological Assessment of Older Adults. In L. Poon (ed.), *Aging in the 1980's: Selected Contemporary Issues in the Psychology of Aging.* Washington, D.C.: American Psychological Association, 1980.

23. Gurland, B. J., et al. The assessment of cognitive function in the elderly. *Clin. Geriatr. Med.* 3:53, 1987.

24. Hedrick, S. C., Katz, S., and Stroud, M. W., III. Patient assessment in long term care: Is there a common language? *Aged Care Services Rev.* 2(4): 3, 1980/81.

25. Hodgson, J. H., Jr., and Quinn, J. L. The impact of the triage health care delivery system upon client morale, independent living and the cost of care. *Gerontologist* 20:364, 1980.

26. Kahn, R. L., et al. Brief objective measures for the determination of mental status in the aged. *Am. J. Psychiatry* 117:326, 1960.

27. Kane, R. A., and Kane, R. L. *Assessing the Elderly:*

28. Katz, S., et al. Active life expectancy. *N. Engl. J. Med.* 309:1218, 1983.

29. Katz, S., et al. Studies of illness in the aged. The index of ADL: A standardized measure of biological and psychosocial function. *J.A.M.A.* 185: 94, 1963.

30. Kay, D. W. K. Epidemiology and Identification of Brain Deficit in the Elderly. In C. Eisdorfer and R. O. Friedel (eds.), *Cognitive and Emotional Disturbance in the Elderly: Clinical Issues.* Chicago: Year Book, 1977.

31. Kerski, D. Post-geriatric evaluation unit follow-up: Team vs non-team. *J. Gerontol.* 42:191, 1987.

32. Lawton, M. P. Assessing the Competence of Older People. In D. Kent, R. Kastenbaum, and S. Sherwood (eds.), *Research, Planning and Action for the Elderly.* New York: Behavioral Publications, 1972.

33. Lawton, M. P., and Brody, E. Assessment of older people: Self-maintaining and instrumental activities of daily living. *Gerontologist* 9:179, 1969.

34. Moore, J. T. Functional disability of geriatric patients in a family medicine program: Implications for patient care, education, and research. *J. Fam. Prac.* 7:1159, 1978.

35. Nelson, E. Functional health status level of primary care patients. *J.A.M.A.* 249:3331, 1983.

36. Robinson, B. E., et al. Validation of the functional assessment inventory against a multidisciplinary home care-team. *J. Am. Geriatr. Soc.* 34:851, 1986.

37. Rubenstein, L. Z. Geriatric assessment: An overview of its impacts. *Clin. Geriatr. Med.* 3:1, 1987.

38. Rubenstein, L. Z., Abrass, I. B., and Kane, R. L. Improved care for patients on a new geriatric unit. *J. Am. Geriatr. Soc.* 29:531, 1981.

39. Rubenstein, L. Z., et al. Effectiveness of a geriatric evaluation unit. *N. Engl. J. Med.* 311:1664, 1984.

40. Schuman, J. E., et al. The impact of a new geriatric program in a hospital for the chronically ill. *Can. Med. Assoc. J.* 118:639, 1978.

41. Sloane, P. D. Nursing home candidates: Hospital inpatient trial to identify those appropriately assignable to less intensive care. *J. Am. Geriatr. Soc.* 28:511, 1980.

42. Somers, A. R. Long-term care for the elderly and disabled: A new health priority. *N. Engl. J. Med.* 307:221, 1982.

43. Teasdale, T. A., et al. A comparison of placement outcomes of geriatric cohorts receiving

A Practical Guide to Measurement. Lexington, MA: Lexington Books, 1981.

care in a geriatric assessment unit and on general medicine floors. *J. Am. Geriatr. Soc.* 31:529, 1983.

44. U.S. Department of Health, Education and Welfare, Public Health Service, Office of Health Research, Statistics, and Technology, National Center for Health Statistics: Current estimates from the health interview survey: United States 1978. In *Vital and Health Statistics,* Series 10, No. 130. DHEW Publ. No. (PHS) 80-1551. Washington, D.C.: U.S. Government Printing Office, 1980.

45. U.S. Department of Health, Education and Welfare, Public Health Service, Office of Health Research, Statistics and Technology Administration: *Health United States,* 1979. DHEW Publ. No. (PHS) 80-1232. Washington, D.C.: U.S. Government Printing Office, 1980.

46. Warshaw, G. A., et al. Functional disability in the hospitalized elderly. *J.A.M.A.* 248:847, 1982.

47. Williams, M. E. Outpatient geriatric evaluation. *Clin. Geriatr. Med.* 3:175, 1987.

48. Williams, T. F. Comprehensive functional assessment: An overview. *J. Am. Geriatr. Soc.* 31:637, 1983.

49. Williams, T. F. Integration of geriatric assessment into the community. *Clin. Geriatr. Med.* 3:111, 1987.

50. Williams, T. F., et al. Appropriate placement of the chronically ill and aged: A successful approach by evaluation. *J.A.M.A.* 226:1332, 1973.

51. Williamson, J., Lowther, C. P., and Gray, S. The use of health visitors in preventive geriatrics. *Gerontol. Clin.* 8:362, 1966.

52. Williamson, J., et al. Old people at home: Their unreported needs. *Lancet* 1:1117, 1964.

53. Wilson, L. A., Lawson, I. R., and Brass, W. Multiple disorders in the elderly. *Lancet* 2:841, 1962.

53a. Yesavage, J. A., and Sheik, J. I. Geriatric depression scale (GDS): Recent evidence and development of a shorter version. *Clin. Gerontol.* 5:165, 1986.

54. Zawadski, R. T. The long term care demonstration projects: What are they and why they come into being. *Home Health Care Services Q.* 4 (No. 3/4):5, 1983.

55. Zimmer, J. G., Groth-Juncker, A., and McCusker, J. A randomized controlled study of a home health care team. *Am. J. Publ. Health* 75:134, 1985.

56. Zung, W. W. K. A self-rating depression scale. *Arch. Gen. Psychiatry* 12:63, 1965.

5

The Social and Service Context of Geriatric Care

TERRIE WETLE

THE SOCIAL CONTEXT and organizational framework of health care determine the experience of illness for the older person and the physician's ability to deliver timely and appropriate care. The social status of the elderly, the changing demographics of health and illness, and evolving social values exert complex pressures on the patchwork of policies, programs, and services that constitute the continuum of care available to older individuals. Perhaps it is possible in other aspects of medicine to care adequately for patients by attending primarily to pathophysiology, but the successful practice of geriatric medicine requires an understanding of the broader context in which illness occurs and care is provided. This chapter reviews service use by older persons, discusses the influence of selected social events on utilization behaviors, describes the continuum of care used by an aged population, and outlines the programs and resources for geriatric care.

Service Use Among the Elderly

Elderly individuals are more likely to use health care services than other age groups. Although comprising only 12 percent of the population, older persons account for 39 percent of all acute hospital bed days, use 25 percent of all prescription drugs, and account for 30 percent of the overall $425 billion health care expenditure and more than 50 percent of the $124 billion federal health budget [1]. This disproportionate use of health resources by elderly Americans, though notable, should not be regarded as unfair or unjustified. The escalating disease burden accompanying aging (see Chap. 3) produces the accelerated need for and use of health care. For example, in 1979 older people with chronic activity limitations had 8.7 visits to a physician and 41.2 hospitalizations per 100 compared with 4.3 physician visits and 14.8 hospitalizations per 100 elderly with no activity limitations [2]. Moreover, the chronic nature of many of the diseases prevalent among the aged requires repeated contacts with the health care system. Only 8.6 percent of older persons' visits represented a first visit to that physician, and a return visit was scheduled at 72 percent of visits [1].

SOCIAL SUPPORTS

Use of institutional services such as hospitals and nursing homes is also more frequent among older persons. In addition to the obvious relationship between health status and hospital or nursing home use, more subtle factors are also at play. The availability of family members to provide care at home decreases with age. Elderly individuals, particularly women, are likely to be widowed, and for the very old, children may themselves be aged. Divorce and geographic

TABLE 5-1. *Labor force participation rates of women*

Year	Age 25–34	Age 35–44	Age 45–54
1947	32%	36%	33%
1957	36%	43%	47%
1967	42%	48%	52%
1977	60%	60%	56%
1987	73%	73%	65%
1997	80%	81%	74%
2007	81%	83%	75%

SOURCE: U.S. Bureau of Labor. Presentation by Thomas Maloney to Working Group on Health Policy and Aging, Harvard Medical School, May 20, 1986.

separation may weaken family ties, and the entry of women, particularly middle-aged women, into the paid labor force has reduced their availability to provide care. Table 5-1 illustrates the increasing proportion of women in the labor force in each successive cohort from 1947 to 1987 and also shows projections into the future. These factors interact with increased prevalence of disease to increase demand for geriatric services.

FAMILY CAREGIVING

Although the concept of social supports encompasses neighbors and friends, it is usually family members who are the responsible caregiving agents, providing substantial physical, emotional, social, and economic support to elderly relatives [3]. The amount of involvement and the nature of the services provided depend on economic resources, family structure, quality of relationships, and other competing demands on family time and energy [4]. It has been estimated that as much as 80 percent of home health care for the elderly is provided as informal support (as opposed to purchased services) by family members [5]. This care is provided both to elders living with adult children and to those living in their own homes. As might be expected, older people who live with adult children tend to be poorer and in worse functional condition than those residing in their own homes [6]. The amount of care provided by the family may range from minimal assistance such as periodic checking-in to elaborate full-time care. Sex roles and female longevity converge so that women are more likely to be

both receivers and givers of care. Women typically provide more direct care for chronically ill parents and parents-in-law than do men [3,7]. Several studies indicate that there may be a slow trend toward more egalitarian views of gender roles in caregiving [3,8], although these attitudinal changes are more pronounced in women than in men.

Several changing social patterns are leading to a decreased availability of adult children to provide care. The increasing entry or reentry of middle-aged and older women into the paid labor force deprives dependent older persons of a major source of informal support [9]. The increased prevalence of separation and divorce is another. Cicirelli [10] compared adult children in intact and in disrupted families (those who were divorced, widowed, or remarried) and observed that those in intact families perceived more filial obligation, higher parental needs, and more responsibility for caregiving. Nonetheless, increasing numbers of elderly persons are closely involved with family members, and increasing proportions of families have elderly relatives; 40 percent of those aged 55 to 59 have at least one living parent, as do 20 percent of those aged 60 to 64 [11].

Spouses are major providers of care for the frail elderly. Adult children frequently provide care to mildly or moderately impaired elders, whereas severely disabled elders are more likely to be cared for by a spouse [12]. Johnson and Catalano [13] view marriage as the most viable, comprehensive, and long-term support available in old age. There are, however, several considerations related to spousal caregiving. As a group, "caregiving" couples are disproportionately below the poverty level and usually include a caregiver with poor health [14]. As with children, spouse caregivers experience considerable stress [15], and one longitudinal study revealed that caregiving spouses' health deteriorated in 50 percent of cases examined [13]. Another study of wives caring for disabled husbands identified the wives as "generally worried, frustrated, sad, resigned, and impatient" [14].

Social supports are an important factor in predicting use of health services. The availability of family caregivers plays a salient role in delaying, if not preventing, institutionalization of the chronically ill older person [4,16,17,18]. It has been argued that the provision of supportive services to family caregivers would enhance their willingness and ability to provide care [19]. These supportive services are of two types— those that *support* family caregivers, and those that *supplement* family caregiving. Services that support caregiving include technical assistance in learning new skills, counseling, family mental health services or personal supports, and a variety of respite or emergency caretaking services. For the most part, these services are provided directly to the caregiver, although some (i.e., respite services) involve the elder as well. Services that supplement family care include personal care, home health, adult day care, meals programs, and social services. Supportive services are particularly important in relieving caregiver stress related to efforts to respond to multiple demands, provide care to children and other family members, and deal with feelings of social isolation, restricted mobility, decreased life satisfaction, and anger toward family members who are not participating in care [20,21,22,23].

SOCIAL SUPPORTS AND HEALTH

Social supports have also been shown to have an impact on health status [24]. Several community-based studies demonstrate that social isolation or lack of support is consistently associated with increased mortality risk for white males [25,26,27,28,29], but only the Alameda County study [26] shows an increased mortality risk for women associated with social isolation. Studies of nonwhite groups show markedly weaker effects [25,26]. Although these community studies all demonstrate that social ties are related to mortality, the strength of the association varies dramatically among subpopulations and is reduced when covariates, particularly biologic risk factors, are controlled for [24]. The way social networks influence health is under study. It has been argued that one such influence is the buffering effect against the changes brought about by negative life transitions such as widowhood, retirement, and the departure of children [30,31].

Health and illness behaviors of the aged also influence the way health services are used (see Chap. 3). Satisfaction with lower levels of health as well as misinterpretation of symptoms of illness as a natural part of the aging process directly influence whether or not, and the way in which, symptoms are reported [32]. Failure to report symptoms is especially dangerous given the structure of the American health care system, which, though excellent, waits passively for the individual to activate care by seeking out a provider and accurately reporting symptoms and conditions. It is incumbent on health professionals, therefore, to understand these behaviors, to encourage reporting of symptoms or functional changes, and to respond to such reports with aggressive diagnostic approaches.

LIFE TRANSITIONS

Other social factors also influence health and illness behaviors of older persons. For most elderly, late life is a period of transition and adjustment to loss. These transitions include retirement, relocation, death of spouse, family members, and friends, and the loss of former levels of physical health and function. Referring to the Holmes and Rahe [33] scale of stress associated with life change, each of these transitions correlates with the subsequent development of physical and mental health problems. Yet elderly persons are surprisingly resilient to the many challenges they face.

Retirement is frequently the first major transition faced by older persons. A number of studies have reported a negative impact from retirement, estimating that about a third of individuals experience difficulty adjusting to their changed circumstances [34]. The major areas of adjustment relate to reduced income and self-reported decline in health. However, the circumstances surrounding the retirement itself determine the presence and severity of adjustment problems. Some people choose to retire and look forward to leaving boring or unpleasant work situations and enjoying increased leisure time. Others are forced to retire because of health reasons or job loss. These factors explain to some degree the different physical and mental health outcomes experienced by retirees [35]. It is argued that preparation for retirement and the availability of counseling for families and individuals who experience difficulties will ameliorate most problems of retirement [36].

Relocation is another type of transition faced by older persons. An individual or family unit may experience several housing transitions in later years, including sale of the family residence to move into smaller quarters when the "nest is emptied," a move into a smaller home with the death of a spouse, a move into senior housing to minimize the burden of upkeep, and finally, for about 20 percent, the move into a nursing home. There continues to be controversy in the literature about "relocation trauma" [37,38,39]. Those who respond poorly to a move are more likely to be male, living alone, socially isolated, poor, and of low morale [40]. Two important factors have been shown to mediate the stress of moving—the degree of perceived control over the event and the degree of predictability of the new environment. When a move is perceived as voluntary, there is less stress and less negative impact. In like manner, the more prepared the elder is for the new location, including visits prior to the move, the less stress will surround the move itself [41]. Families should be encouraged to acquaint the older person with the new setting well in advance of the moving date. For the cognitively impaired aged, a move away from familiar surroundings may trigger a substantial increase in functional dependence and disruptive behaviors. Awareness of increased vulnerability of the demented in this situation may help families and staff cope during the period of adjustment.

Bereavement is a complex phenomenon that changes many aspects of elders' lives [36]. Loss of companionship on the death of a spouse may be accompanied by a reduction in financial resources, loss of a caretaker, decline in social interaction, and change in social status [42]. Loss of a spouse has different effects on men and women. Men, for example, tend to have higher mortality rates in the two years following death of spouse than do women. On the other hand, elderly men are much more likely to remarry after the death of a spouse than are women. Health care providers should be alert to symptoms of stress and depression during the grieving period. A rush to treat feelings of sadness with antidepressant medications should be avoided because of potential interference with the important "grief-work" of the adjustment process. On the other hand, counseling and supportive services, such as "widow-to-widow" groups, may ease difficult transitions and en-

hance adjustments to new roles and life circumstances [43]. But prolonged and pathologic grief usually requires psychiatric evaluation and treatment (see Chap. 26).

These are just a few of the important adjustments faced by older persons. The knowledgeable health care provider will include questions about recent life events and other aspects of the living situation as a regular part of the patient assessment (see Chap. 4). This information can identify potential health risks and may also suggest a need for referrals to other professionals and social services. The knowledge that a frail elder lives alone, as do 30 percent of those over 65, [44] causes concern that no one will observe new symptoms or abrupt changes in function that signal the onset or worsening of illness requiring evaluation and treatment. Because the physician is frequently the first professional to become aware of an older patient's need for care beyond the treatment of disease, an awareness of the full continuum of services available for older persons is imperative. This continuum of care is described in the next section.

Continuum of Care Used by the Elderly

The array of health services needed by older persons is complex and fragmented. Specific types of services have different funding sources, regulatory agencies, eligibility requirements, and geographic distribution. Nonetheless, there is general agreement on the basic components of the continuum of care [4] (Fig. 5-1). Services range from those provided in the home to those provided in the community and further, to those provided only on an inpatient basis. This schema simplifies the actual service system as it exists in most communities but provides a framework for the following discussion of specific services.

ACUTE CARE HOSPITALS

The acute care hospital is the final common pathway for most older people requiring care. The first hospitals were primarily of a religious and charitable nature and provided a place of refuge for the sick and the poor. The earliest American hospitals were actually infirmaries in poor houses, and it was not until the early 1900s that hospitals evolved into physician workshops

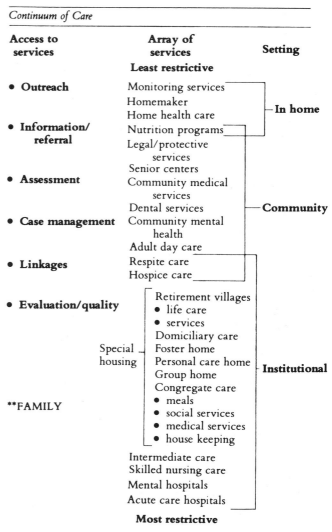

Continuum of Care

Access to services	Array of services	Setting
	Least restrictive	
• Outreach	Monitoring services	
	Homemaker	
	Home health care	In home
• Information/ referral	Nutrition programs	
	Legal/protective services	
	Senior centers	
• Assessment	Community medical services	
	Dental services	Community
• Case management	Community mental health	
	Adult day care	
• Linkages	Respite care	
	Hospice care	
• Evaluation/quality	Retirement villages • life care • services	
	Domiciliary care	
Special housing	Foster home	
	Personal care home	Institutional
	Group home	
	Congregate care • meals • social services • medical services • house keeping	
**FAMILY		
	Intermediate care	
	Skilled nursing care	
	Mental hospitals	
	Acute care hospitals	
	Most restrictive	

FIGURE 5-1. *Continuum of care for the elderly. (From T. Wetle.* Handbook of Geriatric Care. *East Hanover, NJ: Sandoz, 1982.*

for all types of patients [45]. There are more than 6,800 hospitals in the United States today, and they admit more than 36 million patients per year [46], of whom 30 percent are over the age of 65. Older individuals are more likely to be admitted to the hospital than any other age group, with 400.4 discharges per 1,000 elderly in 1985 [1] (Table 5-2).

Although the Medicare prospective payment system (defined later in this chapter) was expected to move elderly patients out of the hospital more quickly, it should be noted that declining lengths of stay are occurring in other age groups as well. Nonetheless, elders tend to

stay in the hospital substantially longer (8.7 days on average) than younger patients.

There are concerns, however, that the new incentives proved by the diagnosis-related groups (DRG) system of reimbursement are changing the acute care hospital in ways that may have harmful effects on older patients. First, efforts to economize in the hospital through "doing better by doing less" [47] have led to reductions in nursing staff and the substitution of less expensive licensed practical nurses (LPNs) and

TABLE 5-2. *Hospital discharges by age and year*

AGE GROUP	DISCHARGES/1,000 POPULATION (HEALTH INTERVIEW)			DISCHARGES/1,000 POPULATION (HOSPITAL SURVEY)		LENGTH OF STAY		
	1964	1980	1985	1979	1984	1964	1980	1985
17–44	162	105	76	152	132	6.5	6.8	5.7
45–64	146	165	162	192	183	10.7	9.4	8.0
65+	190	277	281	361	400	12.1	10.0	8.7

Source: U.S. Department of Health and Human Services, National Center for Health Statistics. *Health, United States—1986.* DHHS Publication No. (PHS)87-1232. Washington, D.C.: U.S. Government Printing Office, 1986. (Based on statistics from the National Health Interview Survey and the National Hospital Discharge Survey.)

nursing aides for registered nurses. Another administrative response that may have a more positive impact on elderly patients is vertical integration [48], in which the hospital consolidates an array of services beyond those included in traditional hospital care. By developing, purchasing, or contracting for services outside the hospital (e.g., home health and nursing homes), the discharge planning problems of patient placement are addressed, marketing is enhanced, and, in some cases, profits occur [49]. It has been argued that vertical integration provides an opportunity to manage patient care better by controlling necessary services and therefore ensuring access. A major concern is that hospital-based programs are more expensive than those of equivalent services based elsewhere. Organizational issues aside, the most frequently voiced concern is that older persons are being discharged "sicker and quicker," placing new burdens on home health agencies, nursing homes, and families. The trend of decreasing lengths of stay started several years ago and is expected to accelerate, resulting in the need for additional staff training, more intensive and sophisticated technology, and more hours of service by home health agencies.

Hospitals are undergoing other changes in response to the evolving demographics of their patient populations. They are recruiting nurses and physicians with special training in geriatrics, developing geriatric consultation services and assessment units, and designing special units for the treatment and rehabilitation of older patients.

MENTAL HOSPITALS

Although state mental hospitals were once a major source of care for the elderly, particularly those suffering from dementing illness, major changes during the past decade have reflected the policy of deinstitutionalization. Since 1955, bed capacity in state and county mental hospitals has decreased 70 percent [50]. Although bed capacity in private mental hospitals and in general hospital psychiatric units increased somewhat during this period, there was a net loss in available beds. Elderly admissions to state and county mental hospitals decreased from 35,000 in 1970 to 20,000 in 1980. The decrease in rate of admissions per 100,000 older persons in the population fell more dramatically, from 172.3 in 1970 to 78.0 in 1980 [1]. During the same period, admissions to private psychiatric hospitals increased from 10,000 to 14,000 per year. Unfortunately, for many older persons with mental illness, deinstitutionalization has translated into "reinstitutionalization" as patients have been transferred from state mental hospitals into nursing homes, which have been termed the "new back wards in the community" [51]. For others, the deinstitutionalization movement meant release into the community, in which the only care, if available at all, came from poorly coordinated and underfunded community-based programs. It is possible that current policies of cost containment for nursing home expenditures and cutbacks in community-based programs may lead once again to increased use of state hospitals for care of the mentally ill and cognitively impaired [52].

NURSING HOMES

Nursing homes are defined as facilities that provide nursing care as their primary and predominant function. Nursing homes tend to be classified according to their certification status as providers of care in the Medicare and Medicaid programs. In general, there are three types of certification: skilled nursing facility (19.2 percent of all nursing homes), intermediate care facility (31.6 percent), facilities that have both skilled and intermediate beds (24.2 percent), and facilities that are not certified (25 percent) [53]. The definitions of each type of facility are complex and run for several pages in the regulations. In brief, a skilled nursing facility (SNF) provides services to individuals who require care from skilled nursing or rehabilitation personnel on a daily basis. Patients in an intermediate care facility (ICF) require health care and related services that are more than room and board but less than those included in SNF care and that can only be provided in an institution.

Since the passage of the Medicaid legislation in 1965, there has been an increase in the number and size of nursing homes, resulting in large increases in the number of beds available (Table 5-3). The rate of nursing home use by the elderly has doubled, from 2.5 percent in 1966 to the current 5 percent of those over the age of 65 [54]. The typical nursing home resident is very old, white, female, and widowed. Risk of nursing home admission increases with age and with dependency in activities of daily living. Only 1.4 percent of persons aged 65 to 74 are in nursing homes compared with 21.6 percent of those over the age of 85 (Table 5-4). Moreover, a larger proportion of those over 85 *with* a functional dependency are institutionalized (61 percent) compared with younger persons with similar functional dependencies (24 percent of those aged 65 to 74) [55].

Although major efforts have been made to improve the quality of nursing home care, cases

TABLE 5-4. *Percentage of persons having activities of daily living (ADL) dependency and percentage of persons in nursing homes, by age*

AGE GROUP	(1) PERCENT HAVING ADL DEPENDENCY*	(2) PERCENT RESIDING IN NURSING HOMES	(3) RATIO BETWEEN (2) AND (1)
45–64	1.2	0.3	0.24
65–74	3.5	1.4	0.40
75–84	11.3	6.4	0.56
85+	35.1	21.6	0.61

*These include all persons who either reside in a nursing home or reside in the community and are dependent in one or more activities of daily living.
SOURCE: Combined data from the 1977 National Nursing Home Survey and the 1977 National Health Interview Survey (unpublished data) as reported by P. Fox. *Long Term Care: Background and Future Directions.* Publication No. HCFA 81-20047. Washington, D.C.: U.S. Government Printing Office, 1981.

of fraud and abuse, haphazard enforcement of regulations, and collusion and conflict of interest among public officials continue to be documented. Concern continues regarding staff turnover, patient neglect, and the absence of active physician participation [56]. On the other hand, nursing home administrators point to problems of overwhelming paper work and inadequate and inconsistent public reimbursement strategies [57].

Several developments point to cautious optimism for the nursing home sector. New attention has been directed toward the nursing home by public and private organizations. The National Institute on Aging and the Robert Wood Johnson Foundation have supported the development of teaching nursing homes [58], which are designed to provide sites for the conduct of clinical and health services research, the teaching of geriatric medicine, and the development of demonstration programs of excellence. There has been a steady trend toward professionalization of nursing home administrators and improvement of management. Perhaps most important, public policymakers have begun to consider changes in reimbursement strategies to improve staffing and to reward desirable outcomes for nursing home residents.

TABLE 5-3. *Percent distribution of nursing and related care homes by bed size 1969–1980*

BED SIZE	1969 (%)	1980 (%)
25–49	38.7	20.8
50–74	27.0	22.9
75–99	14.2	16.3
100–199	16.9	32.5
200+	3.2	7.5
Total residents	759,343	1,329,000

SOURCE: U.S. Department of Health and Human Services, National Center for Health Statistics. Trends in nursing and related homes and hospitals: United States, selected years 1969–1980. *Vital and Health Statistics* 14(30): 4, 1984.

HOUSING

Types of special housing for the elderly vary widely. "Life care" programs are the most comprehensive arrangements, providing a range of services from independent apartments through skilled nursing care. Although most life care communities are on a single campus, other models provide services at a variety of sites. More details regarding the financing of such projects are provided in the insurance section of this chapter. *Congregate care* refers to housing arrangements in which older persons live in individual apartments or rooms in which selected services are available. This arrangement differs from life care communities in that the residents do not own their own housing unit and there is no commitment to provide care over time as the resident's needs change. *Foster, domiciliary, and personal care homes* generally offer room, board, and some supervision. It is important to note that housing options, particularly those that provide supervision, are woefully inadequate in most communities. Current government policy has resulted in major cutbacks in construction of federally subsidized housing, and the unmet demand continues to increase.

HOSPICES

Hospice care offers a set of services intended to improve the quality of life for terminally ill patients [59]. A major goal of hospice care is to enable patients to live the remainder of their lives as comfortably and peacefully as possible, preferably in their own homes. There is a strong emphasis on interdisciplinary teams and the use of *polypharmacy* to minimize physical and emotional suffering [60]. Hospice avoids "heroic" interventions, provides palliative care for the patient, and offers support to the patient and the family during the process of dying. A Medicare hospice benefit is now available, but as of October 1985, only 233 programs had been certified to deliver hospice services under Medicare reimbursement, in part because many programs were unwilling to take the financial risks of providing care after benefits ceased. The impact of hospice care on patient satisfaction, service utilization, and costs is still being determined. Kane and colleagues [61] have demonstrated positive effects of a Veterans Administration hospice program on patient satisfaction and feelings of involvement in care but no reduction in the use of inpatient hospital days or overall costs of care. Brooks [62], using data from

Medicare part A and Blue Cross insurance claims, showed a decrease of 50 percent in hospital days, a ten-fold increase in home care visits, and an overall cost savings of about 40 percent. The results from the National Hospice study are more ambiguous, showing clear-cut cost savings from home care-based programs but more limited cost savings from hospital-based hospice programs, and those only for short-stay patients [63,64]. It has been argued that the limited differences observed in the more recent studies are due in part to the adoption of many aspects of the hospice approach by care providers in the general health system.

Hospice care has also been suggested for patients with certain other illnesses even when death is not imminent. For example, this approach has been used with Alzheimer victims in later stages of the disease with positive reactions from staff and families [65].

RESPITE CARE

Respite care refers to a range of services that allows family members time away from caregiving responsibilities. Services range from an in-home visit of a few hours by a volunteer or paid worker through institutional stays of several weeks. The importance of this service, given the considerable stress of providing care to an aged spouse, sibling, or parent, cannot be underestimated. Unfortunately, the availability of respite services is limited in most communities, as is public funding for this care.

COMMUNITY MENTAL HEALTH CENTERS

Community mental health centers provide ambulatory psychiatric care and other services to residents in specified catchment areas. Under the Community Mental Health Centers Act of 1963, centers were encouraged to foster continuity of care, accessibility of services, and community participation [50]. Although community mental health centers were required to provide inpatient care, outpatient care, and 24-hour emergency service, as well as consultation and educational services to the community, restrictions in public funding have limited program development [66]. Community mental health centers have tended to provide services to the elderly in much lower proportions than population statistics indicate such services are needed, leading to inferences of age discrimination by the U.S. Commission on Civil Rights [67]. Several centers, however, have made efforts to develop special outreach programs, nursing home consultation, and other services targeted toward geriatric clients.

ADULT DAY CARE
Adult day care takes two basic forms: the adult day hospital and multipurpose social day care. Both types of day care are designed for individuals who require supervision and/or medical services during the day but who can spend evenings with family members or in other supportive environments. The array of services provided in adult day care varies among programs [68,69] but generally includes meals, transportation, recreation, and monitoring. In addition to these services, adult day hospitals also offer nursing assessment, some rehabilitation, and medication monitoring. Day care programs were initiated as a cost saving alternative to nursing home care, but population-based prospective studies have yet to demonstrate important savings. Nonetheless, these programs serve a sick and dependent group who benefit from services provided [70].

AMBULATORY PHYSICIAN SERVICES
In 1985, older persons on average had 8.3 physician contacts per year [1]. This was up from 6.3 visits in 1981 and 7.6 visits in 1983 [1,71]. Older persons visit physicians more frequently than do middle-aged (6.1 contacts) or younger individuals (4.7 contacts). Eighty-four percent of the elderly have had a physician contact within the last year. Return visits are more common for the elderly (72 percent of visits had a return visit scheduled) compared with young individuals (49 percent had return visits scheduled). Despite the fact that older persons may take longer to provide a full history, to undress, or to respond to questions, 37 percent of visits lasted less than 10 minutes [1]. Four-fifths of physician visits were made in the doctor's office. Black elderly are twice as likely to make hospital outpatient visits (24 percent) compared with white elderly. This statistic is probably related to income, since the poor (those with incomes of less than $10,000) are twice as likely

to use hospital outpatient clinics as are the wealthy [1].

DENTAL SERVICES
Dental services are an important contributor to the overall well-being of the older patient but are nonetheless frequently overlooked (see Chap. 13). Health of the teeth and oral cavity is related not only to appropriate nutritional intake but also to self-concept and morale. Edentulism increases with age, showing a sharp increase among 85-year-olds. Unfortunately, many elders believe that once they have dentures, they no longer need to visit the dentist, and about 40 percent of one sample of elders had dentures that were more than 20 years old [72,73]. Over time, there are increasing numbers of people who reach old age with teeth to care for. It is therefore difficult to understand the exclusion of virtually all preventive and restorative care from Medicare coverage as well as from most private insurance policies marketed to older people. Under these circumstances, it is not surprising that utilization of dental health services is directly related to income level. In a community-based survey of all elderly residents in East Boston, Massachusetts, 36.2 percent of males with incomes greater than $15,000 reported visiting a dentist in the last six months compared with only 14.8 percent of those with incomes less than $15,000 [73]. Nationally, 51.3 percent of individuals over the age of 65 have not visited a dentist in the last two years [1]. Keeping this in mind, examination of the mouth with dentures in *and* out is an important component of the regular physical examination. Because many older people expect to have oral pain and trouble with dentures [72], health professionals should encourage elderly patients to visit a dentist if poorly fitted or painful dentures or other dental problems are observed.

SENIOR CENTERS
Senior centers provide opportunities for social contact and recreational activities. They also serve as a convenient site for health screening, nutrition and education programs, and outreach activities. Although many communities had already developed senior centers or social facilities for elderly, passage of the Older Ameri-

cans Act in 1965 provided the impetus to develop centers in most communities across the country [74]. Organization of senior centers varies from place to place, but most have paid staff whose activities are supplemented by volunteers. Most offer meals on weekdays, and some have extensive health and social services programs, including adult day care [75]. A listing of senior centers is usually available from the local Area Agency on Aging.

NUTRITION PROGRAMS

Nutrition programs are organized into two types of services—congregate or group meals and home-delivered meals. Congregate meals not only contribute to nutritional health but also provide the opportunity for social contact, educational programs, and outreach efforts. It is estimated that congregate meals programs provide hot lunches to about 2.65 million elderly each year [52]. Homebound meals or "meals on wheels" are an important resource for individuals who are unable to shop, prepare meals, or follow special dietary regimens. Most elderly nutrition programs are subsidized under the Older Americans Act, and meals are provided on a "pay as you can" voluntary contribution basis.

HOME HEALTH CARE

Home health care provides a wide range of services, including

Skilled nursing
Occupational, physical, and speech therapy
Medical social services
Physician care
Nutritional/dietary services and meals
Homemaker services
Home health aid services
Respiration therapy
Intravenous therapy
Medical supplies, drugs, and medical appliances

The actual care provided to an individual client, the person who gives the care, and the length of care depend not only on the patient's needs but also on the restrictions and rules of the funding agency [59]. Generally, home care is provided by five types of agencies—public, non-profit (such as Visiting Nurses Associations), hospital-based, proprietary, and combination agencies. Both parts A and B of Medicare cover home health care (see below under Medicare for program definitions and eligibility), but there are several restrictions on elgibility that are discussed later in this chapter. Despite these restrictions, Medicare expenditures for home care have grown at an annual rate of 20 percent to about $2.3 billion (3.3 percent of benefit payments) in 1985 [76]. Medicaid is less restrictive in its eligibility requirements once the client meets the Medicaid income and assets guidelines. Expenditures from all sources for services for home care are expected to grow from $9 billion in 1985 to $16 billion in 1990 [77].

Physicians have played a central but ambiguous role in the home care system. On the one hand, for all public and most private insurers, physicians must certify a care plan to permit services to be paid for. Frequently, however, the care plan is initiated, developed, and managed by someone other than the sign-off physician. There are, however, increasing numbers of physicians who are working in home care programs as patient advocates and care providers, and geriatricians argue that the time-honored house call should be a regular part of geriatric care [78,79]. The growth of the home care system provides an important resource in management of care of elders.

MONITORING SERVICES

Monitoring services are intended to keep in touch with chronically impaired or frail persons living at home. These can include organized active services, such as telephone networks or friendly visitors, or they may occur as byproducts of other services including home-delivered meals or homemaker services. A variety of innovative programs have been developed, such as having a letter carrier knock at the door to check on an older person who has failed to activate a signal that all is well. More ambitious monitoring efforts have been suggested for elders who are at increased risk for negative health events, including those who are over age 75, living alone, recently bereaved, recently hospitalized, incontinent, immobile, and/or cognitively impaired [80]. Several large-scale studies have been launched to determine the cost-effectiveness of formal surveillance/monitoring programs under Medicare reimbursement [81].

ACCESS TO SERVICES

This impressive array of services is useful only if the patient learns about and is able to receive particular needed services. Sometimes in the course of regular caregiving problems are discovered beyond the range of care provided by the physician; alternatively, older patients and their families seek assistance in deciding which services are most appropriate and how they can be arranged. This task may be time-consuming for busy physicians, who may not know what services are available or how to obtain them. Fortunately, assistance is available in many communites.

Outreach programs are designed to identify and connect with individuals with unmet needs. These diverse programs may be found under a variety of auspices. Most communities have an Area Agency on Aging (AAA), which provides outreach services, directly or under contract, or keeps an updated listing of agencies, that provide outreach in the community. Outreach programs differ in the way services are provided. In some communities, door-to-door surveys are conducted to identify individuals at high risk of dependency and/or institutionalization. Other programs seek clients at senior centers, community centers, or other gathering places.

Information and referral services are run by a variety of community agencies, including the AAA, the community mental health center, the public health department, the Easter Seal Society, and the American Cancer Society, to name a few. The purpose of an information and referral service is to answer service-related questions, to make appropriate referrals to service providers, and, ideally, to follow up on the referral to determine whether appropriate services have been received. This service requires frequent updating of resource files and personnel who are well informed and sensitive about the special problems of older people. Hospital discharge planners are frequently quite knowledgeable about who provides information and referral and the quality of the services provided.

Comprehensive assessment is crucial for matching clients with the most appropriate services. Although health and illness may be the primary focus of the physician, a number of other factors interact with health to determine the exact service package that is most appropriate, including function, social supports, personal and economic resources, and client and family preferences. Assessment is discussed in Chapter 4 of this text.

Case management entails the development of an individualized care plan based on comprehensive assessment. The case manager, after careful consideration of the needs of the client in conjunction with personal and community resources, develops a plan of care with the client. The case manager coordinates delivery of the formal services and follows up to determine that the client received the appropriate services as planned. The case manager also monitors the status of the client, changing the service package as required by improvement or decline in function or by changes in the client's social supports. Although positive patient outcomes of client satisfaction and increased access to services have been observed in case management demonstrations, large-scale studies such as the National Long-Term Care Channeling Demonstration Project have failed to demonstrate differences in cost of care or rates of institutionalization, hospitalization, or mortality [82,83].

This continuum of services needed and used by the elderly is financed by an array of federal, state, and private programs. Frequently, several sources contribute to reimbursement of a single type of service as well as to the multiple services required by many older persons. The major programs that support geriatric care are described in the next section.

Financing Health Care

The cost of geriatric health care is a substantial burden for public programs and for the elderly themselves. Per capita spending on health services is 3.5 times greater for elderly persons ($4,200 in 1984) than for those under the age of 65 [2]. Overall health care expenditures for the elderly were $119.9 billion in 1984 [84]. Out-of-pocket expenditures by the aged have risen from $966 in 1980 to $1,526 in 1984 and are projected to be $2,583 in 1990 [85]. Out-of-

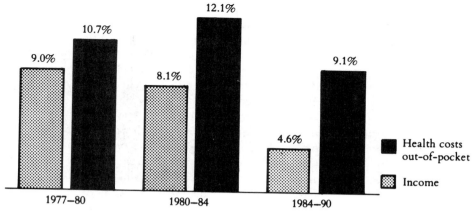

FIGURE 5-2. *Income and health cost increases for the aged (percent increases). (From Select Committee on Aging, U.S. House of Representatives.* America's Elderly at Risk. *Publication No. 99-508, Washington, D.C.: U.S. Government Printing Office, 1985.)*

pocket expenditures are increasing faster than income, and the aged will expend 18.9 percent of their income for health care costs in 1990 (Fig. 5-2). Overall, older persons pay for 38 percent of health care costs out of pocket. Projections suggest that in 1990 they will pay for 15 percent of their hospital costs, 52 percent of physician costs, 55 percent of nursing home costs, and 66 percent of other costs such as dental services and eyeglasses [85].

HISTORIC CONTEXT OF PUBLIC PROGRAMS

Development of public responsibility for financing geriatric care has been a slow and complex process. Although historically public hospitals have provided some care to the indigent aged and state mental hospitals provided care to certain chronically impaired elders, a comprehensive public insurance or service program for the full continuum of care required by older persons has yet to be developed. Since 1966, the major public payors for geriatric care have been the Medicare and Medicaid programs (Titles XVIII and XIX of the Social Security Act). The current package of benefits provided under these two programs is best understood in the context of the many compromises that led to the passage of the bill in 1965. The Kerr-Mills Bill (Public Law 86-778), a precursor to Medicaid, was offered by conservative congressional

leaders in 1960 as a way of avoiding passage of more sweeping Medicare legislation. In theory, Kerr-Mills, a partnership between the states and the federal government, was expected to cover the 2.4 million elders then receiving Old Age Assistance as well as an additional 10 million medically indigent people with a range of services that included hospitalization, physician and nursing care, dental care, and drugs. In practice, implementation was limited. By 1963 only 32 states had operational programs, and most of these were very restricted [86]. As medical care became more expensive and increasing proportions of the non-old were covered by health insurance, public pressure grew for some kind of comprehensive insurance for older Americans.

The Medicare legislation proposed by President John F. Kennedy in 1961 and resubmitted in 1965 was limited to hospital and nursing home costs for aged patients. This was consonant with the political strategy of liberal democrats to get a "foot in the door" with a modest program that then could be incrementally expanded into comprehensive national health insurance. In a surprising response, the conservative members of Congress, under the leadership of Wilbur Mills, proposed a "layer cake" bill combining hospital insurance, voluntary insurance for physician services, and an expanded Kerr-Mills program for the indigent aged. The rationale for this act was tripartite. First, it was assumed that the passage of some sort of Medicare legislation was inevitable. Second, by suggesting this form of legislation, the conservatives could move out of a role of obstructing health care, and third, at the same time, they could make further incremental "add-ons" by the liberals politically unfeasible [86].

Medicare and Medicaid were signed into law in 1965. The programs were intended to maintain and improve access to mainstream health care for the elderly and the medically indigent. Mindful of political pressures from the organizations representing the health professions and institutions, care was taken to write regulations to avoid interfering with the ongoing health care system. Modeled closely after the existing federal insurance program, which had been designed for a younger population, emphasis was placed on reimbursement of hospital and institutional services.

Benefits and financing of the various current programs addressing health care of the aged are described in more detail below.

MEDICARE

Hospital Insurance

Hospital insurance (part A) is one of two types of insurance offered by the Medicare program. The second is supplemental medical insurance (part B). Part A is provided without premiums to elderly individuals who qualify for social security or railroad retirement benefits and is available to other persons aged 65 and over upon payment of a premium ($226 per month). Part A, financed by payroll taxes with cost sharing via deductibles and copayments, covers

four kinds of care: (1) inpatient hospital care; (2) medically necessary inpatient care in a skilled nursing facility; (3) home health care; and (4) hospice care. Approximately 26.9 million elderly and 2.9 million nonelderly disabled were covered by part A, generating payments of $41.5 billion in 1984 [87,88].

Payment for part A services is a shared responsibility between the beneficiary and the Medicare program. The basic formula for copayments has remained stable since the initiation of the program, but the actual amounts paid by beneficiaries have increased dramatically (Fig. 5-3). Beneficiary responsibility is closely tied to what is termed a "benefit period." A benefit period begins with hospital admission and continues until the beneficiary has been out of the hospital or other facility providing skilled services for 60 consecutive days. For the first 60 days of the benefit period, the beneficiary is responsible only for a single deductible payment, currently equal to $520 ($40 in 1966 at the initiation of the Medicare program). For days 61 through 90, the beneficiary pays one-fourth of the deductible (currently $130 per day) and is then responsible for payment of the remaining days in that benefit period. The

FIGURE 5-3. *Medicare copayments as a portion of elderly income (calculated as the median income of a beneficiary aged 65 to 69). (From Harvard Medicare Project.* Medicare: Coming of Age. *Cambridge: Center for Health Policy and Management, John F. Kennedy School of Government, 1986.)*

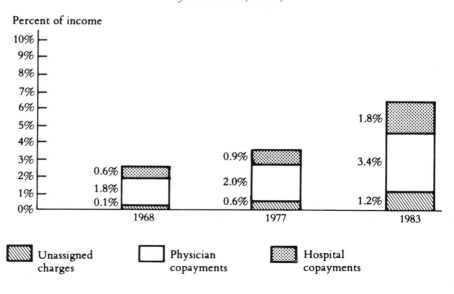

beneficiary has an additional 60 life-time reserve days, which can only be used once and for which the beneficiary pays $260 per day [89].

Medicare payment for hospital services is based on a prospective payment system implemented in 1983. Designed to control rapidly escalating costs of hospital care, payment is determined by the diagnosis-related group (DRG) to which the patient is assigned rather than by charges for services provided. This new system provides strong financial incentives to the hospital to provide services efficiently and to discharge the patient as quickly as possible. As expected, since the implementation of the DRG system, there has been a more accelerated decrease in length of stay than was projected from historic trend lines. Contrary to expectations, there has also been a decrease in admission rates, contributing to the lowest hospital occupancy rates across the country since data have been available [90].

Medicare part A will also pay for inpatient care in a certified skilled nursing facility if rather restrictive requirements are met, including certification by a physician that the patient requires skilled nursing care or rehabilitation on a daily basis. The nursing home stay must be preceded by hospitalization, the reason for nursing home services must be related to a condition treated in the hospital, and a utilization review committee or peer review organization (PRO) must not have denied the benefit. If these requirements are satisfied, Medicare will pay for the first 20 days of care in that benefit period. For days 21 through 100, the beneficiary is responsible for a copayment of $62.50 per day [89].

Home health services—part-time or intermittent skilled nursing care, physical therapy, or speech therapy—are provided if the beneficiary is home bound and if a physician develops and certifies a plan of care. It should be noted that this benefit is quite strictly defined, and many elderly with chronic conditions do not qualify for Medicare reimbursement of home health services.

Hospice services are covered by Medicare part A if a doctor certifies that the patient is terminally ill (life expectancy of 6 months or less), *and* the patient chooses to receive care from a hospice instead of standard Medicare benefits,

and care is provided by a Medicare-certified hospice program. Special benefit periods (two 90-day periods and one 30-day period) apply to this service. If the patient still requires hospice care after these benefit periods are over, the hospice is financially responsible for providing any additional needed services. The beneficiary is responsible for a copayment on medications (5 percent of cost of drugs or $5 per prescription, whichever is less) and inpatient respite care (5 percent of cost up to a total of $400).

Supplemental Medical Insurance
Supplemental medical insurance (part B) is a voluntary program, financed by a combination of premiums and general revenue. Part B premiums are currently $17.90 per month (compared with $3 in 1966). In 1984, 29.5 million people were enrolled in the part B program, and $19.5 billion in benefits were paid [1]. Although individuals can choose not to enroll when they become eligible, the premium rate is increased by 10 percent for each year spent out of the program if they enroll at a later date. About 97 percent of the aged covered by part A are also enrolled in part B [90]. Part B pays a portion of the cost of (1) physician services, (2) outpatient hospital care, (3) outpatient physical therapy and speech pathology services, and (4) some home health care services and supplies not covered by part A. There are special limitations on certain types of outpatient care, including mental health services (50 percent of allowed charges or $250 per year, whichever is smaller) and physical therapists in independent practice ($500 allowed charges per year).

Payment for services is made either directly to the beneficiary or to the physician. In either case, the beneficiary is liable for a $75 annual deductible as well as a 20 percent copayment. By filing a claim for reimbursement, the beneficiary will receive 80 percent of "reasonable charges" above the deductible and is responsible for paying the physician whatever additional amount is billed. By "accepting assignment," the physician agrees to accept the carrier's determination of reasonable charges as the full fee and is paid 80 percent of that amount directly by the carrier. The patient is still responsible for 20 percent of the determined "reasonable" fee. Recent controversy regarding the unwillingness of some physicians to accept assignment has led some states to require "mandatory assignment," under which physicians must accept assignment for all Medicare patients if they are to be reimbursed by Medicare at all.

Health maintenance organizations (HMOs) provide an alternative type of care for Medicare beneficiaries [91]. The Tax Equity and Fiscal Responsibility Act of 1982 (TEFRA, HR 4961) allowed HMOs to contract with Medicare to provide coverage to the elderly and to be reimbursed on a prospective, capitated basis. For each Medicare enrollee, plans receive 95 percent of the adjusted average per capita cost (AAPCC) for their geographic region, adjusted for age, sex, institutional, and welfare status of the beneficiaries. Plans are at risk for cost overruns, and any savings must be used to benefit elderly enrollees [92,93]. It has been argued that the HMO has the potential to improve on the fragmented care provided in the fee-for-service sector by improving management of care and providing a wider array of services [94,95]. In general, the elderly have responded favorably to HMO enrollment [96,97] because of the modest premiums charged and the additional services (e.g., prescription drugs, eyeglasses, hearing aids, walkers) provided by most HMOs at low or no cost to the beneficiary. There are concerns, however, about biased selection and quality assurance as some HMOs struggle for financial survival and others are suspected of fraud and abuse [98,99]. As of March, 1986, 119 prepaid plans had signed TEFRA risk contracts, 64 additional applications were awaiting approval, and 4.6 percent of the Medicare population was enrolled in some type of prepaid plan [91].

MEDICAID

In contrast to Medicare, the Medicaid program is a federal-state partnership in which the federal government provides global programmatic guidelines and approximately half of the funding. The intent of the program is to pay for health services for the aged poor, the blind, the disabled, and families with dependent children. Reimbursement for four types of care is required under the federal guidelines: (1) inpatient and outpatient hospital care; (2) laboratory and x-ray services; (3) physician services; and (4) skilled nursing care for persons over age 21, and home health services. States may also choose to provide certain optional services, including prescriptions, dental services, eyeglasses, and intermediate level nursing home care. Eligibility requirements are determined by each state but must include cash assistance recipients (e.g., Supplemental Security Income) as well as certain groups of poor children and pregnant women. States may optionally extend eligibility to other groups, such as the "medically indigent" (defined as those with income of no more than 133 percent of the poverty level) or those who have incurred medical expenses at least equal to the difference between their income and the applicable income standard [1]. The range of services provided and eligibility requirements vary widely from state to state [74,100]. In fiscal year 1984, 3.2 million elderly received Medicaid benefits. In fiscal year 1985, the federal government paid $21.7 billion from general revenues for the total Medicaid program, and states contributed $17.8 billion [1].

Medicaid is the major public payor for long-term care, contributing about 42 percent of the $35.2 billion spent for nursing home services in 1985 [76]. Expenditures for nursing home care account for 34 percent of the Medicaid budget [101]. In order for elders to qualify for Medicaid reimbursement for such services, they must "spend down"—i.e., pay for care from their own resources until they meet income and asset-related eligibility requirements for the state in which they live. Although the Medicaid program was intended to serve the poor, the high cost of long-term care rapidly brings a majority of elders into this category if they require chronic care. Because income is inversely related to age, but risk of institutionalization increases with age, the older the individual, the more likely he or she is to become Medicaid eligible (Fig. 5-4).

It has been estimated that of elderly individuals who live alone in the community and enter a nursing home in Massachusetts, 63 percent will qualify for Medicaid in three months, 83 percent by one year, and 91 percent by two years [102]. The estimates are only slightly better for a married person who enters a nursing home. Unfortunately, the impact of "spending down" on the spouse living in the community (i.e., spousal

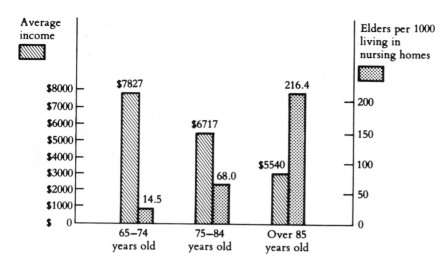

FIGURE 5-4. *Costs and resources for long-Term care: average income and institutionalization rates, by age of beneficiary. (From Harvard Medicare Project.* Medicare: Coming of Age. *Cambridge: Center for Health Policy, John F. Kennedy School of Government, 1986.)*

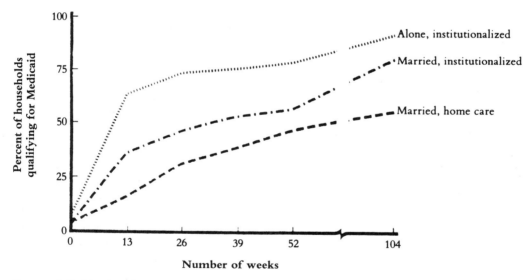

FIGURE 5-5. *Number of weeks required for Massachusetts elderly to spend down income and assets to approximate Medicaid eligibility, 1984 (population aged 66 or over). (From D. J. Friedman and E. Socholitzky. Blue Cross and Blue Shield of Massachusetts, 1985. In Select Committee on Aging, U.S. House of Representatives.* America's Elderly at Risk. *Publication No. 99-508. Washington, D.C.: U.S. Government Printing Office, 1985.)*

impoverishment) is devastating. At best, Medicaid offers an imperfect safety net and only for those in severe need (Fig. 5-5).

VETERANS ADMINISTRATION

Another major public provider of geriatric care is the Veterans Administration (VA). Charged by Title 38 of the United States Code to establish and maintain a health care system to benefit veterans, the VA has developed a set of facilities and benefit programs that serve both veterans suffering "injury or disease incurred or aggravated in the line of duty" (service-connected disability) and those without such disabilities [103]. Between 1980 and 1990, the proportion of elders in the veteran population will more than double, and the absolute number will reach more than seven million in 1990. Their numbers will peak at almost nine million in the year 2000, when two out of three males over the age of 65 will be veterans [104]. Services are provided on a space-available basis, and priority goes to veterans with service-connected disabilities. In response to the growing numbers of older veterans, several geriatric programs have been implemented by the VA. In addition to services provided in 172 VA hospitals, 16 domiciliaries, and 99 nursing home units, the VA supports state veterans nursing homes and hospitals and contracts for care in community hospitals and nursing homes [104]. The VA has also launched several innovative programs to serve older veterans, including geriatric evaluation units (GEU), geriatric research, education and clinical centers (GRECC), and hospital-based home care programs. Recently, the VA's role as a provider of health care has come under increased scrutiny, and cost-conscious suggestions have been made to change or reduce services provided and to cut the VA budget [105,106]. Others have suggested expanding the array of services delivered to older veterans, noting that the VA has unique opportunities to provide a full range of managed care services [107,108]. Given a relatively static budget with increasing demands for service, the continuing evolution of geriatric care in the VA is uncertain.

PRIVATE INSURANCE

The enactment of Medicare and Medicaid legislation some 20 years ago was in part a response to the failure of the marketplace to adequately provide for geriatric health care. Since that time, the private sector has begun to pay much more attention to the large market segment composed of those over 65. A wide array of private insurance products is now marketed to elderly individuals, most taking the form of "medigap" insurance, which pays for some or all of Medicare deductibles and copayments. About two-thirds of the elderly have purchased private supplemental insurance [2]. Income and race influence whether or not an aged individual has private health insurance; 75 percent of white aged persons with incomes above $7,000 in 1980 had private insurance, whereas only about 20 percent of nonwhite aged people with incomes below $7,500 had private insurance [2]. However, if Medicaid is taken into consideration as a form of supplemental coverage, race and income differences are minimized. It should be kept in mind, however, that one-fourth of the poor elderly—those for whom deductibles and copayments are most onerous—have no supplemental coverage [2] (Fig. 5-6). In addition to the inability of poor elderly to pay for insurance, other concerns have been raised regarding the private sector. Reports of fraudulent marketing practices, low payout rates, and confusion among the elderly regarding services covered have been documented in congressional hearings [85], and many states have taken action to regulate medigap insurance more closely.

Very few of the supplemental products cover services such as long-term home health or nursing home care because benefits tend to be tied to Medicare definitions of eligibility and covered services. Recently, a number of private insurers have begun to develop and market long-term care insurance. It has been estimated that the premium for coverage of nursing home and home health care with a limited fixed benefit would be about $50 per month for a 70-year-old [101]. It remains to be seen whether elderly or their family members will be willing to pay the relatively high premiums required for those of advanced age or, alternatively, to enroll at younger ages far in advance of probable need for services when lower premiums are available.

One type of long-term care insurance that takes a rather unusual form is the life care community [109]. Although individual plans differ,

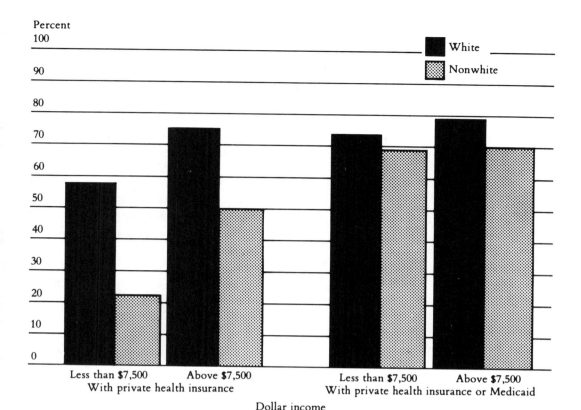

Percent

FIGURE 5-6. *Proportion of elderly with private health insurance or with private health insurance or Medicaid. (Data from National Medical Care Utilization and Expenditures Survey, 1980. In T. Rice and J. Gabel. Protecting elderly against high health costs.* Health Affairs *Fall:5–21, 1986.)*

the usual configuration is for the elder to buy into a residential facility and to pay a monthly fee for an array of fixed services (e.g., grounds-keeping, meals, housekeeping) and additional services as needed (home health aide, visiting nurse, nursing home care). Although some early plans experienced financial difficulties, there are several successful models now in operation. Life care communities differ in the amount of "up-front" money required, in arrangements for providing needed services, and in the amount, if any, that is returned when the resident dies or chooses to leave the community.

OLDER AMERICANS ACT

Since its enactment in 1965, the Older Americans Act has evolved from a program of small grants and research projects to a network of 57 state units on aging (including U.S. territories and Indian tribes), more than 660 Area Agencies on Aging, and thousands of community agencies [54]. Spending in 1987 amounted to approximately $1.2 billion. The primary purpose of the act is to coordinate and/or deliver the following services at the community level: information and referral, outreach, transportation, senior centers, nutritional programs, advocacy, protective services, senior employment, ombudsman programs, and supportive services. In addition, Older Americans Act monies support research and training.

TITLE XX

Title XX of the Social Security Act authorized reimbursements to states for social services, including a variety of home health and home-maker services of benefit to the frail elderly. These monies have now been shifted to the Social Services Block Grant (SSBG) program, which is designed to "prevent or reduce inappropriate institutional care by providing for community-based care." Since 1981, states have not been required to make public reports on how these monies are spent, including types of services or persons served. Because this is a block grant to respond to competing needs from several populations, it is not possible to estimate the benefit to older people. The appropriation level for this program has been constant at $2.7 billion since 1984 [54].

SOCIAL SECURITY

Although Social Security is not usually considered a health program, the provision of a basic pension system provides resources to the elderly that are frequently used to pay for many health care needs. There are two types of income payments to the elderly, Old Age and Survivors Insurance (OASI, Title II) and Supplemental Security Income (SSI, Title VI). The "floor of protection" provided by this program enables older individuals to live independently in later years. It has been argued that the passage of Title II of the Social Security Act (OASI) gave impetus to the growth of the nursing home industry, in that older people remained in the community, moving to room and board homes as their functional dependency increased. As residents of these homes needed more assistance, these homes developed into "board and care" facilities and eventually into the nursing homes we know today [57]. SSI provides a guaranteed minimum income to the aged, blind, and disabled. For the elderly, SSI replaced the state-run old-age assistance programs, which varied widely across the country in eligibility and benefits. Under SSI, income and asset limits determine eligibility for a monthly payment of $336 for individuals and $502 for couples [54]. The low income limits ($4,080 for an individual and $6,120 for a couple) have been criticized, as has the policy of counting gifts as incomes. The Social Security OASI program is financed through an "earmarked" payroll tax to which both employers and workers contribute, and pension payments are determined by the individual's earning history. The SSI program is financed through general revenues.

Conclusion

Although several other programs provide benefits to the elderly that might conceivably affect health, we have discussed the major resources available. Great strides have been made toward improving services for older Americans. The current network of health and social services provides the basis for a true continuum of care. However, as has been suggested in the preceding descriptions of the strengths and weaknesses of public and private programs, much has yet to be done. A well-informed physician, alert to the multiple needs of elderly patients and willing to assist in the negotiation of an imperfect system, is a true asset. The ultimate goal, of course, is not only a longer life but also a better life for older persons.

References

1. United States Department of Health and Human Services, Public Health Service. *Health—United States, 1986.* Publication No. PHS-87-1232, Washington, D.C.: U.S. Government Printing Office, 1986.
2. Rice, T., and Gabel, J. Protecting the elderly against high health care costs. *Health Affairs* 5(3):5, 1986.
3. Brody, E. M., et al. Women's changing roles and help to elderly parents: Attitudes of three generations of women. *J. Gerontol.* 38(5):597, 1983.
4. Brody, S. J., Poulshock, S. W., and Masciocchi, C. F. The family caring unit: A major consideration in the long-term support system. *Gerontologist* 18(6):556, 1978.
5. National Center for Health Statistics. Home care for persons 55 and over, United States, July 1966–June 1968. *Vital and Health Statistics,* 10(73). Publication Number HSM72-1062. Washington, D.C.: U.S. Government Printing Office, 1972.
6. Fendetti, D. V., and Gelfond, D. E. Care of the aged: Attitudes of white ethnic families. *Gerontologist* 16:545, 1976.
7. Shanas, E. Social myth and hypotheses: The case of family relations of old people. *Gerontologist* 19:3, 1979.
8. Thornton, A., and Freedman, D. Changes in the sex role attitudes of women, 1962–1977: Evidence from a panel study. *Am. Sociolog. Rev.* 44:831, 1979.
9. United States Department of Labor, Bureau of Labor Statistics. Labor force by sex, age and race. *Earnings and Employment* 28:167, 1981.
10. Cicirelli, V. G. A comparison of helping behavior to elderly parents of adult children with intact and disrupted marriages. *Gerontologist* 23:619, 1983.

11. National Retired Teachers Association—American Association of Retired Persons. *National Survey of Older Americans*, No. 6. Washington, D.C.: American Association of Retired Persons, 1981.
12. Getzel, G. S. Helping elderly couples in crisis. Paper presented at the 1981 meeting of the Gerontological Society of America, Toronto, Canada.
13. Johnson, C., and Catalano, D. A longitudinal study of family supports to peer elderly. Paper presented at the 1982 meeting of the Gerontological Society of America, Boston, MA.
14. Fengler, A., and Goodrich, N. Wives of elderly disabled men: The hidden patients. *Gerontologist* 19:175, 1979.
15. Cantor, M. Strain among caregivers: A study of experience in the United States. *Gerontologist* 23:597, 1983.
16. Maddox, G. L. Families As Context and Resources in Chronic Illness. In S. Sherwood (ed.), *Long Term Care: A Handbook for Researchers, Planners and Providers.* New York: Spectrum, 1975.
17. Branch, L. G., and Jette, A. M. A prospective study of long term care institutionalization among the aged. *Am. J. Public Health* 72:1373, 1982.
18. Branch, L. G., and Stuart, N. Towards a dynamic understanding of the care needs of the non-institutionalized elderly. *Home Health Care Services Q.* 6(1):25, 1985.
19. Wetle, T., and Evans, L. Serving the Family of the Elder Veteran. In T. Wetle and J. Rowe (eds.), *Older Veterans: Linking VA and Community Resources.* Cambridge: Harvard University Press, 1984.
20. Cohen, P. M. A group approach to working with families of the elderly. *Gerontologist* 23(3):249, 1983.
21. Robinson, B. C. Validation of a caregiver's strain index. *J. Gerontol.* 38(3):344, 1983.
22. Soldo, B., and Myllyluoma, J. Caregivers who live with dependent elderly. *Gerontologist* 23:605, 1983.
23. Clark, N. M., and Rakowski, W. Family caregivers of older adults: Improving helping skills. *Gerontologist* 23:637, 1983.
24. Berkman, L. F. Social networks, support, and health: Taking the next step foward. *Am. J. Epidemiol.* 123(4):559, 1986.
25. Schoenbach, V. J., Kaplan, B. H., and Fredman, L. Social ties and mortality in Veans County, Georgia. *Am. J. Epidemiol.* 123(4):577, 1986.
26. Berkman, L. F., and Syme, S. L. Social networks, host resistance and mortality: A nine-year followup study of Alameda County residents. *Am. J. Epidemiol.* 109:186, 1979.
27. House, J. S., Robbins, C., and Metzner, H. L. The association of social relationships and activities with mortality: Prospective evidence from the Tecumseh Community Health Study. *Am. J. Epidemiol.* 116:123, 1982.
28. Blazer, D. G. Social support and mortality in an elderly community population. *Am. J. Epidemiol.* 115:686, 1982.
29. Rubberman, W., Weinblatt, E., and Goldberg, J. D. Psychosocial influences on mortality after myocardial infarction. *N. Engl. J. Med.* 311:552, 1984.
30. Palmore, E. Total chance of institutionalization among the aged. *Gerontologist* 16:504, 1976.
31. Wan, T. H. *Stressful Life Events, Social Support Networks, and Gerontological Health.* Lexington, MA: Lexington Books, 1982.
32. Levkoff, S. E., Cleary, P. D., and Wetle, T. Differences in the appraisal of health between aged and middle-aged adults. *J. Gerontol.* 42(1):114, 1987.
33. Holmes, T. H., and Rahe, R. H. The social readjustment rating scale. *J. Psychosom. Res.* 11:213, 1967.
34. Kasl, S. V. Changes in Mental Health Status Associated with Job Loss and Retirement. In J. W. Barnett (ed.), *Stress and Mental Disorder.* New York: Raven, 1979.
35. Kasl, S. V. The Impact of Retirement. In C. L. Cooper and R. Payne (eds.), *Current Concerns in Occupational Stress.* New York: Wiley, 1980.
36. Levkoff, S., Green, L. W., and Hansel, N. K. Changes in the cycle of life style and aging: Implications for health promotion. *Special Care in Dentistry* May–June:130–134, 1984.
37. Kasl, S. V. Physical and mental health effects of involuntary relocation and institutionalization: A review. *Am. J. Public Health* 62:377, 1972.
38. Pastalan, L. A. Environmental Displacement: A Literature Reflecting Old-Person Environment Interactions. In G. D. Rowls and R. J. Ohta (eds.), *Aging and Milieu: Environmental Perspectives on Growing Old.* New York: Academic, 1983.
39. Borup, J. Relocation mortality research: Assessment, reply, and the need to refocus on the issues. *Gerontologist* 23:235, 1983.
40. Bourestrom, N., and Pastalan, L. A. Effects of relocation on the elderly. *Gerontologist* 21:4, 1981.
41. Liberman, M. A. Adaptive Process in Late Life. In N. Datan and L. Ginsberg (eds.), *Life Span Developmental Psychology: Normative Life Crises.* New York: Academic, 1975.
42. Lopata, H. Z. Widowhood: Societal Factors in Life Span Disruptions and Alternatives. In N.

Datan and L. Ginsberg (eds.), *Life Span Developmental Psychology: Normative Life Crises*. New York: Academic, 1975.

43. Danish, S. J. Human Development and Human Services: A Marriage Proposal. In B. L. Iscoe and C. C. Spielberger (eds.), *Community Psychology in Transition*. New York: Halstead Press, 1977.

44. American Association of Retired Persons. *A Profile of Older Americans—1986*. Washington, D.C.: AARP, 1987; Atchley, R. C. *The Sociology of Retirement*. New York: Halstead Press, 1979.

45. Kovner, A. R. Hospitals. In S. Jonas (ed.), *Health Care Delivery in the United States* (3rd ed.). New York: Springer, 1986.

46. American Hospital Association. *Hospital Statistics*. Chicago: American Hospital Association, 1984.

47. Kovener, J., and Palmer, J. Implementing the Medicare prospective pricing system. *Health Care Financial Management* 13(9):74, 1983.

48. Sankar, A., Newcomer, R., and Wood, J. Prospective payment: Systemic effects on the provision of community care for the elderly. *Home Health Services Q.* 7(2):93, 1986.

49. Brody, S., and Magel, J. Diagnosis related groups: An overview. *Center for the Study of Aging Newsletter* 6(2):6, 1983.

50. Koran, L. M., and Sarfstein, S. S. Mental Health Services. In S. Jonas (ed.), *Health Care Delivery in the United States* (3rd ed.). New York: Springer, 1986.

51. Schmidt, L. J., et al. The mentally ill in nursing homes: New back wards in the community. *Arch. Gen. Psychiatry* 34:687, 1977.

52. Wetle, T. (ed.). *Handbook of Geriatric Care*. East Hanover, NJ: Sandoz, 1982.

53. United States Department of Health, Education and Welfare. The national nursing home survey: 1977 summary for the United States. *Vital and Health Statistics*. Publication No. PHS 79-1794. Washington, D.C.: U.S. Government Printing Office, 1979.

54. Special Committee on Aging, United States Senate. *Developments in Aging, 1986*. Vol. 1. Washington, D.C.: U.S. Government Printing Office, 1986.

55. Fox, P. *Long Term Care: Background and Future Directions*. Publication No. HCFA 81-20047. Washington, D.C.: U.S. Government Printing Office, 1981.

56. Wetle, T., and Pearson, D. A. Long Term Care. In S. Jonas (ed.), *Health Care Delivery in the United States* (3rd ed.). New York: Springer, 1986.

57. Vladek, B. *Unloving Care: The Nursing Home Tragedy*. New York: Basic Books, 1980.

58. Butler, R. N. The teaching nursing home. *J.A.M.A.* 245(14):1435, 1981.

59. Barhydt-Wezenar, N. Home Care and Hospice. In S. Jonas (ed.), *Health Care Delivery in the United States* (3rd ed.). New York: Springer, 1986.

60. Liegner, L. M. St. Christopher's Hospice, 1974. *J.A.M.A.* 234(10):1047, 1977.

61. Kane, R. L., et al. Hospice role in alleviating the emotional stress of terminal patients and their families. *Med. Care* 23(3):189, 1985.

62. Brooks, C. H., and Smyth-Staruch, K. Hospice home care cost savings to third-party insurers. *Med. Care* 22(8):691, 1984.

63. Mor, V., and Kidder, D. Cost savings in hospice: Final results of the National Hospice Study. *Health Serv. Res.* 20:407, 1985.

64. Birnbaum, H. G., and Kidder, D. What does hospice cost? *Am. J. Public Health* 74(7):689, 1984.

65. Volicer, L. Need for hospice approach to treatment of patients with advanced progressive dementia. *J. Am. Geriatr. Soc.* 34:655, 1986.

66. Estes, C. L., and Wood, J. B. A preliminary assessment of the impact of block grants on community mental health centers. *Hosp. Community Psychiatry* 35:1125, 1984.

67. United States Commission on Civil Rights. *The Age Discrimination Study*. Publication No. 005-000-00190-1. Washington, D.C.: U.S. Government Printing Office, 1979.

68. Weissert, W. Adult day care programs in the United States: Current research projects and a survey of 10 centers. *Public Health Rep.* 92(1):49, 1977.

69. Sherwood, S., Morris, J. N., and Ruchlin, H. S. Alternative paths to long term care: Nursing home geriatric day hospital, senior center and domiciliary care options. *Am. J. Public Health* 76(1):38, 1986.

70. Weissert, W. Seven reasons why it is so difficult to make community-based long term care cost effective. *Health Serv. Res.* 20(4):424, 1985.

71. United States Department of Health and Human Services. Current estimates from the National Health Interview Survey: United States 1981. *Vital and Health Statistics*. PHS 82-1569, 10(141). Washington, D.C.: U.S. Government Printing Office, 1982.

72. Hunt, R. J., et al. Edentulism and oral health problems among rural elderly Iowans: The Iowa 65+ rural health study. *J. Am. Public Health Assoc.* 75(10):1177, 1985.

73. Cartwright, W. S., et al. Self reported use of dental, hospital and nursing home services. National Institute on Aging, USDHHS, Publication No. 86-2443. Washington, D.C.: U.S. Government Printing Office, 1986.

74. Harrington, C., et al. Effects of state Medicaid policies on the aged. *Gerontologist* 26(4):437, 1986.

75. Holmes, M. B., and Holmes, D. *Handbook of Human Services for Older Persons.* New York: Human Sciences Press, 1979.

76. Waldo, D. R., Levitt, K. R., and Lazenboy, H. National health expenditures—1985. *Health Care Financing Review* 8(1):1, 1986.

77. Frost and Sullivan. *Home Health Care Products and Services: Markets in the United States.* Report no. A1120. New York: Frost & Sullivan, 1983.

78. Burton, J. The house call: An important service for frail elderly. *J. Am. Geriatr. Soc.* 33:291, 1985.

79. Koren, M. J. Home care—who cares? *N. Engl. J. Med.* 314(4):917, 1986.

80. Besdine, R. W., and Wetle, T. Surveillance of high risk geriatric patients. A paper prepared for the 1981 White House Conference on Aging. Washington, D.C.: National Institute on Aging, 1981.

81. Piktialis, D. Medicare policy toward preventive services: A demonstration approach. *Gerontologist* 26:110A, 1986.

82. Mathematica Policy Research. *Channeling Effects on Hospital, Nursing Home and Other Medical Services.* Plainsboro, NJ: Mathematica, 1986.

83. Mathematica Policy Research. *Channeling Effects on Formal Community Based Services and Housing.* Plainsboro, NJ: Mathematica, 1987.

84. Waldo, D., and Lazenby, H. C. Demographic characteristics and health care use and expenditures by the aged in the United States. *Health Care Financing Review* 6:1, 1984.

85. Select Committee on Aging, U.S. House of Representatives. *Abuse in the Sale of Health Insurance to the Elderly in Supplementation of Medicare: A National Scandal.* Publication No. 95-160. Washington, D.C.: U.S. Government Printing Office, 1978.

86. Marmor, T. R. The Congress: Medicare Politics and Policy. In A. P. Sindler (ed.), *American Political Institutions and Public Policy: Five Contemporary Studies.* Boston: Little, Brown, 1969. Pp. 3–66.

87. Social Security Administration. Social Security programs in the United States. *Social Security Bull.* 49(1):5, 1986.

88. United States Department of Health and Human Services. *Your Medicare Handbook.* Publication No. HCFA-10050. Washington, D.C.: U.S. Government Printing Office, 1985.

89. Colton, W. Blue Cross, Blue Shield of Massachusetts. Office of HMDs and Special Programs. Personal communication, May 1987.

90. Gornick, M., et al. Twenty years of Medicare and Medicaid: Covered populations use of benefits and program expenditures. *Health Care Financing Review,* Ann. Suppl.:13–59, 1985.

91. Langwell, K. M., and Hadley, J. P. Capitation and the Medicare program: History, issues, and evidence. *Health Care Financing Review,* Ann. Suppl.:9–19, 1986.

92. Iglehart, J. Medicare turns to HMOs. *N. Engl. J. Med.* 312(2):132, 1985.

93. Gillick, M. R. The impact of health maintenance organizations on geriatric care. *Ann. Intern. Med.* 106:139, 1987.

94. Bonanno, J. B., and Wetle, T. HMO enrollment of Medicare recipients: An analysis of incentives and barriers. *J. Health Policy, Politics and Law* 9:41, 1984.

95. Rubenstein, L. Z., and Kane, R. L. Geriatric assessment programs: Their time has come. *J. Am. Geriatr. Soc.* 33:646, 1985.

96. Freeborn, D., and Pope, C. Health status, utilization, and satisfaction among enrollees in three types of private health insurance plans. *Group Health* 3(1):4, 1983.

97. Group Health News. Survey shows HMO-demonstration projects serve elderly well. *Group Health News* 26(1):1, 1985.

98. Fischer, L. A. Medicare turns to HMOs: A caveat. *N. Engl. J. Med.* 312:1131, 1984.

99. Heinz, J. *Medicare and HMOs: A first look, with disturbing findings.* Minority Staff Report, Special Committee on Aging, United States Senate, April 7, 1987.

100. Newcomer, R. J., Benjamin, A. E., and Sattler, C. E. Equity and Incentives in State Medicaid Program Eligibility. In C. Harrington (ed.), *Long Term Care of the Elderly: Public Policy Issues.* Beverly Hills, CA: Sage Publications, 1983.

101. Meiners, M. R., and Trapnell, G. R. Can the elderly afford long-term care insurance: Premium estimates for prototype policies. *Med. Care* 22(10):901, 1984.

102. Select Committee on Aging. U.S. House of Representatives. *America's Elderly at Risk.* Publication No. 99-508. Washington, D.C.: U.S. Government Printing Office, 1985.

103. Bonnano, J. Legislation Regarding Health Care for the Older Veteran. In T. Wetle and J. Rowe (eds.), *Older Veterans: Linking VA and Community Resources.* Cambridge: Harvard University Press, 1984.

104. Mather, J. An Overview of Veteran's Administration and Its Services for Older Americans. In T. Wetle and J. Rowe (eds.), *Older Veterans: Linking VA and Community Resources.* Cambridge: Harvard University Press, 1984.

105. Congressional Budget Office. *Veterans Administration Health Care: Planning for Future Years.*

Washington, D.C.: U.S. Government Printing Office, 1984.

106. Lindsay, C. Veterans Benefits and Services. In E. McAlister (ed.), *Agenda for Progress: Examining Federal Spending*. Washington, D.C.: Heritage Foundation, 1981.

107. Schlesinger, M., and Wetle, T. The elder veteran: New directions for change. *Health Affairs* 5(2):60, 1986.

108. Wetle, T., and Rowe, J. *Older Veterans: Linking VA and Community Resources*. Cambridge: Harvard University Press, 1984.

109. Branch, L. G. Continuing care retirement communities: Self insuring for long term care. *Gerontologist* 27(1):4, 1987.

6

Ethical Issues

TERRIE WETLE

THE TRADITIONAL LITERATURE of values and ethics has paid little attention to the elderly in general or to geriatric health in particular. Beginning in the late 1970s, however, an explosion of interest in the ethics of aging, as documented by articles in the professional and popular literatures, has occurred [1]. Two major issues have fueled much of the discussion—"do not resuscitate" orders and the distribution of scarce resources, either as rationing health care or as intergenerational equity. Yet a much broader range of issues is directly relevant to geriatric care, and an effort is made in this chapter to suggest a taxonomy of such issues, identifying a selected array of questions and problems from the point of view of the provider of care. The organizational structure for this taxonomy begins with the individual patient and then moves on to the family, service providers, and the system of care.

Elderly at Ethical Risk

The first question to be addressed is whether there are any ethical issues that are unique to geriatric care. Once beyond childhood, should age in itself have any influence on the ethical considerations of clinical decision making? Other than circumstances in which physical or mental impairment precludes an elder's ability to make decisions, should not the same ethical

considerations that apply to young and middle-aged adults also apply to the elderly? Although it has been argued that age should not influence the ethics of health care, a variety of societal beliefs and circumstances converge to place the elderly at special risk in the decision-making process [2]. Although there are societal values that give elders a revered status (e.g., honor thy father and mother, filial responsibility), negative traits and behavior commonly identified with old age abound, and evidence of ageism is readily available [3,4]. Although it is true that the elderly as a group are more likely to suffer chronic conditions, to be cognitively impaired, and to be dependent, heterogeneity among individuals increases with age, and the assumption that to be old is to be sick, demented, and dependent is incorrect and discriminatory for a majority of individuals. Several studies indicate that negative stereotypes of elderly patients persist [5,6,7,8]. Ageism affects not only the personal interactions between patients and their caregivers but also the formulation of policy, the design of social programs, and the provision of health and social services [9,10]. Spiraling health care costs, accelerated by changing demographics, have refocused public attention on the one group for whom there is relatively comprehensive public health insurance—the elderly. Efforts to contain costs have changed many of the incentives in the delivery of care, reduced the availability of crucial services, and caused providers to question the fairness of resource distribution among generations. The convergence of these factors places the elderly at risk and adds responsibilities for providers to take special care in considering the ethical components in clinical decision making.

Ethical Issues Pertaining to the Individual

Numerous characteristics of older people interact directly with values that influence the organization and delivery of care. In recent years, a primary consideration in medical ethics has been the locus of control for decision making, and increasing emphasis has been placed on the right of the individual to participate in treatment decisions. The constitutional right to privacy has been interpreted by the courts to include the right of adults in general to make health care decisions [11]. Such a right for older persons in particular is supported by language in the Older Americans Act, the Federal Council on Aging's Bicentennial Charter for Older Americans, and the Nursing Home Patient's Bill of Rights. The Older Americans Act ensures older persons (among other rights) "freedom, independence, and the free exercise of individual initiative in planning and managing their own lives" [12]. The Federal Council on Aging's statement expands on this concept by adding ". . . this should encompass not only opportunities and resources for persons planning and managing one's life-style, but support systems for maximum growth and contributions . . ." [13]. The Nursing Home Patient's Bill of Rights declares that each patient should be "fully informed . . . (and allowed) to participate in the planning of his medical treatment" and be ". . . treated with consideration, respect, and full recognition of his dignity and individuality" [14].

An ethical dilemma arises in the translation of these values into practice. *Autonomy* refers to the individual's right to make decisions that are voluntary and intentional and not the result of coercion, duress, or undue influence. Gadow [15] divides the exercise of personal autonomy into two levels: *agency,* which is the freedom to decide among all options, and *action,* which is the freedom to carry out the course of action

chosen. This is similar to Dworkin's [16] conceptualization of *authenticity* (motives for action are one's own) and *independence* (freedom of action). In a more complex model, Collopy [17] distinguishes among five types of autonomy. *Direct versus delegated autonomy* refers to decisions and actions made by the individual versus the delegation of those decisions and activities to another person. *Competent versus incapacitated autonomy* focuses on the decisional capacity of the individual making decisions. *Authentic versus inauthentic autonomy* moves beyond competency and capacity to examine whether the choice is "authentic" given the individual's personal history and values. *Immediate versus long-term autonomy* recognizes that choices made now may interfere with autonomous action in the future. Efforts to protect long-term autonomy are sometimes used to justify overriding individual choices in the shorter term. Finally, Collopy makes a distinction between *autonomy as a negative right versus autonomy as a positive right.* As a negative right, autonomy demands freedom from interference; as a positive right, support and enhancement are required.

For older persons, the freedom to *choose among options* is potentially constrained by three factors. First, the elderly as a group are more likely to suffer limitations in their capacity to make decisions due to impaired cognitive ability. These cognitive impairments may be a result of mental illness, stroke, dementia, or other mental or physical problems that alter a person's consciousness of the surroundings. Second, the range of options may be constrained by lack of information or available resources. Third, the aged patient may not be allowed to make choices because of assumptions (correct or not) about ability to participate in such decisions. In like manner, the opportunity to *act on choices* may also be constrained by limited personal resources and well-documented gaps in the current system of services.

An important constraint on autonomous behavior is the organization of the health care system and the behavior of care providers. Only recently has any attention been paid to autonomy as a patient's right. In Parson's [18] classic description of the "sick role," patients have certain privileges and obligations because they are sick. One of the privileges is to be free of responsibility for one's own state of health, and obligations include a duty to seek technically competent help, trust the doctor, and comply with the medical regimen. Brody [19] argues that in the traditional concept of the doctor-patient relationship, the patient is passive and dependent, and the physician is granted autonomy and professional dominance. He cites several arguments for why this imbalance of power pertains, including the physician's superior scientific knowledge [20,21], the patient's psychological barriers to understanding information or making decisions [22,23], and the physician's belief that presenting patients with information is too time-consuming, expensive, or anxiety-provoking [24,25].

A counter-trend toward increased patient participation is noted by the publication of a *Patient's Bill of Rights* by the American Hospital Association [26] in 1972 and *The Rights of Hospital Patients* [27] by the American Civil Liberties Union in 1975. These booklets listed formal entitlements, including access to "privileged" information and patient participation in medical decisions. Interest in patient autonomy accelerated with increased emphasis on the concept and process of informed consent. Traditionally, from a legal perspective, consent from the patient was required before initiating any form of treatment [28], but before the 1960s, little attention was paid to the nature of that consent. The Natanson versus Kline case in 1960 held that the physician had a duty to inform the patient of the nature and risks of treatment and that acting on consent from an inadequately informed patient was negligent [29]. In subsequent cases, the courts acknowledged that this new standard constituted a change in practice by subjecting physicians to judicial review, not only for techniques and outcomes of treatment but also for the quality of interactions with patients [28].

Several criticisms of informed consent procedures have special relevance for older persons. Current cohorts of elderly may have expectations of patient behavior that, because of past experience, do not include an active role in decision making. Moreover, lower levels of educational experience and sensory impairments may make it more difficult for older persons to understand and process the technical information included in many consent forms.

Stanley and colleagues [30] found that elderly patients showed significantly poorer comprehension of consent information than did younger patients. They argued that special care should be taken to present information to older patients in a manner that is understandable and not overwhelming. Greenfield and colleagues [31] demonstrated that review by the patient of medical records and coaching in how to ask physicians questions or negotiate medical decisions actually improved patient effectiveness in eliciting information and participation in decisions. Coleman [32], in his editorial on "terrified consent," asserted that overemphasis on potential negative outcomes may deflect the patient from needed care. Moreover, it has been argued that the emphasis on individual autonomy should be modulated by attention to other important values such as beneficence, paternalism, safety of the individual, and common good [10,15,33]. Research into the relative importance of autonomy compared with other values indicates substantial heterogeneity of opinion among community-dwelling elders [34], as well as among elders in nursing homes [35,36].

There is a subset of older persons for whom special ethical issues arise; these are elders with impaired cognitive function. They present unique caregiving problems because of symptoms that may include impaired memory; disorientation; poor judgment; inappropriate, unpredictable, or dangerous behavior; and need for constant surveillance [37]. Additionally, capacity to participate in care decisions may fluctuate over time. Several thorny issues are involved in the determination of competence. First, it should be noted that competency is a legal concept, and all individuals are presumed by law to be competent until determined otherwise by a judicial hearing [38]. In the clinical setting, competency takes on a variety of meanings, and McCullough [39] argues that an individual is not *broadly* competent or incompetent; instead, one is competent for specific tasks.

There are several standards for determining competence. Legal and medical scholars have described patients as functionally competent if they can "make a choice," arrive at a "reasonable outcome" [40], or address "emotionally neutral issues in a reasonable fashion" [41]. For the most part, the greater the risk related to the decision, the more stringent the standard of competence. Generally, every effort should be made to assist even the most minimally competent individual to understand the nature of his or her disease, the likely risks of intervention, and the prognosis with and without interventions and to elicit a preference for action. The President's Commission for the Study of Ethical Problems in Medicine and Biomedical and Behavioral Research [42] stated that "incapacity [should] be treated as a disqualifying factor in the small minority of cases," and that to "the extent feasible, people with no decision-making capacity should still be consulted about their own preferences out of respect for them as individuals."

There will be some elderly who are so impaired that they are unable to participate in treatment decisions, and in these cases a hierarchy of standards should be used in the decision-making process. Most preferable are *advance directives*, provided by the individual while competent, which declare preferences regarding future treatment. These advance directives may be informal letters or written statements or legal documents such as living wills [42]. For most patients, such clear, written statements of preference are not available, and the physician will need to rely on reports from family, friends, or other caregivers regarding past statements or behaviors that indicate what the patient's preferences would be in the current circumstances if they were competent. Using this *value history* or sedimented life preferences [43], the principle of *substituted judgment* is used to determine the appropriate course of action. Substituted judgment means that the decision-maker tries to make the decision that the incapacitated patient would have made in these circumstances were he or she still competent. When the value history is not adequate to apply the principle of substituted judgment, the principle of the patient's best interest applies. Best interest decisions are least desirable because they disregard individual autonomy and are subject to disagreement about the "true" best interest of the patient. In some cases, the appointment of a guardian to participate in treatment decisions on behalf of the incapacitated individual may be necessary. Efforts to address the special ethical concerns of cognitively impaired elders have begun to develop creative approaches to decision making, including durable powers of attorney, living wills, and other advance directives [44,45].

Ethical Issues Pertaining to the Family

Care of aging family members, particularly the chronically impaired, raises difficult issues for families. Shifts in dependency relationships are likely to occur as a family member becomes progressively impaired, producing changes in patterns of interaction within the family and calling into question power relationships and accustomed roles. Families often struggle with the difficult question of balancing the autonomous wishes of the impaired family member against concerns for his or her personal safety and well-being [46].

There is also confusion about what is considered appropriate support from family members for individuals with substantial care needs. Contrary to popular opinion, families are not rushing to dump impaired elders in nursing homes. It is estimated that 80 percent of home care is provided by family members, usually wives, daughters, and daughters-in-law, sometimes at great cost to their own personal health and the well-being of the family [47,48,49, 50,51]. Daniels [52] has identified important tensions in intergenerational responsibilities among families at the societal level. What can a society reasonably expect a family to provide? What does one generation "owe" another? Just as individual and societal expectations influence enactment of laws and social programs, social policy has changed the expectations of individuals and families regarding individual responsibility to impaired family members [53,54]. Furthermore, changes in employment, particularly the entry of increasing proportions of middle-aged and late middle-aged women into the labor force, have reduced the availability of women at home to provide care to impaired family members [55]. The desire to contain costs has provoked consideration of efforts to shift more of the burden of geriatric care back to individuals and families. Family members who provide care to chronically impaired spouses or parents are more likely to suffer from a variety of stress-related problems including alcohol and drug abuse, depression, divorce, and physical diseases thought to have strong psychosomatic components [50,56,57].

There are also concerns regarding involvement of family members in difficult health care decisions. Although it has been the common practice for physicians to turn to family members when the patient is unable to participate in decision making, by 1986 only a dozen states had enacted statutes providing clear legal authority for family members to make such decisions [45]. Individual family members frequently disagree on the most appropriate course of action. In some states, certain family members are given priority by law when disagreements occur; other states require unanimity. In turning to a family member to provide consent for clinical interventions or participation in research, care must be taken to explain the standard by which the family member is to offer advice. Are they being asked to respond as they believe the patient would respond if able (substituted judgment), or are they being asked to respond in the best interest of the patient? Warren and colleagues [58], in studying consent by proxy for participation in research, noted that 31 percent of proxies who believed that the *patient* would have *refused* consent actually gave consent for participation in the project. When asked why they gave consent, many stated that they perceived participation to be in the patient's best interest. Clarifying the task at hand may enhance the ability of the family member to participate in difficult decisions, decrease their discomfort, and clarify information provided to the professional caregiver.

Ethical Issues Pertaining to Service Providers

Providers of geriatric care are confronted daily with value conflicts and ethical dilemmas, though they are often unaware of the ethical issues involved in their day-to-day work [59]. Most often these dilemmas are the result of a conflict of values, professional standards, and fiscal and regulatory constraints. These conflicts are highlighted by Thomasma's [33] identification of (and dissatisfaction with) the various models for viewing the patient/physician relationship (the concepts are equally descriptive for other care-providing professions). These models include the *legalistic* model (provider/client), the *economic model* (provider/consumer), the *contractual model,* and the *religious* model (a covenant between provider and client). He argues that each of these models has been developed to combat the *paternalism model,* in which action is taken by one person in the best interest of another without his or her consent [60]. There are, however, justifications offered for paternalism in geriatric care. Acting in the best interest of an incompetent patient is referred to as *weak paternalism* and is usually considered to be morally acceptable [33,61], if balanced with the patient's wishes as expressed while competent. *Strong paternalism,* the direct violation of a competent patient's wishes, has traditionally been considered morally unacceptable. Perry [61] argues that there are some circumstances in which strong paternalism may be justified, including efforts to ensure future autonomy or to withhold information that is irrelevant to the decision at hand and that might in fact lead to a decision that is detrimental to the patient's best interests. It is further argued that many patients expect care providers to make decisions for them and have, either implicitly or explicitly, delegated autonomy.

Paternalism is frequently practiced in geriatric care and is justified in a variety of ways, the most common being the inability of the patient client to participate in decisions. Unfortunately, inability to make decisions is often assumed, even with evidence to the contrary. In research using clinical vignettes, physicians and nurses justified decisions to withhold treatment based on an elderly patient's "preexisting dementia," even though the case clearly stated that this 80-year-old man had "clear cognitive function" [62]. In some circumstances clients unnecessarily lose the ability to make decisions as a result of being deprived of the opportunity to make decisions, a condition referred to as *learned helplessness* [63,64].

Institutional settings involve special ethical risks. The very nature of nursing homes, for example, reinforces negative feelings of dependence, encourages learned helplessness, and deprives the individual of making all but the most trivial of decisions. Furthermore, few nursing home residents actually choose the physician responsible for their care. The limited involvement of physicians in institutional care makes it unlikely that the physician and patient will even know one another, let alone develop a trusting relationship [65]. Besdine [66] and others [67] have suggested processes through which patients and their families, as well as nursing home staff, can become more effectively involved in the decision-making process. Patient's rights groups and professional organizations are also working to improve the involvement of residents in decision making [44].

Difficult calculus is required to balance individual autonomy with the wish to protect geriatric patients from harm. Gadow [15] suggests that clients must be assisted in developing and exercising self-determination. She argues that the principle of autonomy does not force patients to participate in decisions but rather ensures for them the option and assistance needed to participate if they so choose. Caregivers may find themselves in the position of engaging in paternalism to restore the client's capacity for autonomy. For example, a social worker and nurse in a home care agency may forcibly bring a client into the hospital to be given proper treatment and to restore competence. Unfortunately, the guidelines of professional ethics are often unclear in such complex and difficult cases; they vary from one agency to the next as well as among different professions. Destructive misunderstandings and "turf battles" arise from the miscommunication of values and intents among professionals [46]. There are several specific decisions that are quite likely to involve ethical issues. These include discharge planning, decisions to withhold treatment, and decisions concerning the provision of nutrition to severely disabled persons.

DISCHARGE PLANNING

Misunderstandings surround difficult decisions about placement and discharge planning [68, 69]. Public policy has produced incentives for early discharge of hospitalized patients at the same time that resources for community services face limitations. Impaired elders who wish to remain in the community pose difficult problems for care planners and providers trying to balance support of self-determination with

concerns for the safety of the client and those who live nearby. In extreme circumstances, the legal system may be drawn into the decision through involuntary commitment procedures. More often, family members and health care professionals resort to subterfuge, "white lies," or simple direct action to place the impaired older person in a nursing home or other institutional setting against his or her expressed wishes. The ethical dilemmas surrounding such actions require further study and consideration before global directives or guidelines are promulgated. Communication among professional groups is particularly important in this arena because of differences in perceptions of appropriate roles and responsibilities. An attorney, for example, might take an adversarial approach, in his or her view *protecting* the client from "incarceration." A physician may place primary emphasis on providing a protective and rehabilitative setting in which health and function may be restored. A social worker, from a third perspective, might see the *family* as the client and work toward a resolution that maximizes the well-being of the entire family [46].

"DO NOT RESUSCITATE" ORDERS AND DECISIONS TO WITHHOLD TREATMENT

Just as decisions to treat or provide services to an unwilling client pose value conflicts, so too do decisions to withhold treatment or care. The most widely publicized of these decisions is the "do not resuscitate" (DNR) order. The moral justification for DNR grows out of three principles: autonomy, do no harm, and acting in the best interest of the patient [70]. Standards for entering a DNR order in the patient's chart include having and documenting a full discussion with the competent patient or the incompetent patient's family [70,71,72]. It has been observed, however, that such discussions often do not take place, and that when they do the physician's perception may not agree with the patient's stated preference [73]. Moreover, the entry of DNR in a patient's chart has been shown to result in withholding other forms of treatment and care [74], and although possibly clinically and ethically justified, the lack of clarity in chart notes leads to confusion and dissatisfaction among nursing staff required to carry out the orders.

Decisions to withhold other forms of treatment also require specific attention in the decision-making process. Members of the advisory panel on Life-Sustaining Technologies and the Elderly for the Office of Technology Assessment suggest principles (Fig. 6-1) to be considered in making health care decisions with and for older persons [75]. Besdine [72] offers a model process of decision making in regard to nursing home residents, differentiating among decisions not to resuscitate, not to hospitalize, and not to treat. He emphasizes the importance of involving all members of the health care team, including the family and the resident, even when the resident has impaired decisional capacity.

Several patient characteristics have been shown to correlate with the entry of a DNR order and decisions to withhold other forms of treatment [4]. As one might expect, severity of

FIGURE 6-1. *Principles in decision making regarding the use of life sustaining technologies for elderly persons as developed by OTA's advisory panel. (From Office of Technology Assessment. Life Sustaining Technologies and the Elderly. OTA-BA-306. Washington, D.C.: U.S. Government Printing Office, 1987).*

An adult patient who is capable of making decisions has the right to decline any form of medical treatment or intervention. However, an individual does not necessarily have a right to unlimited medical treatment or intervention.

Decisions regarding the use of life-sustaining treatments must be made on an individual basis and should never be based on chronological age alone. Chronological age per se is a poor criterion upon which to base individual medical decisions; however, age may be a legitimate modifier regarding appropriate utilization of life-sustaining medical technologies.

Diagnosis alone is a poor criterion for decisions about the use of life-sustaining technologies. Because of the great variability among patients with the same diagnosis, patient assessment must also include measures of functional impairment and severity of illness.

Cognitive function is an important marker of the quality of life.

The courts are not and should not be the usual route or determinant for making decisions about the use of life-sustaining technologies or for resolving the dilemmas these technologies may create.

There is little need or room for federal legislation concerning the initiation, withholding, or withdrawal of specific life-sustaining technologies.

There is a major need for a clear, workable definition of the appropriate role of surrogates in health care decision making, including the nature of their responsibilities and their suitability to make decisions.

There is a need to recognize that a process exists, or should exist, for making decisions about the use of life-sustaining technologies. The process described by the President's Commission for the Study of Ethical Problems in Medicine and Biomedical and Behavioral Research could serve as a model.

A physician or other health professional who does not want to follow the wishes of a patient who is capable of making decisions regarding his or her treatment should withdraw from that case.

Socioeconomic status should not be a barrier to access to health care, including life-sustaining interventions.

There is an important need for education of the public and health care providers regarding the nature and appropriate use of life-sustaining technologies.

There is a specific need for improved clinical information that would predict the probability of a critically or seriously ill patient's survival, functional status, and subsequent quality of life.

There is a wide range of medical and legal disagreement and varying levels of emotional strain and moral conflict about the appropriate use of life-sustaining technologies. The great heterogeneity of the American population makes consensus difficult and increases the likelihood of formal institutional decision-making procedures.

disease, diagnosis of carcinoma, and poor prognosis are related to DNR orders. Other characteristics observed to be related are more ethically problematic and include age of patient, dementia, multiple suicide attempts, and violent crimes committed by the patient [76]. Quality of life is an important consideration in DNR and other decisions to withhold treatment, and the Canadian Law Reform Report justifies considerations not only of quantity of life but also of quality of life in making treatment decisions [77]. Interestingly, Pearlman's research indicates that quality of life is used as a justification both by physicians who choose to *provide* and physicians who choose to *withhold* treatment for the same patient [78]. Part of the problem involves the multiple definitions and subjective interpretations attached to the term *quality of life*. At one end of the continuum are definitions that emphasize "fulfillment of personal goals," ability to lead a "normal life," and "social utility" [79]. At the other are definitions that depend on the difference between "having a life" and "being alive" [80]. Many definitions emphasize the patient's subjective satisfaction (or suffering) with his or her own personal life and situation, and others recognize the pitfalls of trying to judge the quality of life of another [78,81]. Although there is general acknowledgement of the sanctity of life, most ethicists recognize that clinical catastrophes can so constrain a person's quality of life that that life is no longer worth living [66]. These evaluative judgments may be strongly influenced by prejudices regarding culturally valued attributes or capacities [62,82,83]. Conscious and unconscious biases regarding social worth, relative value, and the meaning and value of life are a part of such determinations. Furthermore, the specter of ageism is likely to slip in unnoticed [84].

The language we use in referring to the individual who requires care is heavily value-laden and communicates a great deal about our own assumptions and biases. The person may be called client, patient, consumer, resident, dependent, or recipient. Each term implies certain characteristics and relationships with care providers. The phrases used to describe patients may be even more graphic: *gomer* ("get out of my emergency room"), *dirtball, gork, crock,* or *spos* ("subhuman piece of shit"), and have been observed to apply to patients who present more difficult diagnostic, therapeutic, and behavioral problems [7]. This insulting and dehumanizing terminology is not intended to be heard by the patient or the public and is often a part of the "gallows humor" exhibited by workers in highly stressful circumstances [85,86,87]. But the message of this language, whether intended to be humorous or not, is that this patient can be dealt with differently (less humanely) and that the usual rules of clinical care may not apply. Other terms used with elderly patients (*sweetie, dearie, grandpa*) may be less obviously offensive but nonetheless may carry unintended messages that rob the patient of dignity and self-respect.

FEEDING AND NUTRITIONAL SUPPORTS

One category of decisions to withhold treatment receives special attention—withholding nutritional supports such as enteral (nasogastric, gastrostomy, and jejunostomy) feedings and parenteral nutrition and hydration. Although it has been argued that nutritional supports should be viewed no differently than other forms of medical treatment [88,89,90, 91,92], some ethicists and clinicians view feeding and nutrition as quite different in several ways [93,94,95,96,97]. The controversy arises from several areas of disagreement including the symbolic meaning of food [88,94], distinctions between ordinary and extraordinary treatments [89], the impact on physician/patient trust [96], and concerns about the "slippery slope" issue of where withholding treatment stops [93]. Although guidelines outlining appropriate circumstances and processes for withholding food have been promulgated by several groups including the President's Commission for the Study of Ethical Problems in Medicine and Biomedical and Behavioral Research, the American Medical Association's Council on Ethical and Judicial Affairs, the Office of Technology Assessment's panel on Life-Sustaining Technologies and the Elderly, as well as through legal precedent [90,98,99,100], debate continues on this emotionally charged topic.

Most ethicists and clinicians agree that a competent patient has the right to refuse nutritional supports [91,101]. This can be accomplished by a competent patient either by (1) expressing such a wish when faced with the decision or by (2) expressing such a preference for future decisions by the execution of an advance directive such as a living will or durable power of attorney [91]. Much more controversy surrounds decisions to withhold nutrition from patients who are not able to participate in the decision [102]. Annas [91] agrees with the court in the Claire Conway case [90] that a legal guardian should be able to order the withholding or withdrawal of any medical treatment, including artificial feeding if it can be demonstrated (1) that the patient would want such an action or (2) that such an action would be consistent with the best interests of the patient in the sense that the burden of continued treatment outweighs any reasonably hoped-for benefits. This argument follows that of the President's Commission, which holds that treatment decisions should be based on a weighing of burden versus benefit [89]. Lynn and Childress [88] argue that nutrition can ethically be withheld if the effort is futile, if there is no possibility of benefit, or if the burden is disproportionate to the benefits obtained from feeding.

The process involved in such decisions is important [72]. Careful attention must be given to gathering and sharing information with those involved in the decision process. The goals of therapy, including nutritional supports, as well as the potential burdens of such interventions are central considerations [102]. Goals may include relief of hunger or thirst, prolongation of life, avoidance of complications of dehydration or malnutrition, and symbolic "nurturing." Burdens may include the pain and discomfort related to the intervention, complications such as aspirational pneumonias or other infections, or prolonged suffering related to other diseases and conditions. The decision process should be well documented, and the implementation of the decision should be agreed on by those responsible for daily care. Ongoing, careful attention to the hygiene and comfort of the patient should be ensured [72]. Concerned clinicians should recognize that at present there continue to be differences of opinion regarding the appropriateness of such decisions and should be sensitive to the concerns of caregivers who may find the withholding of nutrition or other treatments morally objectionable.

System-Wide Ethical Issues

Value considerations determine the distribution of resources within the health service system, influence the enactment of laws and enforcement of regulations, and provide the framework for policy making. Mechanisms for the distribution of resources are biased in a variety of ways. First, public monies are more likely to be spent for medical and technical services than for social services; more likely to pay for institutional services in hospitals and nursing homes than for services that keep elders in their own homes; and more likely to pay for later, more intrusive interventions than for earlier interventions that support the client, family, and other informal caregivers [103]. An important ethical consideration is whether these biases accurately reflect societal values. On what basis do we distribute scarce health and social service dollars? How much do we hold the individual responsible to pay for needed care, and do we require spending down to the poverty level before public support is made available?

Service providers frequently find themselves in conflict with social policy. Physicians may be required by their hospitals to consider economic issues in the decisions to admit, treat, or discharge patients. Care managers for community-dwelling elders may be forced to balance programmatic goals and funding constraints against the needs and wishes of clients. Nurses may find themselves trapped between residents' interests and the administrative or regulatory constraints of the nursing home in which they work. These ethical dilemmas are not easily resolved. There are those who argue that tensions such as these are necessary, particularly in circumstances in which societal and professional policies have yet to be clearly formulated [104]. Unfortunately, the current mood of budget constraint and cost containment has increased the pressures away from the best interests of geriatric patients. Although data on the impact of recent budget decisions have yet to be collected in the United States, we can draw from the experience of other countries. In his careful analysis of the impact of budgetary constraints on the use of renal dialysis in the United Kingdom, Halper [105] notes that the impact of cost containment involves "sacrifices not only from prosperous physicians and inefficient hospitals, but also from vulnerable patients." Budgetary concerns may indeed change the standards of practice, with unfortunate results for patients and clients.

The entry of for-profit organizations into the health and social service system raises yet another set of ethical issues. Young [106] provides the following list of threats posed by for-profit health care: inefficient customers (those with inadequate resources) are excluded; unprofitable services are phased out; profitable services are overused; voluntary, philanthropic home health agencies face unequal competition; and the traditional mission of hospitals and other health-related facilities will change. Wikler [107] provides his own outline of concerns about a health care system that is an "investor owned, large-scale, corporate activity": (1) that for-profit care will cost more, be less accessible to the poor, and be of lower quality; (2) that the integrity of the medical profession will be compromised; (3) that there will be a redistribution of power; and (4) that this model is not morally and philosophically suitable for health care. It should be noted that these changes are not limited to the for-profit sector; Wikler continues by pointing out that the nonprofit sector is "increasingly characterized by largeness, vertical and horizontal integration" and is not unlike the for-profit institutions in many respects. During this time of radical evolution, long-accustomed "rules of doing business" are changing as the incentive structure moves away from an emphasis on ensuring access to care and toward an emphasis on efficiency and cost containment. It must be recognized that cost-benefit analysis and budgetary efficiencies are not "value free" [84]. Perhaps the time has come to recall and emphasize the societal values that underlie Medicare, Medicaid, the Older Americans Act, and other social programs.

Another system-wide ethical issue is age discrimination, a deeply rooted social value. A variety of rights and responsibilities, privileges, and prohibitions are directly related to chronological age. In our society, children are not required to work but are also not allowed independence from parents. In like manner, adults are allowed a level of personal autonomy not granted to children, including the freedom to choose their work, residence, and spouse and to consume certain controlled substances such as alcohol and tobacco. Although these examples may seem trivial, the importance of age in determining appropriate behavior so permeates our culture that we are often unaware of its impact. Unfortunately, negative characteristics ascribed to age, or ageism, also influence the delivery of geriatric care. The Civil Rights Commission [108], under the leadership of Arthur Flemming, discovered evidence of inappropriate age discrimination in the Medicaid program (e.g., prior approval for dental and other services), in community health centers (e.g., targeting for services and populations served), in community mental health centers (e.g., lack of outreach to elders, populations served, and lack of knowledge about geriatric care), and in vocational rehabilitation services (e.g., eligibility requirements).

An important consideration in the analysis of age discrimination is intergenerational equity [109,110]. Many social and health programs use age as a criterion for eligibility, and the elderly have received benefits due to age status. Some analysts view with alarm the relative distribution of public resources among the elderly and other age groups [111]. Others point out that the aged have been used as a scapegoat in public policy conflicts [112]. Kingson and colleagues [113], in a careful analysis, argue that the distributional balance among generations is complex and dynamic and that we all have a stake in the well-being of the elderly as well as the health of children. Much of the concern about distribution of resources is based on misinformation and misunderstanding and centers on the risk that rather simple-minded comparisons of public spending for old and young will be used to justify budget-cutting of programs for the elderly rather than to focus on the more important issue of whether public monies are spent appropriately, efficiently, and with a proper balance among social programs and other types of spending.

CONCLUSION

At first glance it might seem paralyzing to consider each and every ethical issue arising in the delivery of geriatric care. But awareness and discussion of these issues frequently save the time, costs, and human suffering resulting from inappropriate decisions. Bringing these considerations into the bright light of open discussion will clarify issues and illuminate choices. Decision making will not be easy, in part because the "right path" is not clearly marked and in part because the choices are often a tragic selection of the lesser of several evils. Yet open consideration of ethical issues and their underlying values will improve the quality of the decisions made, leading not only to better lives for older persons but also to increased satisfaction for the providers of their care.

References

1. Cassel, C. K., Feier, D. E., and Traines, M. L. Selected bibliography of recent articles in ethics and geriatrics. *J. Am. Geriatr. Soc.* 34(5):399, 1986.
2. Wetle, T. Ethical Aspects of Decision Making For and With the Elderly. In M. B. Kapp, H. E. Pies, and A. E. Doudera (eds.), *Legal and Ethical Aspects of Health Care for the Elderly.* Ann Arbor: Health Administration Press, 1986.
3. Butler, R. N. Ageism: Another form of bigotry. *Gerontologist* 9:243, 1969.
4. Wetle, T. Age as a risk factor for inadequate treatment. *J.A.M.A.* 258(4):516, 1987.
5. Kogan, N. Beliefs, attitudes and stereotypes about old people: A new look at some old issues. *Res. Aging* 1:11, 1979.
6. Bennet, R., and Eckman, J. Attitudes Toward Aging: A Critical Examination of Recent Literature and Implications for Future Research. In C. Eisdorfer and M. P. Lawton (eds.), *The Psychology of Adult Development and Aging.* Washington, D.C.: American Psychological Association, 1973.
7. Liederman, D. B., and Gisso, J. A. The Gomer phenomenon. *J. Health Soc. Behav.* 26:222, 1985.
8. Grouse, L. D. Dirtball. *J.A.M.A.* 247(22):3059, 1982.
9. Butler, R. N. *Why Survive? Being Old in America.* New York: Harper & Row, 1975.
10. Wetle, T. Ethical issues in long term care of the aged. *J. Geriatr. Psychiatry* 18(1):63, 1985.
11. See for example *Tune v. Walter Reed Army Medical Center,* 602 F. Suppl. 1452 (D.D.C. 1985); *Bartling v. Superior Court,* 147 Cal. App. 3d 1006, 195 Cal. Rptr. 220 (1984); *John F. Kennedy Memorial Hospital v. Bludworth,* 452 So. 2d 921 (Fla. 1984) as reported in American Association of Retired Persons. *A Matter of Choice: Planning Ahead for Health Care Decisions.* Washington, D.C.: American Association of Retired Persons, 1986.
12. Older Americans Act, Public Law 89-73, July 14, 1965 and as amended, Public Law 95-65, July 11, 1977.
13. Administration on Aging. *Federal Council on Aging Bicentennial Charter.* Washington, D.C.: Department of Health and Human Services, 1976.
14. Nursing Home Patient's Bill of Rights. See *Code of Federal Regulations,* 20 CFR 405.1121 (K) and 45 CFR 249.12 (a)(1)b, 1974.
15. Gadow, S. Medicine, ethics, and the elderly. *Gerontologist* 20(6):680, 1980.
16. Dworkin, G. Autonomy and behavior control. *Hastings Center Report* 6(1):23, 1976.
17. Collopy, B. J. *The Conceptually Problematic Status of Autonomy.* A monograph prepared for the Retirement Research Foundation. New York: Fordham University, 1986.
18. Parsons, T. *The Social System.* New York: Free Press, 1951.
19. Brody, D. S. The patient's role in clinical decision-making. *Ann. Intern. Med.* 93:718, 1980.
20. Gill, D. G. Limitations Upon Choice and Constraints Over Decision-Making in Doctor-Patient Exchanges. In E. B. Gallagher (ed.), *The Doctor-Patient Relationship in the Changing Health Scene.* Washington, D.C.: U.S. Department of Health, Education and Welfare, 1976.
21. Waitzkin, H., and Stoeckle, J. D. The communication of information about illness. *Adv. Psychosom. Med.* 8:180, 1972.
22. Freidson, E. *Profession of Medicine.* New York: Dodd, Mead & Co., 1970.
23. Jackson, D. L., and Younger, S. Patient autonomy and "death with dignity": Some clinical caveats. *N. Engl. J. Med.* 301:404, 1979.
24. Mechanic, D. *Medical Sociology.* New York: Free Press, 1978.
25. Tagliacozzo, D. L., and Mauksch, H. O. The patient's view of the patient role. In E. G. Jaco (ed.), *Patients, Physicians and Illness.* New York: Free Press, 1972.
26. American Hospital Association. *Patient's Bill of Rights.* Chicago: American Hospital Association, 1972.
27. Annas, G. J. *The Rights of Hospital Patients: American Civil Liberties Union Handbook.* New York: Avon Books, 1975.
28. Kaufmann, C. L. Informed consent and patient decisionmaking: Two decades of research. *Soc. Sci. Med.* 17(21):1657, 1983.
29. *Natanson v. Kline.* 187 Kansas 393, 350 P. 2d 1093 (1960). See case summary in J. Katz, *Experimentation with Human Beings.* New York: Russell Sage, 1972.
30. Stanley, B., et al. The elderly patient and informed consent. *J.A.M.A.* 252(10):1302, 1984.

31. Greenfield, S., Kaplan, S., and Ware, J. Expanding patient involvement in care. *Ann. Intern. Med.* 102:520, 1985.

32. Coleman, L. L. Terrified consent. *Physician's World* May:607, 1974.

33. Thomasma, D. Beyond paternalism and patient autonomy: A model of physician conscience for the physician and patient relationship. *Ann. Intern. Med.* 98:243, 1983.

34. O'Brien, J., and Whitelaw, N. *Analysis of Community Based Alternatives to Institutional Care for the Aged.* Portland, OR: Institute on Aging, 1973.

35. Wagner, A. Cardiopulmonary resuscitation in the aged. *N. Engl. J. Med.* 310(7):1129, 1984.

36. Wetle, T., Levkoff, S., and Cwikel, J. Research in nursing homes: Ethics and methods. *Gerontologist* 26:30A, 1986.

37. Brody, E., Lawton, P., and Liebowitz, B. Senile dementia: Public policy and adequate institutional care. *Am. J. Public Health* 74(12):1381, 1984.

38. Appelbaum, P. S., and Roth, L. H. Clinical issues in the assessment of competency. *Am. J. Psychiatry* 138:1462, 1981.

39. McCullough, L. B. Medical care for elderly patients of diminished competence: An ethical analysis. *J. Am. Geriatr. Soc.* 32:150, 1984.

40. Roth, L. H., Meisel, A., and Lidz, C. W. Tests of competency to consent to treatment. *Am. J. Psychiatry* 134(3):270, 1977.

41. Abernathy, V. Compassion, control and decisions about competency. *Am. J. Psychiatry* 141(1):53, 1984.

42. President's Commission for the Study of Ethical Problems in Medicine and Biomedical and Behavioral Research. *Making Health Care Decisions.* Vol. I. Washington, D.C.: U.S. Government Printing Office, 1983.

43. Dubler, N. N. Some Legal and Moral Issues Surrounding Informed Consent for Treatment and Research Involving the Cognitively Impaired Elderly. In M. B. Kapp, H. E. Pies, and A. E. Doudera (eds.), *Legal and Ethical Aspects of Health Care for the Elderly.* Ann Arbor: Health Administration Press, 1985.

44. Harris, S. Protecting residents' rights. *Am. Health Care Assoc. J.* 8(1):3, 1982. See also *Questionably Competent Long Term Care Residents—Problems and Possible Solutions.* Washington, D.C.: American Health Care Association, 1982.

45. American Association of Retired Persons. *A Matter of Choice: Planning Ahead for Health Care Decisions.* Washington, D.C.: American Association of Retired Persons, 1986.

46. Wetle, T. Long term care: A taxonomy of issues. *Generations* 10(2):30, 1985.

47. Brody, S., Poulshock, W., and Masciocchi, C. The family caring unit: A major consideration in the long-term support system. *Gerontologist* 18(6):556, 1978.

48. Brody, E. Aging Parents and Aging Children. In P. Ragan (ed.)., *Aging Parents.* Los Angeles: University of California Press, 1979.

49. Brody, E. Women in the middle and family help to older people. *Gerontologist* 21:471, 1981.

50. Brody, E. Parent care as a normative family stress. *Gerontologist* 25(1):19, 1985.

51. Comptroller General of the United States. *Report to Congress on Home Health: The Need for a National Policy to Better Provide for the Elderly.* USGAO HRD-78-19. Washington, D.C.: U.S. Government Printing Office, 1977.

52. Daniels, N. Equity of access to health care: Some conceptual and ethical issues. *Milbank Memorial Fund Q.* 60(1):51, 1982.

53. Lopata, H. *Widowhood in an American City.* Cambridge: Schenkman, 1973.

54. Field, M. *The Aged, the Family and the Community.* New York: Columbia University Press, 1972.

55. Soldo, B. The living arrangements of the elderly in the near future. An unpublished paper prepared for the Conference on The Elderly of the Future. National Academy of Sciences, Annapolis, Maryland, 1979.

56. Archbold, P. Impact of caring for an ill elderly parent of the middle-aged or elderly offspring caregiver. Paper presented at the 31st Annual Meeting of the Gerontological Society, Dallas, Texas, 1978.

57. Cantor, M. Strain among caregivers: A study of the experience in the United States. *Gerontologist* 23:597, 1983.

58. Warren, J. W., et al. Informed consent by proxy. *N. Engl. J. Med.* 315(18):1124, 1986.

59. Lo, B., and Schroeder, S. Frequency of ethical dilemmas in a medical inpatient service. *Arch. Intern. Med.* 141:1062, 1981.

60. Childress, J. Paternalism and Health Care. In W. Robison and M. Pritchard (eds.), *Medical Responsibility.* Clifton, NJ: Humana Press, 1979.

61. Perry, C. B., and Applegate, W. B. Medical paternalism and patient self-determination. *J. Am. Geriatr. Soc.* 33(5):353, 1985.

62. Wetle, T., and Levkoff, S. Attitudes and Behaviors Toward Elder Patients in the VA System. In T. Wetle and J. Rowe (eds.), *Older Veterans: Linking VA and Community Resources.* Cambridge: Harvard University Press, 1984.

63. Avorn, J., and Langer, E. Induced disability in nursing home patients: A controlled trial. *J. Am. Geriatr. Soc.* 30:1, 1982.

64. Langer, E. The Illusion of Incompetence. In L. Perlmutter and R. Monty (eds.), *Choice and Perceived Control*. New York: Lawrence Erlbaum Associates, 1979.

65. Wetle, T., and Pearson, D. Long Term Care. In S. Jonas (ed.), *Health Care Delivery in the United States* (3rd ed.). New York: Springer, 1986.

66. Besdine, R. Decisions to withhold treatment from nursing home residents. *J. Am. Geriatr. Soc.* 31:606, 1983.

67. Lynn, J. Ethical issues in caring for elderly residents of nursing homes. *Primary Care* 13(2):295, 1986.

68. McCullough, L. B., and Soldo, B. J. Protective paternalism in long-term care placement. A paper presented at the Annual Scientific Meeting of the Gerontological Society of America, Toronto, Canada, 1981.

69. Dubler, M. M., and Zuckerman, C. *Discharge Planning for Elderly Patients of Diminished Capacity*. New York: Montefiore Hospital, 1986.

70. Lee, M. A., and Cassel, C. K. The ethical and legal framework for the decision not to resuscitate. *West. J. Med.* 140(1):117, 1984.

71. Rabkin, M. T., Gillerman, G., and Rice, N. R. Orders not to resuscitate. *N. Engl. J. Med.* 295(7):364, 1976.

72. Besdine, R. Decisions to withhold treatment from nursing home residents. *J. Am. Geriatr. Soc.* 31(10):602, 1983.

73. Bedell, S. E., and Belbanco, T. L. Choices about cardiopulmonary resuscitation in the hospital. *N. Engl. J. Med.* 310(17):1089, 1984.

74. Bedell, S. E., et al. Do not resuscitate orders for critically ill patients in the hospital: How are they used and what is their impact. *J.A.M.A.* 256(2):233, 1986.

75. Office of Technology Assessment. *Life Sustaining Technologies and the Elderly*. OTA-BA-306. Washington, D.C.: U.S. Government Printing Office, 1987.

76. Farber, N. J., et al. Cardiopulmonary resuscitation (CPR): Patient factors and decision making. *Arch. Intern. Med.* 144:2229, 1984.

77. Curran, W. J. Quality of life and treatment decisions: The Canadian Law Reform Report. *N. Engl. J. Med.* 310(5):297, 1984.

78. Pearlman, R., and Jonsen, A. The use of quality-of-life considerations in medical decision making. *J. Am. Geriatr. Soc.* 33(5):344, 1985.

79. Edlund, M., and Tancredi, L. R. Quality of life: An ideological critique. *Perspect. Biol. Med.* 28(4):591, 1985.

80. Kushner, T. Having a life versus being alive. *J. Med. Ethics* 1:5, 1984.

81. Thomasma, D. C. Ethical judgments of quality of life in the care of the aged. *J. Am. Geriatr. Soc.* 32(7):525, 1984.

82. Eisenberg, J. Sociological influences on decision-making by clinicians. *Ann. Intern. Med.* 90:957, 1979.

83. Crane, D. *The Sanctity of Social Life: Physicians' Treatment of Critically Ill Patients*. New York: Russell Sage Foundation, 1975.

84. Avorn, J. Benefit and cost analysis in geriatric care. *N. Engl. J. Med.* 310(20):1294, 1984.

85. Goffman, I. *The Presentation of Self in Everyday Life*. Garden City, NJ: Doubleday, 1959.

86. Coser, R. L. Some social functions of laughter: A study of humor in a hospital setting. *Human Relations* 12:171, 1959.

87. Fox, R. C., and Lief, H. I. Training for Detached Concern in Medical Students. In H. Lief, V. F. Lief, and N. Lief (eds.), *The Psychological Basis of Medical Practice*. New York: Harper & Row, 1963.

88. Lynn, J., and Childress, J. F. Must patients always be given food and water? *Hastings Center Report* 13:17, 1983.

89. *President's Commission for the Study of Ethical Problems in Medicine and Biomedical and Behavioral Research: Deciding to Forego Life Sustaining Treatment*. Washington, D.C.: U.S. Government Printing Office, 1983.

90. In re *Conroy*, 486 A. 2d 1209 (NJ 1985).

91. Annas, G. J. Fashion and freedom: When artificial feeding should be withdrawn. *Am. J. Public Health* 75(6):685, 1985.

92. Dresser, R. S., and Boisaubin, E. V. Ethics, law and nutritional support. *Arch. Intern. Med.* 145:122, 1985.

93. Callahan, D. On feeding the dying. *Hastings Center Report* 13:22, 1983.

94. Siegler, M., and Weisbard, A. Against the emerging stream: Should fluids and nutritional support be discontinued? *Arch. Intern. Med.* 145:129, 1985.

95. Meilaender, G. On removing food and water: Against the stream. *Hastings Center Report* 14:11, 1984.

96. Derr, P. G. Nutrition and hydration as elective therapy: Brophy and Jobes from an ethical and historical perspective. *Issues Law Medicine* 2(1):25, 1986.

97. Uddo, B. J. The withdrawal or refusal of food and hydration as age discrimination: Some possibilities. *Issues Law Medicine* 2(1):29, 1986.

98. Paris, J., and Reardon, F. Court responses to withholding or withdrawing artificial nutrition and fluids. *J.A.M.A.* 253:2243, 1985.

99. Olins, N. J. Feeding decisions for incompetent patients. *J. Am. Geriatr. Soc.* 34(4):313, 1986.

100. Curran, W. J. Defining appropriate medical

care: Proving nutrients and hydration for the dying. *N. Engl. J. Med.* 313(15):940, 1985.

101. Watts, D. T., Cassel, C. K., and Hickam, D. H. Nurses' and physicians attitudes toward tube feeding decisions in long term care. *J. Am. Geriatr. Soc.* 34:607, 1986.

102. Lo, B., and Dornbrand, L. Guiding the hand that feeds: Caring for the demented elderly. *N. Engl. J. Med.* 311:402, 1984.

103. Fox, P. *Long-Term Care: Background and Future Directions.* U.S. Department of Health and Human Services, Health Care Financing Administration. HCFA-81-20047. Washington, D.C.: U.S. Government Printing Office, 1981.

104. Burt, R. *Taking Care of Strangers: The Rule of Law in Doctor-Patient Relations.* New York: MacMillan, 1979.

105. Halper, T. Life and death in the welfare state: End stage renal disease in the United Kingdom. *Milband Memorial Fund Q.* 63(1):52, 1985.

106. Young, Q. The danger of making serious problems worse. *Business and Health* Jan/Feb:32, 1985.

107. Wikler, D. Forming an ethical response to for-profit health care. *Business and Health* Jan/Feb:25, 1985.

108. United States Commission on Civil Rights. *The Age Discrimination Study.* 005-000-00190-1. Washington, D.C.: U.S. Government Printing Office, 1979.

109. Minkler, M. Generational equity and the new victim blaming: An emerging public policy issue. *Int. J. Health Serv.* 16(4):539, 1986.

110. Clark, P. G. The social allocation of health care resources: Ethical dilemmas in age-group competition. *Gerontologist* 25(2):119, 1985.

111. Preston, S. H. Children and the elderly in the U.S. *Sci. Am.* 251(6):44, 1984.

112. Binstock, R. H. The aged as scapegoat. The Donald P. Kent award lecture, presented at the annual meetings of the Gerontological Society of America in Boston, MA, 1982.

113. Kingson, E. R., Hirshorn, B. A., and Cornman, J. M. *Ties that Bind: The Interdependence of Generations.* Washington, D.C.: Seven Locks Press, 1986.

7

Abuse, Neglect, and Inadequate Care

TERRENCE A. O'MALLEY
TERRY T. FULMER

ABUSE AND NEGLECT are terms with legal ramifications that have been used to describe elderly persons who manifest signs of trauma, unattended medical problems, poor hygiene, or malnutrition; who live in substandard or dangerous housing; or who report verbal abuse, battering, exploitation, abandonment, denial of rights, forced confinement, or other types of personal harm at the hands of family, neighbors, or professional caretakers [1–5]. Abuse and neglect are parts of a larger sociomedical issue, that of inadequate care of the elderly (Fig. 7-1). They represent an "illness" characterized by the failure of the individual's support system to meet his or her needs or the exacerbation or creation of those needs by the support system. These needs include assistance with the activities of daily living and basic requirements for food, shelter, and clothing, and for protection.

Reliable estimates of the prevalence of abuse and neglect are not available because of the lack of uniform definitions. However, approximately 4 percent of the nation's elderly are estimated to be victims of abuse and neglect as defined by the existing state reporting statutes, and substantially more exist whose needs for care are not being adequately met. Abuse and neglect have been identified in all socioeconomic strata, in urban and rural populations [6], and in all races and religious denominations. There do not appear to be any demographic determinants of inadequate care. An annotated bibliography of many of the important studies is available [7].

Definitions

Many definitions have been proposed for abuse and neglect of the elderly (Table 7-1). Although there are major similarities among these definitions, they do not overlap enough to permit them to be used interchangeably. These definitions emphasize the relationship between the elderly person and a caretaker and focus on the caretaker's acts of omission and commission and on the intentionality of those acts.

Although these definitions adequately cover the range of observations subsumed under the concept of abuse and neglect, it is important to remember that abuse and neglect comprise only part of the larger segment of inadequate care given to elderly persons for reasons other than the actions or omissions of a caretaker. From the geriatrician's perspective, it is important to resolve the problem of inadequate care from any cause, not just that resulting from caretakers' actions. In this regard, the concepts of abuse and neglect are too restrictive [8] and should be replaced by the term *inadequate care.* Within this context, definitions of abuse and neglect that we have found useful are based on the concept of inadequate care resulting from a mismatch between the elderly person's care

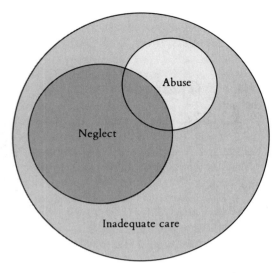

FIGURE 7-1. *The universe of inadequate care. (From T. Fulmer and T. A. O'Malley.* Inadequate Care of the Elderly: A Health Care Perspective on Abuse and Neglect. *New York: Springer, 1987.)*

needs and the services received. These definitions focus on the unmet care needs of the elderly person rather than on the behavior of the caretaker or system.

ABUSE: Active intervention by a caretaker such that unmet needs are created or sustained with resultant physical, psychological, or financial injury.

NEGLECT: Failure of a caretaker to intervene to resolve an important care need despite awareness of available resources [9].

There have been several attempts to divide abuse and neglect into discrete subgroups to better describe and understand their characteristics. One approach has been to separate cases into categories based either on the type of abuse noted (battering, financial crises, psychological problems) or on the kind of professional that is likely to deal with the problem (physical abuse—physicians, nurses; financial exploitation—social workers, lawyers; psychological abuse—social workers). Another method has been to look at cases that manifest only limited aspects of abuse and neglect. One such study [10] used a telephone survey to obtain reports of battering, verbal abuse, and neglect as defined by the individual. The results were reports of

elderly persons who were predominantly victims of spouse abuse. Still other workers have tried to develop categories based on the relationship between the care needs of the elderly person and the amount of caretaking services being provided [11]. The consequences of the many overlapping definitions of abuse and neglect and the resulting lack of widely used categories are that interventions are not consistent [12], and it is difficult to generalize from the results of research.

Theories

An excellent review of the theories advanced to explain causation and guide effective intervention in cases of abuse and neglect is available [13]. The most clinically relevant theories fall into the following five groups.

IMPAIRMENT OF THE OLDER PERSON

Drawing a parallel with child abuse, in which dependency appears to be a factor in abuse, it has been proposed that as dependency increases, the risk of abuse increases [2]. No studies have yet been done that demonstrate that abused elderly persons have a greater degree of dependency than nonabused elderly. In fact, abuse is found frequently in elderly persons who have no dependencies. This theory probably is more applicable to cases of neglect; however, it is likely that while dependency might be a necessary condition for neglect, it is not a sufficient condition.

PSYCHOPATHOLOGY OF THE ABUSER

Abnormal behavior by a psychologically impaired individual has been proposed as one mechanism of abuse. Abusive sociopathic behavior can result from drug or alcohol abuse or from inherent psychopathology. No studies have conclusively demonstrated that abuse is due to psychiatric derangement of the abuser. There are, however, a small number of cases in which violence against an elderly person occurs for no apparent reason and in which the abuser is psychiatrically impaired. "Nonnormal caretakers" have been described [14] as individuals who are responsible for abuse or neglect because they are unable to assume a proper caretaking role owing to mental retardation or dis-

TABLE 7-1. *Definitions of elder abuse*

SOURCE	DEFINITION
O'Malley, Segal, and Perez (1979), adapted from Connecticut Department of Aging	*Abuse:* The willful infliction of physical pain, injury, or debilitating mental anguish; unreasonable confinement; or deprivation by a caretaker of services that are necessary to maintain mental and physical health.
Block and Sinnott (1979)	1. *Physical abuse:* malnutrition; injuries, e.g., bruises, welts, sprains, dislocations, abrasions, or lacerations. 2. *Psychological abuse:* verbal assault, threat, fear, isolation. 3. *Material abuse:* theft, misuse of money or property. 4. *Medical abuse:* withholding of medications or aids required.
Douglass, Hickey, and Noele (1980)	1. *Passive neglect:* being ignored, left alone, isolated, forgotten. 2. *Active neglect:* withholding of companionship, medicine, food, exercise, assistance to bathroom. 3. *Verbal or emotional abuse:* name-calling, insults, treating as a child, frightening humiliation, intimidation, threats. 4. *Physical abuse:* being hit, slapped, bruised, sexually molested, cut, burned, physically restrained.
Lau and Kosberg (1979)	1. *Physical abuse:* direct beatings; withholding personal care, food, medical care; lack of supervision. 2. *Psychological abuse:* verbal assaults, threats, provoking fear, isolation. 3. *Material abuse:* monetary or material theft or misuse. 4. *Violation of rights:* being forced out of one's dwelling or forced into another setting.
Wolf and Pillemer (1984)	1. *Physical abuse:* the infliction of physical pain or injury, physical coercion (confinement against one's will), e.g., slapped, bruised, sexually molested, cut, burned, physically restrained. 2. *Psychological abuse:* the infliction of mental anguish, e.g., called names, treated as child, frightened, humiliated, intimidated, threatened, isolated. 3. *Material abuse:* the illegal or improper exploitation and/or use of funds or other resources. 4. *Active neglect:* refusal or failure to fulfill a caretaking obligation, including a conscious and intentional attempt to inflict physical or emotional stress on the elder; e.g., deliberate abandonment or deliberate denial of food or health-related services. 5. *Passive neglect:* refusal or failure to fulfill a caretaking obligation, excluding a conscious and intentional attempt to inflict physical or emotional distress on the elder; e.g., abandonment, nonprovision of food or health-related services because of inadequate knowledge, laziness, infirmity, or disrupting the value of prescribed services.

SOURCE: From T. Fulmer and T. A. O'Malley. *Inadequate Care of the Elderly: A Health Care Perspective on Abuse and Neglect.* New York: Springer, 1987.

ordered thinking. Such individuals have been forced by circumstances to assume a caretaking role for which they are incompetent.

TRANSGENERATIONAL VIOLENCE

Theories of transgenerational violence describe families in which violence is a learned behavior and is the norm for intrafamily communications [15]. Children learn to use violence from parents as part of their interpersonal relationships and in turn use it in their relations with their parents when power relationships change. Anecdotal reports of violent families are common. However, contrary to the prediction of these theories, one case-controlled study [16] showed no increase in child abuse among children who were abusing their parents.

STRESSED CARETAKER

Theories about stressed caretakers emphasize the relationship between stress on the caretaker and abuse and neglect of the elderly. Many caretakers of elderly parents report symptoms of stress, anxiety, and depression [2,17]. It has been proposed that life crises could trigger abuse [18]. There have been no controlled studies that have shown abusing caretakers to be under greater stress than those who provide exemplary care, and other studies have suggested that interventions directed at reducing caretaker stress may not be effective [16]. Caretaker stress appears to be neither a necessary nor sufficient condition to trigger abuse. It is, however, a common accompaniment to abusive situations, and its treatment provides a useful way to develop a supportive relationship with the individual responsible for the abuse or neglect.

EXCHANGE THEORY

The exchange theory looks at the relationship between the abuser and the victim and predicts that abuse will continue as long as the abuser derives some net gain from it [19]. If the exchange becomes negative because of fear of sanctions, lack of psychic or material benefit, guilt, or increased difficulty in perpetrating it, then the abuse will stop. This theory fits well with current observations on the beneficial effect of interventions that only decrease the elderly person's social isolation (increase the abuser's risk of sanctions) and do not materially affect other aspects of the abuse situation. The high incidence of monetary gain as a motive in abuse also fits well with this scheme.

LIMITATIONS OF THEORIES

With the exception of the exchange theory, which has implications for a wide range of interventions, these theories are more useful for identifying elders potentially at risk for abuse and neglect than for defining interventions. Despite the advances made in proposing theories to explain abuse and neglect, there remains a fundamental theoretical issue: the utility of separating family violence into categories on the basis of the age or marital status of the victim (which is done now with child, spouse, and elder abuse) or using other categories such as the manifestations of abuse or the categories listed previously. None of these approaches adequately provides a framework for under-

standing abuse and neglect of the elderly. No one construct has been proposed that allows an explanation of the similarities and differences of child, spouse, and elder abuse. Abuse and neglect of the handicapped, which extends across age and marital categories, is an example of the inability of our current theories and definitions to provide a broad framework of understanding. To a great extent, the current categorical approaches to these problems and our theoretical constructs have been determined by the legislative response to the sequential identification of aspects of family violence. Abuse and neglect of the elderly may not be the appropriate terms to describe this social problem [20].

Diagnosing Abuse and Neglect

Elderly persons experiencing abuse, neglect, and inadequate care usually present with signs of unattended medical problems, poor hygiene, malnutrition, dehydration, and unexplained trauma. Often it is not possible to determine whether the manifestations of inadequate care result from the natural progression of an underlying disease or involve the actions or omissions of a caretaker [21]. It is easier to identify inadequate care and acute problems that require intervention than it is to determine the role of the caretaker in their genesis or continuation and thereby to establish the diagnosis of abuse or neglect.

Other elderly persons report episodes of abuse that do not have physical manifestations. These include financial mismanagement and exploitation, threats of punishment, verbal harassment, unreasonable confinement, denial of rights, and sexual abuse. Unfortunately, elderly persons rarely divulge information concerning abuse owing to embarrassment, mistrust of health care professionals, or fear of reprisal, separation, or institutionalization.

Diagnosis of abuse or neglect usually rests with the observation of a manifestation of inadequate care and an assessment of the elderly person's social situation, ability to provide self-care, and needs for assistance. Table 7-2 lists commonly reported manifestations of abuse, neglect, and inadequate care. The presence of one or more of these signs does not establish the

TABLE 7-2. *Signs of abuse, neglect, and inadequate care*

Contusions	Decubiti
Lacerations	Untreated but previously
Abrasions	diagnosed medical
Fractures	problems
Sprains	Dehydration
Dislocations	Misuse of medications
Burns	Malnutrition
Oversedation	Freezing
Anxiety	Poor hygiene
Over- or undermedication	Depression

SOURCE: Adapted from T. A. O'Malley, et al. Identifying and preventing family-mediated abuse and neglect of elderly persons. *Ann. Intern. Med*, 98:998, 1983.

TABLE 7-3. *Physical indicators of abuse not shared with neglect*

Unexplained bruises and welts:
  Face, lips, mouth
  Torso, back, buttocks, thighs
  In various stages of healing
  Clustered, forming regular patterns
  Reflecting shape of article used to inflict (electric cord, belt buckle)
  On several different surface areas
  Regularly appear after absence, weekend, or vacation
Unexplained burns:
  Cigar, cigarette burns, especially on soles, palms, back, or buttocks
  Immersion burns (sock-like on feet, glove-like on hands, doughnut-shaped on buttocks or genitalia)
  Patterned like electric burner, iron, etc.
  Rope burns on arms, legs, neck, or torso
Unexplained fractures:
  To skull, nose, facial structure
  In various stages of healing
  Multiple or spiral fractures
Unexplained lacerations or abrasions:
  To mouth, lips, gums, eyes
  To external genitalia
Sexual abuse:
  Difficulty in walking or sitting
  Torn, stained, or bloody underclothing
  Pain or itching in genital area
  Bruises or bleeding in external genitalia or in vaginal or anal areas
  Venereal disease

SOURCE: From T. Fulmer and T. A. O'Malley. *Inadequate Care of the Elderly: A Health Care Perspective on Abuse and Neglect*. New York: Springer, 1987.

diagnosis; it should, however, alert the clinician to that possibility.

Manifestations that suggest abuse rather than neglect or inadequate care are listed in Table 7-3.

Based on earlier studies it has been possible to identify groups of elderly persons who appear to be at higher than average risk for abuse, ne-

TABLE 7-4. *Elderly persons at risk for abuse or neglect*

1. Those with accelerating care needs because of progressive or unstable conditions such Alzheimer's disease, parkinsonism, or severe strokes that exceed or will soon exceed their caretaker's ability to meet them.
2. Those with family members having a history of criminal or violent behavior.
3. Those with a family history of child or spouse abuse.
4. Those whose caretakers manifest signs of stress such as depression, anxiety, or "burn-out."
5. Those who abuse drugs or alcohol or who live with family members who do.
6. Those whose caretakers are under sudden increased stress, for example, due to loss of job, health, or spouse.
7. Those who reside in an institution with the reputation of providing inadequate care.

SOURCE: Adapted from T. A. O'Malley, et al. Identifying and preventing family-mediated abuse and neglect of elderly persons. *Ann. Intern. Med*. 98:998, 1983.

glect, or inadequate care (Table 7-4). All elderly persons who manifest any of the listed signs should be questioned to determine whether they belong to one of these high-risk groups. Conversely, any elderly person who is discovered to be a member of one of these high-risk groups should be questioned about their care needs, and manifestations of inadequate care should be carefully sought.

Screening instruments have been developed and tested to assist emergency room nurses to identify and assess more sensitively and accurately elderly persons experiencing abuse or neglect. Formal instruments are an important aid in the identification of these individuals [22–26].

Treatment and Outcome

A complete discussion of the issues of intervention can be found in other references [13,27]. An important difference between elder abuse and child abuse, with which it is often compared, is that the elderly person is presumed to be competent to make his or her own decisions. This fundamental difference changes the professional's approach to intervention from prescription to negotiation. The elderly person has the right to refuse access, interview, or intervention and in practice often does. Difficult issues include gaining access to the elderly person, assessing the risk of imminent harm, negotiating with reluctant or nonvoluntary clients, setting goals of intervention, determining competency, and choosing an intervention strategy.

GAINING ACCESS

Early studies showed that nearly 40 percent of elderly suspected of being abused or neglected refused any further assessment or intervention [1]. Most of the barriers were internal to the elderly person and included embarrassment, fear of reprisal or change, loss of autonomy, and skepticism regarding medical or social service interventions. Successful access requires the ability to identify the elderly person's concerns about the process of assessment. It also requires an ability to develop a working relationship with the individual responsible for the abuse or neglect so that they can assist with the task of gaining access to the elderly person [27].

RISK OF IMMINENT HARM

The risk of imminent harm exists whenever elderly persons experience life-threatening illness or injury, live in unsafe environments where injury may occur, or are at risk for serious injury at the hands of someone who has unimpeded access to them and has injured them before. The presence of the risk of imminent harm determines the pace of intervention and the urgency of more complete assessment. Frequently, the most acceptable and effective intervention is to arrange for acute hospitalization even if the elderly person's problems are not predominantly medical.

IDENTIFYING CARE NEEDS

Needs for care arise from ongoing medical or psychological problems, alterations in functional status, unsafe environments, and acts of omission and commission of caretakers. Assessment of care needs proceeds at a pace commensurate with the risk of harm to the elderly person occasioned by the care need. Because elderly persons often under-report illness and disability, it is more important to observe the elderly person's functional capabilities than it is to accept his or her reported abilities. Observation of the elderly person's living situation is also important. Frequently, information must also be obtained from other family members or neighbors to gain a more complete picture of the elderly person's situation. Standardized multidimensional assessment instruments help to promote effective and uniform assessment of care needs [28].

NEGOTIATING WITH RELUCTANT CLIENTS

Because the elderly person controls the process of intervention, the health care professional can only negotiate and not prescribe interventions. Further discussion of these skills is available [29,30].

GOALS OF INTERVENTION

Because abused elderly persons control the process of intervention, they also control the goals of intervention. The powerlessness of the professional to influence this process in the usual ways is a source of great frustration, which persists despite the promulgation of many abuse-reporting laws, some of dubious constitutionality [31]. Contrary to what one might think, the goal of intervention is usually not to eradicate abuse or neglect completely but instead to achieve a level that the elderly person finds tolerable balanced by his or her wishes for autonomy, interaction with family, and avoidance of uncertain alternatives. In a sense, the elderly person has the "right to be abused" if he or she so chooses [9]. The professional's role is to persuade against exercising this right.

COMPETENCY

The issue of competency is commonly encountered because of the substantial prevalence of dementia in the "old-old" and in many elderly who experience inadequate care. Elderly persons who are not competent to make decisions regarding the management of finances, property, or personal care are usually afforded some degree of protection by the courts through the use of conservatorship or guardianship. A determination of incompetency requires a court hearing, and the burden rests on those who would have the elderly person deemed incompetent.

Determining incompetency can be difficult, although guidelines exist [32]. The essential characteristic of competency is the ability to comprehend the consequences of one's decisions. The courts usually provide the "least restrictive alternative" so that the elderly person can maintain the greatest degree of autonomy consistent with safety. In this regard, conservatorship extends only to the management of the elderly person's assets, whereas guardianship includes decisions about personal care as well as consent for medical treatment or admission to a long-term care facility. Although family members are occasionally appointed as guardians, courts are reluctant to grant guardianship to individuals who have a major personal financial interest in the outcome of care. Often, less formal methods are used by families to help simplify the management of financial affairs such as joint bank accounts and powers of attorney. Although most such arrangements are maintained appropriately for efficiency, there is ample room for misappropriation of funds. If guardianship is established, then intervention plans are negotiated with the elder's guardian, which usually results in more complete resolution of abuse or neglect but at the cost of limiting the elder's autonomy.

INTERVENTION STRATEGIES

Intervention strategies have been developed empirically and with little testing. They include altering the dependency of the elderly person by providing medical and mental health services, altering the behavior of the abusing or neglectful caretaker through training or counseling, reducing stress on the caretaker by providing home care services to relieve the burden of caretaking, enhancing protective measures such as physical barriers or legal sanctions, and separating the elderly person from the source of abuse by hospitalization, institutionalization, or removal of the abuser [33].

Many studies have noted that abuse and neglect are longstanding patterns of interaction and that immediate intervention is not necessary except in the case of imminent harm. Additionally, most studies have shown that most abused elderly persons would rather receive inadequate care living with their families than excellent institutional care. These two observations guide most interventions because the competent elderly person has control over the content and timing of interventions. As a practical matter, most cases of abuse or neglect fall into two broad categories: cases in which the care needs of the elderly person are so abundant that priority is given to obtaining resources to

meet those needs for care, and cases in which the care needs of the elderly person are modest and priority is given to separating the abuser from the elderly person [9].

The choice of intervention strategy is determined by the willingness of the elderly person to permit intervention and by the relative priorities of meeting needs for care or separation. There are very few studies that describe the outcome of interventions. There is agreement, however, that separation of the elderly person from the source of abuse is the most effective intervention when accepted. Separation usually results in the institutionalization of the elderly person [11,16]. Intervention results in complete or major resolution of the abuse in approximately three-quarters of cases. The reason for the effectiveness of interventions other than separation is not clear. However, the exchange theory offers the best explanation for resolution when the social isolation of the abused elder is reduced [19].

Because patient assessment and intervention require the skills of home care, social work, nursing, and medicine, representatives of these four professions usually make up the multidisciplinary teams charged with managing abuse cases [34]. Legal counsel is also helpful in pursuing guardianship, obtaining emergency court orders to ensure separation of the abuser and elderly person, and giving advice about the requirements of any applicable abuse-reporting laws. Given the complexity of these cases, a multidisciplinary team approach is essential and is the most widely used model.

Ethical Issues

Table 7-5 lists some of the ethical issues that are frequently encountered in these cases. Some have to do with the professional's responsibility to his or her clients, some with the locus of decision making, and some with the rights of the elderly person. Management of these cases needs to be guided by the principles of seeking "the least restrictive alternative" to abuse or neglect, respecting the elderly person's rights, and adhering to the elderly person's priorities. These principles often conflict with the professional's perception of what needs to be done and are discussed extensively elsewhere [35].

TABLE 7-5. *Ethical issues in abuse and neglect of the elderly*

STAGE	ETHICAL ISSUE
Identifying cases	Purpose of identification
	Effect of labeling
	Primum non nocere
Reporting cases	Confidentiality
	Labeling
Gaining access	Right to privacy
	Responsibility if access refused
Intervening	Paternalism
	Self-control versus dependency
	"Right to be abused"
	Incompetency
Follow-up	Contact versus abandonment
	Minimized risk
	Free and informed consent

SOURCE: Adapted from T. Fulmer and T. A. O'Malley. *Inadequate Care of the Elderly: A Health Care Perspective on Abuse and Neglect.* New York: Springer, 1987.

ISSUES OF CASE REPORTING

Conflicts are inherent in the professional's responsibility for the welfare of his or her client, the confidentiality of communications between them, and the provisions of abuse-reporting laws that mandate the filing of reports of suspected abuse or neglect. Because of the potential for harm to the elderly person if the label "abuse" is applied carelessly, the professional should be constrained by the dictum *primum non nocere* and consider the risks of case reporting if the act of reporting has the potential for making intervention more difficult or less likely to succeed.

ISSUES OF ACCESS AND INTERVENTION

Many questions continue to elude clear answers. At what point does the elderly person's right to privacy take precedence over the professional's responsibility to act in the perceived best interests of the client? Is it appropriate to use subterfuge to gain access to the elderly person to present options for improving the elder's care so that he or she can make an informed decision? At what point is it ethical to accept the elderly person's decision to endure inadequate care despite the availability of alternatives? The issue of paternalism and the elderly person's right to self-determination present the most intense conflicts in the issue of intervention. Most ethicists come down on the side of giving precedence to informed self-determination but not as an excuse to abandon an elderly person who remains at risk for further harm [36].

ISSUES OF ONGOING CARE

Do professionals have a right to withdraw from participation in the care of abused elders who do not wish to follow their recommendations? Is the provision of inadequate care by the professional acceptable if that is all that the client will permit? What does informed consent mean if the potential outcomes of an intervention cannot clearly be forecast? In practice, ongoing contact with the elderly person is important even if it is far less than the professional finds acceptable. The expectation, however unrealistic, is that as the relationship grows between the elderly person and the professional, more substantive interventions can be negotiated. Each case raises its own series of ethical issues, which can usually be resolved by keeping the patient's rights foremost and by taking a long-term perspective on case management.

Conclusion

Abuse and neglect are quintessential geriatric problems. The geriatrician needs an understanding of the norms of aging and the contribution of the patient's environment to his or her well-being, an awareness of the full array of supportive services that are available, the sensitivity to confront difficult ethical dilemmas, the ability to negotiate with patients, and the capacity to work as part of a multidisciplinary team. It is likely that abuse, neglect, and inadequate care will become more frequent due to the inexorable increase in the number of elderly persons and a corresponding decrease in available caretakers.

There is no question that abuse and neglect of the elderly exist as problems and that they are important. At issue, however, is whether the consequences of defining these forms of family violence as criminal acts are worth the expenditures of money and energy required by this approach. Given the difficulties inherent in defining abuse and neglect and in putting these definitions into practice, it appears that these problems are not well managed by legalistic approaches. The solution to these problems on a societal level will be as much political as sociomedical. Problems currently subsumed under the labels of abuse and neglect must be redefined so that a national consensus can be established for their resolution [20]. Abuse and neglect are too narrow and too poorly defined to serve as the political focus for improving the care of the elderly. Ensuring minimum standards of income, medical care, housing, and nutrition for the elderly, and developing incentives for families to care for their aging relatives will be parts of the solution. Ultimately, abuse and neglect will diminish when society places a higher value on the well-being of its elders.

References

1. O'Malley, H. C., et al. *Elder Abuse in Massachusetts: A Survey of Professionals and Paraprofessionals.* Boston, MA: Legal Research and Services for the Elderly, 1979.
2. Block, M. R., and Sinnott, J. D. (eds.). *The Battered Elder Syndrome: An Exploratory Study.* College Park, MD: University of Maryland Center On Aging, 1979.
3. Hickey, T., and Douglass, R. L. Mistreatment of the elderly in the domestic setting: An exploratory study. *Am. J. Public Health* 71:500, 1981.
4. Rathbone-McCuan, E. Elderly victims of family violence and neglect. *Soc. Casework* May:296, 1980.
5. Tomita, S. K. Detection and treatment of elderly abuse and neglect: A protocol for health care professionals. *Phys. Occup. Ther. Geriatr.* 2:37, 1982.
6. Hageboeck, H., and Brandt, K. *A Summary Report of Rural/Urban Abuse of the Elderly in Scott County, Iowa.* Iowa Gerontology Model Project. Iowa City: University of Iowa, 1981.
7. Johnson, T. F., O'Brien, J. G., and Hudson, M. F. *Elder Neglect and Abuse: An Annotated Bibliography.* Westport, CT: Greenwood Press, 1985.
8. O'Malley, T. A. Abuse and neglect—The wrong issue? *Pride Inst. J. of Long-Term Care* 5(4):25, 1986.
9. O'Malley, T. A., et al. Identifying and preventing family mediated abuse and neglect of elderly persons. *Ann. Intern. Med.* 98:998, 1983.
10. Pillemer, K., and Finkelhor, D. Prevalence research. *Elder Abuse Report* 2(4):1, 1986.
11. O'Malley, T. A., et al. Categories of family mediated abuse and neglect of elderly persons. *J. Am. Geriatr. Soc.* 32(5):362, 1984.
12. Phillips, L. R., and Rempusheski, V. F. Making decisions about elder abuse. *Social Casework* 67(3):131, 1986.
13. Pillemer, C. N., and Wolf, R. (eds.). *Elder Abuse: Conflict in the Family.* Dover, MA: Auburn House, 1986.
14. Lau, E., and Kosberg, J. I. Abuse of the elderly by informal care providers. *Aging* 229:5, 1979.
15. Strauss, M., Gelles, R., and Steinmetz, S. *Behind Closed Doors.* New York: Anchor Press/Doubleday, 1981.
16. Wolf, R. S., Godkin, M. A., and Pillemer, K. A. *Elder Abuse and Neglect: Final Report from Three Model Projects.* Worcester, MA: University Center on Aging, 1984.
17. Zarit, S. H., Reever, K. E., and Bach-Peterson, J. Relatives of the impaired elderly: Correlates of feelings of burden. *Gerontologist* 20:649, 1980.
18. Douglass, R. L., Hickey, T., and Noele, C. *A Study of Maltreatment of the Elderly and Other Vulnerable Adults.* Ann Arbor, MI: University of Michigan, Institute of Gerontology, 1980.
19. Pillemer, K. A. Social isolation and elder abuse. *Response* 8(4):2, 1985.
20. Callahan, J. J. Guest editor's perspective. *Pride Inst. J. of Long-Term Care* 5(4):2, 1986.
21. Fulmer, T. T., and Ashley, J. Neglect: What part of abuse? *Pride Inst. J. of Long-Term Care* 5(4):18, 1986.
22. Falconi, D. Assessing the abused elderly. *J. Geriatr. Nurs.* 8(4):208, 1982.
23. Ferguson, D., and Beck, C. H.A.L.F.—A tool to assess elder abuse within the family. *Geriatr. Nurs.* Sept/Oct:301, 1983.
24. Fulmer, T. Elder abuse assessment tool. *Dimension Crit. Care Nurs.* 3(4):216, 1984.
25. Fulmer, T., and Cahill, V. Elder abuse: A study. *J. Geriatr. Nurs.* 10(12):16, 1984.
26. Fulmer, T., Street, S., and Carr, K. Abuse of the elderly: Screening and detection. *J. Emerg. Nurs.* 10:131, 1984.
27. Fulmer, T., and O'Malley, T. A. *Inadequate Care of the Elderly: A Health Care Perspective on Abuse and Neglect.* New York: Springer, 1987.
28. Kane, R. A., and Kane, R. L. *Assessing the Elderly: A Practical Guide to Measurement.* Lexington, MA: Lexington Books, 1981. Pp. 209–246.
29. Murdach, A. D. Bargaining and persuasion with nonvoluntary clients. *Soc. Work* Nov:458, 1980.
30. Knapp, M. B. Adult Protective Services: Convincing the Patient to Consent. In M. B. Knapp, H. E. Pies, and A. E. Doudera (eds.), *Legal and Ethical Aspects of Health Care for the Elderly.* Ann Arbor: University of Michigan, Health Administration Press, 1986. Pp. 231–244.
31. Thobaben, M., and Anderson, L. Reporting elder abuse: It's the law. *Am. J. Nurs.* 85(4):371, 1985.
32. Roth, L. H., Meisel, A., and Lidz, C. W. Tests of

competency to consent to treatment. *Am. J. Psychiatry* 134:279, 1977.

33. U.S. Department of Health and Human Services. Family Violence: Intervention Strategies. DHHS Pub. No. [OHDS] 80-30258. Washington, D.C.: U.S. Government Printing Office, 1980.

34. Carr, K., et al. An elder abuse assessment team in an acute hospital setting. *Gerontologist* 26(2): 115, 1986.

35. Wetle, T. T. Ethical Aspects of Decision Making for and with the Elderly. In M. B. Knapp, H. E. Pies, and A. E. Doudera (eds.), *Legal and Ethical Aspects of Health Care for the Elderly*. Ann Arbor: University of Michigan, Health Administration Press, 1986. Pp. 258–267.

8

Nutrition

NAOMI K. FUKAGAWA
VERNON R. YOUNG

THIS CHAPTER reviews generally how the aging process in the adult who is free of significant clinical disease might bring about changes in the utilization of nutrients. In addition, current estimates of the nutrient requirements in older adults are briefly described. The significant increase in numbers of elderly persons in the United States and technically developed nations makes it especially important to explore the aspects of metabolism and nutrition in human subjects. Unfortunately, there has been little detailed scientific inquiry in this field. Of the approximately 50 nutrients that are essential in human nutrition, few have been specifically investigated as to their metabolism and requirements during advancing age in humans [1].

Biochemical and Physiologic Changes During Aging and Their Possible Nutritional Significance

Numerous biochemical and physiologic changes of potential nutritional importance occur with aging. At the molecular, subcellular, and cellular levels, alterations include changes in DNA concentration and gene dosage of ribosomal RNA in various tissues, ultrastructural changes in the mitochondria and in the degree of cross-linking in collagen, and tissue accumulation of pigmented inclusion bodies. The composition of cell and subcellular membrane changes during senescence includes changes in the binding sites for hormones and complex changes in the activities of enzymes. In some organs, such as the kidney and central nervous system, the number of cells is reduced with advancing age [2].

Many organs and organ systems show alterations in function with advancing age that may have a direct influence on the utilization of nutrients. Variables associated with the maintenance of internal environment under resting conditions, such as fasting blood glucose, show little or no consistent age-related change. However, there is a marked decline in maximal organ performance, and the rate at which various indices of physiologic function return to a resting level after stimulation is reduced by aging. Whether such alterations imply an altered capacity to regulate the nutrient supply to cells following changes in nutrient intake is not known. However, such considerations have important practical implications with respect to the frequency and levels of nutrient intake necessary for maintenance of adequate nutritional status in the aged individual. The importance of such effects is underscored, for example, by the finding that the nocturnal rise in urinary calcium excretion in postmenopausal women is greater than that observed in premenopausal women [3].

The central importance of the gastrointestinal

99

tract in nutrient utilization relates in part to the fact that the level and nature of food ingested may be modulated by gastrointestinal function; for example, cancer in the gastrointestinal tract may result in obstruction, reduced food and nutrient intake, and anorexia. The physiologic changes in intestinal function that occur with aging are reviewed in Chapter 33 and are not repeated here.

Organ and Whole Body Metabolism
NUTRIENT LEVEL IN BODY FLUIDS

After absorption from the intestinal lumen, nutrients are transported across the mucosal epithelium and enter the circulation where their utilization and fate depend on the metabolic status of body organs. Transport of nutrients between the various organs and into cells involves the participation of a number of different mechanisms, ranging from the movement of molecules in free solution and simple diffusion across a semipermeable membrane to the binding of nutrients to specific carrier molecules in serum, as for transferrin and iron or for the transcobalamins and vitamin B_{12}, and their passage across cell membranes by active transport or carrier-mediated systems.

Information on blood and tissue levels of nutrients provides some clues to the utilization of essential dietary nutrients, but few reports have appeared in which these levels are considered critically as a function of adult age. For many constituents (e.g., sodium, potassium, bicarbonate, magnesium, total protein, albumin, inorganic phosphate) there may be little change with age, but for others such as urea, creatinine, calcium, alkaline phosphatase, and uric acid, changes may occur. Accurate interpretation of the nutritional significance of levels of nutrients in blood, or their metabolites and compounds, that reflect the activities of metabolic pathways in which these nutrients function awaits the development of adequate age-adjusted guidelines.

BODY COMPOSITION IN RELATION TO NUTRIENT UTILIZATION

Cross-sectional and longitudinal studies indicate a decline in lean body mass (or body cell mass) with advancing human age. Although the

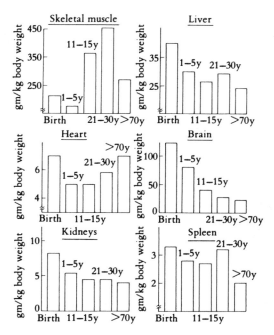

FIGURE 8-1. *Relative proportion (gm/kg of body weight) of major organs at various stages of life in humans. (Drawn from V. Korenchevsky.* Physiological and Pathological Ageing. *New York: Hafner, 1961.)*

contribution made by each of the major body organs to this reduction is not precisely known, postmortem studies indicate that skeletal muscles account for a significant, and perhaps major, proportion of the decline in body protein content [4]. Figure 8-1 shows that during early growth and development, the skeletal muscles account for an increasing contribution to total body weight, amounting to about 45 percent of body weight in the young adult. However, with time, muscle mass continues to decline, decreasing to approximately 27 percent of total body weight by age 70. Atrophy of skeletal muscles is a prominent clinical feature of advancing old age.

The decline in muscle mass with advancing adult age may be predicted to have an influence on nutrient utilization and perhaps overall nutritional health. The etiology of the loss of lean body and muscle mass is not known, but it has been suggested that the decline in physical activity may be of causal significance. Thus, active middle-age men have a higher body cell mass than inactive men [5]. Also, a program of moderate physical activity in elderly persons has been shown to result in favorable effects on body nitrogen content [6].

Older humans not only have increased proportions of total adipose tissue [7] but also many are obese when the standard criterion of an increase of more than 20 percent over ideal body mass is applied. Based on this criterion, the percentage of obesity ranges from 25 to 41 percent among males and from 25 to 54 percent among females [8]. Two caveats must be kept in mind when evaluating these results: (1) the decrease in height with aging has not been considered in this analysis of the prevalence of overweight and obesity, and thus this analysis tends to overestimate the numbers of obese within the population, and (2) all of the studies were conducted before the recent revision in the actuarial statistics for ideal height and weight. For these reasons, Frisancho [9] recently developed new standards for assessing the nutritional status of the elderly, based on data from the first and second National Health and Nutrition Examination Surveys.

Nutrient Requirements and Allowances

Little is known about the nutritional requirements of those who are healthy but very old. The number and variety of required nutrients are unchanged with age but the quantity of any single nutrient may be modified.

RECOMMENDED DIETARY ALLOWANCES

Because the minimum requirements for a nutrient to maintain health vary among apparently similar individuals, the recommended dietary allowances (RDAs) are designed to be adequate to meet the nutritional needs of practically all healthy persons within a particular population. The question of the extent of the variation in nutrient needs among individuals is of particular importance, therefore, in the development of appropriate dietary standards. In healthy populations of adults, this variation is assumed to be normally distributed, and the mean requirement plus two standard deviations above the mean is now considered to be a reasonable objective for establishing an RDA. This level of intake should be sufficient to cover the requirements of about 97.5 percent of the population.

The situation differs for energy requirements, and the RDA for energy is based on the average requirements for the population. Intakes of nutrients providing energy either well above or well below the individual's true requirements would result eventually in a deterioration of health, and it is assumed that most individuals select diets providing energy intakes that meet or approximate their actual needs. Thus, the average energy requirement is given as a guideline rather than as a recommendation for the intake level that would suit those few individuals in a population whose energy requirements are much higher than the mean.

Table 8-1 summarizes the most recent RDAs for adults as proposed by the U.S. Food and Nutrition Board [12]. It should be noted that insufficient information is available on human requirements on which to make reliable recommendations for all of the known essential nutrients. Accordingly, the Food and Nutrition Board has proposed a range of intakes that is considered safe and sufficient to meet the physiologic needs for those nutrients for which RDAs have not been determined. These intake ranges are also given in Table 8-1.

It must be emphasized strongly that the recommended allowances are amounts considered sufficient for the maintenance of health in nearly all adults. Recommendations are concerned with health maintenance, and they are not intended to be sufficient for therapeutic purposes. Thus, they are not designed to cover the additional requirements that may occur during and after recovery from infection or under conditions of malabsorption, trauma, metabolic disease, or other significant stress. The possible benefits that might occur with considerably higher intakes of individual nutrients in a variety of clinical situations are not relevant to RDAs, and proposals for very much higher intakes of nutrients than those proposed in Table 8-1 as a normal dietary practice cannot be justified for healthy old people on the basis of current information.

FACTORS AFFECTING NUTRIENT REQUIREMENTS

In addition to the possible influence of adult age per se, nutritional status and nutrient requirements in humans are affected by various factors.

TABLE 8-1. *RDAs and estimated safe and adequate daily dietary intakes of selected vitamins for adults of 51 years and older*[a]

	MEN	WOMEN
Weight (lb)	154	120
Height (in.)	70	64
Recommended dietary allowances (RDAs)		
Energy (kcal)	2400	1800
Protein (gm)	56	44
Fat-soluble vitamins		
Vitamin A (μgRE)[b]	1000	800
Vitamin D (μg)[c]	5	5
Vitamin E activity		
(mg α-TE)[d]	10	10
Water-soluble vitamins		
Vitamin C (mg)	60	60
Folic acid (μg)	400	400
Niacin (mg NE)[e]	16	13
Riboflavin (mg)	1.4	1.2
Thiamin (mg)	1.2	1.0
Vitamin B_6 (mg)	2.2	2.0
Vitamin B_{12} (μg)	3.0	3.0
Minerals		
Calcium (mg)	800	800
Phosphorous (mg)	800	800
Iodine (μg)	150	150
Magnesium (mg)	350	300
Zinc (mg)	15	15
Safe and adequate intakes		
Vitamin K (μg)	70–140	
Biotin (μg)	100–200	
Pantothenic acid (mg)	4–7	
Copper (mg)	2.0–3.0	
Manganese (mg)	2.5–5.0	
Fluoride (mg)	1.5–4.0	
Chromium (mg)	0.05–0.2	
Selenium (mg)	0.05–0.2	
Molybdenum (mg)	0.15–0.5	
Sodium (mg)	1100–3300	
Potassium (mg)	1875–5625	
Chloride (mg)	1700–5100	

[a] These intakes are designed to be sufficient for the maintenance of good nutrition in practically all *healthy* persons. Diets should be based on a variety of common foods to provide other nutrients for which human requirements have been less well defined. Further details regarding these allowances are described in *Recommended Dietary Allowances* (9th ed.). Food and Nutrition Board, National Research Council, National Academy of Sciences, Washington, D.C., 1980.
[b] Retinol equivalents; RE = 1 μg retinol or 6 μg carotene.
[c] As cholecalciferol; 10 μg = 400 IU vitamin D.
[d] α-tocopherol equivalent; 1 mg D-α-tocopherol = 1 α-TE.
[e] One niacin equivalent (NE) is equal to 1 mg niacin or 60 mg tryptophan.
SOURCE: From E. A. Young (ed.). *Nutrition, Aging and Health.* New York: Liss, 1986.

TABLE 8-2. *Agent, host, and environmental factors that influence nutrient and nutritional status in the elderly*

Agent (dietary) factors
  Chemical form of nutrient
  Energy intake
  Food processing and preparation (may increase or decrease dietary needs)
  Effect of other dietary constituents
Host factors
  Old age
  Sex
  Genetic makeup
  Pathologic states
    Drugs
    Infection
    Physical trauma
    Chronic disease, cancer
Environmental factors
  Physical (unsuitable housing, inadequate heating)
  Biologic (poor sanitary conditions)
  Socioeconomic (poverty, dietary habits and food choices, physical activity)

SOURCE: V. R. Young. Diet and Nutrient Needs in Old Age. In J. A. Behnke, C. E. Finch, and G. B. Moment (eds.), *The Biology of Aging.* New York: Plenum, 1978.

These are listed in Table 8-2 according to host, environmental, and agent (dietary) factors [10]. The importance of these factors, interacting in complex ways, for different individuals makes a definition of the quantitative nutrient requirements of the elderly individual a difficult task.

Not everyone of the same age, body build, and sex has the same requirement; these differences may be due in part to variations in genetic background. In relation to practical human nutrition, it is generally thought that the effects of various environmental, physiologic, psychologic, and pathologic influences are of greater importance in determining variability in nutrient needs among individuals. For example, the growing infant or child requires higher nutrient intakes per unit of body weight than does the young adult. Therefore, nutrient needs are relatively high during the early growth and developmental phase of life, declining as adulthood is approached. However, other than for energy, for which the daily requirement declines due to lowered physical activity, it is uncertain whether the requirements for essential nutrients change in the healthy individual with the progression of the adult years. On the basis of quite limited knowledge, the nutrient needs in healthy aged subjects do not appear to differ significantly from those of young adults. Nevertheless, a characteristic of aging is increased disease incidence and morbidity, and these are conditions that appear to be far more important than age per se in determining practical differences between young adults and elderly people in their need for nutrients.

Numerous dietary factors determine the amounts of a particular nutrient sufficient to meet the body's needs. For example, all forms of dietary iron are not equally available, and the type of diet and composition of individual meals influence the availability of the iron consumed. Another factor of particular importance in our considerations of diet and nutrient needs during old age is the effect of stressful stimuli, such as those arising from infection or physical trauma or even those of psychological origin. Thus, early in an infectious episode there is an increased rate of synthesis of immunoglobulins and other proteins. This stage is followed by a net catabolic response that results in increased losses of body nitrogen and of some vitamins and minerals and in decreases in blood levels of these nutrients. Furthermore, acute or chronic gastrointestinal infection may interfere with absorption of nutrients. The net result is depletion of body nutrients followed by a physiologic increase in the need for nutrients during the recovery phase to promote recovery and to compensate for the earlier losses. However, although it is appreciated that acute and chronic infections and other stressful stimuli, including anxiety, pain, and physical trauma, generally increase the requirements for many essential nutrients, there are inadequate quantitative data to help determine how much nutrient intakes should be increased to meet the additional demands created by these conditions, which may be frequent in elderly people.

Finally, various drugs may have profound effects on nutrient requirements by decreasing nutrient absorption or by altering the utilization of nutrients (Table 8-3). The effects of drugs on nutrient requirements depend on the dose and period of administration; furthermore, multiple administration of drugs may have synergistic effects, thus increasing nutrient needs further. Reduced appetite is a frequent consequence of drug therapy and will exaggerate the effects of drug treatment on the individual's nutritional

TABLE 8-3. *Drugs that may induce nutrient deficiency*

TYPE OF DRUG	EXAMPLES	NUTRIENTS AFFECTED
Antibiotics	Neomycin	Protein, fat, calcium
Anticonvulsants and sedatives	Diphenylhydantoin Phenobarbital Glutethimide Diphosphonates	Vitamins D and K Folic acid, calcium
Antiinflammatory agent	Phenylbutazone	Folic acid
Antitubercular agent	Isoniazid	Vitamin B_6, niacin
Chelating agents	D-Penicillamine EDTA	Iron, calcium, magnesium, zinc, copper
Cholestyramine		Fat-soluble vitamins, iron, vitamin B_{12}
Corticosteroids	Prednisone Cortisone	Vitamin D, ascorbic acid, vitamin B_6
Diuretics	Chlorthiazide	Potassium, magnesium
Estrogens	Ethinyl estradiol Mestranol Conjugated estrogens	Vitamin B_6, folic acid
Ethanol		Thiamine, vitamin B_6, folic acid, magnesium, zinc, protein
Mineral oil		Fat-soluble vitamins

SOURCE: R. E. Shank. Nutrition Principles. In R. Andres, E. L. Bierman, and W. R. Hazzard (eds.), *Principles of Geriatric Medicine.* New York: McGraw-Hill, 1985.

status, particularly if the diet is marginal in adequacy to begin with. Mention of alcohol (ethanol) might be made here because nutritional deficiency is often seen in alcoholics. Although it is due in part to an inadequate diet, ethanol interferes with the absorption and/or utilization of various nutrients, thereby effecting higher nutrient needs than those required by healthy individuals.

SPECIFIC CONSIDERATION OF DIET AND NUTRIENT REQUIREMENTS IN THE AGED

A broad range of conditions that accompany old age may have important effects on the nutritional status of the elderly. A listing of such factors is given in Table 8-4 [11].

Physical and mental disabilities affect a person's mode of living, which in turn may lead to

TABLE 8-4. *Factors that may lead to inadequate nutrition in the elderly*

Depression
Loneliness, psychological problems
Physical disability: immobility at home, poor vision, arthritis
Disease: infection, cancer, and other chronic illnesses
Malabsorptive and gastrointestinal disorders and discomfort
Poverty
Mental deterioration
Inadequate knowledge of dietetic principles: food fads, poor dietary habits
Alcoholism
Medications
Increased requirements

SOURCE: Adapted from A. N. Exton-Smith. Nutritional Problems of Elderly Populations. In W. W. Hawkins (ed.), *Nutrition of the Aged.* Quebec: Nutrition Society of Canada, 1978.

changes in dietary pattern and a deterioration of nutritional status. Underlying medical problems, emotional disturbances, loneliness, and poverty are all factors that may reduce the desire or ability to consume an adequate, well-balanced diet, and these are common causes for inadequate nutrition in elderly people. Energy requirements are reduced with inactivity, and adequate intake of other essential nutrients may not be met without a change in the dietary pattern toward foods of increased nutrient density. This problem may be compounded by the decrease in taste sensitivity that occurs with old age, and the poor health of the oral tissues that may restrict selection of foods to those that are bland, soft, and readily masticated. The net result is a further worsening of the condition of the oral tissues and an increase in the intensity of the vicious cycle leading to nutrient depletion, one that produces a reduced capacity to respond favorably to infection and disease, which in turn produces a gradual deterioration in health.

Vulnerable groups of old people therefore must be identified, and a means must be developed for improving nutrient intakes. Only a small percentage of the elderly population may be affected, and many elderly individuals will never experience nutritional deficiencies. However, with the increasing numbers of elderly persons in our society, a small percentage translates into many lives.

The following sections briefly review specific areas of nutrient requirements and metabolism.

Energy Metabolism and Utilization
BASAL ENERGY EXPENDITURE

Daily energy expenditure is the sum of basal energy metabolism, a small loss composed of the heat increment after food ingestion and that associated with physical activity. Basal or resting energy metabolism represents the combustion of substrates required to meet the energy needs of the metabolic processes involved in maintaining cell function and integrity and the mechanical processes necessary for survival. Synthetic processes (protein, nucleic acid, lipid, and urea synthesis, and gluconeogenesis), transport processes (including the pumping of ions to maintain ion gradients within cells and organelles), and mechanical processes (involving muscular activity) all require energy inputs. These are obtained from high-phosphate compounds such as adenosine triphosphatase (ATP) and guanosine triphosphate (GTP) that are generated during the oxidation of energy-yielding substrates. Various nutritional, physiologic, and pathologic factors alter the activities of these processes and the types and sources of substrate used for supplying their energy needs.

The basal metabolic rate (BMR) falls with increasing adult age. This decline appears to be due to the loss of cell mass rather than to a reduction in the metabolic activity of body tissues, since there is little decline in basal metabolic rate when the latter is expressed per unit of body cell mass [13]. However, because of the importance of the brain, liver, and muscle in total body energy metabolism, it is to be expected that alterations in the relative mass of these organs will lead to differences in the contribution made by each of them to total body energy expenditure during advancing adult age.

In support of this, Tzankoff and Norris [14, 15] examined the relationships between basal oxygen consumption and creatinine excretion, the latter as an index of muscle mass, in adults of varying ages. They observed an age-dependent linear relation between basal oxygen and creatinine excretion and calculated the contribution made by nonmuscle tissue to basal oxygen con-

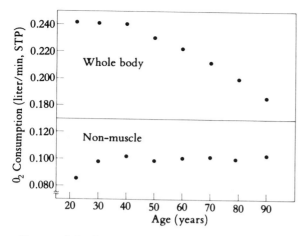

FIGURE 8-2. *An estimate of the age-related changes in oxygen consumption by the skeletal muscles and nonmusculature tissues in men at various stages of adult life. STP-standard temperature and pressure. (From S. P. Tzankoff and A. H. Norris. Effect of muscle mass decrease on age-related BMR changes.* J. Appl. Physiol. *43:1001, 1977.)*

TABLE 8-5. *Estimated mean energy intakes necessary for healthy men and women in the United States*

AGE (YEARS)	WEIGHT (KG)	HEIGHT (CM)	ENERGY NEEDS (MEAN)	KCAL (RANGE)
Men
25–50	70	178	2700	2300–3100
51–75	70	178	2400	2000–2800
76+	70	178	2050	1650–2450
Women
23–50	55	163	2000	1600–2400
51–75	55	163	1800	1400–2200
76+	55	163	1600	1200–2000

SOURCE: Food and Nutrition Board, National Research Council, National Academy of Sciences. *Recommended Dietary Allowances* (9th ed.). Washington, D.C.: U.S. Government Printing Office, 1980.

sumption. As shown in Figure 8-2, nonmuscle consumption showed no age-related changes, indicating that the loss of muscle mass may be responsible for the age-related decrease in BMR.

Table 8-5 offers a guide for estimating energy needs for males and females of various ages who are relatively inactive. The figures represent the estimated mean energy intakes necessary for healthy men and women of different ages in the United States. A totally sedentary or bedridden person may require fewer calories, whereas the very active may need additional calories.

FUEL SOURCES

The major sources of energy in mammalian tissues are glucose, fatty acids, ketone bodies, amino acids, and lactate. The pattern of fuel sources changes markedly if food is withheld for longer than the usual overnight fast [16]. Hence, for a fast that lasts for two or three days or longer, glucose oxidation is decreased, as is gluconeogenesis. In parallel with the diminished glucose metabolism, mobilization of triglycerides from adipose tissue and utilization of fatty acids in peripheral tissues, particularly muscle, are increased, and the brain utilizes ketone bodies as its principal fuel source if the fast is continued. This pattern of change in fuel utilization during short- and long-term fasts is accompanied by alterations in substrate availability and hormonal balance and is achieved, in part, by the regulatory effects of ketone bodies on protein turnover and amino acid oxidation in peripheral tissues. Whether individuals maintain a capacity similar to that characteristic of young adults to effectively bring about these changes in the pattern of fuel utilization when dietary energy intake is reduced is not clear.

LIPIDS

Lipids contribute a significant proportion of the total dietary energy intake. There is a specific need for essential fatty acids, which are involved in the maintenance of membrane composition, fluidity, and function and also serve as precursors of a class of "local" hormones, the prostaglandins and thromboxanes. These hormones have diverse actions involving, for example, gastric secretion, blood platelet function, and nervous system activity.

Most available data on changes in lipid metabolism and utilization during aging are derived from studies in experimental animals. Investigations in humans are less extensive, and most have been concerned with measurement of blood lipid levels. These studies are often cross-sectional, and since elevated levels of certain lipid moieties are risk factors for death from cardiovascular disease, the elderly may be viewed as "survivors" and thus represent a selected group. Even longitudinal studies may be difficult to interpret in view of the marked secular changes in diet and exercise that have occurred during the past several decades. Nonetheless, presently available data indicate that the circulating levels of low-density lipoproteins, which are associated with increased risk of atherosclerosis, increase with age, whereas levels of high-density lipoproteins, which appear to offer protection against atherosclerosis, do not change with age. Alteration of lipid levels by diet, exercise, weight reduction, or administration of medications is of uncertain value in the elderly and seems particularly out of place in the very old. Thus, the appropriate management of the patient with abnormal circulating lipoprotein levels must take into account the patient's age, capacity to comply with the recommended regimens, and likelihood of benefit.

Since adipose-tissue lipids serve as an important source of fuel, the effects of aging on the capacity for mobilization of fatty acids from these depots are of interest. In the rat there is a reduction in hormone-stimulated fat mobilization with progressive aging, and this may be the case in humans as well [17]. Whether this implies a diminished capacity in the aged individual to adapt successfully to a deficient energy intake remains to be determined and is clinically relevant in view of the increased frequency of periods of short- and longer-term food restriction in the aged due to infectious episodes, physical trauma, and psychological stress. However, initial studies [18] indicate that, at least during a brief fast lasting for two or three days, there is no impairment in the mobilization of triglyceride from adipose tissue in healthy elderly subjects. The possible impact of superimposed infection or other stressful stimuli on the mobilization of energy from the adipose reserves in elderly compared with young adult subjects must now be explored in view of the fact that fasting is often associated with such stressful conditions.

Because of its high caloric density (9 cal/gm), fat may in certain situations serve as a useful tool in the management of elderly patients who are emaciated from disease or injuries. The large number of fat calories packed into small volumes of nutrient supplements may assist in the rapid rehabilitation of elderly persons, who frequently have difficulty managing large volumes of nourishment.

In general, the aged tend to consume a higher percentage of their food intake as fat (42.8 percent for males and 38.1 percent for females) than is recommended by the Food and Nutrition Board [12]. There are, however, no studies addressing the effect of different long-term diets on mortality and morbidity in the elderly. Clearly, further work needs to be done to determine the optimal intake of fat in the aging population.

PROTEINS

Alterations in energy balance and in fuel metabolism have important consequences for body and tissue protein metabolism and vice versa. Changes in the rate of tissue and organ protein synthesis will lead to alterations in substrate need, particularly because whole-body protein synthesis is thought to account for a significant proportion of basal energy utilization. Skeletal muscles account for about 30 percent of whole-body protein breakdown in young adult men and for about 20 percent in elderly men.

Most studies of the metabolism of individual proteins in human subjects have focused on albumin. A low plasma albumin level is a frequent finding (in the absence of nephrosis and liver disease) in nutritional surveys among the elderly. In a recent study it was reported that albumin synthesis in older subjects is regulated at a lower set-point than in healthy young adults [19], which suggests that the response of albumin metabolism to nutritional repletion in older subjects may differ from that in young adults.

The need for dietary protein has two components—essential (indispensable) amino acids and a utilizable nontoxic source of nitrogen (nonspecific)—for synthesis of the nonessential (dispensable) amino acids. The major quantitative function of dietary protein in the adult is to furnish substrate for maintenance of tissue and organ protein synthesis. In addition, amino acids participate in the synthesis of the purine and pyrimidine moieties of nucleic acids and in the formation of neurotransmitters and other metabolically active molecules such as porphyrins, creatinine, and peptide hormones.

Response of Nitrogen Metabolism to Altered Protein Intake

Body nitrogen losses, after adaptation to a brief period of very low or protein-free feeding (obligatory nitrogen losses), in elderly men are essentially the same as those in young men. However, when expressed per unit of creatinine excretion or per unit of body cell mass, obligatory urinary nitrogen losses are apparently higher in the elderly [21]. These differences in nitrogen output parallel those seen in rates of whole-body protein breakdown (and synthesis) with aging, implying a relationship between whole-body protein turnover and obligatory nitrogen losses.

The effect of aging on nitrogen metabolism may also be examined by comparing the response of nitrogen metabolism in young adults and elderly subjects given differing protein intakes within a submaintenance range of nitrogen intake. Such studies indicate that the mean nitrogen intake necessary to maintain body nitrogen balance in the elderly is greater than 120 mg nitrogen per kilogram per day for women and 110 mg nitrogen per kilogram per day for men. The nitrogen balance response pattern for elderly subjects is similar in qualitative terms to that observed for healthy young adults. Comparisons suggest that the efficiency of dietary nitrogen utilization for maintenance of nitrogen equilibrium might be less in quantitative terms for older subjects [21].

CARBOHYDRATES

Carbohydrate intake provides a ready source of energy to support cellular activities. Excess ingested carbohydrates are easily converted to triglyceride for energy storage in fat deposits.

The influence of age on carbohydrate metabolism is discussed in detail in Chapter 28. In brief, advancing age is associated with slight increases in fasting glucose levels and substantial increases in postprandial glucose levels. These decreases in glucose tolerance are sufficiently consistent to require use of age-related adjusted criteria for the diagnosis of chemical diabetes. Present data indicate that resistance to the effect of insulin on peripheral tissues is the primary physiologic abnormality underlying age-related carbohydrate intolerance.

VITAMIN AND MINERAL METABOLISM

The effects of human aging per se on the utilization of vitamins and minerals remain largely unexplored. The major problems of osteoporosis and of calcium and vitamin D metabolism in relation to human aging are discussed in Chapter 29. B-complex vitamins serve as cofactors and coenzymes in many of the enzyme systems involved in carbohydrate, lipid, protein, and nucleic acid metabolism. Other vitamins, particularly the lipid-soluble vitamins, fulfill specific functions of key metabolic importance such as the glycosylation of proteins (vitamin A), calcium transport and utilization (vitamin D), prothrombin production (vitamin K), and antioxidation (vitamin E). Assessment of overall vitamin nutrition in the elderly population is difficult and complex. There are few controlled and comprehensive studies in humans related to micronutrient metabolism. Although adult age may influence the plasma levels of some vitamins, such as vitamin B_6 and vitamin C, interpretation of the biochemical, physiologic, and nutritional significance of such findings is difficult at present. The following sections briefly review current knowledge and recommendations for vitamins and minerals for the elderly population.

Calcium and Phosphorus

Calcium and phosphorus metabolism and its relationship to human aging are extensively discussed in Chapters 28 and 29.

Magnesium

Magnesium is found in most foods, vegetables being relatively rich sources. It is an essential component of many enzymes and plays a role in maintaining electrical potential in nerves and muscle membranes. Deficiency rarely occurs as a consequence of inadequate dietary intake but is seen not infrequently in elderly persons who are alcoholic, have disorders producing increased intestinal losses and/or malabsorption, or take medications causing increased losses (e.g., diuretics). Recently, magnesium depletion has been implicated in aggravating potassium depletion and interfering with potassium repletion [22]. The RDA is 350 mg per day for men and 300 mg for women. It is likely that many older persons with limited appetite and poor food intake are more likely than younger adults to deplete stores of exchangeable magnesium and manifest deficiency if chronic illness intervenes.

Trace Elements

The RDAs include levels of daily intakes required for iron, zinc, and iodine, but copper, manganese, fluoride, chromium, selenium, and molybdenum are also required. Table 8-1 lists safe and adequate intakes for each of these. Other minerals, such as cobalt, nickel, vanadium, and silicon, might be listed, but requirements for these in humans, particularly the elderly, have not been established. Three of the trace minerals—iron, zinc, and selenium—deserve some comment in relation to the nutrient needs and health of older persons.

IRON

The RDA for iron in elderly men and women has been set at 10 mg. The reduced food intake and changes in the gastrointestinal tract that are commonly associated with aging may affect the availability and absorption of food iron. Although a number of studies have found altered iron absorption in the elderly, recent better controlled studies suggest that heme iron and absorption of ferrous sulfate are unaffected by aging [23]. Iron turnover studies suggest that iron loss is either the same or slightly decreased in the elderly compared with the young. Practically speaking, advantage should be taken of the factors known to enhance iron absorption (e.g., the heme iron component of meats and other foods of animal origin is more completely absorbed than the nonheme iron in vegetables and cereals, and the presence of ascorbic acid in a feeding will increase the utilization of nonheme iron).

ZINC

Zinc deficiency in humans may lead to anorexia, impaired immune function, poor wound healing, and possible altered taste acuity. The RDA for zinc is 15 mg, a quantity greater than that found in the diet of many older persons [24]. Studies suggest that zinc levels decline with age [25], possibly as the result of chronic, longterm marginal zinc intake. Marginal zinc levels may be further aggravated by illnesses resulting in excessive losses (e.g., diabetes mellitus, alcoholism, intestinal malabsorption). The zinc present in animal foods is more fully absorbed than that in vegetable sources. Furthermore, dietary fiber and phytates may impair zinc absorption. Since an antagonism between zinc and copper in experimental animals has been proposed, increases in dietary zinc should not be prescribed without consideration of the intake of copper.

SELENIUM

Selenium is an essential component of one mammalian enzyme, glutathione peroxidase. Part of its potential relationship to aging may be inferred from its ability, like that of vitamin E, to inhibit lipid peroxidation. Selenium and selenium-containing amino acids appear to function in decomposing hydrogen peroxides and scavenging free radicals, thus maintaining the stability of lipid-containing biologic membranes [26]. The correlation between glutathione peroxidase activity and selenium concentrations in erythrocytes is high; and some studies suggest that the elderly have lower selenium levels and glutathione peroxidase activity than the young. However, further investigation is warranted to determine the relationship between selenium intake and biologic aging.

VITAMINS

Suter and Russell recently reviewed vitamin requirements of the elderly [27], and a brief summary is provided here. RDAs for vitamins were established for adults in two age categories: 25 to 50 years and 51 years and over. It is uncertain, however, that the nutrient needs of a 25-year-old are the same as those of a 50-year-old or that the needs of a 51-year-old are the same as those for a 90-year-old. Clearly, more knowledge needs to be acquired before linkages between specific nutrients and chronic disease patterns can be established, especially in regard to vitamin nutrition in the elderly.

Fat-Soluble Vitamins

VITAMIN A

From the point of view of elderly persons, the main functions of vitamin A are its role in dark adaptation, maintenance of epithelial integrity, and hemoglobin synthesis. A significant decline in light threshold with aging has been demonstrated; however, this does not correlate with serum vitamin A levels and is not changed by vitamin A administration. Similarly, follicular hyperkeratosis, a classic sign of vitamin A deficiency, is often seen in elderly subjects, but it appears to be due more commonly to poor hygiene than to vitamin A deficiency in this group [28]. There is no evidence that plasma concentrations of vitamin A or its absorption is affected by aging [27]. Vitamin A deficiency does occur with increased frequency among alcoholics and in those with chronic gastrointestinal disorders, and a small percentage of elderly institutionalized patients were deficient in vitamin A. Furthermore, a number of drugs including mineral oil, neomycin, and cholestyramine may interfere with vitamin A absorption.

Vitamin A exists in foods as retinol, the preformed vitamin, or as carotene, which as provitamin A is converted to retinol during or after absorption in the intestinal mucosa. An amount of 0.3 µg retinol represents one international unit (IU) of vitamin A activity. Retinol is found in animal food products, especially in liver and dairy products, whereas carotenes occur in vegetables and fruits, especially those that are dark green or yellow in color. Carotenoids are not completely absorbed or fully converted to retinol; their biologic activity is only from one-sixth to one-twelfth that of the preformed vitamin. The typical American diet contains about equal proportions of vitamin A activity derived from retinol and from carotenoids. The RDA is 1,000 µg retinol for men and 800 µg for women.

Vitamin A deficiency is manifest by night blindness, xerophthalmia, and dry, hyperkeratotic skin. Infectious diseases and febrile episodes can cause rapid loss of hepatic stores, the liver being the primary organ of storage; diarrheal disease or other pathologic processes causing intestinal malabsorption may also result in hypovitaminosis A.

It has been suggested that vitamin A and its precursor, carotene, may be protective against cancer. In addition, vitamin A and other retinoids have been tested as cancer chemotherapeutic agents. These findings have led to great enthusiasm among health faddists and others for "prophylactic" consumption of megadoses of vitamin A. Vitamin A is the second most commonly used nutritional supplement. In contrast to the rarity of symptoms of vitamin A deficiency in the elderly, vitamin A toxicity is seen more commonly. Symptoms of hypervitaminosis A, which may occur after long-term ingestion of doses of 50,000 IU or more a day, includes headaches, liver dysfunction, leukopenia, general malaise, loss of hair, and hypercalcemia [29]. Carotene is also available as a "health" pill, and patients ingesting excessive doses of this nutrient may present with yellow discoloration of the skin.

Vitamin E

Dietary sources of vitamin E include vegetable oils, margarine, whole-grain cereals, fruits, and vegetables. Deficiency is a rare occurrence in clinical experience. The RDA is 8 mg delta-alpha-tocopherol daily for older women and 10 mg for older men. There is little or no evidence from clinical trials to support the frequently reported claims that ingestion of large supplements of vitamin E will prevent or modify the course of heart disease.

Vitamin K

The fat-soluble vitamin K (phylloquinone) is necessary for the maintenance of normal prothrombin activity as well as clotting factors VIII, IX, X, and possibly V. Vitamin K is present in most vegetables, particularly green leafy vegetables. Intestinal bacteria produce another form of the vitamin, K_2. Both forms are converted to menadione in the intestine prior to absorption. Deficiency is likely to occur when disease interferes with fat absorption or following long-term use of antibacterial drugs. A recommended allowance is not given for vitamin K; however, the requirement appears to be in the range of 1 to 2 µg per kilogram of body weight per day.

Water-Soluble Vitamins

As noted earlier, socioeconomic, educational, and disease factors among the elderly are also the principal causes of water-soluble vitamin deficiency. However, water-soluble vitamin deficiency problems among the elderly have no proven relation to biologic aging per se. Obtaining valid documentation of the influence of water-soluble vitamin supplementation is virtually impossible, and hence, many older Americans may be spending their scarce financial resources for water-soluble vitamin supplements for which there is no scientific or medical benefit. However, improper meal preparation practices may result in loss of labile vitamins (as well as minerals and trace elements), which, when compounded by decreased food intake and possible nutrient-drug interactions, may indeed lead to clinically manifest water-soluble vitamin deficiency syndromes.

VITAMIN B$_{12}$

Except for totally vegetarian diets, the usual patterns of food intake in the United States afford a sufficiency of vitamin B$_{12}$. The RDA is 3 μg. Deficiency is almost always due to malabsorption caused by lack of the specific binding glycoprotein, intrinsic factor. Vitamin B$_{12}$ and other cobalt-containing compounds, cobalamines, which have vitamin B$_{12}$ activity, serve as coenzymes in the methylation of homocysteine to form methionine, the regeneration of folate from 5-methyltetrahydrofolate, the synthesis of succinyl coenzyme A, and the formation of amino acids and fatty acids.

Pernicious anemia is both a cause and a manifestation of vitamin B$_{12}$ deficiency. The megaloblastic changes in the bone marrow and blood respond promptly to parenteral administration of cyanocobalamin in appropriate doses, but neurologic manifestations are not as readily nor as fully corrected. Once begun, vitamin B$_{12}$ therapy must be continued throughout the life of the patient. Many drugs, such as alcohol, neomycin, colchicine, cholestyramine, and clindamycin, can interfere with B$_{12}$ absorption and metabolism.

VITAMIN C

Vitamin C, or ascorbic acid, plays a role in the synthesis of collagen and a variety of other functions. The 1980 RDA for adults is 60 mg per day for both sexes. When a dietary source is lacking, perifollicular and gingival hemorrhage occur, and wound healing and resistance to infection may be impaired. The full-blown deficiency state is scurvy.

Citrus fruits are the richest sources of vitamin

C, but other fruits, potatoes, and vegetables also contribute. Older persons who may depend on reconstituted juices should be aware that vitamin C is rapidly oxidized and loses much of its activity within a day or two of storage in the refrigerator.

Recent articles in the news media have proclaimed the usefulness of large supplements of vitamin C in the prevention and treatment of upper respiratory infections and for other health benefits. There is little experimental evidence to support these claims. Both Chalmers [30] and Sauberlich [31] in their reviews concluded that megadoses of vitamin C were worth neither the effort nor the risk. The risks of megadoses of vitamin C include rebound scurvy when high doses of ascorbic acid are reduced to the RDA, reduced vitamin B$_{12}$ absorption, false-negative fecal occult blood results leading to delayed detection and possibly erroneous management of the pathology involved, oxalic acid renal calculi, hemolytic anemia in patients with glucose 6-phosphate dehydrogenase deficiency, and excessive absorption of dietary iron. Despite the fact that the RDA is only 60 mg, vitamin C is the dietary supplement most frequently used by the elderly.

There is no direct evidence for altered vitamin C absorption with age, and age trends in tissue vitamin C levels are inconsistent. Hence, at present megadoses of vitamin C seem unwarranted and may be accompanied by significant health hazards.

FOLATE

The principal functions of folate and related compounds are their use as coenzymes in the transport of single carbon atoms. Therefore, folate is essential for the synthesis of nucleic acids and for the metabolism of certain amino acids. Deficiency leads to impaired cell division and protein synthesis. The major clinical manifestation is megaloblastic anemia, which must be differentiated from vitamin B$_{12}$ deficiency.

The 1980 RDA is 400 μg per day for adults. Folate is found in many foods, especially liver, leafy vegetables, fruits, and yeast. There are no consistently demonstrated age-related changes in folate metabolism or absorption. Deficiency often results from intestinal malabsorption or excessive alcohol intake. Drugs that inhibit

DNA synthesis (e.g., 5-fluorouracil, methotrexate) are folate antagonists, and others may interfere with absorption (e.g, Dilantin and neomycin).

VITAMIN B_6

Vitamin B_6, a collective term for pyridoxine, pyridoxal, and pyridoxamine, is widely distributed in food but is sensitive to heat and ultraviolet light. Good sources are liver, meats, fish, and whole-grain cereals. In the form of pyridoxal phosphate, it functions as a coenzyme in various aspects of amino acid and protein metabolism. Requirements vary directly with levels of protein intake. The RDA is 2.2 mg for male adults and 2.0 mg for females. Despite evidence from human and animal studies for age-related changes in vitamin B_6 metabolism, there are presently insufficient data to suggest an alteration in the B_6 RDA with age [27].

Certain drugs have an important influence in vitamin B_6 status. Deficiency occurs in 20 to 30 percent of alcoholics. Isoniazid increases urinary excretion. Cycloserine and hydralazine are B_6 antagonists. Finally, provision of B_6 supplements to patients with parkinsonism treated with levodopa reduces the effectiveness of this therapy and should be avoided.

THIAMIN

The 1980 RDA for thiamin for the elderly is 1.2 mg per day for males and 1.0 mg per day for females. Thiamin (vitamin B_1) as the pyrophosphate serves as a coenzyme in a number of metabolic reactions, specifically in the oxidative decarboxylation of alphaketoacids and in transketolase activity in the pentose-phosphate pathway. Whole-grain cereals and enriched bread are good sources of thiamin. Temperatures above $100°C$ cause substantial destruction of the vitamin in foods. Requirements are limited to the quantity of carbohydrate and/or food calories consumed. The RDA is 0.5 mg per 1000 kcal. Alcoholism is a major cause of deficiency in the elderly.

RIBOFLAVIN

Vitamin B_2, or riboflavin, functions as the prosthetic group of flavoproteins, which have vital roles in biologic oxidation. The most important sources are milk and other dairy products, organ meats (liver, heart, and kidney), whole-grain products, eggs, and green, leafy vegetables. Vitamin B_2 is heat stable but is destroyed by exposure to light. The RDA is 0.6 mg riboflavin per 1000 kcal and a minimum intake of 1.2 mg daily, implying that older persons with calorie intakes of less than 2000 kcal should make special efforts to ensure adequate intake.

Deficiency of riboflavin rarely occurs alone or without evidence of other B vitamin defects. In the elderly, the most likely cause of deficiency is low intakes. There is no proven evidence of altered riboflavin absorption with age. Clinical signs of riboflavin deficiency are not pathognomonic (e.g., angular stomatitis, chelosis, glossitis, and seborrheic dermatitis) and may occur with other nutrient deficiencies. Hence, it is advisable to provide therapeutic amounts not only of riboflavin but also of iron and other water-soluble vitamins if deficiency is suspected. Biochemical evidence of deficiency is achieved when glutathione reductase activity of erythrocytes is reduced and the activity of the enzyme is stimulated when flavin adenine dinucleotide (FAD) is added to the test system.

NIACIN

Niacin activity exists in foods as nicotinic acid or nicotinamide and functions as a coenzyme in a number of key metabolic reactions such as tissue respiration processes, glycolysis, and fat synthesis. Important food sources include enriched breads and cereals, peas, beans, nuts, meats, fish, and liver. Niacin is relatively stable and is influenced little by storage or cooking of foods.

A portion of the human requirement for niacin is met by synthesis from the essential amino acid tryptophan. In usual diets, about 50 percent of niacin is provided as the preformed vitamin in foods and 50 percent as the precursor, tryptophan. As a general guide, most animal proteins contain 1.5 percent tryptophan, whereas vegetable proteins contain about 1 percent. The protein in corn is particularly low in tryptophan (0.6 percent).

The RDA for niacin takes into consideration the dual sources of the vitamin and are thus expressed as niacin equivalents. The RDA is related to energy intake and is estimated on a basis of 6.6 niacin equivalents per 1000 kcal.

Pellagra is the disorder produced by niacin deficiency; it may evolve in alcoholics or patients with chronic gastrointestinal disease resulting in absorptive defects. Nicotinic acid, but not nicotinamide, has the properties of a vasodilator and causes flushing of the skin and pruritus. Taken in large quantities, nicotinic acid may cause gastrointestinal distress and liver damage.

OTHER WATER-SOLUBLE VITAMINS

There is no established RDA for biotin, which is involved in the metabolism of fat and carbohydrate. Part of the requirement for biotin is met by the microflora of the intestine. Estimates of adequate intake range from 100 to 200 μg daily.

Pantothenic acid functions as a component of coenzyme A, which plays a role in many essential metabolic processes. It is present in most foods, and the usual daily intake is about 7 to 10 mg daily.

Both pantothenic acid and biotin are often included in vitamin supplements, but further data need to be gathered vis-à-vis the appropriateness of the 1980 safe and adequate intake recommendations for these nutrients, especially in the elderly.

Finally, many species of animals have a dietary requirement for choline, but evidence in humans is not yet definitive. Choline is consumed in the form of lecithin, which is present in many foods, particularly eggs, liver, soybeans, and peanuts. The average American diet provides approximately 300 mg daily. In addition, the human body has the capacity to synthesize choline. Investigation is now being conducted to determine the possible therapeutic role of choline supplements in memory disorders because choline is utilized in the synthesis of the neurotransmitter acetylcholine.

Summary

Although the majority of the elderly are not undernourished, they represent a vulnerable segment of the population. Their nutritional balance can be easily disturbed by illnesses, decreased mobility, or increased economic hardship. Hence, it is essential that health care providers pay attention to assessing the nutritional status of the elderly. If we are to reduce morbidity in the aged, thereby achieving associated reductions in recurrent hospitalization and institutionalization, it is essential in preventive medicine in the elderly to pay attention to nutritional needs.

References

1. Shank, R. E. Nutritional Characteristics of the Elderly: An Overview. In M. Rothstein and M. L. Sussman (eds.), *Nutrition, Longevity and Aging.* New York: Academic Press, 1976.
2. Finch, C. E., and Hayflick, L. (eds.). *Handbook of the Biology of Aging.* New York: Van Nostrand Reinhold, 1977.
3. Nordin, B. E. C., et al. Calcium and Bone Metabolism in Old Age. In. L. A. Carlson (ed.), *Nutrition in Old Age.* Uppsala, Sweden: Swedish Nutrition Foundation, 1972.
4. Korenchevsky, V. *Physiological and Pathological Ageing.* New York: Hafner, 1961.
5. Brozek, J. Changes in body composition in man during maturity and their nutritional implications. *Fed. Proc.* 11:784, 1985.
6. Sidney, K. H., et al. Endurance training and body composition of the elderly. *Am. J. Clin. Nutr.* 30:326, 1977.
7. Allen, G., et al. Total body potassium and gross body composition in relation to age. *J. Gerontol.* 15:348, 1960.
8. Rossman, J. The Anatomy of Aging. In J. Rossman (ed.), *Clinical Geriatrics* (2nd ed.). Philadelphia: Lippincott, 1979.
9. Frisancho, A. R. New standards of weight and body composition by frame size and height for assessment of nutritional status of adults and the elderly. *Am. J. Clin. Nutr.* 40:808, 1984.
10. Young, V. R. Diet and Nutrient Needs in Old Age. In J. A. Behnke, C. E. Finch, and G. B. Moment (eds.), *The Biology of Aging.* New York: Plenum Press, 1978.
11. Exton-Smith, A. N. Nutritional Problems of Elderly Populations. In W. W. Hawkins (ed.), *Nutrition of the Aged.* Quebec: Nutrition Society of Canada, 1978.
12. Food and Nutrition Board, National Research Council, National Academy of Sciences. *Recommended Dietary Allowances* (9th ed.). Washington, D.C.: U.S. Government Printing Office, 1980.
13. Shock, N. W. Energy Metabolism, Caloric Intake and Physical Activity of the Aging. In L. A. Carlson (ed.), *Nutrition in Old Age.* Uppsala, Sweden: Swedish Nutrition Foundation, 1972.

14. Tzankoff, S. P., et al. Effect of muscle mass decrease on age-related BMR changes. *J. Appl. Physiol.* 43:1001, 1977.
15. Tzankoff, S. P., et al. Longitudinal changes in basal metabolism in man. *J. Appl. Physiol.* 45:536, 1978.
16. Cahill, G. J. Starvation in man. *Clin. Endocrinol. Metab.* 5:397, 1976.
17. Masoro, E. J., et al. Nutritional probe of the aging process. *Fed. Proc.* 39:3178, 1980.
18. Klein, S., et al. Palmitate and glycerol kinetics during brief starvation in normal weight young adult and elderly subjects. *J. Clin. Invest.* 78:928, 1986.
19. Gersovitz, M., et al. Albumin synthesis in young and elderly subjects using a new stable isotope methodology: Response to level of protein intake. *Metabolism* 29:1075, 1980.
20. Briker, M. L., et al. A study of endogenous nitrogen output of college women, with particular reference to use of the creatinine output in the calculation of the biological values of the protein of egg and sunflower seed. *J. Nutr.* 44:553, 1951.
21. Uauy, R., et al. Human protein requirements: Nitrogen balance response to graded levels of egg protein in elderly men and women. *Am. J. Clin. Nutr.* 31:771, 1978.
22. Whang, R. Magnesium deficiency: Pathogenesis, prevalence, and clinical implications. *Am. J. Med.* 82 (Suppl. 3A):24, 1987.
23. Marx, J. J. M. Normal non-absorption and decreased red cell iron uptake in the aged. *Blood* 53:204, 1979.
24. Sandstead, H. H., et al. Zinc nutriture in the elderly in relation to taste acuity, immune response, and wound healing. *Am. J. Clin. Nutr.* 36:1046, 1982.
25. Morley, J. E. Nutritional status of the elderly. *Am. J. Med.* 81:679, 1986.
26. Tappel, A. L. Free radical lipid peroxidation damage and its inhibition by vitamin E and selenium. *Fed. Proc.* 24:73, 1965.
27. Suter, P. M., et al. Vitamin requirements of the elderly. *Am. J. Clin. Nutr.* 45:501, 1987.
28. Watkin, D. M. *Handbook of Nutrition, Health, and Aging.* Park Ridge, NJ: Noyes Publications, 1983.
29. Brin, M., et al. Some preliminary findings on the nutritional status of the aged in Onondaga County, New York. *Am. J. Clin. Nutr.* 17:240, 1965.
30. Chalmers, T. C. Effects of ascorbic acid on the common cold. An evaluation of the evidence. *Am. J. Med.* 58:532, 1975.
31. Sauberlich, H. E. Ascorbic Acid. In R. E. Olson (ed.), *Nutrition Reviews: Present Knowledge in Nutrition.* Washington, D.C.: Nutrition Foundation, 1984. P. 260.

Suggested Reading

Albanes, A. A. *Nutrition for the Elderly.* New York: Alan R. Liss, 1980.
Exton-Smith, A. N., et al. *Metabolic and Nutritional Disorders in the Elderly.* Bristol, England: John Wright & Sons, 1980.
Munro, H. N. Nutrition and ageing. *Br. Med. Bull.* 37:83, 1981.
Watkin, D. M. Nutrition for the Aging and Aged. In R. S. Goodhart and M. E. Shils (eds.), *Modern Nutrition in Health and Disease.* Philadelphia: Lea & Febiger, 1978.
Young, V. R., et al. Human Aging: Protein and Amino Acid Metabolism and Implications for Protein and Amino Acid Requirements. In G. B. Moment (ed.), *Nutritional Approaches to Aging Research.* Boca Raton, FL: CRC Press, 1982. Pp. 47–81.

9

Medications and the Elderly

Jerry Avorn

THE REMARKABLE PROGRESS in the last decade in fields ranging from molecular biology to clinical research has provided the health care system with an unprecedented armamentarium of powerful, effective new therapies for treating both the acute and chronic illnesses common in old age. However, these tools have proved to be a double-edged sword: Our increasing capacity to affect the most basic cellular mechanisms brings with it both the power to treat disease and the potential for important adverse effects, particularly in the elderly. The wise use of medications in this age group requires an intimate understanding of their mechanism of action coupled with an understanding of the changes in physiology that occur with aging. In addition, the increasing numbers, complexity, and cost of recently developed agents have given added importance to the nonpharmacologic aspects of their use. These nonpharmacologic aspects involve issues such as physician prescribing patterns, patient compliance, and policy-level issues associated with the development, testing, and reimbursement of our expanding arsenal of therapies.

This chapter begins by considering the physiologic aspects of geriatric pharmacology. Although the properties of specific agents for specific illnesses are considered in detail in the chapters addressing specific organ systems and conditions, this chapter addresses the use of medications in the elderly in general. The aging patient will be discussed in light of the absorption, distribution, metabolism, and excretion of medications (pharmacokinetics), and emerging insights into changes in the cellular response to various medications, partially determined by alterations in drug-receptor interactions (pharmacodynamics), are considered as well. The clinical effects of these changes will be discussed in light of the physiologic changes that occur in various organ systems with aging as well as the increased likelihood of drug-drug and drug-disease interactions in this age group. Specific attention will be given to the definition and detection of adverse drug effects in the elderly.

The psychosocial aspects of medication use are also of paramount importance in geriatrics. This chapter therefore also considers recent research on patterns of physician prescribing as well as compliance with therapeutic regimens by elderly patients. Persons over 65 consume nearly a third of all prescription medications, although they comprise only 12 percent of the population. Because of the physiologic changes noted above, the elderly are also at markedly greater risk of drug side effects. The final sections of this chapter therefore address the important policy issues that face the health care system and the individual clinician in relation to the development and testing of new medications to benefit the elderly, current approaches to post–marketing surveillance of medications for possible toxicity, and reimbursement for medications in a rapidly changing system of health care delivery and financing. Each section addresses the implications of current knowledge and recent research for the practicing clinician.

Pharmacology

PHARMACOKINETICS

Even in healthy elderly, the normal aging process creates important changes in many of the phenomena included under the heading of pharmacokinetics: absorption, distribution, metabolism, and excretion. Given the importance of these changes, which occur even in the absence of disease, the additional disordered physiology associated with specific disease states can create major perturbations in the actions of many commonly used drugs.

Absorption

A number of changes have been well documented in the aging gastrointestinal system: the increasing frequency of gastric achlorhydria, reduced gastric motility, and reduced blood flow to the splanchnic bed. However, these changes tend not to be of great importance in affecting the absorption of medications. The preponderance of evidence indicates that there is generally no clinically important reduction in drug absorption resulting from changes associated with normal aging. For a few agents, such as chlorazepate, which require acid hydrolysis in the stomach to be transformed into the metabolically active form, marked achlorhydria can result in a diminution of drug effect, but this is uncommon. Of course, like all patients, the elderly remain susceptible to problems of absorption associated with simultaneous ingestion of incompatible compounds, such as antacids taken concurrently with antibiotics that they can adsorb.

Distribution

One important consideration often given little attention in drug therapy of the elderly is the fact that the current cohort of elderly tend to be smaller in size than are younger cohorts. Although most of this is a secular effect associated with growing up earlier in the twentieth century rather than an aging effect, it is nonetheless an important difference that should be taken into consideration in calculating dosages of various medications for the elderly. Because this consideration is rarely made, the use of standard "adult" regimens in elderly patients actually results in an *increase* in milligram per kilogram administered to older patients [1].

Other changes affecting the distribution of drugs in the elderly do have a basis in age-related physiologic changes. In many species, including humans, there is a loss of skeletal muscle mass with advancing age, combined with an increase in fatty tissue. Thus, the percentage of total body weight that is lean body mass declines as the proportion of total body weight occupied by fat rises. These changes have important implications for drug distribution. The *volume of distribution* is a theoretical space occupied by a given compound in the body and depends on the solubility of that compound in water versus lipid spaces, among other factors. Thus, medications that are highly lipid soluble (such as the benzodiazepines) will have a higher volume of distribution in an elderly patient than in a comparable younger patient of the same weight. Conversely, medications that are primarily soluble in water (i.e., muscle) spaces, such as lithium, will have a smaller volume of distribution in a 70-kg, 80-year-old person than in a 70-kg, 30-year-old. Since the serum half-life of any drug is directly proportional to its volume of distribution in a given subject, an increase in volume of distribution will result in a prolongation of drug effect [2] (see below).

Many drugs exist in the circulation bound to serum proteins, often albumin. There is a small decrease in serum albumin concentration with advancing age (see Chap. 3), but this is usually modest and does not result in drug-binding changes of major clinical importance. However, important aberrations in drug effect can be seen with pathologically low levels of serum albumin, sometimes seen in malnourished or chronically ill elderly patients. When this occurs, binding of medications can be compromised, and the potential for toxicity can increase. It is also important to bear in mind that many serum drug levels measure the *total* concentration of drug per unit of serum volume, regardless of whether the drug is bound or unbound. Thus, a "normal" drug level in an older patient with inadequate protein binding can be falsely reassuring. (There are other reasons why "normal" serum drug levels can be misleading even in the absence of changes in serum proteins; these are discussed below.)

Metabolism

For many medications, metabolism in the liver is the main route of drug deactivation. Important changes have been found in the capacity of the liver to metabolize medications in old age. These changes are present in healthy elders, and the effect is of course greater in patients with primary or secondary hepatic dysfunction. Phase I metabolism appears to be the most impaired with advancing age. Phase I includes processes such as oxidation, hydroxylation, and phosphorylation. By contrast, there appears to be relative sparing of the phase II metabolic processes, such as conjugation (transformation of the substance into its sulfate, glucuronide, and so forth). This distinction is important in choosing among various available medications within a class, since those that require only conjugation will be metabolized and thus cleared more readily than those that require more complex forms of phase I metabolism by the aging liver [3].

In addition, the aging process is associated with a diminution in liver size and hepatic blood flow. As a result, those medications that have "first pass" metabolism as an important component of their clearance will have higher serum levels in older than in younger patients.

It is important to point out that although serum transaminases are commonly (and incorrectly) considered "liver function tests," normal transaminase levels in the blood do not indicate normal liver function, particularly in an elderly patient. Absence of elevation of these enzymes indicates simply that there is no ongoing destruction of hepatocytes, although the liver may or may not be adequately performing its metabolic functions. Even tests more properly considered measures of hepatic synthetic function, such as the prothrombin time, can be preserved in the face of loss of hepatic capacity to metabolize medications normally.

Excretion

For many compounds, excretion by the kidneys is the main route of elimination from the body. Here, too, there are important changes attributable to aging itself, which are exacerbated by any illness that decreases renal function further (see Chap. 18) [4]. Thus, for medications such as cimetidine or digoxin, whose main clearance is through the kidney, toxic levels can accumulate if account is not taken of this decrement in renal function that is so commonly seen in the elderly. Similarly, active metabolites produced in the liver may also depend on the kidney for excretion and will accumulate in the presence of reduced renal function.

As with hepatic function, it is inappropriate to assume normal renal function on the basis of commonly used laboratory tests. Patients with inadequate levels of protein (nitrogen) intake may not present an adequate urea load to the kidney to demonstrate an increase in the blood urea nitrogen (BUN); the same is true of patients with severe liver disease, who cannot metabolize the ingested protein to urea. Likewise, patients with markedly diminished muscle mass (as is common in the elderly) may not present enough of a creatinine load to the kidney to demonstrate its inability to clear this substance. Actual measurement of creatinine clearance is a much more reliable guide to renal function, but this somewhat cumbersome test is often considered impractical in many settings. A two- to four-hour timed urine sample may provide a reasonable estimate of renal function when a full 24-hour collection is not feasible.

Serum Half-Life

The serum half-life of a medication ($t_{1/2}$) is equal to the volume of distribution for that medication in a given individual (multiplied by a constant), divided by the clearance of that medication in that subject, generally through the liver and/or kidney:

$$t_{1/2} = \frac{V_d \times k}{Cl}$$

Thus, it can be seen from the above formula that a medication that has an increased volume of distribution in the elderly (such as any drug soluble in lipid tissues) will have a prolonged serum half-life in the elderly. The same will be true of any medication with diminished clearance because of hepatic or renal impairment. A medication that is both lipid soluble and has impaired clearance will have a particularly prolonged duration of action [5].

PHARMACODYNAMICS

Although the pharmacokinetic considerations described above form the basis of classic pharmacology, in recent years considerable progress has been made in the field of pharmacodynamics, which considers the effect of medications at the cellular level, apart from their absorption, distribution, metabolism, and excretion [6]. Insights from research in pharmacodynamics have produced findings that make the task of a clinician even more difficult. For at the same time that pharmacokinetic factors (such as impaired hepatic and renal function or changes in volume of distribution) are conspiring to create higher levels of drug that persist longer, for many commonly used agents receptors in the elderly are actually *more* sensitive to each molecule of drug than they are in the young. The mechanism of this is not well understood, but it appears that even if the wise clinician reduces the dose or the frequency of administration of a given medication to achieve the "ideal" level of drug in serum, such "normal" levels will produce a more intense drug effect in many end organs in the elderly. It should be noted that this increased receptor sensitivity will create an enhanced drug effect in target organs and nontarget organs alike. For example, receptors in the central nervous system are more sensitive to a number of agents in the elderly, even drugs whose "target" organs are not in the central nervous system. Thus, increased adverse effects as well as increased efficacy (or toxicity) in the target organs themselves can be expected in the aged because of these pharmacodynamic changes [7].

Conversely, for some medications there appears to be a decrease in receptor sensitivity with advancing age. These medications include the beta-adrenergic agents, both agonist and antagonist. Evidence indicates that higher doses of both isoproterenol and propranolol are needed in older patients to produce an acceleration or

deceleration of the heart [8]. It is not known why these receptors appear to lose sensitivity with aging while other receptors appear to gain in sensitivity.

CLINICAL CONSEQUENCES

The foregoing pharmacologic considerations have important consequences in clinical practice. First, they provide both a rationale and an added emphasis for the ubiquitous message that medications be kept to the minimum number necessary to treat important clinical problems. Understanding of the magnified drug effect seen in the elderly makes it clear why therapies that are not clearly indicated should be considered with great skepticism. It also underlines the wisdom of periodically reviewing each patient's medication regimen regularly (at least every six months) and making an ongoing attempt to eliminate any drugs that may not be making an important therapeutic contribution.

A very careful medication history is one of the simplest and yet most neglected aspects of the geriatric examination (see Chap. 3). Attention must also be paid to medications that the patient may have received from another physician or even from friends and family. The patient may be reluctant to discuss these, but no history is complete without a detailed inquiry into such "extracurricular" therapies. In addition, with the increasing trend for once-prescription medications to become available over-the-counter (diphenhydramine and ibuprofen are two important examples), a detailed inquiry into self-medication through this route must also be undertaken. The fact that some preparations are available without prescription creates the unfortunate misconception in the minds of many patients (and occasionally their physicians) that they are unlikely to produce toxicity, even in the elderly. However, because of the considerations noted above, it is quite possible for a patient to experience a wide variety of symptoms, often severe, related to such therapies. Of particular concern is the range of anticholinergic side effects (constipation, blurry vision, dry mouth, urinary retention, confusion) that can occur with the antihistamines that are ubiquitous in over-the-counter remedies for colds, allergic symptoms, and insomnia.

With time, many patients experience an accretion of medications to their regimen, much like the formation of coral on a reef. Since many of these may appear to be treating potentially dangerous conditions (such as the antiarrhythmics, anticonvulsants, or digoxin), the physician is often anxious about discontinuing them. This problem is particularly difficult in the absence of ongoing primary care, in which the original decision to begin a particular drug was made by another, presumably for a good reason, but often with little available documentation. It therefore requires considerable bravery to "strip down" a regimen containing such potentially life-saving therapies. However, a growing body of research indicates that this is precisely what can and should be done. Digoxin, phenytoin, and thiazide diuretics have been subjected to careful studies of withdrawal in patients who did not have an ongoing apparent need for them [9]. In these series, the vast majority of these therapies could be withdrawn with no adverse effects. Patients who demonstrated continuing need for medication could be restarted on their regimen with relatively little difficulty.

It is often falsely assumed that if a patient is feeling well his or her medication regimen should not be challenged. This is an unwise assumption for two reasons. First, it is often the case that a patient who is "stable" will nonetheless feel considerably better if the physician withdraws an unnecessary medication that may have been causing a subtle side effect such as fatigue or depression. This may be apparent only in retrospect once the offending agent has been removed. Second, every unnecessary medication can be viewed as a "time bomb" that may damage the patient at some point in the future when an intercurrent illness, even as mild as gastroenteritis, further reduces an already impaired capacity to clear the drug and precipitates toxicity [10].

Adverse drug effects are a common cause of hospitalization among the elderly [11]. Although this is sometimes the result of inevitable toxicity of essential medications in appropriate doses, it is quite often preventable through assiduous "pruning" of the therapeutic regimen at regular intervals. A high index of suspicion should be maintained for any symptom in the elderly as a possible adverse drug effect, particularly for all central nervous system symptoms, ranging from memory loss to changes in affect. Adverse effects can also present as virtually any known somatic complaint. Because symptoms caused by drug toxicity are among the simplest and most gratifying conditions to treat in geriatrics, their existence should be suspected frequently, and a cautious trial off the offending agent should be attempted whenever clinically feasible. If therapy for the underlying condition is mandatory, another agent in the same or a similar therapeutic class may produce the desired effect with less toxicity. Occasionally (see below), nonpharmacologic alternatives may work as well, with less risk of adverse effects.

Psychosocial Aspects of Medication Use in the Elderly

Pharmacologic considerations represent only one part, albeit a very important part, of the complex process of drug therapy in the elderly. A great deal of medication use in this age group is heavily shaped by the prescribing habits of physicians and the medication-taking practices of patients, both of which have been the subject of considerable research.

THE DECISION TO PRESCRIBE

Considerable evidence indicates that the prescribing choices of physicians are determined in part by scientific considerations and in part by other factors. Important among these is the well-intentioned desire to offer some help to the patient even in the absence of evidence from randomized controlled studies indicating efficacy. There is a particularly great temptation when the physician is faced, as is often the case in geriatrics, with one or more degenerative diseases for which there do not exist completely satisfactory therapies, such as Alzheimer's disease, arthritis, or situational depression and other life problems. Pushing the physician in the same direction is the plethora of promotional material presented by pharmaceutical companies in an attempt to encourage use of products addressing these and similar complaints. Thus, the writing of a prescription fulfills a number of situational demands, even in the absence of a particularly effective therapy: It enables the physician to feel that he or she is offering a science-based solution to the patient, preserves the therapeutic alliance, and reassures both patient and family that the physician is making every effort to address the clinical problem [12]. An argument has even been made that if the placebo effect is a "real" physiologic phenomenon mediated by endorphins, then therapies based on faith alone can be truly effective even in the absence of any pharmacologic activity [13].

However, there are important considerations that run counter to these trends and favor the avoidance of medication use unless it is grounded in good efficacy data and specific clinical need. First is the possibility that *any* medication can contribute to the development of an adverse drug reaction in this patient population, for the reasons outlined in the preceding sections. It is particularly unfortunate when the adverse effect, whether a transient loss of alertness or a femoral fracture, is the result of a therapy that was not truly indicated in the first place [14].

Second is the issue of cost. Because medications are not covered by Medicare or by most other insurance plans, drugs are one of the highest out-of-pocket health care expenses for the elderly [15]. Each new prescription can have a major impact on the household budget of a nonaffluent elderly patient, and yet most evidence indicates that cost is not a factor that is considered by physicians in making prescribing decisions. (Often this is because physicians are unaware of the actual cost to the patient of most commonly used medications.)

A third factor in favor of restrained prescribing practices is associated with a more subtle issue, that of "medicalization." According to this view, excessive reliance on prescription medications to address a variety of problems creates the misimpression that these problems can be addressed only with the intervention of the physician. This impression may be false for several reasons. First, for many patients, non-pharmacologic approaches or simple over-the-counter remedies may be very effective for the treatment of problems often brought to the primary care physician, such as insomnia, the mild chronic pain of arthritis, or nonspecific gastro-intestinal discomfort. Second, the prescription

of a medication (often a psychoactive drug) may "label" a problem such as loneliness, boredom, nervousness, or reactive depression as one having an inherently medical basis requiring pharmacologic intervention by the physician rather than as a life problem that could more effectively and appropriately be addressed by psychosocial interventions [16]. However, access to other forms of life intervention is difficult and may yield little in the way of results, whereas access to medical care is socially sanctioned, publicly funded, and culturally acceptable. These factors, coupled with the economic disincentives that physicians sometimes believe are associated with refusing to offer a patient a prescription, make it unlikely that such non-drug approaches will become much more widespread than they are at present.

Nonetheless, as concern mounts about cost in all aspects of medical care and awareness of the need for restrained prescribing in geriatrics becomes somewhat more pervasive, several promising approaches are being developed to reduce unnecessary drug use in this population. Several randomized controlled studies have shown that academic "detailing"—that is, outreach education in physicians' offices by clinicians working under the auspices of medical schools—can sizably reduce overuse of medications in several settings [17]. Benefit-cost analysis has indicated that these programs can yield savings far in excess of program costs for any agency responsible for reimbursement of prescription costs [18]. This approach has now been extended to the nursing home setting as well. The entry of health maintenance organizations and other reimbursement authorities into the once-insulated doctor-patient dyad of drug-prescribing and drug-taking may well add a new variable that will undoubtedly have positive as well as negative clinical outcomes.

THE DECISION TO COMPLY WITH A PRESCRIBED REGIMEN

The realization that a very large proportion of prescriptions are never taken as directed (or at all) by patients has raised concern about the frequency of the phenomenon of noncompliance among the elderly. Initially, it was believed that those over 65, with their increased burden of visual impairment, functional incapacity, and memory disorders, would be particularly prone to failure to take medications as directed. This failure was seen as a major barrier to effective management of both acute and chronic illness, although some authors, more concerned with the high frequency of inappropriate prescribing for this age group, have argued that "intelligent noncompliance" by skeptical elderly patients may be one of the most effective forms of preventive medicine in this age group.

However, more careful research has revealed that the main predictor of noncompliance is the number and complexity of individual medication regimens prescribed rather than age itself, a fact obscured by the frequent coexistence of old age and multiple medications [19]. This observation provides yet another reason to keep drug regimens as lean and as simple as possible in the elderly. A variety of devices are available to make the often complex task of taking the right medication at the right time more manageable [20]. These range from simple plastic containers with three or four compartments for each time of the day, seven days a week, to sophisticated electronic reminder devices that beep at the patient if a dose has been missed.

Considerable attention has been paid to the appearance of medications, particularly the fact that so many drugs of very different properties are manufactured as either "little white pills" or "big white pills." This problem has caused some to suggest that drug-prescribing take into account the physical appearance of various possibly interchangeable agents, so that the regimen is visually understandable by the patient. The problem is compounded by the fact that the distinctive colors of capsules are often a part of the protected trademark for a given brand of medication. Thus, if a physician or pharmacist switches the patient to a generic version of the exact same therapy, the appearance of the capsule may change dramatically, causing considerable consternation. Attempts to standardize the appearance of capsules for all preparations of the same chemical entity have been met with resistance by manufacturers of the trade name product, who have argued that such similarity of appearance would constitute an unfair infringement on their patent rights.

Policy Considerations

Because of the enormous clinical and economic importance of medications used by the elderly, they are the subject of intense debate among policymakers and regulators—deliberations that ultimately affect every physician and patient. Areas under intense current scrutiny include procedures for testing newly discovered medications on aged patients, widespread surveillance of older patients for adverse drug effects once a medication has been marketed, and reimbursement for medications used by the elderly.

THE ELDERLY AND THE PROCESS OF DRUG DEVELOPMENT

Surprisingly, it is only recently that consideration has been given to the need to test newly discovered medications on older patients prior to marketing. In general, the Food and Drug Administration (FDA) has not required that any patients over age 65 routinely be included in the premarketing clinical trials of medications submitted for approval [21]. Because of the high cost of such clinical trials and because of the perceived need to bring drugs to market as quickly as possible, manufacturers have in turn preferred younger, less complicated patients in whom to test the efficacy of new products without the interference that would result from multiple coexisting illnesses and other therapies. Although this makes it possible to pass larger numbers of subjects through clinical trials with greater speed and efficiency, the approach obviously runs the risk of missing important drug-disease or drug-drug interactions that may well occur in multiply impaired patients who often comprise the largest proportion of patients actually taking these medications once they are approved for widespread use. A classic case in point is benoxaprofen (Oraflex), a nonsteroidal antiinflammatory drug marketed in the United States in the early 1980s, which was tested primarily on nonelderly patients prior to approval. Evidence began to accumulate that because of its long half-life it was creating renal and hepatic toxicity in older patients, who were less able to clear the drug rapidly, and its use was implicated in a number of deaths. The drug was voluntarily removed from the market by its manufacturer in 1983. As a result of this and other problems, in the mid-1980s the FDA began to consider a series of recommendations for the systematic inclusion of elderly patients in clinical trials of medications destined for use by the elderly, before they are approved for marketing [22]. Progress on this point has been slow, and at the time of this writing no guidelines are yet in place.

Closely related to the issue of approval is that of product labeling, an area over which the FDA likewise has jurisdiction. Such labeling appears in all promotional materials and is commonly referred to in the *Physician's Desk Reference,* a compendium of such labeling information. Although a number of manufacturers have in recent years voluntarily included statements alerting prescribers to particular considerations in the use of certain medications in the elderly, no systematic or coherent requirements exist in this regard. One of the most striking examples of this is the labeling for the most commonly prescribed brand of digoxin. Although specific mention is given to special considerations associated with the use of digoxin in children, in pregnant women, and in nursing mothers, no mention is made of the particular issues surrounding use of this medication in the elderly, who are its most frequent users [23]. There is some reason to believe that product liability suits, naming manufacturers as defendants in cases in which adverse drug effects in the elderly were not adequately described in the product information, may prove to be a powerful if bizarre way of addressing this informational lacunae.

References

1. Campion, E. W., et al. Overmedication of the low-weight elderly. *Arch. Intern. Med.* 147:945, 1987.
2. Greenblatt, D. J., Sellers, E. M., and Shader, R. I. Drug therapy: Drug disposition in old age. *N. Engl. J. Med.* 306:1081, 1982.
3. Vestal, R. E. (ed.). *Drug Treatment in the Elderly.* New York and Sydney, Australia: Adis Press, 1982.
4. Rowe, J. W., et al. The effect of age on creatinine clearance in man. *J. Gerontol.* 31:155, 1976.
5. Schmucker, D. L. Aging and drug disposition: An update. *Pharmacol. Rev.* 37:133, 1985.
6. Lakatta, E. G. Age-related alterations in the cardiovascular response to adrenergic mediated stress. *Fed. Proc.* 39:3173, 1980.
7. Reindenberg, M. M., et al. Relationship between diazepam dose, plasma level, age, and central nervous system depression. *Clin. Pharmacol. Ther.* 23:371, 1978.
8. Vestal, R., Wood, A., and Shand, D. Reduced beta-adrenoreceptor sensitivity in the elderly. *Clin. Pharmacol. Ther.* 26:818, 1979.
9. Hutt, S. M., and Mackintosh, A. Discontinuation of maintenance digoxin therapy in general practice. *Lancet* 2:1054, 1977.
10. Everitt, D. E., and Avorn J. Drug prescribing for the elderly. *Arch. Intern. Med.* 146:2393, 1986.
11. Williamson, J., and Chopin, J. M. Adverse reactions to prescribed drugs in the elderly: A multicentre investigation. Age Ageing 9:73, 1980.
12. Mapes, R. (ed.). *Prescribing Practice and Drug Usage.* London: Croom Helm, 1980.
13. Brody, H. *Placebos and the Philosophy of Medicine.* Chicago: University of Chicago Press, 1977.
14. Ray, W. A., et al. Psychotropic drug use and the risk of hip fracture. *N. Engl. J. Med.* 316(7):363, 1987.
15. U.S. Senate Special Committee on Aging. Drug costs and the elderly. Congressional Record. Washington, D.C.: U.S. Government Printing Office, 1987.
16. Lennard, H. *Mystification and Drug Misuse.* San Francisco: Jossey-Bass, 1978.
17. Avorn, J., and Soumerai, S. B. Improving drug-therapy decisions through educational outreach: A randomized controlled trial of academically based "detailing." *N. Engl. J. Med.* 308:1457, 1983.
18. Soumerai, S. B., and Avorn, J. Economic and policy analysis of university-based drug "detailing." *Med. Care* 24:313, 1986.
19. German, P. S., et al. Knowledge and compliance with drug regimens among the elderly. *J. Am. Geriatr. Soc.* 30:568, 1982.
20. Eraker, S. A., Kirscht, J. P., and Becker, M. H. Understanding and improving patient compliance. *Ann. Intern. Med.* 100:258, 1984.
21. Avorn, J. Drug policy in the aging society. *Health Affairs* 2(3):24, 1983.
22. Temple, R. FDA Clinical Guidelines for Studying Drugs in the Elderly. In S. R. Moore and T. W. Teal (eds.), *Geriatric Drug Use—Clinical and Social Perspectives.* New York: Pergamon Press, 1985.
23. *Physician's Desk Reference* (41st ed.). Oradell, NJ: Medical Economics Co., 1987. Pp. 791–795.

10

Anesthesia and Surgery in the Elderly

GRAYDON S. MENEILLY
JOHN W. ROWE
KENNETH L. MINAKER

ALTHOUGH THE ELDERLY comprise only 11 percent of the population, they undergo between 20 and 40 percent of all surgical procedures and account for 50 percent of surgical emergencies and 75 percent of operative deaths [1]. Even more elderly patients will undergo surgery as more sophisticated and safe anesthetic and surgical techniques become available and aggressive postoperative care reduces morbidity and mortality. Because geriatric patients often carry significant burdens of disability and disease, correct management involves individualized assessment of the risks and benefits. This chapter reviews the special features of preoperative assessment and postoperative care of the elderly patient.

Surgical Risk and Age

Prior to 1960, surgery was frequently avoided in the elderly because operative mortality rates were two to five times higher in the aged than in the young [2, 3], often reaching 20 percent or higher [4]. This early experience is difficult to evaluate because the reported studies did not separate elective from emergency procedures and often failed to assess the severity of underlying disease. Currently, elective surgical mortality in the aged is generally reported as 10 percent or less [5, 6, 7], with one study [8] reporting an elective surgical mortality of 2.3 percent in patients over age 90. Emergency surgery still carries a mortality three or four times higher than that of elective surgery.

Although early studies identified age as an independent risk factor for surgical mortality, this finding is not supported by recent studies that employ precise quantitation of illness burden and sophisticated statistical analyses. Boyd et al. [9] found that in 350 patients over age 50 who underwent colon resection, mortality correlated with the number of underlying pathologic processes and not with age. In Djokovic's series [10] of 500 consecutive surgical procedures in patients over age 80, age was not a risk factor for operative mortality up to age 95.

Although not an independent risk factor for operative mortality, age increases operative cardiac morbidity. Increasing age enhances the risk of postoperative congestive heart failure (CHF) after noncardiac surgery [11] and stroke following coronary surgery. Pulmonary complications are related more to operative site and underlying disease than to chronologic age [2, 12].

Although the elderly have a higher morbidity and mortality than younger patients, the increased risk is generally due to underlying disease. The restrictions in physiologic reserve due to aging are well adjusted for by modern anesthetic techniques and perioperative care. Underlying disease and not chronologic age should be the major criterion for assessing operative risk [2, 3].

The extended life expectancy of the aged and the prolonged natural history of some surgical diseases often make a surgical approach to cure a more attractive alternative than chronic morbidity, even in the very elderly patient. At age 65, American males can expect to live another 14 years, and females can expect to live another 18 years. Even at advanced age, such as age 85, mean life expectancy approaches six years, and at age 90 it approaches five years. This information has to be weighed against the natural history of the disease for which surgery is being considered.

Preoperative Evaluation and Preparation

RISK ASSESSMENT

Preoperative assessment aims to define the present functional status and quality of life of the patient, to identify special vulnerabilities for perioperative morbidity, and to develop a plan for proper preoperative preparation and postoperative management. Complications of specific operations should be anticipated and postoperative education and rehabilitation planning initiated prior to surgery.

This assessment is often a team effort. Starting with a physician sensitive to geriatric problems, social service and nursing assessment add immeasurably to the preoperative and postoperative care of the patient, facilitating safe discharge home. With this assessment in hand, the surgeon can decide whether to operate.

The preoperative evaluation of an elderly person should follow a standard format (Table 10-1). The cornerstone is the history and physical examination. Since postoperative complications are most likely to involve cardiac and pulmonary systems, they must receive special emphasis. As discussed in Chapter 4, atypical or nonspecific symptoms and signs in these systems are particularly frequent in the elderly [13]. For example, a patient with myocardial ischemia may not complain of chest pain but rather of fatigue or shortness of breath. It is also critical to obtain a careful drug history for both over-the-counter and prescription drugs. A nutritional history is valuable given the 10 to 20 percent prevalence among the elderly of borderline nutritional status. A standardized test of

TABLE 10-1. *Preoperative assessment of the elderly patient*

Cardiopulmonary symptoms and signs
Drugs—prescription and over-the-counter
Nutritional status
Mental status
Functional assessment
Selected laboratory tests

TABLE 10-2. *American Society of Anesthesiologists physical status scale*

CLASS	PHYSICAL STATUS
I	Normal healthy individual
II	Patient with mild systemic disease
III	Patient with severe systemic disease that is not incapacitating
IV	Patient with incapacitating systemic disease that is a constant threat to life
V	Moribund patient who is not expected to survive 24 hours with or without operation
E	Added to any class patient undergoing emergency surgery

mental status such as the mini-mental state examination identifies patients at risk for postoperative confusion while providing a baseline for postoperative mental status testing. Functional assessment predicts rehabilitative needs, particularly after orthopedic procedures. Laboratory evaluation should include a complete blood count; glucose, albumin, electrolyte, blood urea nitrogen, and creatinine measurements; urinalysis; electrocardiogram; and chest x-ray. Skinfold measurements and other biochemical measures of nutritional status, an exercise tolerance test, pulmonary function tests, or arterial blood gas measurements may be required in selected cases.

Based on these preliminary evaluations, an assessment of overall risk can be obtained. Two methods of formally estimating overall risk are in use. The American Society of Anesthesiologists (ASA) criteria remain the best tool (Table 10-2), stratifying patients into five clinical classes that predict mortality in both elective and emergency surgery. The ASA scale adjusts for age by not permitting an elderly person to receive a class I designation. The classification has been validated in patients over age 80, yielding a spread of risks from less than 1 percent in class II patients to 25 percent in class IV patients [10].

Recently, interest has developed in the use of invasive preoperative assessment with a Swan-Ganz catheter to develop a more quantitative measure of surgical risk in old age. DelGuercio and Kohn [14] assessed 148 consecutive patients over 65 who had been cleared for surgery by a general internist. A high prevalence of clinically unsuspected cardiopulmonary abnormalities was found in their patients, and poorer hemodynamics were linked to higher mortality. There were no deaths in patients (13.5 percent) with normal hemodynamics. Patients with moderate impairment (65 percent) had a 9 percent mortality. Twenty-three percent of patients had severe impairment, and all patients in this group who underwent surgery died. There was a good correlation between ASA class and physiologic parameters as well as operative mortality, and it is unclear whether invasive monitoring was a better predictor of operative mortality or could reduce morbidity and mortality when compared with a careful history and physical examination, selected laboratory tests, and ASA classification by an experienced anesthetist. Thus, while potentially helpful, preoperative invasive monitoring should not become routine for the elderly. However, as discussed later, patients felt to be at high risk should have a Swan-Ganz catheter and an arterial line placed in the operating room, and these should be kept in place until stability is established in the recovery room.

Cardiovascular System

Cardiovascular complications are very common in the perioperative period. Normative age-related changes in cardiovascular function and the high prevalence of vascular and coronary disease make the elderly particularly susceptible to cardiac complications. The patient should be carefully questioned about a history of myocardial infarction, angina, and congestive heart failure, which carry an increased risk of perioperative myocardial events.

The presence of elevated jugular venous pulses, a third heart sound, or other signs of congestive heart failure are critical to assessing cardiac risk because congestive heart failure often worsens postoperatively. Murmurs are very common in the elderly, and although often hemodynamically insignificant, they may suggest the need for antibiotic prophylaxis. If significant valvular disease is suspected clinically, an echocardiogram is indicated because patients with significant aortic stenosis require a Swan-Ganz catheter to guide perioperative fluid management. Pulmonary crepitations do not always represent congestive heart failure, particularly if they are medium or coarse and are heard early in inspiration, but instead may indicate areas of pulmonary fibrosis. Pedal edema in the elderly is often due to venous stasis and in the absence of other findings is not a reliable sign of congestive heart failure.

Specific techniques for estimating cardiac risk in the elderly have proved valuable. Based on experience in 1,001 patients undergoing noncardiac surgery, Goldman [11] developed a four-category scale consisting of clinical and laboratory parameters that predict postoperative cardiovascular morbidity and mortality (see Tables 10-3 and 10-4). The strongest predictors were a third heart sound or raised jugular venous pressure and a recent myocardial infarction. Age over 70 was an independent risk

TABLE 10-3. *Estimation of cardiac risk in noncardiac surgery (Goldman score)*[a]

RISK CONDITION	POINTS
Third heart sound (S3) or jugular venous distension on preoperative physical examination	11
Myocardial infarction in the previous six months	10
Premature ventricular beats greater than five per minute documented at any time	7
Rhythm other than sinus or presence of premature atrial contractions on last preoperative electrocardiogram	7
Age over 70 years	5
Emergency operation	4
Intraperitoneal, intrathoracic, or aortic site of surgery	3
Evidence of important aortic valvular stenosis	3
Poor general medical condition[b]	3

[a]Patients are divided into four risk categories based on their score: I: 0–5 points, II: 6–12, III: 13–25, IV 26.
[b]As evidenced by electrolyte abnormalities (K < 3.0 mEq/L, HCO_3 < 20 mEq/L), renal insufficiency (blood urea nitrogen > 50 mg/dl, creatinine > 3.0 mg/dl), abnormal blood gases (PO_2 < 60 mm Hg, PCO_2 > 50 mm Hg), abnormal liver status (elevated serum glutamic-oxaloacetic transaminase (SGOT) or signs at physical examination of chronic liver disease) or any condition that has caused the patient to be chronically bedridden from noncardiac causes.
SOURCE: Adapted from Goldman, L. et al. Multifactorial index of cardiac risk in noncardiac surgical procedures. *N. Engl. J. Med.* 297:845, 1977.

TABLE 10-4. *Cardiac risk index*

CLASS	POINT TOTAL	NO OR ONLY MINOR COMPLICATIONS (N = 943)	LIFE-THREATENING COMPLICATIONS [a] (N = 58)	CARDIAC DEATHS (N = 19)
I (N = 537)	0–5	532 (99)[b]	4 (0.7)[b]	1 (0.2)[b]
II (N = 316)	6–12	295 (93)	16 (5)	5 (2)
III (N = 130)	13–25	112 (86)	15 (11)	3 (2)
IV (N = 18)	> 25	4 (22)	4 (22)	10 (56)

[a]Documented intraoperative or postoperative myocardial infarction, pulmonary edema, or ventricular tachycardia.
[b]Figures in parentheses denote percentages.
SOURCE: Adapted from Goldman, L., et al. Multifactorial index of cardiac risk in noncardiac surgical procedures. *N. Engl. J. Med.* 297:845, 1977.

factor predicting postoperative complications, particularly congestive heart failure. Patients who had had a myocardial infarction within six months had a 37 percent risk of serious complications and a 23 percent mortality versus a 2.5 percent mortality if the myocardial infarction had occurred more than six months previously.

Gerson et al. [15] evaluated 100 patients over the age of 65 scheduled for major elective and abdominal thoracic surgery with history, physical examination, laboratory screening, electrocardiogram, chest x-ray, ASA criteria, Goldman index, and resting and exercise radionuclide ventriculogram. Failure to raise the heart rate above 99 beats per minute during two minutes of supine exercise on a bicycle ergometer was the most powerful predictor of perioperative cardiac complications, followed closely by ASA criteria and the Goldman criteria.

Patients who have a normal history, physical examination, and electrocardiogram and are at low risk by the Goldman index need not undergo a preoperative exercise tolerance test. However, those undergoing major abdominal or thoracic surgery who are at high risk by the Goldman criteria or have signs or symptoms of significant cardiovascular disease should undergo an exercise tolerance test. The rate-pressure product (heart rate times systolic blood pressure) at onset of symptoms during the exercise tolerance test cautions the anesthetist to maintain heart rate and blood pressure values below this level during surgery to limit the risk of an ischemic event.

Prophylaxis for asymptomatic ventricular or supraventricular arrhythmias or frequent unifocal premature ventricular contractions is not indicated, although these patients should have cardiac monitoring perioperatively [16]. Unstable angina and symptomatic arrhythmias must be controlled preoperatively, and antianginal and antiarrhythmic medications should be continued right up to the time of surgery. Unstable angina carries as great a risk for cardiac complications as a recent myocardial infarction. Patients with congestive heart failure are less likely to decompensate in the perioperative period if the failure is well controlled prior to surgery. However, excessive diuresis should be avoided to prevent hypotension under anesthesia and postoperative renal complications.

Hypertension
Forty percent of patients over age 65 are hypertensive. Well-controlled or mild hypertension (diastolic less than 110 mm Hg) does not increase intraoperative risk (Goldman criteria), but severe, uncontrolled hypertension (diastolic over 140 mm Hg, systolic over 200 mm Hg) carries an increased risk of myocardial infarction and should be controlled preoperatively. Surgery need not be delayed to control mild hypertension [11]. There is no need to control isolated systolic hypertension if systolic values are less than 200 mm Hg. Antihypertensive drugs should be continued up to the time of surgery, particularly clonidine and beta-blockers because preoperative discontinuation may induce rebound hypertension or angina.

Pulmonary Disease
Patients with symptoms, signs, or clinical histories suggesting disease in the pulmonary system should be further evaluated with pulmonary function tests and arterial blood gas determina-

tion, especially if thoracic or upper abdominal surgery is planned. Routine chest x-ray is not valuable in young asymptomatic patients [17]. A recent study [18] in patients over age 60 undergoing elective surgery showed that the prevalence of abnormal chest films was very high. Thirty percent of patients at low risk for cardiovascular disease by history and physical examination had clinically significant chest x-ray abnormalities that either influenced the decision to operate, required further workup, or increased the likelihood of postoperative complications. In otherwise low-risk patients, the presence of an abnormal chest x-ray doubled the risk of postoperative complications from 10 to 20 percent. Additionally, a preoperative chest x-ray would have been useful for comparison in 10 percent of patients who developed a postoperative pulmonary complication. Thus, a preoperative chest x-ray should be obtained routinely before surgery in all patients over the age of 65 except for the most minor operations.

Patients at high risk for pulmonary complications [19] include those with carbon dioxide retention (PCO_2 more than 45 mm Hg), PO_2 less than 60 mm Hg, FEV_1 less than 2 liters or 75 percent of predicted, FEV_1 to FVC ratio of less than 0.65, smokers, and any patients with a history or physical findings suggestive of pulmonary disease. A slight decrease in PO_2 with age or an increase in the arterioalveolar oxygen tension gradient up to 20 mm Hg by the age of 80 is normal and should not increase risk. Normal preoperative PO_2 for the aged can be estimated by the formula $PO_2 = 100 - 0.34 \times age$ [20].

Patients with respiratory disease should be taught breathing exercises and incentive spirometry preoperatively and should receive chest physiotherapy. To be beneficial, cigarette smoking cessation must occur at least two weeks prior to surgery, and early cessation of smoking should be encouraged whenever possible. Bronchodilators can improve bronchospasm prior to surgery, and antibiotics should be used to treat active pulmonary infection.

Venous Thrombosis
Subcutaneous heparin is useful for the prevention of deep venous thrombosis in thoracoabdominal surgery in the elderly but is not effective in orthopedic surgery, where the incidence of deep venous thrombosis after hip or knee replacement approaches 50 to 75 percent. Newer anticoagulant regimens, such as adjusted subcutaneous heparin [21], warfarin [22], dihydroergotamine/heparin [23], and low-molecular-weight heparin [24], prevent venous thrombosis in orthopedic surgery.

Renal Function and Fluid Management
Patients at high risk for perioperative renal complications include those with a raised blood urea nitrogen or creatinine and a history of long-standing hypertension, renal disease, or diabetes. These patients should have a 24-hour urine test or at least several timed hourly urine collections to assess renal function adequately. Extracellular fluid status can be assessed by orthostatic vital signs, jugular venous pulse, tissue turgor, or the response of urine output to a brief infusion of normal saline. Patients with volume depletion should be repleted preoperatively to reduce the risk of renal complications and perioperative hypotension. Because many elderly individuals have an impaired thirst mechanism [25], this symptom cannot be relied on as a marker of extracellular fluid volume status. In patients with marked volume depletion or other risk factors for renal complications, a Swan-Ganz catheter should be placed to aid fluid management perioperatively. Since the senescent kidney has a blunted ability to conserve salt and water, isotonic fluids should not be restricted in the absence of congestive heart failure or hyponatremia (see Chap. 18). Hypokalemia should be corrected to reduce the risk of arrhythmias.

Nutritional Assessment
Ten to 20 percent of the elderly have borderline nutritional status. Patients at high risk include those who are depressed or demented, those who have recently lost more than 5 percent of body weight, the poor, widowers who have no skills in food preparation, alcohol abusers, and patients who are immobile or isolated [26]. In addition, a serum albumin level of less than 3.0 gm/dl is associated with an increased risk of postoperative complications [12]. Malnourished patients with hip fractures are more likely to have low body temperatures on admission, and hypothermia is felt to predispose these pa-

tients to falls and fractures because of attendant confusion and impaired coordination [27]. Malnourished patients are also particularly prone to certain postoperative complications such as skin breakdown [28], impaired wound healing, and infection.

Age-adjusted criteria have not been developed for many nutritional parameters. Skinfold thickness and muscle mass decrease with age in normal elderly subjects, and there is an increased prevalence of cutaneous anergy. Transferrin and albumin may be reduced by chronic disease in the absence of malnutrition. Nonetheless, recent studies [29] suggest that these parameters should remain within the normal range for healthy free-living individuals. All patients who are at high risk by history, who appear emaciated or malnourished on physical examination, or who have a serum albumin of less than 3.0 gm/dl should have a skinfold thickness, mid-arm circumference, transferrin level, and total lymphocyte count performed. Patients with reduced skinfold thickness and mid-arm circumference, decreased levels of transferrin and other biochemical parameters, and a total lymphocyte count of less than 1,000 should be considered malnourished. Retinol-binding protein and prealbumin levels are recently developed tests that may be better markers of nutritional adequacy than albumin because they more accurately reflect recent changes in nutritional status. Patients with evidence of malnutrition should have aggressive nutritional supplementation prior to surgery to attain normal nutritional status and reduce the risk of postoperative complications. Details of nutritional intervention are covered in Chapter 8.

Diabetes

Diabetes is common in older people and is apt to decompensate under the stress of surgery. No preoperative intervention is necessary in patients with diet-controlled diabetes with a fasting blood sugar level of less than 180 mg/dl or a two-hour postprandial sugar level of less than 250 mg/dl. Patients on oral hypoglycemic medications should discontinue these two days prior to surgery, and patients on long-acting insulin should continue this up to but not including the morning of surgery. Patients with blood glucose levels above 300 mg/dl can be controlled with injections of regular insulin every six hours. Because the renal threshold for glucose increases with age, urine glucose measurements are less useful, and the insulin dose should be based on a fingerstick or venous glucose measurement. There is no need to reduce the blood sugar level below 200 mg/dl. For a detailed discussion of the management of insulin and glucose therapy in insulin-dependent diabetics on the day of surgery, the reader is referred to other sources [30]. If blood sugar remains below 300 mg/dl postoperatively in diet-controlled diabetics or patients on oral hypoglycemic drugs, no therapy is indicated, and oral agents can be restarted as soon as the patient is able to drink. Patients with blood sugar levels over 300 mg/dl can be managed with regular insulin every six hours provided that adequate glucose is given to prevent hypoglycemia.

Antibiotic Prophylaxis

Antibiotic prophylaxis is recommended for many gynecologic, orthopedic, abdominal, cardiothoracic, and vascular procedures, often with a cephalosporin [31]. In addition, antibiotic prophylaxis should be used for dental work or genitourinary and gastrointestinal procedures if cardiac murmurs are present (even if they are hemodynamically insignificant) or if prosthetic joints are in place because the elderly are at risk for bacterial endocarditis and prosthetic joint infections [32]. Prophylactic regimens for gastrointestinal and urologic procedures must be sufficient to cover enterococci. Antibiotic prophylaxis is not recommended for upper gastrointestinal endoscopy without biopsy, liver biopsy, sigmoidoscopy, barium enema, pelvic examination, and dilatation and curettage.

Pharmacology

A drug history is important because certain drugs may affect perioperative complications. For example, a patient on chronic benzodiazepine therapy may exhibit withdrawal symptoms in the postoperative period, or a patient with poor compliance with antianginal medications may decompensate under the stress of surgery. It is important to remember that drugs can also interact adversely with anesthetic agents or cause problems during surgery. Diuretic-induced hypokalemia may yield arrhythmias during surgical stress. Digitalis can also result in arrhythmia, especially if potassium is decreased by hyperventilation-induced alkalosis during surgery. Beta-blockers predispose to bradycardia and hypotension when combined with certain anesthetics that depress the myocardium such as halothane. Agents with anticholinergic properties may predispose to tachycardia with a subsequent increase in myocardial oxygen demand and may also predispose to postoperative confusion.

Functional Assessment

It is essential to assess the general functional status in the preoperative period. Patients with impairment in basic (i.e., bathing, dressing, toileting, walking) and instrumental (i.e., handling finances, shopping, cooking, using the telephone, driving) activities of daily living should be considered at high risk for functional deterioration in the postoperative period and should be treated with aggressive and early physiotherapy and occupational therapy.

Anesthetic Drug Management

In the past, anesthetics contributed significantly to perioperative mortality. Studies before 1960 indicated that up to 20 percent of perioperative deaths were due to anesthetic complications [33]. Anesthetic agents and techniques have improved to the point that in a recent series [10] of 500 patients over age 80, no deaths could be attributed to anesthesia itself. In addition, current data find no association between increased operative time and mortality [10, 11]. Adjustment of anesthetic, analgesic, and paralytic drug management is based on knowledge of age-related alterations of pharmacokinetics and pharmacodynamics (Table 10-5).

Intravenous benzodiazepines and barbiturates are frequently used for the induction of anesthesia. Since metabolism of longer-acting benzodiazepines such as diazepam is up to two times slower in the aged [34], and the elderly are also more sensitive to benzodiazepines, doses should be generally no more than half those employed in the young. The half-life of and sensitivity to the short-acting barbiturate thiopental is also increased with age [35], and induction can be achieved with doses one-third to one-half of the

TABLE 10-5. *Anesthetic drug management in the aged*

PHARMACOKINETIC AND PHARMACODYNAMIC CHANGES WITH AGE	ANESTHETIC AGENTS AFFECTED
Decreased liver blood flow	Lidocaine
Decreased liver metabolism	Thiopental, long-acting benzodiazepines
Decreased renal function	Pancuronium, D-tubocurare
Decreased albumin	Thiopental
Increased body fat	Increased volume of distribution of inhaled anesthetics, thiopental, and benzodiazepines
Increased sensitivity	Narcotic analgesics, benzodiazepines

usual dose for a younger adult and even less if the patient is taking other highly protein bound drugs such as warfarin. Both diazepam and thiopental induce rapid anesthesia because of their high lipid solubility. However, the prolonged half-life of these agents in the elderly may prolong recovery from anesthesia. Midazolam, a shorter-acting benzodiazepine with as rapid an onset of action as diazepam, also has a prolonged half-life in the aged [36] but is less likely to prolong recovery from anesthesia, and many anesthetists favor it as an inductive agent in patients over 65.

Sensitivity to inhalational anesthetics also increases with age. The minimum alveolar concentration (MAC) that prevents response to surgical incision (a measure of anesthetic potency) of halothane and isoflurane [37, 38] decreases approximately 20 percent from age 20 to age 80, indicating decreased requirements of inhalational anesthetic with age. The influence of age on sensitivity to enflurane and methoxyflurane has not been studied, but decreases in MAC are also likely for these agents. The reduction in blood pressure with isoflurane, enflurane, and halothane may be slightly greater in the aged, although individual variability is great [39]. The effects of halothane and enflurane on pulse are not changed with age, but the pulse increase in response to isoflurane is less in the elderly. Age effects on the influence of these agents on cardiac output have not been well assessed.

The elimination of muscle relaxants such as pancuronium and D-tubocurare, which are excreted in the urine, is impaired with age because of decreased renal function, resulting in longer recovery from pancuronium-induced paralysis in the aged [40, 41, 42]. Although the half-life of tubocurare is increased in the aged [43], recovery times from neuromuscular blockade produced by tubocurare and reversed by neostigmine are similar in young and old [44]. There are no reported studies on changes with age in the response to succinylcholine.

A number of studies have suggested that the amount of local anesthetic required for spinal anesthesia is reduced with age, perhaps due to changes in blood flow or the architecture of the spinal canal [45, 46]. The half-life of lidocaine, which is used for local and systemic anesthesia (e.g., suppressing the cough reflex), is markedly prolonged in the aged [47].

Analgesics are used for perioperative sedation and intraoperative and postoperative analgesia. Free levels of meperidine and morphine are increased, and their half-lives are prolonged in the aged [48, 49]. Fentanyl also has a markedly prolonged half-life in the aged [50]. In addition, there may be up to a twofold increase in sensitivity to these agents with advancing age [51]. This suggests that reduced doses, probably half those of young individuals, should be used in the aged in the perioperative period.

The heart rate increase in response to atropine is less in the aged, but the incidence of arrhythmias is increased. Since the half-life of this drug is prolonged in the elderly [52], and central nervous system toxicity may result, its use has been deemphasized in the aged.

OPERATIVE MANAGEMENT
Anesthesia
Premedications should not be given routinely. Barbiturates may cause paradoxical agitation or confusion and are rarely required. Atropine or scopolamine also may induce confusion or aggravate underlying medical disorders such as glaucoma. Analgesics should be given only if pain is present and then in reduced dosages. If sedation is required, shorter-acting benzodiazepines such as triazolam or oxazepam, which are conjugated in the liver and thus do not have an increased half-life in the elderly, should be used.

The choice of anesthesia is best left up to an experienced anesthetist with the pharmacologic caveats noted above. Elderly patients tolerate regional anesthesia very well, and epidural or spinal analgesics are satisfactory for procedures below the waistline, although arthritic changes may make lumbar puncture difficult. Although opinion is divided, certain kinds of surgery, such as repair of a fractured hip, may have a lower mortality with regional anesthesia [53, 54]. The pulmonary changes and complications are similar for local and general anesthesia if higher levels of the spinal cord are paralyzed for procedures in the upper abdomen [19].

General anesthesia is required for surgical procedures above the midabdomen and for lower abdominal procedures if the patient is uncooperative. Induction of anesthesia should be slow to minimize undue stress on the cardiovascular system. A shorter-acting agent such as midazolam in conjunction with fentanyl may be preferable to diazepam or thiopental for induction, as noted earlier. The excessive blood pressure and heart rate responses to intubation may be reduced by premedication or use of inhalational anesthetics. Intubation is generally easier in the elderly because of laxer tissues, although a stiff osteoarthritic neck or poor dentition may be troublesome. Maintenance anesthesia with nitrous oxide and oxygen and muscle relaxant technique has minimal adverse cardiovascular effects.

Several physiologic and pathologic aging changes influence intraoperative management of elderly patients. Baroreflex sensitivity is blunted, and heart rate decreases in response to hypertension and increases in response to hypotension are reduced [55]. There is a reduced blood pressure response to pressor agents [56], a decreased heart rate response to beta-stimulants [57], a decreased response to beta-blockers, and increased sensitivity to hypotensive agents such as nitroprusside [58]. Lability of blood pressure in response to various stimuli is increased. Because of the high prevalence of coronary artery disease, it is important to avoid excessive hypotension or tachycardia. In addition, excessive hypertension can increase myocardial oxygen demand. In the absence of a preoperative exercise tolerance test, rate-pressure product should be kept below 12,000 in patients with severe coronary artery disease, 15,000 for mild coronary artery disease, and 20,000 for healthy elderly [59]. Regarding pulmonary changes, PO_2 decreases and ventilation-perfusion mismatch occur to a greater degree, dictating a higher inspired oxygen concentration during the intraoperative period.

Intraoperative Monitoring

Intraoperative monitoring is essential for complex surgery in the aged. An arterial line should be used in vascular surgery if blood pressure is expected to be unstable and in any procedure where changes in PO_2 or PCO_2 are expected, as in thoracic surgery or when hyperventilation is needed for neurosurgery. There are no reported studies on complications of arterial pressure monitoring in the elderly, but it is probably well tolerated if used for less than 24 hours. A Swan-Ganz catheter should be used if there is moderate or advanced coronary artery disease, significant aortic stenosis, congestive heart failure, recent myocardial infarction, or unstable angina; if the patient is class III or IV by the Goldman criteria; if the circulation is unstable as in sepsis or burns or when there is marked extracellular fluid volume depletion; and in major vascular and cardiac surgery. Because age predisposes to the complications of Swan-Ganz catheterization such as arrhythmia, perforation, or rupture of the pulmonary artery, a Swan-Ganz catheter should not be used for trivial indications. Because of the decrease in glomerular filtration rate with age and the poor prognosis of postoperative renal failure, a urinary catheter should be used in patients with underlying renal disease or dehydration, operations over three hours long, or when alterations in renal blood flow or large fluid shifts may occur (e.g., resection of an abdominal aortic aneurysm). Urine flow should be maintained at greater than 1 ml per kilogram per hour. The elderly have impaired thermoregulatory mechanisms, which may be further impaired by many inhalational anesthetics. Core temperature should be monitored if surgery is long, if large amounts of fluid are given, or if the abdomen or chest is open. If over 300 ml of fluid is to be given, it should be warmed to body temperature.

Recovery Room

Management of the elderly patient in the recovery room and the early postoperative period room must be equally meticulous. The prolonged half-life of drugs such as diazepam and pancuronium may delay recovery from anesthesia and should be anticipated. Protective airway reflexes and cough are impaired, requiring more careful management of the airway to prevent aspiration. Airway closure occurs at higher lung volumes and also predisposes to postoperative infection. The ventilatory responses to hypercarbia and hypoxia are impaired in the elderly, particularly if the level of consciousness is impaired, and the ventilatory pattern should be carefully assessed. In addition, ventilation-perfusion abnormalities are common in the elderly and often become worse in the postoperative period, increasing the likelihood of hypoxia. It is important to remember that restlessness or combativeness in the recovery room is often due to hypoxia rather than to drug effects or pain.

Inspired oxygen tension should be increased in the early postoperative period because of the above considerations. Oxygenation can be monitored noninvasively with an ear oximeter if necessary. Prophylactic ventilation has been recommended for elderly patients after major procedures. However, this increases the risk of pulmonary complications such as pneumonia, and elderly patients should be extubated using the same criteria applied to young patients [60]. In general, weaning from the ventilator after cardiothoracic surgery in the elderly may take 24 hours longer than in young individuals.

Shivering occurs commonly after anesthesia with certain inhalational anesthetics and after long operations. It results in increased tissue oxygen demand and catecholamine release and impaired blood flow to many tissues. It may be appropriate to maintain the cold patient paralyzed and ventilated to prevent shivering while rewarming occurs.

Close attention should be paid to blood pressure, pulse, and rate-pressure product in the recovery room because most serious cardiac complications occur in the first several days. Proper oxygenation should be maintained, and shivering should be prevented as above to protect the myocardium. Proper analgesia will improve breathing and mobility and decrease catecholamine release. We favor meperidine 0.2 to 0.4 mg per kg intramuscularly every one to two hours.

Increases in blood pressure occur frequently after vascular procedures, are often due to pain and/or hypoxia, and will respond to analgesia and O$_2$, but vasodilator therapy with nitroprusside can be used if analgesia fails. Hypotension usually responds to fluid challenge, but pressor agents may be needed. If sedatives are required, short-acting (for example, triazolam) or intermediate-acting (for example, oxazepam) agents should be used in half the usual doses.

Postoperative Complications

The most common postoperative complications in the elderly are cardiopulmonary. Infections, acute renal failure, acute confusional states, nutritional problems, and pressure sores are sufficiently common to merit discussion also. Incontinence, another common problem, is discussed in Chapter 19.

The elderly patient must be monitored very carefully in the postoperative period and examined frequently. The elderly are frequently asymptomatic with such common postoperative complications as myocardial infarction, pulmonary embolus, and pneumonia. Slight fevers, changes in respiration, pulse, blood pressure, or nonspecific symptoms such as fatigue or weakness should be carefully assessed with a history, physical examination, chest x-ray, electrocardiogram, and appropriate laboratory tests. Attention to impaired functional status and early and aggressive rehabilitation are critically important to prevent permanent disability, especially after orthopedic procedures.

CARDIAC MORBIDITY AND MORTALITY

Cardiac complications, most commonly congestive heart failure, myocardial infarction, arrhythmias, and hypotension, account for approximately half of all postoperative deaths in the elderly. The National Halothane Study [61] indicates that the risk for myocardial infarction is greatest during the first five postoperative days and falls dramatically thereafter. As noted earlier, the Goldman criteria predict the risk for perioperative cardiac morbidity and mortality.

Careful questioning for cardiorespiratory symptoms and examination of the heart and lungs are essential. The threshold for obtaining an electrocardiogram should be low and is routine in class III or class IV patients. Antihypertensive, antiarrhythmic, and antianginal medications should be restarted as soon as possible in the postoperative period [16]. New mild hypertension 24 to 48 hours after surgery is probably due to mobilization of intraoperative fluid and can often be managed with diuretics. Postoperative ventricular premature contractions (VPCs) are precipitated by hypoxia, pain, or electrolyte disturbances. Oxygen, sedation, analgesia, and correction of fluid and electrolyte disturbances may be effective in managing ventricular arrhythmias, but if these measures fail, antiarrhythmics, including lidocaine, may be used. Infrequent or unifocal VPCs usually do not require antiarrhythmic treatment, but frequent or multifocal VPCs or those inducing hemodynamic compromise should be treated promptly. As mentioned previously, because of the kinetic changes that occur with age, the dose of lidocaine should be reduced in the elderly.

Postoperative supraventricular tachycardia and other arrhythmias, such as multifocal atrial tachycardia, are frequently due not to underlying heart disease but rather to infection, medication, pain, hypoxia, or electrolyte disturbances [16]. If arrhythmias are persistent despite correction of the above factors, they will often respond to calcium-channel blockers such as verapamil. Antiarrhythmic drugs can usually be discontinued prior to discharge in patients without underlying heart disease.

Although congestive heart failure is due in at least half of cases to intraoperative fluid overload rather than myocardial infarction, serial electrocardiograms and enzyme measurements should be done in all cases. Management depends on whether the congestive heart failure is due to increased preload (increased volume), increased afterload (increased vascular resistance), reduced pump function, or a combination of these factors and is discussed in Chapter 14. Digitalis tends to have a higher risk of complications in the aged patient in the postoperative period and should not be used routinely. Patients should not be committed to long-term therapy based on a single episode of postoperative congestive heart failure because the cardiac failure may resolve after the stress of surgery.

PULMONARY COMPLICATIONS

Common postoperative pulmonary events include pulmonary emboli, respiratory failure, and pneumonia. The age-related physiologic changes reviewed earlier make the elderly patient particularly susceptible to atelectasis and pneumonia. Thus it is not surprising that the risks of pneumonia after surgery are greater in the elderly. In a large series of patients over 70 years old undergoing general surgery Burnett et al. found a 14 percent incidence of bronchopneumonia [62]. Some authors report postoperative mortality associated with pneumonia of more than 50 percent in the elderly. Djokovic et al. [10] reported that 25 percent of patients over age 80 who underwent upper abdominal surgery and 50 percent of patients undergoing thoracic surgery required ventilation for at least 24 hours. Sixty percent of the patients requiring controlled ventilation had colonization of the upper respiratory tract with gram-negative organisms. About 20 percent of ventilated patients developed pneumonia, which was predominantly due to gram-negative organisms. Half of these patients died.

Deep venous thrombosis occurs in 50 to 75 percent of the elderly after orthopedic procedures on the hip or knee. A substantial percentage of these patients develop pulmonary emboli, which are more likely to be fatal in older patients than in their younger counterparts [63].

The management of pulmonary complications has been described earlier in this chapter. Vigorous attempts at earlier mobilization are essential. Adequate control of pain may improve respiratory effort and mobilization. Adequate hydration is important to allow mobilization of secretions. Physiotherapy and incentive spirometry should be used aggressively. Although choice of antiobiotics is dictated by culture results, if an organism is not readily apparent therapy should target gram-negative organisms, the most common cause of postsurgical pneumonia in the elderly.

RENAL COMPLICATIONS

The elderly are vulnerable to postoperative renal complications because of the marked reduction in creatinine clearance with age and their high incidence of diabetes and hypertension. The mortality of postoperative renal failure in the elderly approaches 50 percent. Whenever possible, nephrotoxic drugs such as aminoglycosides should be avoided, and if antibiotics are required, the newer cephalosporins are preferred. Fluid management should be judicious because older patients have a blunted capacity to regulate extracellular volume and are thus at risk for hypovolemia and acute renal insufficiency. A Swan-Ganz catheter may be required for several days in patients with tenuous renal function as a guide to fluid management. Urinary output should be monitored carefully and kept above 30 ml per hour, and fluids should be given to maintain adequate extracellular fluid volume status. Excessive use of hypotonic fluids may result in hyponatremia, a particularly common postoperative complication in the elderly (see Chap. 18).

PRESSURE SORES, NUTRITIONAL PROBLEMS, AND DELIRIUM

The management of pressure sores, nutritional problems, and delirium is covered in detail in other chapters and will be dealt with only briefly here. Pressure sores occur commonly in elderly patients, particularly those who are malnourished or who undergo orthopedic procedures requiring prolonged immobilization. Major risk factors include impaired level of consciousness, volume depletion, restricted mobility or paralysis, incontinence, and pronounced emaciation [64]. The pathogenesis and management of these lesions are covered in detail elsewhere [65] and in Chapter 12. General measures are at least as important as nursing care and topical therapy in the management of these lesions. For example, treatment of anemia and supplemental oxygen in hypoxic patients will improve tissue oxygen delivery, and treatment of malnutrition will speed healing and improve the ability to resist infection.

Approximately 10 percent of the elderly population are likely to have nutritional deficits. Patients with clinical or biochemical evidence of malnutrition should undergo nutritional support early in the postoperative period in an effort to speed wound healing, improve immune function, and decrease the likelihood of pressure sores. Details of nutritional intervention are covered in Chapter 8 and elsewhere [26]. If a malnourished patient will not take in adequate calories orally within two to three days after surgery, a feeding tube should be placed and enteral nutrition begun. Peripheral or central total parenteral nutrition can be used if the patient is unable to tolerate a feeding tube.

There is some evidence that aggressive nutritional support postoperatively is beneficial in the elderly. Lipschitz [66] reported on nine elderly subjects, six of whom were evaluated postoperatively. All patients had biochemical and clinical evidence of malnutrition. Aggressive enteral supplementation returned immune and hematopoietic parameters to normal levels, weight increased, and mental status, appetite, and functional capacity improved.

Delirium occurs very commonly postoperatively. Most studies suggest that the incidence is about 10 percent in general surgical patients over 65 years old but may be as high as 25 percent in patients with hip fractures [67]. The preoperative mental status is helpful as a baseline to establish the degree of confusion. Most cases of delirium are multifactorial in etiology. Drugs, particularly sedatives and agents with anticholinergic properties, are the most common offenders. Other common causes include electrolyte disturbances (especially hyponatremia) and dehydration, infection (especially urinary tract infection and pneumonia), and cardiovascular disorders (especially congestive heart failure and myocardial infarction). The management of this difficult syndrome is covered in Chapter 27 and elsewhere [68].

References

1. Vowles, K. J. D. Surgery for the Aged. In K. J. D. Vowles (ed.), *Surgical Problems in the Aged*. Bristol, England: John Wright & Sons, 1979.
2. Johnson, J. C. The medical evaluation and management of the elderly surgical patient. *J. Am. Geriatr. Soc.* 33:621, 1983.
3. Morh, D. N. Estimation of surgical risk in the elderly: A correlative review. *J. Am. Geriatr. Soc.* 33:99, 1983.
4. Mason, J. H., et al. General Surgery. In F. U. Stanberg (ed.), *The Care of the Geriatric Patient* (5th ed.). St. Louis: Mosby, 1976. P. 217.
5. Linn, B. S., et al. Evaluation of results of surgical procedures in the elderly. *Ann. Surg.* 195:90, 1982.
6. Marx, G. F., et al. Computer analysis of post–anaesthetic deaths. *Anaesthesiology* 39:54, 1973.
7. Palmberg, S., et al. Mortality in geriatric surgery: With special reference to the type of surgery, anaesthesia, complicating disease and prophylaxis of thrombosis. *Gerontology* 25:103, 1979.
8. Adkins, R. B., et al. Surgical procedures in patients aged 90 years and older. *South. Med. J.* 77:1357, 1984.
9. Boyd, J. B., et al. Operative risk factors of colon resection in the elderly. *Ann. Surg.* 192:743, 1982.
10. Djokovic, J. L., et al. Prediction of outcome of surgery and anesthesia in patients over 80. *J.A.M.A.* 242:2301, 1979.
11. Goldman, L., et al. Multifactorial index of cardiac risk in noncardiac surgical procedures. *N. Engl. J. Med.* 297:845, 1977.
12. Garibaldi, R. A., et al. Risk factors for postoperative pneumonia. *Am. J. Med.* 70:677, 1981.
13. Hodkinson, H. M. Non-specific presentation of illness. *Br. Med. J.* 4:94, 1973.
14. DelGuercio, L. R. M., et al. Monitoring operative risk in the elderly. *J.A.M.A.* 243:1350, 1980.
15. Gerson, M. C., et al. Cardiac prognosis in noncardiac geriatric surgery. *Ann. Intern. Med.* 103:832, 1985.
16. Goldman, L. Cardiac complications of non-cardiac surgery. *Ann. Intern. Med.* 98:504, 1983.
17. Tape, T. G., et al. The utility of routine chest radiographs. *Ann. Intern. Med.* 104:663, 1986.
18. Boghosian, S. G. H., et al. Usefulness of routine preoperative chest roentgenograms in elderly patients. *J. Am. Geriatr. Soc.* 35:142, 1987.
19. Tisi, G. M. Preoperative evaluation of pulmonary function. *Am. Rev. Resp. Dis.* 119:293, 1979.
20. Kitamura, H., et al. Postoperative hypoxemia: The contribution of age to the maldistribution of ventilation. *Anesthesiology* 36:244, 1972.
21. Leyvraz, P. F., et al. Adjusted versus fixed-dose subcutaneous heparin in the prevention of deep-vein thrombosis after total hip replacement. *N. Engl. J. Med.* 309:954, 1983.
22. Francis, C. W., et al. Two-step warfarin therapy: Prevention of postoperative venous thrombosis without excessive bleeding. *J.A.M.A.* 249:374, 1983.
23. Comerota, A. J., et al. The use of dihydroergotamine and heparin in the prophylaxis of deep venous thrombosis. *Chest* 89 (Suppl.): 389S, 1986.
24. Turpie, A. G. G., et al. A randomized controlled trial of a low-molecular-weight heparin (enoxaparin) to prevent deep-vein thrombosis in patients undergoing elective hip surgery. *N. Engl. J. Med.* 315:925, 1986.
25. Philips, P. A., et al. Reduced thirst after water

deprivation in healthy elderly men. *N. Engl. J. Med.* 311:753, 1984.

26. Morley, J. E. Nutritional status of the elderly. *Am. J. Med.* 81:679, 1986.

27. Bastow, M. P., et al. Undernutrition hypothermia and injury in elderly women with fractured femur, an injury response to altered metabolism. *Lancet* 1:143, 1983.

28. Pinchcofsky-Devin, G. D., et al. Correlation of pressure sores and nutritional status. *J. Am. Geriatr. Soc.* 34:435, 1986.

29. Burns, R., et al. Nutritional assessment of community-living well elderly. *J. Am. Geriatr. Soc.* 34:781, 1986.

30. Yeston, N. S. Medical Management of the Surgical Patient. In J. Noble (ed.), *Textbook of General Medicine and Primary Care.* Boston: Little, Brown, 1987. Pp. 2203–2222.

31. Kaiser, A. B. Antimicrobial prophylaxis in surgery. *N. Engl. J. Med.* 315:1129, 1986.

32. The infected hip arthroplasty (editorial). *Lancet* 21:557, 1984.

33. Bolander, F. M. S. Deaths associated with anaesthesia. *Br. J. Anaesthesiol.* 47:36, 1975.

34. Klotz, U., et al. The effects of age and liver disease on the disposition and elimination of diazepam in adult man. *J. Clin. Invest.* 55:347, 1975.

35. Christensen, J. H., et al. Pharmacokinetics and pharmacodynamics of thiopentone, a comparison between young and elderly patients. *Anaesthesia* 37:398, 1982.

36. Collier, P. S., et al. Influence of age on the pharmacokinetics of midazolam. *Br. J. Clin. Pharmacol.* 13:602, 1982.

37. Stevens, W. C., et al. Minimum alveolar concentrations of isoflurane with and without nitrous oxide in patients of various ages. *Anesthesiology* 42:197, 1975.

38. Gregory, G. A., et al. The relationship between age and halothane requirement in man. *Anaesthesiology* 30:488, 1969.

39. Krechel, S. W. Inhalation Agents in the Aged. In *Anesthesia and the Geriatric Patient.* Orlando, FL: Grune & Stratton, 1984. Pp. 99–114.

40. Duvaldestin, P., et al. Pharmacokinetics, pharmacodynamics and dose response relationships of pancuronium in control and elderly subjects. *Anesthesiology* 56:36, 1982.

41. McLeod, K., et al. Effects of aging on the pharmacokinetics of pancuronium. *Br. J. Anaesthesiol.* 51:435, 1979.

42. Marsh, R. H. K. Recovery from pancuronium: A comparison between old and young patients. *Anaesthesia* 35:1195, 1980.

43. Matteo, R. S., et al. Pharmacokinetics of d-tubo-curarine in the aged. *Anesthesiology* 57 (Suppl. 3A): A271, 1982.

44. Chmielewski, A. T., et al. Recovery from neuromuscular blockade. A comparison between young and old patients. *Anaesthesia* 33:539, 1978.

45. Park, W. Y., et al. Age and the spread of local anesthetic solutions in the epidural space. *Anesthesiol. Analg.* 59:768, 1980.

46. Bromage, P. R. Aging and epidural dose requirements. *Br. J. Anaesthesia* 41:1016, 1969.

47. Nation, R. L., et al. Lidocaine kinetics in cardiac patients and aged subjects. *Br. J. Clin. Pharmacol.* 4:439, 1977.

48. Mather, L. E., et al. Meperidine kinetics in man: Intravenous injection in surgical patients and volunteers. *Clin. Pharmacol. Ther.* 17:21, 1975.

49. Chan, K., et al. The effect of aging on plasma pethidine concentration. *Br. J. Clin. Pharmacol.* 2:297, 1975.

50. Bentley, J. B., et al. Age and fentanyl pharmacokinetics. *Anesthesiol. Analg.* 61:968, 1982.

51. Bellville, J. W., et al. Influence of age on pain relief from analgesia. *J.A.M.A.* 217:1835, 1971.

52. Virtanen, R., et al. Pharmacokinetic studies on atropine with special reference to age. *Acta Anaesthesiol. Scand.* 26:297, 1982.

53. MacLaren, A. D., et al. Anaesthetic techniques for surgical correction of fractured neck of femur. A comparative study of spinal and general anaesthesia in the aged. *Anaesthesia* 33:10, 1978.

54. Hole, A. Epidural versus general anaesthesia for total hip arthroplasty in elderly patients. *Acta Anaesthesiol. Scand.* 24:279, 1980.

55. Gribbin, B., et al. Effect of age and high blood pressure on baroreflex sensitivity in men. *Circ. Res.* 29:424, 1971.

56. Elliot, H. L., et al. Effect of age on the responsiveness of vascular alpha-adrenoreceptors in man. *J. Cardiovasc. Pharmacol.* 4:388, 1982.

57. Vestal, R. E., et al. Reduced beta adrenoreceptor sensitivity in the elderly. *Clin. Pharmacol. Ther.* 26:181, 1970.

58. Lawson, N. W. A dosage nomogram for sodium nitroprusside-induced hypotension under anesthesia. *Anesthes. Analg.* 55:574, 1976.

59. Robinson, B. F. Relationship of heart rate and systolic blood pressure to the onset of pain in angina pectoris. *Circulation* 35:1073, 1967.

60. Shackford, S. R., et al. Early extubation vs. prophylactic ventilation in the high risk patient: A comparison of post–operative management in prevention of respiratory complications. *Anesthesiol. Analg.* 60:76, 1981.

61. Banker, J., et al. (eds.). *The National Halothane Study: A Study of the Possible Association Between*

Halothane and Post–operative Hepatic Necrosis. Bethesda, MD: National Institutes of Health, National Institute of General Medical Science, 1969.

62. Burnett, W., et al. Surgical procedures in the elderly. *Surg. Gynecol. Obstet.* 134:221, 1972.

63. Morrell, M. T., et al. The post-mortem incidence of pulmonary embolism in a hospitalized population. *Br. J. Surg.* 55:347, 1968.

64. Anderson, K. E., et al. Prevention of pressure sores by identifying patients at risk. *Br. Med. J.* 284:1370, 1982.

65. Reuler, J. B., et al. The pressure sore: Pathophysiology and principles of management. *Ann. Intern. Med.* 94:661, 1981.

66. Lipschitz, D. A., and Mitchell, C. O. The correctability of the nutritional, immune, and hematopoietic manifestations of protein calorie malnutrition in the elderly. *J. Am. Coll. Nutr.* 1:17, 1982.

67. Seymour, D. G., et al. Post–operative complications in the elderly surgical patient. *Gerontology* 29:262, 1983.

68. Lipowski, Z. J. Transient cognitive disorders (delirium, acute confusional states) in the elderly. *Am. J. Psychiatry* 140:1426, 1983.

11

Rehabilitation: Goals and Approaches in Older People

T. FRANKLIN WILLIAMS *

As Phyllis Rubenfeld, President of the American Coalition of Citizens with Disabilities, has pointed out, older persons with disabilities are in double jeopardy—from both the prejudices of ageism and those of "disabilityism" [1]. The attitudes and practices of our society, including our health professions, are pervaded with negative views of old age and negative views of disabled people. Based in part on our own personal fears of old age and on what we now know to be myths about inevitable declines in function with aging, we have expected older people to become "less able," and our response to disability from age or disease has tended to be to provide dependent care, typically in some setting such as a nursing home, rather than to concentrate on restoring independence.

In fact, exactly the opposite views and approaches should characterize our services to older people. As much recent research has documented, older persons who are fortunate enough to be free from major diseases and are pursuing moderately active life-styles have as good cardiac output on standard stress tolerance tests as younger persons [2]. Also, in most older persons mental capabilities are well maintained [3], and in many there is no evidence of decline in

renal function [4]. Further, previously sedentary persons in their sixties and seventies can show as much improvement in maximum aerobic capacity as younger persons achieve with participation in fitness programs, and they also show improved blood lipid profiles and glucose tolerance [5, 6]. It is clear that we should start with the presumption, when an older person presents with a symptom of some loss of function, that some disease or other potentially treatable and reversible external cause of the disorder is present, and *not* that the problem is simply "old age" [7].

Thus, when faced with a condition causing disability or loss of function in an older person, our goal should be to restore as much function as quickly as possible. *The rehabilitation philosophy and approach should be at the heart of geriatric medicine:* "to restore the person to his/her former functional and environmental status, or, alternatively, to maintain or maximize remaining function" [8, 9].

In addition to understanding the potentials for physical and mental functional independence in older persons, physicians and other health professionals must be aware of the impact of attitudes, on the part of the patient as well as family and close friends, on the likelihood of accomplishing rehabilitative goals. As already noted, many people have negative views of themselves and tend to lose even more

* This article was written by Dr. Williams in his private capacity. No official support or endorsement by the National Institutes of Health is intended or should be inferred.

self-esteem when confronted with any disability [10]. Family expectations may be either positive and supportive for rehabilitative efforts, or passively or actively negative, accepting the disability as inevitable and tending to look on rehabilitative therapy as fruitless or even cruel. Dealing effectively with whatever attitudes are present is a part of the professional's job.

Principles of Rehabilitation in Older Persons

The main principles that should be included in the rehabilitative approach to any disability in older persons have been stated in simple terms such as the mnemonic SPREAD [11].

SPecific diagnosis and treatment of the underlying disease(s)

Prevention of secondary disability including that from disuse

Restoration of as much function as possible

ADaptation to persisting impairments by patient, family and environment

To these should be added the necessity for a *rehabilitation team approach*. Older patients' immediate problems are usually complicated by other concomitant disorders as well as behavioral and social issues. The combined skills of a geriatrically competent, rehabilitatively oriented physician, nurse, social worker, physiotherapist, and occupational therapist, and often other professionals such as a nutritionist, dentist, pharmacist, or speech pathologist, must be applied in initial assessment and, through team discussion, in working out the rehabilitation plan. This plan should include:

Prompt treatment for the treatable aspects of the problem(s)

Early ambulation and/or use of all bodily functions possible

Early return to a normal social and physical environment

Follow-up to help ensure continuation or modification of the plan as needed

Use of assistive devices as needed

In some other countries, notably the United Kingdom, Australia, and New Zealand, the geriatric services that have been established in most general hospitals are in fact geriatric rehabilitation services, which include participation of the full range of the rehabilitation professions under the leadership of a geriatrician as a routine aspect of the evaluation and conduct of treatment plans for every patient. Furthermore, this approach carries over into post–acute-hospital "day hospital" services for further rehabilitation therapy and follow-up observation. It would be desirable to see widespread development of such geriatric rehabilitation services in the United States.

Conditions Commonly Producing Disability in Older People

The most common conditions producing significant discomfort and/or disability in older persons in the United States have been identified in national surveys. Table 11-1 presents the chronic conditions reported by persons aged 65 and older living in the community. "Arthritis" was reported by almost half the respondents; hypertension, hearing impairment, and heart

TABLE 11-1. *Number of selected reported chronic conditions per 1,000 persons, by age: United States, 1982*

TYPE OF CONDITION	AGE		
	TOTAL 65 AND OVER	65–64	75 AND OVER
Arthritis	495.8	507.8	476.0
Hypertension	390.4	384.3	400.4
Hearing impairment	299.7	262.0	362.2
Deformity or orthopedic impairment	168.5	172.7	161.5
Chronic sinusitis	151.7	159.1	139.6
Visual impairment	101.1	80.7	134.8
Diabetes	88.9	96.6	76.3
Varicose veins	77.7	79.3	75.2
Hernia of abdominal cavity	75.5	87.8	55.2

SOURCE: National Center for Health Statistics. National Health Interview Survey. *Vital and Health Statistics*, Series 10, No. 150. DHHS Publication No. (PHS) 85-1578. Washington, D.C.: U.S. Government Printing Office, 1985.

TABLE 11-2. *Probability of selected medical conditions (not including sensory impairments) as the first reported cause of chronic disability among disabled persons, 85 years and older, United States, 1982*

CONDITION	PERCENT
Dementia	19.43
Arthritis	16.75
Peripheral vascular disease	14.88
Cerebrovascular disease	12.86
Hip and other fractures	8.81
Ischemic heart disease	1.88
Hypertension	1.38
Diabetes	1.01
Cancer	0.91
Emphysema and bronchitis	0.26

SOURCE: Health Care Financing Administration. Long-Term Care Survey, 1982. Presented by K. G. Manton at Annual Meeting of American Public Health Association, Washington, D.C., 1985.

disease also ranked high, and more than 10 percent reported deformities or orthopedic impairments, visual difficulties, and chronic sinusitis. These represent conditions that the respondents were aware of but do not indicate the degree of disability.

Table 11-2 presents more specific information on major disability among the "oldest old" people—i.e., the first reported causes among persons aged 85 and older who were disabled to the point of needing help from another person daily. Forty percent of persons living in the community among this very old group are this dependent on others. It may be seen that dementia is the most commonly listed principal problem, followed by arthritis, peripheral vascular disease, cerebrovascular disease (stroke), and loss of mobility due to hip and other fractures. Of note is that the major killers of older people, ischemic heart disease and cancer, are not common causes of severe chronic disability. To this list should be added urinary incontinence, which, while not often the primary problem of severe disability, is nevertheless a frequently reported concomitant problem and is one of the major burdens of care precipitating admission to a nursing home.

Rehabilitative Approaches to Specific Common Conditions

The following sections present details of the rehabilitative approach to the conditions com-

monly associated with potential or actual disability in older people; these conditions, if not corrected or improved, may lead to serious loss of independence. Many of the recommended measures are familiar to health practitioners, but it should be helpful to bring them together in relation to rehabilitation for these common problems. More detailed discussions of these disease entities appear elsewhere in this volume.

DEMENTIA

By far the most important step in the care of an older person who is developing a loss of cognitive functions and loss of memory is to conduct a thorough diagnostic evaluation [12, 13], searching for potentially reversible or treatable causes (see Chap. 27). Even when an irreversible form of dementia, such as Alzheimer's disease, is present, important steps can be taken to help achieve some stability of function for patient and family, which can certainly be considered a form of rehabilitation. These steps include establishing and maintaining a familiar environment and regular daily routines for the patient, and supportive and respite services for the caregiving family members. Support groups, such as local chapters of the Alzheimer's Disease and Related Disorders Association, now exist in most communities, and respite services such as day programs and temporary admissions to nursing homes are increasingly available.

OSTEOARTHRITIS

Perhaps the most serious consequences of osteoarthritis, a common symptomatic condition in older people, are the declines in level of daily activity, with resultant secondary disuse atrophy of muscles and further stiffness and limitation of motion in joints—a vicious cycle. The goal of treatment should be fundamentally rehabilitative: to restore full musculoskeletal function and vigor in the patient. The first necessity is relief of pain in the affected joints through use of antiinflammatory drugs, hydrotherapy, and strengthening of supportive muscle groups around the affected joint(s), and the second need is use of prostheses such as canes or braces. If joint pain is not adequately controlled by such efforts, surgical intervention with joint replacement should be considered. The decision on surgery is perhaps the most critical in a patient with intractable hip pain due to osteoarthritis, with resulting important limitation in mobility [14]. Hip surgery under these circumstances, with follow-up physiotherapy for muscle strengthening and ambulation, can be fully restorative of normal functions, and age is not a consideration for recommendation of this choice; if there is no uncontrollable disease or functional loss in some other organ system, the surgery is reasonably safe and effective at any age.

Hip Fracture

Risk factors for falls and hip fractures and measures that may be taken to prevent this severe and relatively common cause of loss of independence in older people are discussed elsewhere in this volume (see Chap. 16). Here we will discuss features and steps that may favor recovery of ambulation and independence following hip fracture.

Certain characteristics of patients have been found to be predictive of eventual independent living. In one recent study [15] of patients recovering from hip fracture it was found that the three features of prior good general health, living with another person or persons (rather than alone), and ability to walk within two weeks postoperatively, gave a 90 percent accurate prediction of being able to live at home independently. Patients who had any two of these three qualities had an 80 percent chance; those with only one of the three, a 50 percent chance; and those with none of the three, only a 12 percent chance of returning home. This study is an example of the observation that it may be the *number* of risk factors (or, in this instance, favorable factors), that determine outcomes in disabling conditions in older persons rather than any single specific factor [16].

Factors in management that are keys to achieving rehabilitation goals include:

Minimizing immobilization, including early surgical correction and immediate ambulation under a physiotherapist's supervision
Emphasizing functionality rather than anatomic perfection
Use of appropriate prostheses—e.g., braces, casts, canes, walkers—to favor early use of the extremities
Continued physiotherapy until maximum functional return has been achieved, and then maintenance therapy under periodic professional guidance

Early use of muscle-strengthening exercises and avoidance of any prolonged period of disuse are critical elements in achieving reasonably quick recovery from hip fracture or any other immobilizing condition, such as stroke. Studies have shown that it typically requires at least two days of exercise activities to regain the strength and function lost in each day of disuse [17].

Even in very old patients with hip fractures, surgical correction followed by rehabilitative therapy can produce impressive recovery. In one recently reported series of 18 such patients aged 91 to 102, 16 survived the immediate postfracture period, 63 percent attained independent ambulation, and 44 percent returned to their own homes. After one year, 12 survived, of whom nine were still functioning independently, although only five were still living at home [18]. Such a survival and functional outcome record at the ages of these patients is probably no different from similarly aged persons without hip fracture.

Stroke

Despite gratifying declines in the incidence of stroke in recent years, due in large part to improved control of hypertension, strokes continue to be a common and often severely disabling problem in older people. Recent data from an ongoing study of a total community of 215,000 persons in England [19] gives some perspective. The incidence of new strokes was found to be 0.47 per 1,000 persons per year among those aged 0 to 64 years, 7.28 per 1,000 per year in those aged 65 to 74 years, and 15.32 per 1,000 per year among those aged 75 or more. Those aged 75 and older had higher early mortality (57 percent within six months, compared to 35 percent for those aged 65 to 74 and 28 percent among those aged 64 and younger). Also, more of the oldest survivors required long-term institutional care—25 percent of those older than 75 compared to 13 percent of those aged 65 to 74 and 2 percent of those less than 65 years old. However, it is interesting to note that, due to the much higher mortality among the oldest group, the actual numbers of persons per 1,000 population in a given age group who were receiving long-term institutional care as a result of strokes was not much larger in the oldest group: 1.65 persons per 1,000 population aged 75 and older entered institutional care within one year after a stroke compared·with 0.62 persons per 1,000 population in the age group 65 to 74.

A number of factors appear to influence the ultimate outcome in stroke victims: the nature of the lesion itself; the premorbid condition of the patient; the specific features of the damage (e.g., degrees of aphasia, spasticity, incontinence, depression or apathy); and the social, economic, and environmental resources or limitations of the patient after the stroke.

The rehabilitation program for a stroke victim should begin as early as possible—within 48 hours of the event—and should increase in intensity as the medical condition stabilizes [20]. The full rehabilitation team should be involved, as described earlier. Attention must be paid to essential life-support measures such as keeping the airway clear. Full passive range of joint motion as well as changing position and skin care to prevent pressure ulcers should be provided by the nursing and physical or occupational therapy staff. Flaccid extremities should be kept in neutral positions with sandbags, rolled towels, or pillows. As much as possible, there should be normal sensory input, particularly by family and friends. Studies have shown the value of early rehabilitative intervention in regaining ability to ambulate and in early discharge [21].

As soon as possible, the stroke patient should be out of bed, in normal clothes, eating at a table, and using the toilet or commode. If there is any aphasia or swallowing difficulty, a speech pathologist should be involved in assessment and therapy. The common and fortunately often temporary intellectual, psychomotor, and mood changes that accompany strokes should be anticipated, taken into consideration in care plans, and interpreted to family members. Strokes, perhaps more than any other problem, call for a comprehensive, sustained team effort by well-prepared professionals in the interests of maximum recovery.

PERIPHERAL VASCULAR DISEASE

Types of peripheral vascular disease that can limit mobility and independence include occlusive arterial disease (including that secondary to diabetes), venous thrombosis and insufficiency, and, less commonly, chronic lymphedema. These problems become more frequent with age and the duration of the underlying pathology. Ambulation may be limited by pain (including intermittent claudication), by ulceration, by edema, and by development of gangrene requiring amputation. Preventive measures, aimed at minimizing vasoconstriction and edema, are again fundamentally rehabilitative in that they are the best hopes for restoration or maintenance of function. Such measures include avoidance of smoking, maintaining normal skin temperature exposure, systematic exercise within tolerance limits, cleanliness, and avoidance of trauma [22]. Reconstructive vascular surgery or angioplasty may be indicated.

HEARING IMPAIRMENT

A decline in hearing is present and progressive, to varying degrees, in almost everyone as he or she grows older: 90 percent of persons aged 85 and older report some loss of hearing [23]. Antecedent factors such as previous prolonged exposure to high noise levels may contribute to the loss, as may current factors such as the side effects of a number of drugs. Hearing loss is among the least treated of the common causes of disability in older persons, and neglect of efforts to determine potentially treatable causes and to use corrective measures to the maximum extent possible unfortunately results in social isolation for many older persons.

When loss of hearing is detected, the person should have the benefit of careful evaluation by an otolaryngologist and audiologist. An appropriate hearing aid should be fitted, and, depending on the degree of loss and the success of correction with the hearing aid, it may be desirable for the patient to have instruction in lip reading. Family members and close associates should be included in the rehabilitative plans and instructed in how they can help the patient through careful elocution and face-to-face speaking.

Many challenges concerning hearing impairment in older people remain, including the need to learn more about causes and possible prevention, the need to develop more technologically advanced hearing aids that can be adjusted to amplify only the frequency ranges lost in a given patient, and better understanding of the psychological impact of deafness on the patient and his or her associates [23].

VISUAL IMPAIRMENT

Thirty to forty percent of persons aged 65 and older report some visual difficulty in such common activities as doing household chores, going up and down stairs, or reading the newspaper [24]. In addition to regular examinations and appropriate treatment when possible for such problems as cataracts and glaucoma, full use should be made of available optical aids. Besides corrective lenses, these aids may include special lighting, magnifying glasses, large print, and special markings at potential danger spots around the home such as steps or corners [24, 25]. Potentially risky activities such as driving a car may need to be proscribed. Ophthalmologists and opticians should be consulted for help in achieving the best approaches to maintain or improve visual function.

CARDIAC DISEASES

Although, as noted above, cardiac diseases are relatively uncommon causes of *severe* dependency in old persons, nevertheless the high frequency of complications of atherosclerotic and other cardiovascular diseases in older persons makes the need for cardiac rehabilitative efforts quite common and potentially rewarding. Use of a systematic cardiac rehabilitation program may be indicated in older patients after cardiac surgery and in other disorders including cor pulmonale, aortic valvular disease, and thyroid heart disease, as well as after an acute cardiac event [26, 27].

Following an acute cardiac event, in older as in younger patients, cardiac rehabilitation should begin in the hospital with progressive ambulation, education of the patient and family about the condition and important life-style practices, and planning for continuing return to activities after discharge. There is no evidence that the return to ambulation and other usual activities needs to be any slower in older patients after myocardial infarction.

Post hospital planning should include a schedule for supervised, active exercise reconditioning followed by plans for long-term maintenance of physical condition. The goal should be to achieve and maintain the best possible aerobic capacity and the extent of daily activity desired by the patient. Although many older persons have persistent anxiety and depression after a coronary event [28], so many persons of all ages have successfully accomplished lifestyle changes—giving up smoking, following a prudent diet, exercising regularly—and have continued to live a satisfying, independent existence that professionals should actively promote these rehabilitative efforts.

URINARY INCONTINENCE

The common problem of urinary incontinence is discussed in detail elsewhere in this volume (see Chap. 19). Here it is simply emphasized that urinary incontinence often accompanies other conditions in which rehabilitative efforts are important such as stroke, hip fractures, and osteoarthritis (in which slower or impaired mobility may convert a tendency toward incontinence into a reality). In all circumstances in which urinary incontinence occurs it is most important that a careful workup be done to identify the pathogenetic mechanism(s) present and that active corrective steps be undertaken. As many recent studies have shown, control or marked improvement of this condition can be achieved in the majority of older patients, and such an accomplishment is always a key contribution to continuing an independent, social lifestyle.

"TOOLS FOR LIVING"

Wolff [29] has used this phrase to refer to the assistive and self-help devices that can help disabled persons of any age manage their environment and daily tasks more successfully. Most professionals know too little about the wide range of such materials that are now available. There are good discussions of this topic in the books edited by Williams [8] and by Brody and Ruff [30]. Medical-surgical supply stores, sales catalogues such as *Comfortably Yours: Aids for Easier Living* (Maywood, NJ 07607), and special catalogues by major department store chains such as Sears, Roebuck and Company, now provide many such resources.

In summary, rehabilitative possibilities should be considered an integral part of the workup and plans for treatment of every older patient who has or is at risk of developing some loss of function. The key principles to be kept in mind are an emphasis on the modifiable aspects of the problem; the necessity for a comprehensive multidisciplinary assessment as a first step, leading to a plan of care with specific rehabilitative goals; the importance of even small gains; and constant attention to and respect for the integrity and sense of worth of each older patient.

References

1. Rubenfeld, P. Ageism and Disabilityism: Double Jeopardy. In S. J. Brody & G. E. Ruff (eds.), *Aging and Rehabilitation: Advances in the State of the Art*. New York: Springer, 1986. Pp. 323–328.
2. Rodeheffer, R. J., et al. Exercise cardiac output is maintained with advancing age in healthy human subjects: Cardiac dilatation and increased stroke volume compensate for a diminished heart rate. *Circulation* 69:203, 1984.
3. Schaie, K. W. (ed.), The Seattle Longitudinal Study: A 21-year Exploration of Psychometric Intelligence in Adulthood. *Longitudinal Studies of Adult Psychological Development*. New York: Guilford, 1983. Pp. 54–135.
4. Lindeman, R. D., Tobin, J., and Shock, N. Longitudinal studies on the rate of decline in renal function with age. *J. Am. Geriatr. Soc.* 33:278, 1985.
5. Seals, D. R., et al. Endurance training in older men and women: I. Cardiovascular response to exercise. *J. Appl. Physiol.* 57:1024, 1984.
6. Seals, D. R., et al. Effects of endurance training on glucose tolerance and plasma lipid levels in older men and women. *J.A.M.A.* 252:645, 1984.
7. Williams, T. F. Geriatrics: The fruition of the clinician revisited. *Gerontologist* 26:345, 1986.
8. Williams, T. F. (ed.). *Rehabilitation in the Aging*. New York: Raven, 1984.
9. Williams, T. F. The future of aging. *Arch. Phys. Med. Rehabil.* 68:335, 1987.
10. Kemp, B. Psychosocial and Mental Health Issues in Rehabilitation of Older Persons. In S. J. Brody and G. E. Ruff (eds.), *Aging and Rehabilitation: Advances in the State of the Art*. New York: Springer, 1986. Pp. 122–158.
11. Hunt, T. E. Practical considerations in the rehabilitation of the aged. *J. Am. Geriatr. Soc.* 28:59, 1980.
12. National Institutes of Health. *Consensus Development Conference on Diagnosis of Dementia*. Bethesda, MD, July 6–8, 1986.
13. Reifler, B. V., and Teri, L. Rehabilitation and Alzheimer's Disease. In S. J. Brody and G. E. Ruff (eds.), *Aging and Rehabilitation: Advances in the State of the Art*. New York: Springer, 1986. Pp. 107–121.
14. Harris, D. M. Joint Replacement in the Elderly. In T. F. Williams (ed.), *Rehabilitation in the Aging*. New York: Raven, 1984. Pp. 199–228.
15. Cedar, L., Svensson, K. B., and Thorngren, K. Statistical prediction of rehabilitation in elderly patients with hip fractures. *Clin. Orthop.* 152:185, 1980.
16. Tinetti, M., Williams, T. F., and Mayewski, R. Fall risk index for elderly patients based on the number of chronic disabilities. *Am. J. Med.* 80:429, 1986.
17. Jones, R. H. Physiological Basis of Rehabilitation Therapy. In T. F. Williams (ed.), *Rehabilitation in the Aging*. New York: Raven, 1984. Pp. 97–110.
18. Kauffman, T. L., Albright, L., and Wagner, C. Rehabilitation outcomes after hip fracture in persons 90 years old and older. *Arch. Phys. Med. Rehab.* 68:369, 1987.
19. Wade, D. T., and Hewer, R. C. Stroke: Associations with age, sex and side of weakness. *Arch. Phys. Med. Rehabil.* 67:540, 1986.
20. Gibson, C. J., and Caplan, B. M. Rehabilitation of the Patient with Stroke. In T. F. Williams (ed.), *Rehabilitation in the Aging*. New York: Raven, 1984. Pp. 145–160.
21. Hayes, S. H. and Carroll, S. R. Early intervention care in the acute stroke patient. *Arch. Phys. Med. Rehabil.* 67:319, 1986.
22. Spittell, J. A., Jr. Rehabilitative Aspects of Peripheral Vascular Disorders in the Elderly. In T. F. Williams (ed.), *Rehabilitation in the Aging*. New York: Raven, 1984. Pp. 283–290.
23. Glass, L. E. Rehabilitation for Deaf and Hearing-Impaired Elderly. In S. J. Brody and G. E. Ruff (eds.), *Aging and Rehabilitation: Advances in the State of the Art*. New York: Springer, 1986. Pp. 218–238.
24. DiStefano, A. F., and Aston, S. J. Rehabilitation for the Blind and Visually Impaired Elderly. In

S. J. Brody and G. E. Ruff (eds.), *Aging and Rehabilitation: Advances in the State of the Art.* New York: Springer, 1986. Pp. 203–217.

25. Kornzweig, A. L. Rehabilitation in Ophthalmology for the Aged. In T. F. Williams (ed.), *Rehabilitation in the Aging.* New York: Raven, 1984. Pp. 229–234.

26. Brammel, H. L. Rehabilitation of the Elderly Cardiac Patient. In S. J. Brody and G. E. Ruff (eds.), *Aging and Rehabilitation: Advances in the State of the Art.* New York: Springer, 1986. Pp. 241–255.

27. Wenger, N. K. Specific Cardiac Disorders. In T. F. Williams (ed.), *Rehabilitation in the Aging.* New York: Raven, 1984. Pp. 265–282.

28. Pathy, M. S., and Peach, H. Disability among the elderly after myocardial infarction: A 3-year follow-up. *J. R. Coll. Physicians London* 14:221, 1980.

29. Wolff, H. S. Introduction: Tools for Living. In J. Bray and S. Wright (eds.), *The Use of Technology in the Care of the Elderly and the Disabled.* Westport, CT: Greenwood, 1980.

30. Brody, S. J., and Ruff, G. E. (eds.), *Aging and Rehabilitation: Advances in the State of the Art.* New York: Springer, 1986.

12

Skin

Tania J. Phillips
Barbara A. Gilchrest

Skin is the interface between humans and their environment that protects the other organs of the body against excessive temperature changes, mechanical injury, ultraviolet irradiation, toxic chemicals, and microbial pathogens. It is also a tactile organ through which individuals receive pleasurable stimuli and assess their physical surroundings. With age, the skin performs each of these vital functions less well. Skin is also readily visible and hence is of great psychologic and social, as well as physiologic, importance. For this reason, the morphologic changes that accompany aging in the skin often affect an individual as greatly as do the functional changes.

Consideration of age-induced changes in the skin is complicated by the fact that the skin is subjected to repeated and often cumulative environmental damage that is difficult to distinguish from true aging. In the minds of the public and many physicians, sun-damaged skin is synonymous with old skin, whereas virtually all skin cancers and most of the cosmetically undesirable changes in cutaneous appearance occur in exposed areas only. In addition, portions of the skin and some of its appendages are very sensitive to hormonal stimulation, so that age-associated hormonal shifts (e.g., puberty and menopause) may produce skin changes not directly attributable to aging itself.

The following sections review the physiologic and underlying morphologic changes that occur in aging skin and discuss the skin lesions that frequently or disproportionately affect the elderly. Detailed, exhaustively referenced reviews of these topics are listed at the end of the chapter under Suggested Reading. References are provided in the text only to recent papers not available from these sources.

Age-Associated Changes in Normal Skin
MORPHOLOGIC CHANGES

The major aging changes in gross morphology of the skin include "dryness" (by which is meant roughness), wrinkling, laxity, uneven pigmentation, and a variety of proliferative lesions.

Epidermis

The most striking and consistent change in biopsies of old skin is flattening of the dermoepidermal junction with effacement of both the dermal papillae and the epidermal rete pegs, shown schematically in Figure 12-1. This flattening results in a tremendously smaller contiguous surface between the two compartments and presumably in less "communication" and nutrient transfer as well as greater ease of dermoepidermal separation.

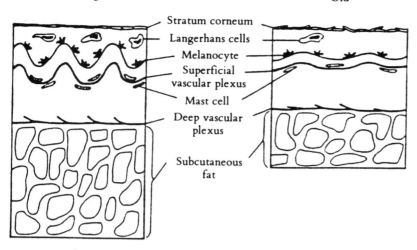

Young   Old

Stratum corneum
Langerhans cells
Melanocyte
Superficial vascular plexus
Mast cell
Deep vascular plexus
Subcutaneous fat

FIGURE 12-1. *Histologic changes in aging normal skin. Schematic drawings emphasize the age-associated flattening of the dermoepidermal junction, loss of dermal and subcutaneous mass, shortened capillary loops, reduced numbers of melanocytes, Langerhans cells, and mast cells. In most body areas, epidermal thickness is approximately 0.1 mm; dermal thicknesses range from 1.0 to 4.0 mm, depending on body site. Melanocyte densities range from 1,000/mm² to 2,000/mm² surface area in most body areas; Langerhans cell density is approximately 500/mm². Reprinted with permission from the American Geriatrics Society, Histologic changes in aging normal skin, by B. A. Gilchrest (Journal of the American Geriatrics Society, 30:139, 1982).*

A decrease of approximately 10 to 20 percent per decade in the density of enzymatically active epidermal melanocytes has been repeatedly documented. It is not known whether the cells truly disappear or simply become undetectable by ceasing to produce pigment, but in either case the body's protective barrier against ultraviolet light is reduced. The number of melanocytic nevi also progressively decreases with age beginning in the third or fourth decade, and pigment cells similarly disappear from hair bulbs.

Langerhans cells are bone marrow–derived immune effector cells that are necessary for allergic sensitization and probably for immune surveillance generally within the epidermis. This population, approximately 3 to 4 percent of epidermal cells in young adult skin, has been noted to decline 20 to 50 percent during adulthood in two studies relying on different quantification techniques [1, 2]. Further reduction, up to 50 percent of the values in sun-protected skin of the same subjects, has been reported in habitually sun-exposed sites [2, 3].

Dermis

Loss of dermal thickness is pronounced in elderly individuals and accounts for the paperthin, sometimes nearly transparent, quality of their skin. The remaining dermis is relatively acelluar and avascular. The marked reduction of the vascular bed, especially the vertical capillary loops that occupy dermal papillae in young skin, is felt to underlie many of the physiologic alterations in old skin discussed in the following section. The marked reduction in the vascular network surrounding hair bulbs and eccrine, apocrine, and sebaceous glands may be responsible for their gradual atrophy and fibrosis with age.

Pacinian and Meissner's corpuscles, cutaneous end-organs responsible for pressure perception and light touch, display progressive disorganization and histologic degeneration with age. Free nerve endings appear not to change substantially.

Appendages

Age-related changes in hair color, density, and distribution are widely recognized. Greying, which is pronounced in about half the population by age 50, is due to progressive and eventually total loss of functional melanocytes from the hair bulb. This process is believed to occur more rapidly in hair than in skin because melanocytes are called on to proliferate and manufacture melanin at maximal rates during the anagen or growth phase of the hair cycle, whereas epidermal melanocytes are relatively inactive throughout their life span. Scalp hair is believed to grey more rapidly than other body hair because its anagen (growth phase) to telogen (resting phase) ratio is considerably greater than that of other body hair. Advancing age is also accompanied by a gradual decrease in number of hair follicles over the entire body, with atrophy and fibrosis of many follicles. Appreciable hair loss on the scalp, commonly called balding, results primarily from the androgen–dependent conversion of the relatively dark, thick scalp hairs to lightly pigmented, short, fine vellus hairs similar to those on the ventral forearm. By age 50 the process is at least moderately advanced in approximately 60 percent of men and noticeable in perhaps 20 percent of women. Since hair density must decrease by at least 50 percent to be clinically detectable, it is apparent that this loss of hair is substantial. Axillary hair is virtually absent in 30 percent of women and in 7 percent of men by age 60, and pubic hair also thins markedly. Remaining scalp and body hairs grow more slowly and may be smaller in diameter.

Eccrine (sweat), apocrine, and sebaceous (oil) glands become smaller, less numerous, and fibrotic throughout the skin, coincident with their reduced activity.

With age, fingernails and toenails develop longitudinal ridges (onychorrhexis), an expression of alternating hyperplasia and hypoplasia of the nail matrix as well as generalized thinning. Frequently traumatized or relatively ischemic nails, usually on the feet, may thicken, as apparent overcompensation for injury.

PHYSIOLOGIC CHANGES

The major functions of the skin known to decline with age are listed in Table 12-1.

Cell Renewal

The epidermis is a continuously self-renewing compartment. Keratinocytes in the basal layer

TABLE 12–1. *Functions of the skin that are known to decline with age*

Epidermal turnover	Immune function
Wound healing	Vascular responsiveness
Injury response	Thermoregulation
Barrier function	Sweat production
Chemical clearance rates	Sebum production
Sensory perception	Vitamin D production

periodically divide and hence supply daughter cells for upward migration through approximately 20 to 30 cell layers to the skin surface, where the then terminally differentiated cells (corneocytes) are shed.

An age-related decrease in epidermal turnover rate of approximately 50 percent between the third and seventh decades has been documented by a study of desquamation rates for these corneocytes at selected body sites [4]. In earlier independent studies relying on intradermal injection of H-thymidine to label cycling basal layer keratinocytes, the labeling index averaged approximately 5.5 percent in adults aged 18 to 25 years but only 3 percent in adults aged 71 to 86 years. Hair and nail growth also depends on cell division in the hair bulb and nail matrix respectively and slows considerably with age. Fingernail linear growth rates decrease approximately 0.5 percent annually, from an average of 0.9 mm per week in the third decade to 0.5 mm per week in the tenth.

In vitro studies of mitogen responsiveness have documented significant losses between newborns and adults and between young adults and old adults for both keratinocytes and dermal fibroblasts [5, 6].

Wound Repair

Wound repair rate declines with age, whether measured in terms of wound closure, collagen deposition, or regeneration of blister roofs (epidermal cell migration and mitosis). Excision of thymine dimers in DNA of ultraviolet (UV)-irradiated cultured dermal fibroblasts has been reported to decrease with age, although more recent and more technically sophisticated studies have failed to find consistent age-associated changes in DNA repair capacity [5, 6]. Comparison between adults below age 35 years and those above age 65 years reveals an approximately 50 percent prolongation with age in the average time required to reepithelialize an experimentally blistered skin site, from 3.5 to 5.5 weeks.

Barrier Function

An age-related decrease in the barrier function of intact stratum corneum has been documented by measuring percutaneous absorption of various substances, although the literature is contradictory and suggests that penetration of polar versus nonpolar compounds may be differently affected by aging [9]. There is a decreased clearance of the absorbed materials from the dermis as well, probably due to alterations in the vascular bed and in the extracellular matrix. These combined changes may render old skin susceptible to irritant and allergic reactions, both of which require local accumulation of the offending substance.

Immune Function

An age-associated decline in cell-mediated immune reactions in the skin has been documented by a decreased positivity rate for skin tests to classic recall antigens such as mumps purified protein derivative and candidin [10], and decreased ease of sensitization to neoantigens such as dinitrochlorobenzene (DNCB). In a study of sensitization to DNCB 69 percent of patients over the age of 70 were sensitized, in contrast to 94 percent of patients under the age of 69 who reacted to the chemical [11]. The decrease in epidermal Langerhans cell number mentioned above may contribute. Also, recent in vitro studies support an age-associated loss of keratinocyte immune function. Epidermal cell-derived thymocyte activating factor (ETAF), a cytokine very similar or identical to interleukin-1 and presumed to amplify T-lymphocyte responses in the skin, has been found to be produced only one-sixth as well by cultured adult keratinocytes as by cultured newborn keratinocytes [12]. These local age-associated changes, compounded by the decline in systemic immune function, undoubtedly contribute to the decreased intensity and positivity rate for cutaneous delayed hypersensitivity reactions and may further predispose the elderly to photocarcinogenesis.

Decreased immunocompetence may also be reflected in the skin of the elderly as a high prevalence of certain chronic infections such as tinea pedis. The tendency in many older patients toward bacterial superinfection of cuts and abrasions, especially on the legs, probably results from compromised tissue perfusion and inherently slow healing in those areas.

Vascular Responsiveness

Decreased vascular responsiveness in the skin of older individuals has been documented by observing vasodilation after application of standardized irritants or ultraviolet light exposure in young and old subjects. Compromised thermoregulation, which predisposes the elderly both to heat stroke and hypothermia, is probably due largely to reduced vasodilation or vasoconstriction of dermal arterioles but is also attributable in part to decreased eccrine sweat production and loss of subcutaneous fat, both of which also occur with advancing age.

The time required for blister formation following topical application of irritant chemicals doubles between young and old adulthood, illustrating another compromise of vascular response to injury (transudation).

Vitamin D Production

An important endocrine function of skin now known to decline with age is vitamin D_3 production. The amount of epidermal precursor, 7-dehydrocholesterol, decreases approximately 75 percent during adulthood, and circulating (serum) levels of 1,25-dihydroxyvitamin D_3 following whole body ultraviolet-irradiation are similarly reduced [13]. Because perhaps 25 to 30 percent of the elderly hospitalized for hip fractures suffer osteomalacia, the result of vitamin D_3 deficiency [14], as well as osteoporosis, this age-associated cutaneous functional loss may directly contribute to their morbidity and mortality.

Sebum Production

The steady decline in sebum production that accompanies advancing age in both men and women appears to be independent of any recognized hormonal change and is better attributable to decreased cell turnover rate in this holocrine gland [15]. The clinical effects of decreased sebum production, if any, are unknown. There is no direct relationship to xerosis.

Sensory Perception

Finally, both nerve conduction velocity and stimulation thresholds for cutaneous fibers and end-organs increase with age, undoubtedly contributing to the risk of mechanical or chemical injury to the skin.

Skin Disorders and the Elderly

PREVALENCE

Certain inflammatory disorders, infections, and neoplasms of the skin increase in prevalence throughout life among otherwise healthy individuals. The best documentation of this fact derives from a 1971–1974 survey of over 20,000 representative noninstitutionalized Americans aged 1 to 74 years in which each person underwent a physical examination and laboratory testing [16]. In the first decade, approximately 15 percent of those surveyed had a dermatologic disorder at the time of examination sufficiently severe to warrant at least one physician visit; in almost all of these individuals, a single problem was present. In contrast, nearly 40 percent of the population aged 65 to 75 years had at least one skin disease of similar severity, and affected individuals averaged more than 1.5 disorders each. Not all dermatologic disorders disproportionately affect the elderly, however. Many common conditions affect young and old adults equally, whereas others are virtually restricted to children and young adults. The disorders discussed here are those that occur more commonly, although certainly not exclusively, in the elderly.

PRINCIPLES OF MANAGEMENT

Management of skin conditions in the elderly must consciously be tailored to their abilities. Many elderly patients live alone, have substantial limitations of motion due to neurologic impairment or arthritis, and experience difficulty applying topical treatments or bathing [17].

Medication errors are also common in this patient group, as discussed elsewhere. Twenty-five to 50 percent of elderly patients fail to take prescribed medications [18], 59 percent make medication errors, and 26 percent make potentially serious errors [19]. It therefore seems prudent to keep treatment regimens as simple as possible. Moreover, the elderly are especially prone to adverse effects from drugs. The incidence of adverse drug reactions is increased two- to threefold in elderly patients. Frequent offenders include some of the more common oral medications employed in dermatology, antihistamines and corticosteroids [20], and these should therefore be prescribed with caution.

XEROSIS

Xerosis, the "dry" or rough quality of skin, may be generalized but is especially common and prominent on the lower legs. The condition may reflect minor abnormalities in the epidermal maturation process and is exacerbated by a low-humidity environment. Affected skin is often pruritic and may show evidence of inflammation, probably as a result of breaks in the stratum corneum with secondary entry of irritating substances into the dermis. The resulting condition is called eczema craquele or winter eczema.

Treatment

The patient should not expose his skin to irritants such as excessive soap and water or disinfectants. Emollients such as petrolatum should be used frequently, especially after bathing when the skin is moist. Creams that contain urea or lactic acid are also helpful and may be more cosmetically acceptable to some patients. Topical steroid ointments provide rapid symptomatic relief of eczema craquele, especially when applied under occlusive dressings.

PRURITUS

Itching is a common complaint in elderly patients. The patient should be carefully examined for any skin eruption that might explain the symptom; in the absence of this, any possible underlying systemic cause such as chronic renal failure, hepatic disease, lymphoma, polycythemia rubra vera, endocrine or metabolic disorder, or drug allergy should be excluded. Bullous pemphigoid is a blistering disorder that may be preceded by generalized pruritus for several months before the blisters appear. However, despite extensive investigation, pruritus is unexplained in at least half of affected patients. In these cases, liberal use of emollients is often of benefit. Systemic antihistamines can be helpful, but should be used cautiously in the elderly.

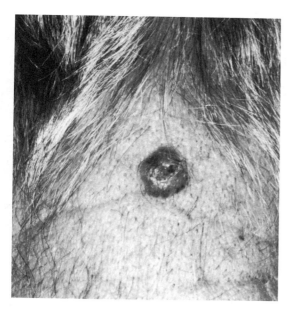

FIGURE 12-2. *Basal cell carcinoma is characterized by a pearly telangiectatic appearance and rolled edge.*

MALIGNANCIES

Malignant neoplasms of the skin increase in incidence throughout adulthood and account for nearly 50 percent of all malignancies reported annually in the United States. By far the most common are basal cell epitheliomas (Fig. 12-2). These are slow-growing, locally invasive, and destructive proliferations of basilar keratinocytes that extend down from the epidermis and characteristically form multiple, nearly spherical masses in the dermis. Clinically, basal cell epitheliomas begin as painless "pearly" or opalescent telangiectatic papules; 90 percent arise on the head or neck and virtually always on a background of markedly sun-damaged skin. The appearance is so distinctive that an experienced examiner can readily diagnose basal cell epithelioma less than 2 mm in diameter. As lesions enlarge, central ulceration and crusting may occur, creating "rodent ulcers," but the epidermis remains intact over many lesions exceeding a centimeter in diameter. Cure rates for small lesions approach 100 percent, utilizing any of several therapeutic modalities (excision, cryotherapy, curettage, or x-irradiation). Large neglected basal cell epitheliomas may be virtually impossible to eradicate and may result in major disfigurement, loss of an eye, or death

from debility and sepsis, although even the largest basal cell epitheliomas rarely metastasize.

Squamous cell carcinomas are overwhelmingly lesions of sun-exposed skin, although these malignancies also occur in sites of chronic inflammation, such as ulcer margins. Lesions usually present as firm, painless, slightly erythematous nodules or plaques. The surface may be scaly or ulcerated. Rate of growth and tendency to metastasize vary with the location and clinical setting of the lesion. The prognosis for squamous cell carcinomas involving a mucous membrane or otherwise unrelated to chronic sun exposure is poor.

Treatment is based on the size and location of the tumor, as well as the setting in which it arises. Electrosurgery, excision, and x-irradiation are commonly employed modalities.

In addition to ultraviolet light, other environmental carcinogens established as causes of cutaneous squamous cell carcinomas include x-irradiation, arsenic, soot, coal tar, and numerous industrial oils. Because such environmental carcinogens are often present in small amounts over long time periods, and because induction time following adequate exposure is usually many years, most squamous cell carcinomas arise in older individuals. In addition, there is evidence in rodents that older animals are more prone to develop skin cancers following a standard challenge than are younger animals.

Actinic keratoses (Fig. 12-3) are extremely common, minimally raised "sandpaper-like" patches in sun-exposed areas that are acknowledged precursor lesions of squamous cell carcinomas but rarely evolve into invasive malignancies. Even those lesions that invade the dermis metastasize in fewer than 3 percent of cases, in contrast to nearly 50 percent for squamous cell carcinoma of the skin in other settings.

Keratoacanthoma (Fig. 12-4) is considered a benign epidermal neoplasm by most authorities. However, histologically and clinically it may resemble squamous cell carcinoma, and its relation to the latter is not well understood. Clinically, it occurs almost exclusively in sun-exposed sites in patients over the age of 50. It enlarges rapidly within a few weeks to form a nodule with a central crater containing a keratin plug. Although spontaneous resolution can occur, keratoacanthoma is usually treated by cu-

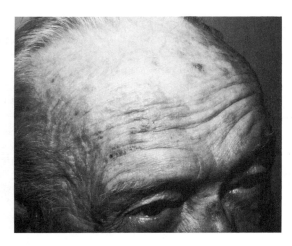

FIGURE 12-3. *Actinic keratoses are rough scaly patches that appear on sun-exposed surfaces.*

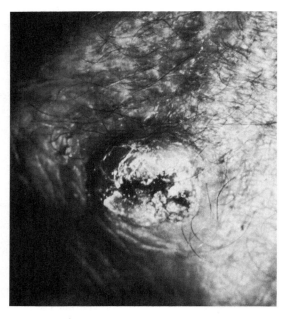

FIGURE 12-4. *A keratoacanthoma is a rapidly growing flesh-colored nodule with a central keratinous plug. It can closely resemble squamous cell carcinoma, both clinically and histologically.*

rettage and cautery or by excision, in part to shorten the duration of these cosmetically distressing lesions and in part out of concern for its malignant potential.

Lentigo maligna is a macular (flat) lesion with irregular brown–black pigmentation and an ir-

regular border that occurs predominantly on sun-exposed areas (cheeks [42 percent] and forehead [19 percent]). The lesions usually enlarge and may gradually become nodular, the latter change heralding conversion to invasive lentigo maligna melanoma. This form of melanoma appears to be relatively indolent, is usually diagnosed while still a relatively thin lesion, and is associated with favorable survival. However, thicker lesions have the same poor prognosis as other categories of melanoma, and all lesions should be regarded as life-threatening. The estimated risk of melanoma in patients with lentigo maligna by the age of 75 is 1.2 percent, and the case fraction of lentigo maligna melanoma among all melanomas is 5 percent [22].

All patients with suspected cutaneous malignancies should be seen by a dermatologist or other physician familiar with their diagnosis and treatment to optimize patient management. Long-term as well as short-term referral is often warranted. Probably as a result of combined environmental and host factors, individuals with a history of cutaneous squamous cell carcinoma or basal cell epitheliomas are at much higher risk of developing a new lesion than are those without a prior history and hence merit as well a careful examination of the entire cutaneous surface at least annually.

HERPES ZOSTER

Herpes zoster ("shingles") is a familiar vesicular dermatomal eruption caused by reactivation of latent varicella virus in the dorsal ganglia of a partially immune host. The disorder has a peak incidence between 50 and 70 years of age and usually affects otherwise healthy individuals, although immunosuppressed patients are at higher risk. The major difference between herpes zoster in the elderly versus that in the young adult is the incidence of postherpetic neuralgia, which increases sharply with age to approximately 40 percent in patients over the age of 60 years. Moreover, duration and severity of the discomfort increase even more markedly with age than does incidence.

Acyclovir, administered intravenously or in high doses orally [23], has been found to be beneficial in reducing discomfort and duration of viral shedding and development of new vesicles during the acute phase of the illness but does not appear to influence the incidence or severity of postherpetic neuralgia [24]. Prednisone, 40 to 60 mg per day or its equivalent administered orally during the active eruption, also appears to reduce both acute symptomatology and the risk of postherpetic neuralgia in elderly patients [25]. Despite the potential adverse effects of a two- to three-week course of corticosteroids in elderly patients, prednisone remains the most widely employed prophylactic treatment against postherpetic neuralgia in high-risk patients. Psychotropic drugs are also reported to be useful in treating postherpetic neuralgia [26].

BULLOUS PEMPHIGOID

Bullous pemphigoid (Fig. 12-5) is a not uncommon blistering disease of the elderly that appears to have an immunologic basis. Complement (C3) and in most cases immunoglobulins are fixed at the dermoepidermal junction of perilesional skin, and circulating anti-basement-membrane antibodies are usually detectable. Histologically, these abnormalities result in subepidermal bullae. Clinically, patients have mixed erosions and intact bullae, arising either from normal-appearing skin or from erythematous macules or urticarial plaques. The process is usually generalized but may be localized to small areas of the body. Untreated patients may remain in good general health for prolonged periods, although infection of denuded skin is a constant threat. Systemic steroids in doses equivalent to prednisone 40 to 60 mg a day are

FIGURE 12-5. *Bullous pemphigoid. There are tense bullae on an erythematous base.*

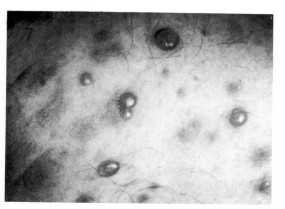

the mainstay of therapy and can be successfully tapered or discontinued after weeks to months in many patients. Immunosuppressants such as cyclophosphamide (Cytoxan) are often employed in elderly patients for their steroid-sparing effect, although they provide little benefit in the first six to eight weeks of therapy. Early diagnosis is critical because extensive disease requires on average longer courses and higher doses of corticosteroids to achieve a remission. Immunofluorescent studies of perilesional skin biopsies are diagnostic.

PSORIASIS

Psoriasis is common in all age groups, and approximately 3 percent of psoriatic patients first develop lesions after age 60 years. In one large survey, 43 percent of patients aged 60 to 74 years first developed psoriasis after age 45 years [27]. In elderly patients bothered by psoriasis a careful drug history should be taken, because many drugs, especially beta-blockers, can precipitate or exacerbate the disease. Sometimes very small doses of oral methotrexate, 5 to 10 mg per week, will control psoriasis in the elderly patient, but liver and renal function (including creatinine clearance) and blood counts must be carefully monitored. Ultraviolet treatment, which entails multiple clinic visits, is often very helpful but may be impractical if the patient has poor mobility. Topical corticosteroids alone are rarely effective in controlling extensive disease.

DECUBITUS ULCERS

The decubitus ulcer or pressure sore is one of the most difficult management problems encountered in geriatric patients and is common among those confined to bed or wheelchair. The lesion is better classified as a systemic rather than a cutaneous disorder because major illness involving at least one and usually several organ systems is invariably present. Indeed, decubitus ulcers are a major problem in clinical medicine precisely because the predisposing factors are of paramount importance and rarely correctable.

The ulcers occur over bony prominences: Statistically, 65 percent occur in the pelvic area and 30 percent on the lower extremeties [28]. Prolonged direct pressure, in excess of the 32 mm Hg average capillary perfusion pressure in the skin, produces tissue anoxia with necrosis of the epidermis and superficial dermis. Transcutaneous oxygen tension over bony prominences when the patient is lying supine is zero. Since pressures up to 70 mm Hg at the sacrum and 45 mm Hg at the heels are generated when the body is supine, it is not surprising that decubitus ulcers may arise after as little as an hour of total immobility. Additional contributing factors in the elderly often include (1) folding of loose lax skin, with compromised blood flow in the larger dermal vessels, as well as increased compression of superficial capillaries; (2) reduced subcutaneous fat, which results in greater local pressure on the skin over bony prominences such as the ischial tuberosities and sacrum; and (3) reduction in baseline cutaneous blood flow by congestive heart failure, atherosclerosis, loss of intravascular volume, or another disorder common in advanced age. Perhaps more important, once an ulcer occurs, healing may be retarded by general inanition, by incontinence with secondary chemical irritation and bacterial infection of the ulcer base, or by inadequate vascular supply of the involved area. These same factors are indeed responsible for the inexorable progression of many decubitus ulcers into the underlying fat, muscle, and ultimately bone.

Prevention, although difficult in high-risk patients, is much easier than cure. Relief of pressure over decubitus ulcers is the most important principle of management. The simplest method is frequent turning of the bedridden patient, at least every two hours. The patient should be regularly turned to a 30-degree inclined lateral position, which has been shown to be superior to the 90-degree lateral position [29]. Air- or fluid-filled mattresses or supersoft support mattresses tend to equalize pressure over the entire area of contact and are thus a great improvement over conventional mattresses. The best of the currently available support surfaces is the ripple mattress, a series of contiguous, 12-cm in diameter, horizontally aligned inflatable tubes. A machine pump repeatedly inflates and deflates the tubes every 5 to 10 minutes in an alternating pattern, so that the patient is supported first by the even-numbered tubes and then by the odd-numbered tubes, and no area is continuously weight-bearing for more than the 5- to 10-minute pump cycle time.

Once a decubitus ulcer is present, in addition to the previously mentioned measures, it is necessary to maintain the ulcer base in as optimal condition for healing as possible. Necrotic tissue creates favorable conditions for bacterial growth and prevents epithelialization of wounds. Necrotic ulcers should therefore be treated aggressively with surgical debridément of any necrotic tissue or eschar.

Underlying osteomyelitis will hinder healing of pressure sores. A recent study suggested that in nonhealing decubiti with a positive bone scan, a bone biopsy and culture should be performed to exclude osteomyelitis [30].

Healing is always slowed by heavy colonization of the ulcer with bacteria, the species depending on body site, patient continence, and recent antibiotic administration. Frequent changes of wet-to-dry saline dressings, at least four times daily, provide gentle debridément and substantially reduce bacterial counts. Routine use of systemic antibiotics is ill-advised because tissue levels are often subtherapeutic in the ulcer bed when sufficient elsewhere to alter bowel and skin flora dangerously. Topical antibiotics also penetrate granulation tissue poorly, may have a direct adverse effect on wound healing, and occasionally induce marked allergic sensitization with its attendant discomfort and risk of cross-reaction to subsequently administered systemic drugs. Antibiotic usage may be justified for two to three days preceding definitive surgical treatment of a decubitus ulcer, however. The choice of antibiotics should ideally be based on a recent culture of granulation tissue excised from the ulcer crater.

General medical conditions that may contribute to impaired ulcer healing include dehydration, anemia, hypoalbuminemia, and poor nutrition. These should be corrected when present. Maintaining a positive nitrogen balance and normal serum protein level may require supplementary feedings. Deficiencies of ascorbic acid and zinc, both implicated in wound healing, should be corrected if present. Finally, surgical closure of decubitus ulcers is often preferable to the extremely slow process of natural healing. Primary closure, grafting, and rotation of a skin flap are excellent procedures in appropriate patients.

Although decubitus ulcers are often considered a chronic problem, it has been shown that adequate nursing care combined with any of several therapeutic regimens can significantly hasten the healing of most of these lesions [31].

VENOUS ULCERS

Venous ulcers are a major source of morbidity in elderly patients. The current prevalence in the United States is not known, but in 1964 an estimated 600,000 patients suffered with stasis ulcers [32], which cost approximately $15,000 per treatment course. Effective management is therefore important both economically and with regard to patient comfort and mobility.

The pathogenesis of venous ulceration is related to incompetence of the valves within the perforating veins connecting the superficial to the deep venous systems in the legs. In normal people, exercise results in a drop in limb venous pressure. In patients with venous disease, the limb venous pressure rises on exertion, with high pressure reflux of blood through the incompetent perforator veins. This results in venous hypertension, a corresponding rise in the intraluminal pressure of the capillary bed, and leakage of fibrinogen into the dermis [33]. Pericapillary fibrin deposition is found in ulcer-bearing skin of patients with postphlebitic changes and liposclerosis, and blood and tissue fibrinolytic activity is depressed in these patients [34]. It is hypothesized that insoluble fibrin complexes form around blood vessels, producing a barrier to the passage of oxygen and other nutrients from the lumen and eventually resulting in ulceration.

Venous ulcers commonly occur on the medial or lateral aspect of the lower limbs. Often edema, hyperpigmentation (due to hemosiderin deposition), eczematous changes, and induration are present in the surrounding skin. Sharply demarcated sclerotic atrophic white plaques stippled with telangiectasia and surrounded by hyperpigmentation are distinctive scars also commonly found in patients with venous insufficiency (atrophie blanche).

All patients with venous ulceration should be examined for systemic disorders that may be contributing to their condition, such as congestive cardiac failure, hypoalbuminemia, or nutritional deficiencies. Peripheral neuropathy, diabetes mellitus, and arterial insufficiency should be excluded. Edema reduction, usually achieved by compression and/or elevation of the affected limb, is the cornerstone of treatment for venous insufficiency. Compression stockings, graduated pressure bandages, or Unna paste boots, applied from toe to knee, have been shown to be effective and inexpensive treatments [35]. Pneumatic compression devices may be used for more rapid reduction of edema [36].

Patients with venous ulceration and stasis dermatitis are at substantial risk of developing allergic contact dermatitis to topical antibiotics or other potential sensitizers applied to the broken skin surface. Chronic low-grade delayed hypersensitivity reactions may impede ulcer healing as well as increase local pruritus and edema. Neomycin ointment, lanolin, and Balsam of Peru are among the most commonly implicated allergens [37]. In any patient in whom allergy is suspected, topical therapy should be discontinued for at least two weeks and the ulcer treated with wet-to-dry saline compresses alone, and if feasible, patch testing should be performed.

Other agents often used topically to treat venous ulcers include aluminum salt solutions, silver nitrate, and acetic acid soaks. Hydrogen peroxide and aqueous Betadine may actually impair wound healing by damaging regenerating epithelium. Frequent wet dressings with normal saline are often very helpful in reducing debris and slough over the ulcer while eliminating this risk. Systemic antibiotics do not appear to enhance wound healing unless cellulitis is present. In a recent randomized clinical trial to evaluate the efficacy of systematically administered antibiotics to heal leg ulcers, there was no statistically significant difference in healing rates or microbial flora between the patients who received systemic antibiotics and those who received only local care for their leg ulcers [38]. Fibrinolytic agents, such as stanozolol, have been shown to be useful in the treatment of patients with lipodermatosclerosis, but effectiveness in the therapy of venous ulceration per se remains to be proved [39].

Results of surgical treatment for underlying incompetent perforating veins have been disappointing [40], although correction of deep venous insufficiency is often successful [41].

In patients with very deep or nonhealing ulcers, local surgical intervention may be required. Split-thickness skin grafts or pinch grafts have been used most extensively. Unfortunately, even following successful "takes," improvement is often short-lived, with 50 percent of previously healed lesions reulcerating after three months in some large series [42].

More recently, sheets of cultured epidermal cells derived from healthy adult donors have been employed in lieu of split-thickness autografts. Preliminary results using this technique are very promising, with an approximately 50 percent success rate and immediate pain relief in a series of 70 elderly patients [43]. The ability to graft ulcers without harvesting donor skin and without administration of general anesthesia may substantially broaden treatment options for patients with this debilitating condition.

PHOTOAGING

Many individuals are distressed by the visible changes in their exposed skin, especially the face. These age-associated changes are now known to be induced by habitual sun exposure and are correctly called photoaging. The medical relevance of this phenomenon is that elderly patients who are judged attractive are more social, have more positive personalities, and are subjectively healthier than those who are objectively less physically attractive [44]. Fortunately, the coarsened, yellow, wrinkled, and irregularly pigmented quality of skin can be prevented by long-term avoidance of sunlight and the use of high-potency (SPF 15) sunscreens. Although prevention is clearly most effective if practiced from childhood, anecdotal evidence suggests that considerable clinical improvement and reversal of histologic changes can be achieved by regular use of sunscreens even after marked actinic damage is present.

Preliminary studies [45] suggest that topical tretinoin (all transretinoic acid or Retin A) can also partly reverse the structural damage caused by excessive sunlight exposure and may therefore be useful in the treatment of aging. New capillary formation, new collagen synthesis, decreased elastosis, regularization of epidermal melanin distribution, and disappearance of premalignant actinic keratoses have all been observed in volunteer subjects after six to nine months of daily tretinoin application. Clinically, improvement is more likely to occur in patients with slight to moderate damage than in those with severe elastosis.

The numerous benign proliferative growths manifested in old skin are so nearly universal that they might be considered part of the normal aging process. In habitually exposed areas such as the face and hands, these changes are compounded by environmental exposure. Patients should be made aware that seborrheic keratoses, lentigens, and indeed most of these unwanted lesions can readily be removed with routine office procedures such as currettage or liquid nitrogen cryotherapy. Because many elderly patients are hesitant to discuss "cosmetic" concerns with their physician, this information should be volunteered.

References

1. Gilchrest, B. A., Murphy, G., and Soter, N. Effects of chronologic aging and UV light on Langerhans cells in human epidermis. *J. Invest. Dermatol.* 85:88, 1982.
2. Thiers, B. H., et al. The effect of aging and chronic sun exposure on human Langerhans cell populations. *J. Invest. Dermatol.* 82:223, 1984.
3. Gilchrest, B. A., et al. Chronologic and actinically induced aging in human facial skin. *J. Invest. Dermatol.* 80:81, 1983.
4. Leyden, J. J., McGinley, K. J., and Grove, G. L. Age-Related Differences in the Rate of Desquamation of Skin Surface Cells. In R. D. Adelman, J. Roberts, and V. J. Cristofal (eds.), *Pharmacological Intervention in the Aging Process.* New York: Plenum, 1978.
5. Gilchrest, B. A. In vitro assessment of keratinocyte aging. *J. Invest. Dermatol.* 81:184S, 1983.
6. Stanulis-Praeger, B. M., and Gilchrest, B. A. Growth factor responsiveness declines during adulthood for human-derived skin cells. *Mech. Aging Devel.* 35:185, 1986.
7. Liu, S. C., Meager, K., and Hanawat, P. Role of solar conditioning in DNA repair response and survival of human epidermal keratinocytes fol-

lowing irradiation. *J. Invest. Dermatol.* 85:93, 1985.

8. Liu, S. C., Parsons, C. S., and Hanawalt, P. C. DNA repair response in human epidermal keratinocytes from donors of different age. *J. Invest. Dermatol.* 79:330, 1982.

9. Roskos, K. V., Guy, R. H., and Maiback, H. I. Percutaneous absorption in the aged. *Dermatol. Clin.* 4(3):455, 1986.

10. Roberts-Thompson, I. C., et al. Ageing: Immune response and mortality. *Lancet* 2:368, 1974.

11. Waldorf, D. S., Wilkens, R. R., and Decker, J. L. Impaired delayed type hypersensitivity in an aging population associated with antinuclear reactivity and rheumatoid factor. *J.A.M.A.* 203:831, 1968.

12. Sauder, D. N., Stanulis-Praeger, B. M., and Gilchrest, B. A. Autocrine growth stimulation of human keratinocytes by epidermal cell derived thymocyte activating factor: Implications for skin aging. *Arch. Derm. Res.* (in press, 1987).

13. MacLaughlin, J., and Holick, M. F. Aging decreases the capacity of the skin to produce vitamin D_3. *J. Clin. Invest.* 76:1536, 1985.

14. Sokoloff, L. Occult osteomalacia in American patients with fracture of the hip. *Am. J. Surg. Pathol.* 2:21, 1978.

15. Downing, D. T., Stewart, M. E., and Strauss, J. S. Changes in sebum secretion and the sebaceous gland. *Dermatol. Clin. North Am.* 4:419, 1986.

16. Johnson, M. L. T., and Roberts, J. *Prevalence of Dermatological Disease Among Persons 1–74 Years of Age: United States.* Advance Date No. 4. Washington, D.C.: U.S. Department of Health, Education and Welfare, 1977.

17. Beauregard, S., and Gilchrest, B. A. A survey of skin problems and skin care regimens in the elderly. *Arch. Dermatol.* 123:1638–43, 1987.

18. Blackwell, B. The drug defaulter. *Clin. Pharmacol. Ther.* 13:841, 1972.

19. Schwartz, D., Wang, M., Feitz, L., et al. Medication errors made by elderly, chronically ill patients. *Am. J. Public Health* 52:2018, 1962.

20. Vestal, R. E., and Dawson, G. W. Pharmacology and Aging: Health in an Older Society. In C. E. Finch and E. L. Schneider (eds.), *Handbook of the Biology of Aging.* New York: Van Nostrand Reinhold Co., 1985. Pp. 744–819.

21. Morris, B. T., and Sober, A. Cutaneous malignant melanoma in the older patient. *Dermatol. Clin. North Am.* 4:473, 1986.

22. Weinstock, M. A., and Sober, A. J. The risk of progression of lentigo maligna to lentigo maligna melanoma. *Br. J. Dermatol.* 116:303, 1987.

23. McKendrick, M. W., et al. Oral acyclovir in acute herpes zoster. *Br. Med. J.* 293:13 Dec 1986.

24. Peterslund, N. A., et al. Acyclovir in herpes zoster. *Lancet* 2:827, 1981.

25. Eaglstein, W. H., Kaatz, R., and Brown, J. A. The effects of early corticosteroid therapy upon the skin eruption and pain of herpes zoster. *J.A.M.A.* 211:1881, 1970.

26. Taub, A. Relief of postherpetic neuralgia with psychotropic drugs. *J. Neurosurg.* 39:235, 1973.

27. Melski, J. W., and Stern, R. S. The separation of susceptibility to psoriasis from age at onset. *J. Invest. Dermatol.* 77:474, 1981.

28. Agris, J., and Spira, M. Pressure ulcers: Prevention and treatment. *Clin. Symp.* Vol. 31, 1979.

29. Seiler, W. O., Allen, D., and Stahlein, H. B. Influence of the 30° laterally inclined position and the 'super-soft' three piece mattress on skin oxygen tension on areas of maximum pressure—implications for pressure sore prevention. *Gerontology* 32:158, 1986.

30. Sugarman, B. Pressure sores and underlying infection. *Arch. Intern. Med.* 147:553, 1987.

31. Freeman, G. Decubitus ulcer warfare: Product vs. process. *Geriatr. Nurs.* May/June, 166, 1984.

32. Dale, W. A., and Forster, J. H. Leg ulcers: Comprehensive plan of diagnosis and management. *Med. Sci.* 15:56, 1964.

33. Browse, N. L., and Burnand, K. G. The cause of venous ulceration. *Lancet* 2:243, 1982.

34. Browse, N. L., et al. Blood and vein wall fibrinolytic activity in health and vascular disease. *Br. Med. J.* 1:478, 1977.

35. Kitihama, A., et al. Leg ulcer: Conservative management or surgical treatment? *J.A.M.A.* 247:197, 1982.

36. Falanga, V., and Eaglstein, W. H. A therapeutic approach to venous ulcers. *J. Am. Acad. Dermatol.* 14:777, 1986.

37. Fraki, J. E., Peltonen, L., and Hopsy-Hava, V. K. Allergy to various components of topical preparations in statis dermatitis and leg ulcer. *Contact Dermatitis* 5:97, 1979.

38. Alinovi, A., Bassissi, P., and Pini, M. Systemic administration of antibiotics in the management of venous ulcers. *J. Am. Acad. Dermatol.* 15:186, 1986.

39. Burnand, K. G., et al. Venous lipodermatosclerosis: Treatment by fibrinolytic enhancement and elastic compression. *Br. Med. J.* 280:7, 1980.

40. Burnand, K., et al. Relation between post–phlebitic changes in the deep veins and results of surgical treatment of venous ulcers. *Lancet* 1:936, 1976.

41. Psathakis, N. Has the 'substitute valve' at the

popliteal veins solved the problem of venous insufficiency of the lower extremity? *J. Cardiovasc. Surg.* 9:64, 1968.

42. Monk, B., and Sarkany, I. Outcome of treatment of venous stasis ulcers. *Clin. Exp. Dermatol.* 7:397, 1982.

43. Phillips, T., et al. Allografts of cultured keratinocytes in clinical practice. *Br. J. Dermatol.* 115:21, 1986.

44. Graham, J. A. The psychotherapeutic value of cosmetics. *Cosmetics Technol.* 5:25, 1983.

45. Kligman, A. M., et al. Topical tretinoin for photoaged skin. *J. Am. Acad. Dermatol.* 15:836, 1986.

Suggested Reading

Fenske, N. A., and Lober, C. W. Structural and functional changes of normal aging skin. *J. Am. Acad. Dermatol.* 15:571, 1986.

Gilchrest, B. A. *Skin and Aging Processes.* Boca Raton, FL: CRC Press, 1984.

Kligman, A. M., Grove, G. L., and Balin, A. K. Aging of Human Skin. In C. E. Finch, and E. L. Schneider (eds.), *Handbook of the Biology of Aging.* New York: Van Nostrand Reinhold Co., 1985. Pp. 820–841.

Montagna, W., et al. Special issue on aging. Proceedings of the 28th Symposium on the Biology of the Skin. *J. Invest. Dermatol.* 73:1, 1979.

13

Oral Cavity

BRUCE J. BAUM

THE ORAL CAVITY serves two critical functions in human biology: the initiation of alimentation and the production of speech. To accomplish these functions, many specialized tissues have evolved in the mouth. The teeth, the periodontium (supporting structures of the teeth including gingiva, periodontal ligament, alveolar bone), and the masticatory muscles exist to initiate mechanical food processing. The tongue is a finely coordinated organ directly involved in eating and speech. Salivary glands provide an exocrine secretion with multiple and important roles. Certain components of saliva lubricate both the oral mucosa, ensuring the competence and integrity of the lining tissue of the mouth, and the ingested food, permitting its transformation into a swallow-acceptable bolus. Saliva contains many hydrolytic enzymes (proteases, nucleases, glycosidases), which initiate the breakdown of complex foodstuffs into nutritionally useful, simpler products, and saliva is also a solvent for tastants, carrying them to taste buds for detection and recognition.

It is also important to realize that the mouth is exposed to the outside world and thus is vulnerable to an almost limitless number of insults. To protect the mouth, exquisite sensory systems have evolved; these include, besides taste, mechanisms for tactile, thermal, textural, and pain discrimination. Saliva too has several special protective roles. For example, saliva contains at least six different antimicrobial proteins (both immune and nonimmune), which modulate oral bacterial and fungal colonization. There are other salivary proteins whose role it is to maintain the functional integrity of the teeth (i.e., remineralize teeth and "repair" incipient caries).

The vast majority of clinical problems associated with the oral cavity are not life-threatening; however, many of these problems may be serious. Unfortunately, insufficient attention is frequently paid to oral health concerns. Yet, as can be surmised from the discussion above, changes in oral function can severely affect an individual's quality of life. Such changes, regardless of etiology, may have a particularly strong impact on the elderly individual. It is the purpose of this chapter to call attention to oral disorders or complaints that are common to older persons and to provide guidance for the clinician in their evaluation and management.

Salivary Glands
PHYSIOLOGY

Salivary glands consist of two major segments, an acinar endpiece (which elaborates the secretory fluid, termed *primary saliva*) and a ductal component (which modifies the primary saliva and carries it to the mouth). There are three bilateral pairs of major salivary glands (parotid, submandibular, sublingual) and many minor glands (e.g., labial, buccal, palatal) scattered throughout the mouth. An acinar endpiece consists of one or two principal cell types (serous or mucous), whereas the duct segment may have four or five cell types.

Reports have indicated that morphologic changes occur in salivary glands with age [1, 2]. Studies of salivary gland function (mostly with parotid glands) demonstrate, however, that diminished output of saliva is not a normal sequela of aging [l3, 4]. Cross-sectional evaluations of generally healthy persons show that older and younger adults are equally competent to elaborate salivary fluid. Furthermore, recent studies of the macromolecular and ionic constituents of saliva suggest that salivary composition does not vary systematically with age [4–6].

PATHOLOGY

Xerostomia, the subjective complaint of oral dryness, is the common "catch-all" condition linked with altered salivary performance. Xerostomia, however, is not a disease. It is a symptom and may or may not be associated with reduced saliva output. Xerostomia may result from many other factors besides low fluid levels, including altered lubricatory proteins, defective sensory receptors, and inadequate cortical integrative functions. Patients with true salivary gland dysfunction present with certain symptoms or signs that are indicative of the condition, including complaints of oral dryness (which is particularly meaningful if it is present during meals and requires frequent fluid intake for relief), difficulty in swallowing or in speaking at length, pain (which may arise from the teeth or the oral soft tissues), and diminished food enjoyment or altered taste. On oral examination a number of signs may be present. In the most dramatic case the mucosa appears atrophic, furrowed, ulcerated, and erythematous; however, the mucosa may appear normal even when glands are dysfunctional. There may be an unexplained recent increase in caries (dental decay), particularly along the gingival margins of the teeth (i.e., cervical versus coronal decay). A lack of moisture may be apparent in the oral cavity, although, since fluid output varies by a

TABLE 13-1. *Categories of xerostomia-inducing drugs**

Analgesic	Antiinflammatory
Anorexic	Antinauseant
Anticholinergic	Antiparkinsonian
Antidepressant	Antipsychotic
Antidiarrheal	Diuretic
Antihistamine	Psychotherapeutic
Antihypertensive	

*This table is an abbreviated form of Table 2 in L. M. Sreebny and S. S. Schwartz. A reference guide to drugs and dry mouth. *Gerodontology* 5:75, 1986. The authors utilized *The Physician's Desk Reference* (1983 through 1986), the New York State Department of Health's publication, *Safe, Effective and Therapeutically Equivalent Prescription Drugs* (6th ed.), and *Drug Facts and Comparisons* (1986) to obtain information on about 400 drugs listing xerostomia (dry mouth) as a side effect. Only major categories are listed. The original reference [49] contains a specific listing, by product and generic names, of all medications reported to induce xerostomia.

factor of about 20 in normal populations, reduced fluid levels may be an unimportant observation.

There are two major etiologic categories to consider. The most common causes of salivary gland hypofunction are iatrogenic [7]. Many medications, commonly taken by older persons, reduce or alter salivary gland performance. These include anticholinergic, antihypertensive, antidepressant, diuretic, and antihistaminic preparations (Table 13-1). Indeed, the oral side effects of such medications often lead to patient noncompliance. Additionally, common forms of oncologic therapy, such as radiation for head and neck neoplasms and cytotoxic chemotherapy, can have direct and dramatic effects on the salivary glands.

The single most common disease affecting the salivary glands is Sjögren's (sicca) syndrome. This autoimmune exocrinopathy usually affects postmenopausal women (about 90 percent prevalence) and occurs in either a primary form (altered salivary and lacrimal function) or a secondary form (altered salivary and lacrimal function plus a connective tissue disease). Between two and four million Americans are estimated to suffer from the condition [8]. In addition, although not frequently seen, many inflammatory and obstructive salivary gland disorders (e.g., bacterial infections, sialoliths, trauma, neoplasms) result in reduced gland function [9].

MANAGEMENT

Initial evaluation of patients should include a careful oral examination, paying special attention to the signs mentioned earlier. The patency of each major salivary gland orifice should be checked, and an attempt should be made to express saliva. When inflammatory or obstructive disorders are suspected, sialography, with retrograde infusion of radiopaque materials into the gland, may be useful. This imaging method is not particularly informative with other causes of salivary gland dysfunction. Objective measurement of salivary gland function should include both basal and stimulated secretory ability [10, 11]. Most often (due to iatrogenic causes or Sjögren's syndrome) it is basal function that is impaired. The presence of some stimulated function (in response to sour lemon taste or mastication) strongly indicates the presence of operational gland parenchymal tissue and has important management implications (see below). A particularly useful diagnostic approach for assessing the presence of water-transporting gland parenchyma is scintigraphic examination with ^{99m}technetium pertechnetate [10, 12]. The radionuclide parallels water movement by the salivary glands [13], and both an uptake phase (which shows the presence of gland parenchyma) and an efflux phase (showing secretion into the mouth) can be visualized. When Sjögren's syndrome is suspected (i.e., all patients with salivary dysfunction for which there is no clear iatrogenic or obstructive etiology), biopsy of the labial minor salivary glands should be performed. This is a relatively easy procedure with minimal patient inconvenience [14], and well-described criteria exist for the histopathologic changes associated with Sjögren's syndrome [15, 16]. Several serologic tests for autoimmune disease should also be performed, including sedimentation rate (Westegren), rheumatoid factor, serum immunoglobulins, and specific extractable nuclear antigens (SS-A [Ro] and SS-B [La]).

The results of evaluation procedures obviously dictate the treatment of patients. If the cause of gland hypofunction is pharmacologic and treatment is warranted because of oral complications, then either reducing medication levels or changing to different preparations can be helpful. Drug-induced dry mouth is usually fully reversible, although cases of long-term sicca symptoms after specific drug therapy have been reported. If patients have deficits in basal secretory rates but show stimulated responses, some functional gland parenchyma is present. Such individuals (including many irradiated and Sjögren's syndrome patients) have been successfully treated with an orally administered parasympathomimetic agent (pilocarpine) in recent trials [17]. Patients with autoimmune disorders exhibiting a salivary exocrinopathy also may respond to systemic antiinflammatory therapy [18]. For patients without gland parenchyma, no salivary or systemic treatment will be helpful because they lack water-transporting salivary epithelial tissues. All patients with salivary hypofunction should have comprehensive and frequent preventive dental care, including frequent prophylaxis and fluoride treatments. There is no excuse for rampant caries rendering such persons edentulous, given the preventive measures available. Whereas effective therapy is available for dental hard tissues, there is no effective therapy for soft tissue complaints (dryness, pain, swallowing difficulty). At present, these can be treated only in an indirect, palliative, and unsatisfactory manner [7]. For example, salivary substitutes are available, but their physical properties are unlike natural saliva, and they are minimally effective. Mouth rinses that include topical analgesics and antimicrobials may help. Patients having or suspected of having Sjögren's syndrome also should be monitored longitudinally for the possible development of an associated connective tissue disease or of a malignant lymphoma [19].

Gustatory Tissues
PHYSIOLOGY

The chemical senses are essential for nutrient selection and food enjoyment. In addition, there is an important, though not often appreciated, protective role of an intact gustatory system in that it allows us to distinguish spoiled (and thus potentially harmful) food items from suitable food. We are able to taste because there are, scattered throughout the tongue, taste papillae (circumvallate, fungiform, foliate), which contain taste buds for detecting and transmitting gustatory cues. Additional taste buds are found on the soft palate and epiglottis. Signals for gustatory responses are transmitted primarily through cranial nerves VII and IX. In a typical clinical or real life setting, it is virtually impossible to exclude olfactory function from taste judgments, and consideration of gustatory dysfunction should include olfactory assessment as well.

Prior to 1940 the number of taste buds in humans was reported to be reduced with increased age [20]; however, several recent reports show no significant loss of taste buds with age in humans, nonhuman primates, and rodents [21–23]. Electrophysiologic recordings from the chorda tympani in old rats do show statistically significant changes when compared with results from young rats [24]; however, these changes are small and of unclear biologic relevance. The peripheral gustatory system is well maintained through old age [25].

There are four basic taste qualities: sweet, salty, sour, and bitter. Recent studies evaluating the ability of healthy adults to detect and order the intensity of tastants representative of these qualities support the concept that with increased age there are only modest, quality-specific changes in these simple gustatory functions [26–28]. Conversely, results from other studies that have evaluated more complicated gustatory tasks, which probably involved additional sensory cues (e.g., olfactory and textural), have shown diminished function among older adults [29]. These results are not surprising, since direct measurement of the ability of adults to recognize odors shows a clear age-associated reduction [30].

PATHOLOGY

There are no good epidemiologic data to describe the frequency of gustatory complaints in the general population, particularly among older persons. Hypogeusia, a reduction in the ability to taste, and dysgeusia, a persistent bad taste in the mouth, have been associated with a range of situations including frank or subtle neuropathy, upper respiratory infections, medication usage, dietary inadequacies, traumatic injury, dental treatment, salivary gland dysfunction, menopause, and a host of systemic diseases. Strong linkage between any of these situations and gustatory malfunction is not well-established. For example, it recently has been shown that persons without any salivary gland function can give normal gustatory responses on objective, four-quality testing [31]. Such patients may in fact complain of reduced food enjoyment, but their complaints point to pain from the contact of food with atrophic or ulcerated mucosal tissues. At present there is no convincing support for gustatory impairment due to loss of a zinc-binding protein in saliva or for a role for zinc in normal gustatory events [32]. Most gustatory complaints in older people are indirect and relate to dental status and poor oral hygiene. Today's elderly have experienced more dental problems (including higher rates of edentulousness) than will probably be experienced by future elderly populations. Good oral hygiene is often difficult for older persons to practice because of reduced manual coordination skills. The presence of a dental or periodontal abscess may often result in purulent material entering the mouth, contributing to a distortion of gustatory signals. The chronic, unpleasant taste sensations often reported to be associated with aging may result from poor oral hygiene, especially on dental prosthetic appliances and about teeth with severe periodontal disease.

MANAGEMENT

The initial step in management of a patient with a gustatory complaint is to obtain a careful history. For example, the complaint may be related to the use of a new medication (the phenomenon of blood-borne taste is recognized), and changing a medication schedule may be beneficial. Complaints also may be associated with a systemic disease whose treatment will lead to resolution of the taste disorder. The clinician should inquire about the pattern of the complaint. Does it exist at all times or is it mostly associated with meals (the latter may suggest a dental disease component)? If a bad taste exists, can it be removed by rinsing the mouth with water (this may also suggest a problem of oral hygiene)? Dental status should be assessed. If it appears that there is no local (i.e., dental, oral hygiene) cause for the complaint, and especially if there is a history of head trauma, upper respiratory disease, or possible neuropathy, a careful cranial nerve examination should be performed to assess cranial nerves VII and IX. Since impaired olfaction should always be considered, cranial nerve I should also be carefully evaluated.

It is difficult to test gustatory function in a clinical setting because many subtleties exist in testing procedures. An accurate and complete assessment of gustatory function may require two to three hours of intense testing. Guidelines for such testing have been reported [27, 28, 33], but the procedures are impractical for the average general or specialty practitioner. Screening procedures that can identify gross gustatory deficits in the four basic taste qualities, can, however, be readily performed and require about 10 minutes. The simplest procedure (which, it must be emphasized, lacks thoroughness and may be misleading) requires the patient to rinse the mouth with water first, then sample an unknown tastant (sucrose, sodium chloride, citric acid [sour lemon], or quinine) dissolved in water, and then identify the taste. This is repeated, with intervening water rinses, for all four tastants. Such a screening procedure may well prove unsatisfactory for diagnosis, and referral for intensive testing may be necessary.

Olfactory function (odor recognition) can and should be tested. This test is fairly simply performed with a prepackaged kit called the University of Pennsylvania Smell Identification Test (UPSIT) [30]. It is a scratch and sniff booklet that can be purchased and stored, requires minimal supervision during administration, is easy to score, and is well standardized.

There are no good specific or effective therapies available for correcting these chemosensory disorders. As noted, when the chemosensory complaint is secondary to local or systemic conditions, successful resolution can be anticipated. Often olfactory disorders may result from airway obstruction, which can be surgically corrected; however, many complaints are untreatable at present. The complaints should nevertheless be documented and the patients reassured that their difficulties result from

measurable sensory deficits. Patients should be followed because these complaints may resolve spontaneously.

Dental and Periodontal Tissues
PHYSIOLOGY

Until recently, older individuals were very likely to finish their lives substantially or fully edentulous. Extensive tooth loss among elders was due primarily to high rates of coronal caries during youth and adolescence or to severe periodontal disease during middle life. However, changes in public health procedures (water fluoridation and patient education in oral hygiene and nutrition) and in the emphasis of dental practice (prevention oriented) in the last 20 years have greatly altered the dental status of the elderly. Coronal caries rates have markedly declined worldwide in response to a number of factors [34]. Whereas 12 to 15 years ago more than 50 percent of persons over 65 years old had no natural teeth [35], initial results of the recent adult oral health survey by the National Institute of Dental Research indicate that for the present population of persons over 65 years, this figure is about 40 percent. More impressive is the observation from this study that among dentate persons over 65 years old, the average number of teeth present is 19, indicating that many elderly are substantially dentate [36]. Tooth retention is becoming the norm among the elderly.

The periodontium, the supporting structure of the tooth, includes the gingiva, alveolar bone, and periodontal ligament. There are few data about these tissues in elderly persons. In part, this lack of information is due to the previous high rates of edentulousness, which meant that there was no need for attention to periodontal health. Given the increasing numbers of dentate older individuals, proper research emphasis should generate data about the periodontium in old age. The data at hand indicate that the elderly have more periodontitis than younger persons [37]. Indeed, data from the adult oral health survey [36] indicate a threefold increase in periodontal attachment loss in persons over 65 years compared with those 18 to 20 years old. However, the periodontal status of current elderly cannot be classified generally as moderate to severe, with active disease requiring surgical management. Instead, it is likely that the periodontal status of an older person represents the accumulation of lesions over a lifetime rather than any increased susceptibility to active disease with age [37].

PATHOLOGY

Both dental caries and periodontal disease are related to the accumulation of bacterial plaque adherent to teeth. Caries may occur on either the coronal (enamel) or the cervical (cemental or root) surfaces of teeth. Coronal caries is typically a disease of children and adolescents, although older persons are still susceptible, particularly in areas adjacent to previously restored surfaces (i.e., recurrent decay) [38]. Coronal caries is strongly associated with the presence of *Streptococcus mutans* in plaque. Cervical caries is a condition most frequently found in older adults. The prevalence of carious lesions on root surfaces in adults over 65 years is about 10-fold greater compared with rates in adults aged 18 to 24 years old [36]. The specific bacterial etiology of cervical caries has not been established, and it is not known if changes in oral microbial flora in older adults account for the high prevalence in this population. One predisposing factor is the loss of periodontal attachment around teeth that occurs with increased age, thus exposing the root surfaces and rendering them susceptible to carious attack.

Adult periodontal disease results from immunopathologic destruction of connective tissue. Bacterial antigens (thought to be primarily from gram-negative species) penetrate the gingival and periodontal tissues and initiate an inflammatory response. Without adequate plaque removal, inflammation continues, resulting in destruction of the soft and hard tissues supporting the teeth. Periodontal disease in adults tends to progress slowly and in an episodic pattern [37]. Initially, gingivitis affects only gingival tissues. Thereafter, alveolar bone and the periodontal ligament are affected. This latter stage weakens support for the tooth and is, by itself, properly called periodontal disease. Senescent changes in the immune system have been suggested to be important in the etiology of periodontal disease. Since immunosenescence primarily affects T-cell function, and periodontal disease is associated with B-cell responses [37, 40], normal immunologic aging may not be important in periodontal disease.

Both caries and periodontal diseases are primarily affected by local oral circumstances, but many medications and systemic diseases may exacerbate these conditions. For example, any medication markedly affecting saliva production will diminish its endogenous protective influence and allow rampant caries to occur. More than 400 commonly prescribed medications are known to reduce saliva production (see Table 13-1) [41]. Particularly well known are psychoactive anticholinergic drugs and antihypertensives. Other examples include phenytoin and cyclosporin, both of which result in considerable gingival hyperplasia in response to local irritants. Also, patients with uncontrolled diabetes mellitus may display an exaggerated inflammatory response with poor healing and may respond poorly to local treatment.

MANAGEMENT

It is important to recognize that increasing numbers of older individuals are keeping their teeth and are therefore at risk for the development of both caries and periodontal diseases. Most of the care for these problems will be rendered by dentists, yet medical practitioners may hear complaints related to dental pain or bleeding gingivae. The emphasis in dental practice today is toward prevention of these diseases. Since bacterial plaque is central to disease development, it is important that good oral hygiene be practiced by older persons. Manual dexterity often is diminished in these individuals, so clinicians should urge patients to have frequent professional oral prophylaxis and to expect good preventive oral care, including fluoride treatments and antimicrobial rinses. Indeed, there has been considerable advance with the availability of the antimicrobial chlorhexidine in an antiplaque rinse. These approaches should allow older persons to maintain most of their dentition for life and be free from the undesirable esthetic, masticatory, and painful sequelae of dental caries and periodontal disease.

Oral Motor Function

PHYSIOLOGY

The oral motor apparatus is involved in several intricately coordinated functions important in everyday life, including speech, mastication, swallowing, and posture. In general, aging is associated with morphologic and biochemical alterations in neuromuscular systems [39, 42], and it is likely that such changes affect units involved in oral functions. Studies of oral motor performance in healthy older persons have revealed no severe impairments in function, but annoying and potentially troublesome functional compromises have been noticed. For example, masticatory muscle performance is reduced among the elderly [25, 43] and can lengthen the time required to prepare a swallow-ready bolus, thus making it more likely that older persons will accept larger-sized food particles for swallow, a possibly dangerous decision [25]. This diminution in masticatory efficiency is further increased among individuals with inadequate dentition. After mastication of food, bolus preparation and translocation (to the pharynx) occur, requiring, besides well-coordinated neuromuscular processing, an intact oral mucosal barrier and salivary lubricatory molecules. For a healthy young adult, the entire oral phase of swallowing takes about 1 to 1.5 seconds to complete with a 5-ml water bolus present. In healthy older persons, this time is approximately doubled [44]. Although in normal circumstances such changes may be of only statistical significance, under unusual conditions, such as in café choking episodes, these "physiologic" perturbations may place the older person at risk.

Several studies have examined in detail speech production in the elderly and have noted that certain changes characteristically occur with increased age [45, 46]. However, among healthy older adults there appears to be no impairment in the ability to produce normal speech. Similarly, we associate many alterations in posture with growing old. In the oral area, drooping of the lower face and lips results not only from loss of supporting hard tissues in edentulous persons, but also, in most elderly, from diminished tone of the circumoral muscles [43]. Aside from esthetic concerns, embarrassing or annoying situations can occur, such as drooling or food spills due to an inability to close the lips completely while eating, speaking, or lying down. Often a loss of circumoral muscle tone may be associated with complaints of excess salivation by an elderly person.

The temporomandibular joint (TMJ), located between the glenoid fossa and the condylar process of the mandible, exhibits a functionally unique combined gliding and hinge-like movement. This is of particular interest because in adults it is often the focus of many craniofacial pain disorders. Although it has been frequently stated that TMJ dysfunction is a common sequela of aging, recent work does not confirm TMJ functional impairment as a normal age-associated event [47].

PATHOLOGY

A variety of pathologic problems are associated with oral motor function in the elderly. The present section does not address frank neurologic disease affecting performance by the orofacial musculature, although it should be recognized that difficulties in speech, mastication, and swallowing may be associated with a variety of neuropathies. The most common local pathologic entities the clinician is likely to encounter are related to disturbances of the masticatory/alimentary system. Symptoms indicative of such disorders include difficulty in swallowing certain foods (especially "dry") with or without a history of episodes of choking or apnea, and pain from the TMJ or masticatory muscles associated with eating or repose.

Complaints related to swallowing are frequently iatrogenic. For example, any treatment affecting salivary gland secretion may have important effects on the oral phase of swallowing, and chronic dysfunction of salivary glands can result in irreversible changes in the pattern and timing of oral swallowing events [48]. Similarly, phenothiazine therapy is often associated with the development of tardive dyskinesia, which may affect swallowing performance and speech and may cause major disorders of movement. In addition, surgical treatment in the head and neck region (e.g., for neoplasms) may severely impair swallowing and other oral motor behaviors.

Pathology associated with the TMJ may be either articular (directly related to the joint itself) or nonarticular (unrelated to joint pathology; e.g., dental, muscular, or psychophysiologic in origin) [49]. Complaints of pain in the TMJ region (joint, paraspinal, and masticatory muscles) may be associated with clicking noises from the joint, limitation of jaw opening, and mandibular deviation on function. Joint abnormalities in elderly persons are most likely related to osteoarthritic degeneration and traumatic events. The most common nonarticular disorder is myofascial pain dysfunction syndrome, which is associated with involuntary jaw-clenching or tooth-grinding as a manifestation of tension.

MANAGEMENT

Initial evaluation of patients with subjective complaints suggestive of oral motor dysfunction should include a detailed history and a careful cranial nerve-based examination of orofacial neuromuscular coordination [43, 50], including testing of cranial nerves V, VII, IX, X, and XII. Any obvious weakness or asymmetry in the oral area is probably a sign of localized neurologic impairment. In assessing the possible etiology of TMJ pain, the presence of joint clicking and the extent of jaw opening (less than 40 mm can be considered abnormal) should be noted. The latter sign seems to be particularly age-associated among nonhealth-care–seeking persons (i.e., the nonpatient population) [47]. If articular pathology is suspected, imaging by radiographs, tomographs, or arthroscopy may be useful. When perturbation of the oropharyngeal phase of swallowing is suspected, noninvasive examination of both wet swallows (with a water bolus) and dry swallows (with only endogenous oral fluids) should be performed using ultrasonography [51]. If speech production appears compromised, speech articulation, rhythm, rate, voice quality, and inflection should be evaluated [10, 46].

If oral motor dysfunction is related to pharmacologic therapy, consideration should be given to alternative therapies or dosage regimens. Similarly, oral motor dysfunction may be a sign of a generalized disorder, and improvement will result from systemic therapy [52]. For patients with diminished muscle mass or muscle tone, and for patients whose problems are secondary to surgery, exercises and alternative means of coping with oral motor functions may be necessary. Referral to a specialist in rehabilitative medicine or to a speech pathologist will probably be quite beneficial. If TMJ pain is suspected to have a dental (e.g., malocclusion) or psychologic cause, the patient should be referred to an appropriate specialist.

Oral Mucosal Lesions

It is impossible, because of space considerations in a text such as this, to provide any substantive description of oral mucosal lesions to which the general physician should be attentive. However, it would be inappropriate not to provide some comment. Although it has been suggested that there are age-related changes in the oral mucosa, there is little firm evidence to support such a conclusion [53]. Certainly individuals with dental prostheses present with a higher frequency of some mucosal lesions (ulcers, hyperkeratoses) than dentate persons. But most concerns about oral mucosal disease in older persons are similar to those for younger adults, and the reader is referred to a comprehensive text dealing with these problems [54]. An important exception to this generalization is the concern in older individuals about oral cancer. Malignancies in the oral cavity appear to be more frequent in older persons and may present in a variety of ways. The reader again is referred to a separate comprehensive text for diagnostic and management considerations of oral cancer [55].

References

1. Andrew, W. Comparison of age changes in salivary glands of man and rat. *J. Gerontol.* 7:178, 1952.
2. Scott, J. Quantitative age changes in the histological structure of human submandibular salivary gland. *Archs. Oral Biol.* 22:221, 1977.
3. Baum, B. J. Evaluation of stimulated parotid saliva flow rate in different age groups. *J. Dent. Res.* 60:1292, 1981.
4. Chauncey, H. H., et al. Parotid fluid composi-

tion in healthy aging males. *Adv. Physiol. Sci.* 28:323, 1981.

5. Baum, B. J., Costa, P. T., Jr., and Izutsu, K. T. Sodium handling by aging human parotid glands is inconsistent with a two-stage secretion model. *Am. J. Physiol.* 246:R35, 1984.

6. Baum, B. J., Kousvelari, E. E., and Oppenheim, F. G. Exocrine protein secretion from human parotid glands during aging: Stable release of the acidic proline-rich proteins. *J. Gerontol.* 37:392, 1982.

7. Baum, B. J., et. al. Therapy-induced dysfunctions of salivary glands. *Spec. Care Dent.* 5:274, 1985.

8. Talal, N. Sicca syndrome. *J. Dent. Res.* 66:672, 1987.

9. Blitzer, A. Inflammatory and obstructive disorders of salivary glands. *J. Dent. Res.* 66:675, 1987.

10. Fox, P. C., et al. Xerostomia: Evaluation of a symptom with increasing significance. *J. Am. Dent. Assoc.* 110:519, 1985.

11. Heft, M. W., and Baum, B. J. Unstimulated and stimulated parotid salivary flow rate in individuals of different ages. *J. Dent. Res.* 63:1182, 1984.

12. Katz, W. A., et al. Salivary gland dysfunction in systemic lupus erythematosus and rheumatoid arthritis. Diagnostic importance. *Arch. Intern. Med.* 140:949, 1980.

13. Fox, P. C., et al. Uptake and secretion of technetium pertechnetate by the rat parotid gland. *Comp. Biochem. Physiol.* 83A:579, 1986.

14. Fox, P. C. Simplified biopsy technique for labial minor salivary glands. *Plast. Reconstr. Surg.* 75:592, 1985.

15. Chisholm, D. M., and Mason, D. K. Labial salivary gland biopsy in Sjögren's disease. *J. Clin. Pathol.* 21:656, 1968.

16. Greenspan, J. S., et al. The histopathology of Sjögren's syndrome in labial minor salivary gland biopsies. *Oral Surg.* 37:217, 1974.

17. Fox, P. C., et al. Pilocarpine for the treatment of xerostomia associated with salivary gland dysfunction. *Oral Surg.* 61:243, 1986.

18. Talal, N., et al. Elevated salivary and synovial fluid β_2-microglobulin in Sjögren's syndrome and rheumatoid arthritis. *Science* 187:1196, 1975.

19. Moutsopoulos, H. M., et al. Sjögren's syndrome (sicca syndrome): Current issues. *Ann. Intern. Med.* 92:212, 1980.

20. Arey, L. B., Tremaine, M. J., and Monzingo, F. L. The numerical and topographical relations of taste buds to circumvallate papillae throughout the life span. *Anat. Rec.* 64:9, 1935.

21. Arvidson, K. Location and variation in number of taste buds in human fungiform papillae. *Scand. J. Dent. Res.* 87:435, 1979.

22. Mistretta, C. M. Aging effects on anatomy and neurophysiology of taste and smell. *Gerodontology* 3:131, 1984.

23. Mistretta, C. M., and Baum, B. J. Quantitative study of taste buds in fungiform and circumvallate of young and aged rats. *J. Anat.* 138:323, 1984.

24. McBride, M., and Mistretta, C. M. Taste responses from the chorda tympani nerve in young and old Fischer rats. *J. Gerontol.* 41:306, 1986.

25. Feldman, R. S., et al. Aging and mastication. Changes in performance and in the swallowing threshold with natural dentition. *J. Am. Geriatr. Soc.* 28:97, 1980.

26. Grzegorczyk, P. B., Jones, S. W., and Mistretta, C. M. Age-related differences in salt taste acuity. *J. Gerontol.* 34:834, 1979.

27. Weiffenbach, J. M., Baum, B. J., and Burghauser, R. Taste thresholds. Quality specific variation with human aging. *J. Gerontol.* 37:372, 1982.

28. Weiffenbach, J. M., Cowart, B. J., and Baum, B. J. Taste intensity perception in aging. *J. Gerontol.* 41:460, 1986.

29. Schiffman, S. Food recognition in the elderly. *J. Gerontol.* 32:586, 1977.

30. Doty, R. L., Shaman, P., and Dann, M. Development of the University of Pennsylvania Smell Identification Test: A standardized microencapsulated test of olfactory function. *Physiol. Behav.* 32:489, 1984.

31. Weiffenbach, J. M., Fox, P. C., and Baum, B. J. Taste and salivary function. *Proc. Natl. Acad. Sci. USA* 83:6103, 1986.

32. Catalanotto, F. A. The trace metal zinc and taste. *Am. J. Clin. Nutr.* 31:1098, 1978.

33. Bartoshuk, L. M. The psychophysics of taste. *Am. J. Clin. Nutr.* 31:1068, 1978.

34. Beck, J. D. The epidemiology of dental diseases in the elderly. *Gerodontology* 3:5, 1984.

35. Baum, B. J. Alterations in Oral Function. In R. Andres, E. L. Bierman, and W. R. Hazard (eds.), *Principles of Geriatric Medicine.* New York: McGraw-Hill, 1985.

36. Carlos, J. P. National Institute of Dental Research Survey of Adult Oral Health. Personal communication, 1986.

37. Page, R. C. Periodontal diseases in the elderly: A critical evaluation of current information. *Gerodontology* 3:63, 1984.

38. Chauncey, H. H., et al. The incidence of coronal caries in normal aging male adults. *J. Dent. Res.* (special issue) 57:148, 1978.

39. McCarter, R. Effects of Age on the Contraction of Mammalian Skeletal Muscle. In G. Kaldor and W. J. DiBattista (eds.), *Aging in Muscles*. New York: Raven, 1978.

40. Walford, R. L., et al. Immunopathology of aging. *Ann. Rev. Gerontol. Geriatr.* 2:3, 1981.

41. Sreebny, L. M., and Schwartz, S. S. A reference guide to drugs and dry mouth. *Gerodontology* 5:75, 1986.

42. Pradhan, S. N. Central neurotransmitters and aging. *Life Sciences* 26:1643, 1980.

43. Baum, B. J., and Bodner, L. Aging and oral motor function: Evidence for altered performance among older persons. *J. Dent. Res.* 62:2, 1983.

44. Sonies, B. C., et al. Durational aspects of the oral phase of swallow in normal aging adults. *Dysphagia* (in press, 1988).

45. Benjamin, B. J. Frequency variability in the aged voice. *J. Gerontol.* 36:722, 1981.

46. Sonies, B. C., Baum, B. J., and Shawker, T. H. Tongue motion in elderly adults: Initial in situ observations. *J. Gerontol.* 39:279, 1984.

47. Heft, M. W. Prevalence of TMJ signs and symptoms in the elderly. *Gerodontology* 3:125, 1984.

48. Hughes, C. V., et al. Oral-pharyngeal dysphagia: A common sequela of salivary gland dysfunction. *Dysphagia* 1:173, 1987.

49. Laskin, D. M. Dental and Oral Disorders. In R. Berkow (ed.), *The Merck Manual*. Rahway, NJ: Merck, 1977.

50. Sonies, B. C., et al. Clinical examination of motor and sensory functions of the adult oral cavity. *Dysphagia* 1:178, 1987.

51. Shawker, T. H., et al. Real-time ultrasound visualization of tongue movement during swallowing. *J. Clin. Ultrasound* 11:485, 1983.

52. Marshall, J. F., and Berrios, N. Movement disorders of aged rats: Reversal by dopamine receptor stimulation. *Science* 206:477, 1979.

53. Hill, M. W. The influence of aging on skin and oral mucosa. *Gerodontology* 3:35, 1984.

54. McCarthy, P. L., and Shklar, G. *Diseases of the Oral Mucosa*. Philadelphia: Lea & Febiger, 1980.

55. Silverman, S. *Oral Cancer*. New York: American Cancer Society, 1985.

14

Cardiovascular System

JEANNE Y. WEI

Pathophysiology
ANATOMIC CHANGES

Aging, in the absence of disease, exerts a clinically significant influence on the structure and function of several aspects of the cardiovascular system. Although many of these changes are reviewed below, the effect of age on regulation of blood pressure is discussed in detail in Chapter 15.

Vasculature

Aging exerts a different effect on each layer and region of the vascular tree [1–3]. Although the proximal portion of the artery tends to demonstrate age changes initially, eventually the entire vessel is involved, with the most extensive changes found distally [3]. The left coronary arteries usually begin to show age changes during youth or mid-adulthood, followed by the right coronary artery, which usually demonstrates age changes after the fifth decade [3].

Aortic mass or lumen size and wall thickness increase with age [1–3]. Because the rate of change of lumen size and wall thickness varies with vascular site, in the elderly there are increases (in renal and carotid arteries) as well as decreases (in aorta and femoral artery) in the ratio of wall thickness to lumen radius in different arteries [3]. Vascular tortuosity also increases significantly with age [4].

In the *intimal* layer, the endothelial cells, homogeneous in cell diameter and configuration in youth, become irregular in size and shape with advancing age [1–3]. As one ages, cells lose their uniform orientation with their long axis parallel to the longitudinal axis of the vessel and become oriented in different directions. The subendothelial layer thickens with age as connective tissue content rises, elastic laminae duplicate (becoming thinned, frayed, and fragmented), and calcium and lipid deposits increase, especially around the internal elastic membrane [1–3, 5, 6].

In the *media,* the most prominent age changes are thickening of the media, elastic fragmentation, and increased calcification. During the first five decades of life, the aortic media thickens by almost 40 percent [1–3]. The time course of change in the media is similar to that in the intima. Elastin fragmentation and calcification occur earlier in the proximal portions of the large arteries and later in the distal segments of the smaller vessels [1–6]. No significant age change has been found in human aortic adventitia [3].

Heart

Although overall heart size is not increased in normal, healthy, elderly compared to younger persons [1, 2, 7, 8], a modest increase in left ventricular wall thickness is seen [1, 2, 8]. In the conduction system, the number of proximal bundle fascicle interconnections between the left bundle and the main bundle decrease slightly with age, and there may be a small age-related reduction in the density of the distal conduction fibers [1, 2, 9]. The atrioventricular node and His bundle show relatively little change.

The number of pacemaker cells in the heart decreases with age. Age-related sinoatrial node cell loss accelerates around the age of 60 years, and by age 75 years only 10 percent of the number of pacemaker cells usually present in the 20-year-old may be seen [1, 2, 9]. Less marked loss of muscle cells with increases in fibrous tissue also occurs in the internodal tracts. The myocardial elastic tissue, fat, and collagen content are either unchanged or slightly increased in the aged, and small focuses of fibrosis appear. The atrial endocardium and the atrial surface of the atrial ventricular valves are often thickened in the elderly [1, 2, 10]. Amyloid deposition has been found in 40 percent of hearts at autopsy from patients over age 65 years [10], and half of these have only minor deposits limited to the atria. Calcification of at least part of the mitral annulus of the aortic valve and conduction system is frequently observed [2, 9, 10].

PHYSIOLOGIC CHANGES IN CARDIAC FUNCTION
Cardiac Function at Rest
The major determinants of cardiac output include heart rate, loading conditions, intrinsic muscle performance, and neurohumoral regulation [1]. Loading conditions influencing cardiac output include cardiac filling (preload) and opposition to left ventricular ejection (afterload). Early diastolic rapid filling rate declines with age [1, 2, 8] and in the 65- to 80-year-old group is about one-half of that observed in the 25- to 44-year-age group [1, 8]. Late diastolic filling, i.e., the atrial contribution to left ventricular inflow (Fig. 14-1), is significantly increased with advancing age [1]. Possible mechanisms for the diminished early diastolic filling include decreased left ventricular compliance, decreased compliance of the mitral valve, and prolonged relaxation [1, 2, 8]. Opposition to left ven-

FIGURE 14-1. *Left ventricular diastolic inflow at the mitral annulus, demonstrated using Doppler time-velocity plots, in a healthy young person aged 23 years (young, left panel) and a healthy elderly person aged 76 years (old, right panel). The early diastolic rapid filling (E) is greater than the later diastolic, atrial-dependent filling (A) in the young, while the opposite is true for elderly individuals as a result of age-related decreases in ventricular compliance (From J. Y. Wei, and B. J. Gersh: Heart disease in the elderly. Cur. Probl. Cardiol. 12:1, 1987.*

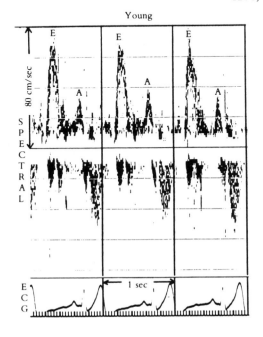

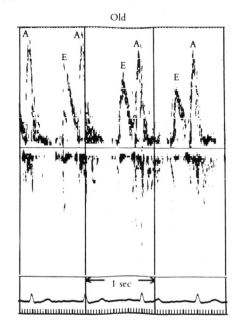

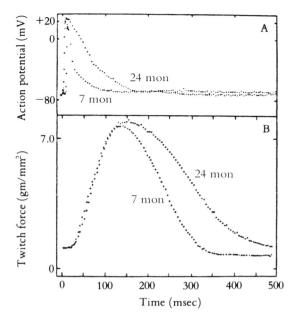

FIGURE 14-2. *Effect of age on simultaneously measured transmembrane action potentials (A) and contractions (B) in rat cardiac muscle. Note that the action potential and contraction duration are both significantly prolonged in senescence. (From J. Y. Wei, H. A. Spurgeon, and E. G. Lakatta: Excitation-contraction in rat myocardiums: Alterations with adult aging. Am. J. Physiol. 246:H784, 1984.)*

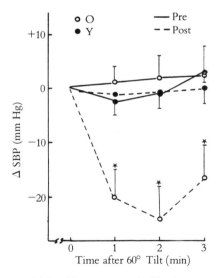

FIGURE 14-3. *Change in systolic blood pressure during upright tilt (60°) in six young (Y) and six old (O) healthy adults before (Pre) and after (Post) modest diuresis. Asterisk indicates significant change from prediuresis values (p < 0.02). (From R. P. Shannon, et al. The effect of age and sodium depletion on cardiovascular response to orthostasis. Hypertension 8:438, 1986.)*

tricular ejection (afterload) increases with age [1–3]. The ascending aorta becomes stiffer, whereas the cross section of the peripheral vascular bed is reduced in the elderly, causing an age-related increase in pulse wave velocity and wave reflection.

Intrinsic muscle performance shows no definite age change in the contractile phase, but there is significant prolongation in the relaxation phase [1, 2, 14]. The duration of active state may be lengthened, and isovolumic relaxation as well as early diastolic relaxation are prolonged with advancing age [1, 2, 8, 14]. Although left ventricular thickening may cause mildly prolonged relaxation [1, 8], similarly thickened left ventricles of younger adult cohorts do not show such prolonged relaxation [1, 2, 14]. Furthermore, there are age changes in the excitation-contraction coupling of the mammalian ventricular myocardium (Fig. 14-2) even in the absence of hypertrophy [14]. Thus, the aged heart has impaired diastolic performance with decreased ventricular compliance and relaxation, leading to impaired filling and higher ventricular pressures. These changes, as discussed later, have major clinical impact.

Sympathetic tone, as reflected in plasma norepinephrine levels, is increased with age [1, 2, 15]. The end-organ responsiveness to beta-adrenergic stimulation, however, is reduced in the heart and peripheral vasculature [1–3]. Whether vascular alpha-adrenergic responsiveness is altered with age in the human is not established, but it appears to be decreased in the conscious rat [1, 16]. The cardiovascular reflex responses to daily activities such as orthostasis (Fig. 14-3), meal consumption, and cough or Valsalva maneuver are attenuated with age [1, 2, 12, 13, 16–18]. This attenuation may be due in part to attenuated baroreflex function [1, 2, 12, 13, 15, 17].

In older animals and humans aortic compliance is decreased while stiffness of the ascending aorta and large vessels is increased [1–3]. This decreased arterial compliance may induce the altered baroreflex function, as noted above [1, 2, 19]. Greater intravascular pressure would be required to stimulate the baroreceptors of a less distensible vessel, thereby raising the baroreceptor threshold and altering its sensitivity [1, 2, 15]. It is not known whether vasodilatory potential decreases with age and precedes the age-related increase in arterial pressure [1].

Local vascular tone may be altered or unchanged with age [1–3, 16]. The aortic relaxation response to beta-adrenergic stimulation may be diminished with age [1–3]. Alpha-adrenergic response may be attenuated in senescence [1, 16].

Aside from catecholamines, circulating neurohumoral factors contributing to cardiovascular homeostasis include renin, angiotensin II, aldosterone, vasopressin, and atrial natriuretic factor (ANF) [1, 2, 20]. Plasma renin levels are decreased with age, mainly due to a reduction in active renin concentration [1, 20]. Plasma angiotensin II and aldosterone levels are also decreased with age [1, 20], the decrement being proportional to the decreased plasma renin activity [20]. Plasma vasopressin may be unchanged or decreased with age at baseline or following a hypovolemic stimulus and is increased with age following a hyperosmotic stimulus [21]. Preliminary studies indicate that plasma ANF levels vary but are generally increased in the elderly.

Although supine resting cardiac output and stroke volume decline with age, upright cardiac output does not decrease [1, 2, 22]. This effect of posture may reflect an age-associated decline in the capacity to increase cardiac output when recumbent due to decreased myocardial compliance and increased diastolic stiffness [1–3]. This notion is supported by the recently reported echocardiographic finding that, despite larger basal left ventricular volumes in older persons, changes in left ventricular end-diastolic and stroke volumes in response to alterations in cardiac preload are diminished in old compared to younger persons [23]. Resting systolic blood pressure rises with advancing age with less prominent increases in diastolic pressure [1, 2, 13, 24]. Whether these age changes reflect genetic or environmental influence(s) or a combination of these factors remains to be elucidated.

Hemodynamics During Exercise

In response to exercise stress, cardiac output normally increases by as much as four- to five-fold [1, 22]. Maximal attainable heart rate during intense physical exercise declines steadily with age [1, 2, 11], though age has little effect on heart rate at submaximal exercise levels. The cardioacceleratory response to various physiologic stimuli (e.g., postural change, cough, Valsalva maneuver) is substantially attenuated with age [1, 2, 12, 13]. The maximal increase in ejection fraction tends to be less in the elderly [1, 2, 11]. For any given increase in cardiac output, the rise in systemic arterial pressure is usually greater, as is the concomitant elevation in pulmonary artery pressure in the elderly [1, 22]. Thus in the aged, exercise-induced increases in cardiac output are accomplished primarily through augmented cardiac filling (preload) and less as a myocardial response to beta-adrenergic stimulation [11]. The ability to handle venous return is hampered by decreases in vascular and myocardial compliance in the elderly [1, 23].

EFFECTS OF EXERCISE TRAINING

With exercise conditioning, the cardiovascular adaptation may be different with age [1, 2, 25–27]. Basal blood pressure may decline in the senescent rat, whereas heart rate may decrease in the young adult, so that the response can be characterized as vasodepressant in the old and cardioinhibitory in younger adult animals [25]. In the absence of cardiac hypertrophy, treadmill exercise conditioning of moderate intensity results in significantly improved myocardial function in the aged rat, with reversal of the age-related prolongation of contraction duration [26]. Exercise conditioning in the aged animal also preserves cardiac muscle function during hypoxia [27].

Although there is a progressive decline in maximal oxygen uptake with age, sedentary older individuals have values that are 10 to 20 percent lower than active persons of the same age [1]. Physically conditioned older persons also have lower body fat, lower blood pressure and resting heart rate, and lower plasma insulin levels and improved physical working capacity compared to old sedentary persons [1, 28]. Apparently, physically active elderly persons also have lower rates of myocardial infarction than age-matched sedentary persons [1, 29].

Epidemiology of Cardiovascular Diseases of the Elderly

Cardiovascular disease is the most common cause of death in older persons, accounting for a major portion of the health care costs in this age group [1, 30]. Mortality due to cardiovascular disease continues to rise through the very old, from 50 percent in those 65 to 74 years old (41 percent heart, 9 percent cerebrovascular) to 65 percent in the over-85-year-old age group (48 percent heart, 17 percent cerebrovascular). Between 80 and 85 percent of cardiac deaths are attributed to ischemic heart disease [1, 30], whereas hypertensive plus rheumatic heart disease deaths comprise about 5 percent. Congestive heart failure accounts for about 6 percent of deaths in the 65- to 69-year-old age group but rises to approximately 15 percent in the over-85-year-old age group [1].

Several studies report a prevalence of heart disease of nearly 50 percent in persons over 65 years. In 1980–1981 over two million Americans aged 65 and over with diagnosed coronary heart disease [1, 30] accounted for six million visits to doctors' offices. Half of all individuals aged 75 years and older saw a physician for coronary heart disease [1, 30]. Heart disease is a major contributor to disability in 20 percent of community-dwelling elderly who require some form of home assistance to avoid institutionalization [1]. Beginning in the fifth decade, the annual incidence of congestive heart failure rises exponentially with increasing age, doubling every 10 years in men and every seven years in women [1]. Congestive heart failure is present in 10 to 20 percent of patients admitted to a geriatric unit in an acute care hospital [1].

Coronary Heart Disease

Coronary atherosclerosis progresses with advancing age, with the severity of disease in men leading that in women by approximately 15 years. Angina pectoris shows a prevalence of about 10 percent in the elderly and is often the first clinical sign of coronary atherosclerotic disease [1].

ANGINA PECTORIS

Angina pectoris is the presenting symptom in over 80 percent of elderly patients with coronary artery disease [1]. In the Coronary Artery Surgery Study (CASS), 50 percent of elderly patients but less than one-third of younger patients presented with unstable angina pectoris [1, 31]. The prevalence of prior myocardial infarction and serum cholesterol levels was similar in older and younger patients in this study, but more of the elderly had hypertension, cerebrovascular disease, congestive heart failure, and diabetes [1, 31]. The elderly also had more multivessel coronary artery disease, left main coronary artery disease, and angiographic and hemodynamic evidence of left ventricular dysfunction [31].

Clinical presentation of angina pectoris in the elderly is usually similar to that in younger patients [1, 31]. Dyspnea rather than pain, however, may be the major complaint. In addition, syncope with exertion, sudden coughing during emotional stress, palpitations with effort, and sweating with exertion are also more commonly observed. Atypical chest pain occurs less commonly in the elderly [1]. Nonanginal causes of chest pain among the elderly include aortic dissection, pericarditis, pulmonary embolism, cervical spine disease, and abdominal emergencies.

Diagnosis of angina pectoris depends in large part on the history [1]. Physical examination in elderly patients with angina pectoris is often nonspecific [1]. The resting electrocardiogram may show ST–T wave changes that are nonspecific, especially when associated with increased QRS voltage compatible with left ventricular hypertrophy [1, 31]. In elderly patients who are able to exercise to increase heart rate to at least 60 percent of the predicted maximum, the use of rest and exercise thallium-201 myocardial imaging may be helpful in delineating areas of decreased coronary perfusion during exercise-induced ischemia [1].

The *management* of angina consists of two main approaches: (1) helping to change the patient's lifestyle to accommodate a reduced level of activity, and (2) providing therapy—medical and surgical—to maintain the level of activity desired by the patient [1]. Increasingly, the elderly are remaining more active than their predecessors, so that aggressive medical and/or surgical therapy is now frequently considered

[1]. For the past six years at Boston's Beth Israel Hospital, over 25 percent of the patients undergoing coronary bypass graft surgery have been 65 years or older, and over 17 percent of all patients undergoing cardiac surgery have been 70 years or older [1]. In prescribing the appropriate medical regimen, it is important to keep in mind that decreased renal function as well as decreased hepatic perfusion and drug metabolism result in higher plasma drug levels in the elderly, who are also often more prone to adverse drug effects. Nitrates are effective and are usually well tolerated [1, 32]. Hypotension and headaches may occur, however, and nitrate tolerance may develop [1, 32]. In some instances, the calcium channel-blocking agents may be preferred over certain beta-blockers because calcium antagonists may exert less inotropic suppression at the usual clinical doses [32]. On the other hand, postural hypotension and impaired atrioventricular node conduction and/or heart block may occur following calcium antagonist administration [32].

The six-year survival results of medical management of angina in elderly patients with normal coronary arteries, one-vessel disease, or two-vessel disease with good ventricular function has been reported to be fairly good, with 86 percent, 76 percent, and 69 percent survival, respectively [1, 30, 31].

ACUTE MYOCARDIAL INFARCTION

Approximately 10 percent of patients with unstable angina pectoris will develop acute myocardial infarction. In patients aged 70 years and over with myocardial infarction, the male-to-female ratio is nearly equal, whereas in younger myocardial infarction patients, men outnumber women nearly three to one [1]. Remote myocardial infarcts are common in the elderly, occurring in 10 percent of men and five percent of women over age 65 years. The average annual incidence of acute myocardial infarction in those over age 65 years is approximately 15 to 20 per 1000 individuals [1]. The elderly patient may present with symptoms other than chest pain or dyspnea, including confusion, syncope, stroke, vertigo, weakness, abdominal pain, persistent vomiting, and even cough. Sudden onset of intense dyspnea is often the dominant symp-

tom of acute infarction in advanced old age. Whereas chest pain may be a less common presenting symptom in some older patients, syncope may be slightly more common. Myocardial infarction tends to occur at rest and during sleep more frequently in elderly than in younger patients [1]. There may be an increased incidence of smaller, non-Q wave infarcts in older patients [1].

In addition to differences in the clinical presentation of acute myocardial infarction in elderly patients, the serum cardiac system enzyme profile may also be altered with advancing age [1, 33, 34]. With an acute infarct, the finding of an elevated serum concentration of the myocardial fraction of creatine kinase (CK-MB isozyme) with a normal total plasma creatine kinase level occurs twice as often in patients aged 70 years and over than in younger patients [33]. These events usually occur in concert with several other changes associated with acute myocardial infarction and probably represent definite myocardial injury, which should be considered part of the spectrum of nontransmural, non-Q wave myocardial infarction [33, 34]. Whether a lower total creatine kinase level in the elderly represents a small infarct, a decreased number of myocytes or myofibers in the myocardium, altered creatine kinase isozyme distribution (perhaps an increased MB fraction), or other changes (such as increased collateral blood supply or recanalization) in the older heart remains to be determined [1, 33–35].

A higher percentage of elderly infarct patients have a history of systemic arterial hypertension [1]. Elevated systolic blood pressure (>160 mm Hg) is associated with increased mortality and morbidity from ischemic heart disease [1, 30]. In addition, the elderly have a higher frequency of complications, including atrial arrhythmias, heart block, and conduction defects as well as cardiogenic shock, pulmonary edema, cardiac rupture, hypovolemia, and right-sided heart failure during the acute infarct period [1]. The in-hospital mortality may be substantially higher (usually over 20 percent), and the length of hospital stay in those who survive the acute event may be longer [1, 34]. The recovery/rehabilitation period also tends to be prolonged in older patients. In a recent study, patients aged 80 years and over had a 67 percent in-hospital mortality, compared to 15 percent in patients 79 years and younger [34].

Management

The management of elderly patients with acute myocardial infarction should be prompt and aggressive when indicated [1]. Recently developed intravenous thrombolytic therapy and invasive medical procedures include cardiac catheterization with angiography, intraaortic balloon counterpulsation, intracoronary thrombolytic therapy, and/percutaneous transluminal coronary angioplasty. The incidence of complications associated with each of the procedures tends to rise with advancing age [1]. Therefore, although these more aggressive therapeutic interventions have been performed with excellent results in patients in their sixties, seventies, and eighties and over [1, 36], and although advanced age should not be an absolute contraindication, one should be aware of the increased risks when treating older patients.

Elderly patients with papillary muscle rupture or ventricular septal defect complicating acute myocardial infarction should be considered for prompt surgical repair after hemodynamic stabilization, provided no other contraindications for surgery are present [1, 37–39]. The incidence of failed insertion of intraaortic balloon counterpulsation catheters (due to tortuous vessels and atherosclerosis) and of associated complications from this procedure may be substantially higher in the elderly [1, 31]. In older patients with postinfarction cardiogenic shock with surgically remediable lesions such as ventricular septal defect (Fig. 14-4), papillary muscle rupture, or pump failure, advanced age does not preclude a successful surgical result, and the long-term outcome may be excellent [1, 38–40].

THROMBOLYTIC THERAPY

Thrombolytic therapies (intracoronary or intravenous) are being increasingly utilized to treat a greater number of elderly patients presenting within the first few hours after an acute myocardial infarction [1, 36]. Although no data from a prospective study are available for comparison of results in elderly versus younger patients, the overall results of reperfusion in the elderly may be somewhat less successful than in younger patients [36]. When patients in cardiogenic shock or pulmonary edema are excluded from comparison, however, the percentage of successful reperfused patients over and under age 65 years may be equal [36]. The average pretherapy left ventricular ejection fraction in the elderly was decreased to a level similar to that in younger individuals, but it was less likely to increase following successful revascularization compared with young patients [36]. Further studies are needed to define the benefits of this intervention in elderly patients.

LIDOCAINE PROPHYLAXIS

The issue of prophylactic lidocaine administration in elderly infarct patients is not clearly settled [1]. The incidence of primary ventricular fibrillation is lower in patients over age 65 [1], and there is little information about lidocaine's efficacy in such patients. Decreased hepatic perfusion and metabolism of the drug, together with increased central nervous system (CNS) drug sensitivity, place the elderly at greater risk for significant lidocaine toxicity [1, 32], and an acute confusional state, lethargy, and seizures may occur more frequently in elderly patients receiving lidocaine at the usual dosage. However, because it clearly reduces primary ventricular fibrillation and is more than 80 percent effective in treating ventricular arrhythmias during acute myocardial infarction in younger patients, the tendency is to recommend lidocaine prophylaxis for the aged. To adjust for the reduced plasma volume (8 percent) and increased body fat (35 percent) as well as for the twofold prolongation of lidocaine's plasma half-life in the elderly [1], the loading dose should be reduced to one-half to two-thirds of the usual amount, and the maintenance dose should be kept under 25 μg/kg/minute. Lidocaine prophylaxis against primary ventricular fibrillation should be discontinued 24 hours after the acute infarct. If high-grade ventricular ectopy is present, however, lidocaine therapy may be continued at the lowest effective maintenance dose.

Management. During the acute myocardial infarction period, lidocaine is the drug of choice for premature ventricular contractions [1]. Beta

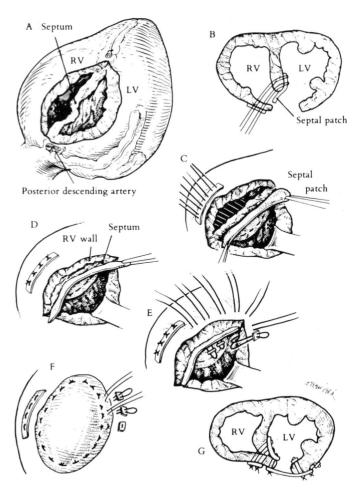

A Septum

RV

LV

Posterior descending artery

B

RV   LV

Septal patch

C

Septal patch

D   Septum

RV wall

E

F

G

RV   LV

blockers such as propranolol may be successful against ventricular ectopic beats associated with increased sympathetic activation, such as reversible ischemia or anxiety. However, the negative inotropic effects and CNS side effects of some beta blockers may preclude their use in certain elderly patients. Procainamide may accumulate in serum levels in older patients owing to age-associated decreases in renal clearance and excretion [1, 41]. The active metabolite of procainamide, *N*-acetyl procainamide (NAPA), has fewer associated untoward effects such as the development of antinuclear antibodies, but it may accumulate to potentially toxic levels in patients who have poor kidney function [41].

CARDIAC REHABILITATION

Prolonged bed rest and inactivity, especially among elderly patients, contribute to the se-

FIGURE 14-4. *Repair of postinfarction inferior ventricular septal defect. A. Septum and defect viewed through excised infarction. B,C. Sutures placed through septum, Teflon felt patch, and free wall of right ventricle. D. Patched septum transposed to right. E. Sutures placed around defect in ventricular wall. F,G. Overlying patch tied in place and reinforced by 4-0 polypropylene sutures. (RV = right ventricle; LV = left ventricle.) (From R. M. Weintraub, et al. Repair of post-infarction VSD in the elderly: Early and long-term results.* J. Thorac. Cardiovas. Surg. *85:191, 1983.)*

rious complications of thrombophlebitis, pulmonary embolism, and cardiac and respiratory deconditioning, as well as negative nitrogen and potassium balance [1]. The physician should institute early, gradual ambulation, followed by progressive levels of activity during convalescence. In prescribing an exercise regimen for the elderly postinfarct patient, it is important to remember the following: Careful and gradual progression during training is imperative;

warm-up must be slow and careful to ensure an appropriate increase in deep-muscle temperature and to help prevent muscle injuries; cooldown after exercise must be performed slowly. Elderly persons should continue some very light exercise, such as walking or unloaded pedaling for a short time after active exercise. Static stretching techniques also are effective in preventing muscle injury [1].

DISCHARGE PLANNING

Discharge planning from the hospital should be formulated with special attention given to the patient's socioeconomic status, emotional needs, personal support systems (both formal and informal), and physical environment in the home. Too often, unanticipated gaps in medical or nonmedical care at home result in further compromise in the elderly patient's weakened condition and an early (and avoidable) return to the hospital.

Postmyocardial Infarction Beta-Adrenergic Blockage

Beta-blockade therapy may be associated with a reduction in long-term mortality in elderly survivors of acute myocardial infarction [1, 30, 42]. Metoprolol, propranolol, and timolol have been shown to significantly *decrease* postinfarction mortality in older patients compared with age-matched patients who received placebo (Fig. 14-5). There was no major age difference in patient complaints, side effects or withdrawal from study [42]. It is recommended, therefore, that elderly patients be considered for beta-adrenergic blockade therapy following acute myocardial infarction [1, 30, 32, 42].

Coronary Bypass Surgery in the Elderly

The mean age of patients in the United States undergoing coronary artery bypass surgery (CABG) is rising each year [1, 43], and in 1980 the number of patients over the age of 65 undergoing CABG had increased fivefold compared to 1975 [43]. It must be noted, however, that data from randomized trials for coronary artery disease involve a younger population and that there are no randomized trial data for patients aged 65 years and older. Several explanations for the increased frequency of coronary bypass surgery in older patients exist: (1) older but active patients with angina are an expanding seg-

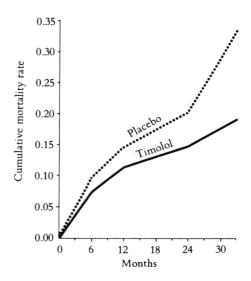

FIGURE 14-5. *Life table cumulative mortality curves for all cause mortality in patients 65–75 years old receiving timolol or placebo. (From T. Gundersen, et al. Timolol-related reduction in mortality and reinfarction in patients aged 65–75 years surviving acute myocardial infarction. Circulation 66: 1179, 1982.)*

ment of our population, (2) many such patients have severely symptomatic coronary disease, and (3) techniques of coronary bypass surgery have steadily improved with the successful application of this technique to subgroups of patients at higher risk, including the elderly.

PATIENT CHARACTERISTICS

Older patients undergoing revascularization tend to be "sicker" than their younger counterparts. A CASS Registry study compared preoperative characteristics in 1,086 patients aged 65 years and older undergoing isolated CABG with the same characteristics in 7827 younger patients [1, 31, 43]. Elderly patients were more symptomatic, with a higher incidence of unstable angina and a prior history of cardiac failure, and had a higher prevalence of associated medical diseases including diabetes, cerebrovascular disease, hypertension, peripheral vascular disease, and chronic lung disease. There was a higher incidence of left main coronary artery disease, triple vessel disease, and abnormal left ventricular function in older patients [43].

PERIOPERATIVE MORTALITY AND MORBIDITY

Perioperative mortality is higher in the elderly. In the CASS Registry study (Fig. 14-6), peri-

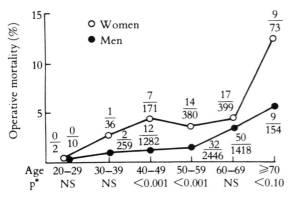

FIGURE 14-6. *Operative mortality according to age and sex for 1,061 women and 5,569 men. Chi-square for trend with increasing age (years): men p < 0.001; women, NS. (From J. W. Kennedy, et al. Clinical and angiographic predictors of operative mortality from the Collaborative Study in Coronary Artery Surgery (CASS). Circulation 63:793, 1981.)*

operative mortality in those aged 65 years and older was 5.2 percent, significantly higher than the 1.9 percent in young patients [1, 43]. Mortality increased with advancing age: For patients aged 65 to 69 years, it was 4.6 percent; for patients aged 70 to 74 years, it was 6.6 percent; and for patients aged 75 years or more, it was 9.5 percent [43]. Nonetheless, even in the older population, the recent trend has been toward a reduction in perioperative mortality [1, 43]. Clinical features of older patients at lower risk included the presence of stable angina, absence of heart failure, absence of current cigarette smoking, and most important, absence of more than one associated medical disease. As with younger patients, surgical mortality was increased in the presence of left ventricular dysfunction and/or cardiomegaly and significant left main coronary artery disease [1, 43].

Perioperative morbidity is higher in the elderly. In a series of patients aged 70 years and older, frequent nonfatal complications included stroke, psychoses, conduction disturbances, pulmonary emboli, and supraventricular arrhythmias [1, 43]. The mean duration of hospital stay after CABG in the CASS Registry study was 11.4 days in patients under 65 years, 12.9 days in those aged 65 to 69, 14.0 days in patients aged 70 to 74 years, and 16.5 days in patients aged 75 years and older.

LONG-TERM SURGICAL RESULTS

Mortality. Cumulative six-year survival of patients aged 65 years and older in the CASS Registry study was 83 percent compared to 91 percent in younger patients [43]. This difference was mainly attributable to the higher perioperative mortality in older patients. With increasing age, even within the older age group, long-term survival declines. Five-year survival (including perioperative mortality) was 84 percent in patients aged 65 to 69 years, 80 percent in those aged 70 to 74 years, and 70 percent in patients aged 75 years and older. Among 30-day survivors, five-year survival was 88 percent, 85 percent, and 77 percent, respectively, for the three age groups. Major predictors of long-term mortality (in perioperative survivors) were indices of left ventricular dysfunction and the number of associated medical diseases. In older patients without left ventricular dysfunction or other medical diseases, five-year survival was almost 90 percent. Others have reported similar five-year survival rates, ranging from 80 to 85 percent [1, 43].

Functional Outcome. Regarding recurrence of angina, older patients in the CASS Registry study fared as well as younger patients, although angina relief was more sustained in men than in women [43]. It appears, therefore, that the symptomatic benefits from coronary artery bypass surgery are similar in older and younger patients, although this may relate in part to reduced levels of activity in the elderly. Documentation of the efficacy of coronary artery bypass and the relief of angina in the elderly is also evident from other studies [1, 30, 43].

COMPARATIVE STUDY OF MEDICAL AND SURGICAL THERAPY IN PATIENTS 65 YEARS OR OLDER

A nonrandomized study from the CASS Registry compared the results of coronary artery bypass with medical therapy alone in 1491 patients aged 65 years and older [43]. Cumulative six-year survival (Fig. 14-7) in the entire series (adjusted for the major differences in preoperative variables) was 79 percent in the surgical group and 64 percent in those treated medically (P < 0.0001). Relief of chest pain was also more prominent in those treated surgically.

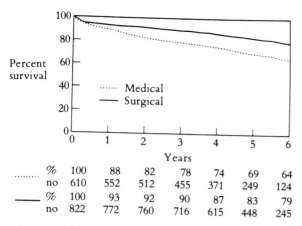

....	%	100	88	82	78	74	69	64
	no	610	552	512	455	371	249	124
———	%	100	93	92	90	87	83	79
	no	822	772	760	716	615	448	245

FIGURE 14-7. *Cumulative six-year survival in surgical and medical groups for entire series, adjusted for left ventricular wall motion score, congestive heart failure score, number of diseased vessels, number of associated medical diseases, and age at baseline angiography. (p < 0.0001; log rank statistics = 36.485) (From B. J. Gersh, et al. Comparison of coronary artery bypass surgery and medical therapy in patients 65 years of age or older. A nonrandomized study from the Coronary Artery Surgery (CASS) registry. Reprinted, by permission of* The New England Journal of Medicine *[313:217, 1985].)*

Multivariate analysis suggested an independent beneficial effect of surgery on survival. Among 234 "low-risk" patients with mild angina, relatively well preserved left ventricular function, and absence of left main coronary disease, survival was no different between surgically and medically treated patients, being 82 and 83 percent, respectively.

Thus, the current status of coronary artery surgery is such that the procedure can be effectively applied to the older population, with an increased but acceptable risk. In selected patient populations, excellent late survival and functional relief can be expected. Many elderly patients with symptomatic coronary disease comprise a "high-risk" group who may receive substantial benefits from coronary bypass surgery, and their survival may be prolonged by this procedure, particularly because many may tolerate "maximal" medical therapy poorly [1].

Percutaneous Transluminal Coronary Angioplasty
An increasing number of patients aged 65 years or older with coronary artery disease are now undergoing percutaneous transluminal coronary angioplasty (PTCA) procedures [1]. Because of the higher morbidity and mortality as well as the longer hospitalization in elderly patients undergoing revascularization surgery, PTCA has important potential applications in this age group. In the National Institutes of Health PTCA registry there were 786 patients over age 60, and of these, 140 were 70 years or older. Seventy-four percent of the 786 patients had functional class III or IV angina pectoris. Single vessel disease was present in 70 percent, multivessel disease in 26 percent, and left main coronary disease in 4 percent. PTCA was successful in 56 percent of the patients under 60 years and in 62 percent of those 60 years or older. The incidence of myocardial infarction was similar in those over and under age 60 years. The overall mortality was 2.2 percent in those over age 60 compared with 0.8 percent in the under-60 years group. Thus, PTCA success rates in the elderly are comparable to those in younger patients, and the mortality with the procedure, although higher, is not different from that seen with bypass surgery [1, 44]. Newer developments and technical advances should increase the success rate and lower the mortality in elderly patients [44].

Optimism for the role of PTCA in the elderly also grows from other recent reports [45, 46]. The primary success rate was reported at 93 percent for younger and 91 percent for elderly (70 years and older) patients [45]. Two percent of older subjects sustained myocardial infarction, and 1 percent required emergency bypass surgery. The combination of advanced age and the presence of triple vessel disease contributed to increased late mortality (7 percent) after an initially successful procedure [45]. With increased experience and technical refinement, it is anticipated that multilesion PTCA may be performed in selected elderly patients with high primary success rate and relatively low procedural risk [44–46].

Congenital Heart Disease
Several congenital cardiac lesions do not preclude survival to old age. The classic diagnostic clinical findings associated with congenital

heart lesions may be obscured or confounded in older patients by concomitant age-related changes or other diseases. Valvular lesions affecting the very old are either initially mild congenital lesions, lesions that develop in late life due to age-related processes, or a combination of these factors. As internists and cardiologists become increasingly aware of the safety, usefulness, and availability of recently developed noninvasive cardiac imaging techniques, the identification of congenital heart disease will probably increase in frequency in elderly patients.

ATRIAL SEPTAL DEFECT

Although most elderly patients with intracardiac shunt lesions have minor defects, the major medical problem is one of differential diagnosis and antibiotic prophylaxis against infective endocarditis. Patients with atrial septal defects (ASD) are the exception [1, 47]. Old patients with ASD often present with congestive heart failure and atrial arrhythmias, and the diagnosis of ASD may be missed. Patients with ASD often manifest pathophysiologic consequences of volume overload of the right heart and circulation. When the atrial left-to-right shunt increases the volume of the pulmonary circulation by two or more times that of the systemic circulation, right ventricular hypertrophy and pulmonary vascular prominence and plethora result. These features are usually considered the classic signs of atrial septal defect. Ordinarily, pulmonary atrial pressures remain at normal or slightly above normal levels, and many elderly ASD survivors have modestly to moderately elevated pulmonary artery pressures [47]. Those who develop severe reactive pulmonary hypertension (about 15 percent of all patients with ASD) tend to do so in their twenties to forties and usually do not survive to old age [1, 47]. Severe pulmonary hypertension (pulmonary artery pressures above 60 mm Hg) with atrial septal defect, however, has been observed not infrequently in the very old. In a study of patients aged 60 years or older, 18 of 56 (32 percent) had peak systolic pulmonary artery pressures of 60 mm Hg or greater [47]. These patients tended to have a poorer functional class and an increased incidence of atrial fibrillation.

Diagnostic clinical findings in elderly patients are usually not different from those in younger individuals (i.e., exaggerated precordial motion, a widely split and "fixed" second heart sound, a right-sided S_4, a pulmonic systolic ejection murmur, incomplete or complete right bundle branch block with first-degree atrioventricular block on electrocardiogram, and dilated main and pulmonary arterial branches with pulmonary plethora on chest x-ray). The echocardiogram (M-mode and two-dimensional) may reveal enlarged right ventricular chamber dimensions and paradoxical motion of the interventricular septum. Contrast echocardiography may demonstrate an intracardiac communication at the atrial level, and Doppler studies may reveal the presence of an interatrial flow signal [1].

Elderly patients with atrial septal defect may be asymptomatic or may have some disability. They often present with symptoms of congestive heart failure. Dyspnea and heart failure may be precipitated by atrial arrhythmias (atrial flutter or fibrillation), which occur with increased likelihood in ASD patients. Because heart failure typically involves the right ventricle, elevated central venous pressure, hepatomegaly, peripheral edema, and fatigue are often present.

The treatment for ASD is usually surgical. The operative risk, although slightly higher in the elderly, is very low unless severe pulmonary hypertension is present. In a large study conducted at the Mayo Clinic of 66 older patients (mean age 65 years) who underwent surgical repair for ASD, postoperative deaths occurred in four, all of whom also underwent other surgical procedures at the same operation [47]. Both early and late postoperative arrhythmias tend to be increased in elderly patients [1, 47]. Abnormal right ventricular function may not revert to normal in old patients after ASD repair, but the long-term benefits of surgical repair of an atrial septal defect may be otherwise excellent [1, 47].

COARCTATION OF THE AORTA

A common adult congenital cardiovascular disease lesion, coarctation of the aorta usually becomes manifest in early and mid adult life (90 percent of patients were under age 40 years in a recent report of 234 patients) but may rarely be diagnosed in very late life [1, 47, 48]. The diagnosis and treatment of this lesion in the elderly are similar to that in younger adults. Older patients with coarctation of the aorta frequently present with hypertension. In addition to congestive heart failure, other complications including infective endocarditis, cerebrovascular accident, and aortic dissection may occur. Coarctation is associated with a bicuspid aortic valve (which may cause valvular aortic stenosis in the elderly) in 10 to 15 percent of patients [1, 48, 49]. Over half of the patients who undergo surgical repair improve postoperatively [48, 49]. Although the operative risk is higher in older patients, surgery should be undertaken if possible because the expected outcome following repair is positive and there is a high likelihood of severe morbidity and/or premature mortality without corrective surgery.

INTERVENTRICULAR SEPTAL DEFECT

Elderly patients rarely present with unrepaired congenital ventricular septal defects (VSD) of substantial size because if the defect is significant and the left-to-right shunt is large, pulmonary vascular disease would usually have developed, making survival to old age unlikely. Therefore, a VSD in the elderly patient is usually tiny and has a small left-to-right shunt; it does not require surgery, and prophylactic antibiotic therapy against infective endocarditis may be the only medical therapy needed. Management of older patients who develop acquired VSD following an acute myocardial infarction was discussed in the previous section on coronary heart disease.

PATENT DUCTUS ARTERIOSUS

Although a rare entity in the very old, patent ductus arteriosus (PDA) has been diagnosed in an occasional elderly patient. A continuous murmur at the base of the heart is compatible with this diagnosis. Echocardiography and Doppler studies may be performed to evaluate possible etiologies for the continuous murmur [1, 50]. In symptomatic elderly patients with PDA and a large left-to-right shunt, surgical therapy (closure of PDA) should be recommended. In those with small left-to-right shunts in whom the major risk is infective endocarditis or in those with sizeable left-to-right shunts without pulmonary vascular disease, the poten-

tial benefits of surgery must be weighed against the increased operative risk of dissection and hemorrhage at surgery in this age group (due to extensive atherosclerosis and markedly friable tissue around the ductus).

CYANOTIC HEART DISEASE

Cyanosis in the elderly is usually due to pulmonary disease. It must be noted, however, that diagnoses of pulmonary valve stenosis and, less frequently, tetralogy of Fallot have been made in the elderly. As more patients continue to survive into later years, mainly as a result of improved surgical repair techniques, it is anticipated that more physicians will find unusual cases of congenital heart disease (primarily postoperative) in their geriatric patient population. In pulmonary valve stenosis, the diagnosis may be made noninvasively using echocardiography, and the valvular gradient may be estimated using Doppler techniques. Surgery should be recommended, if at all, for symptomatic patients only, because little information is available on surgical benefits versus risk for this age group [1]. Adult patients with unrepaired tetralogy of Fallot rarely survive beyond the third or fourth decade, but those with successful surgical correction will begin attaining the geriatric age range in the near future. The very late problems associated with surgical corrective procedures for these and other cardiac anomalies await definition in the elderly.

Ebstein's disease may rarely be diagnosed in an elderly patient. Supraventricular tachycardia and tricuspid insufficiency are the major complications. Tricuspid regurgitation may be quantified by two-dimensional Doppler echocardiography. If cyanosis with right-to-left shunt develops, surgical therapy should be considered.

Valvular Heart Disease
AORTIC VALVE DISEASE
Aortic Stenosis
DIAGNOSIS
Aortic stenosis can be difficult in elderly patients because certain classic clinical features may be obscured or confounded by concomitant changes due to aging. Although systolic murmurs occur in 60 to 80 percent of elderly [1,

51], most are benign and are due to aortic valve sclerosis (thickening and calcification of the aortic leaflets as a result of long-term wear and tear). A small percentage of elderly patients with systolic murmurs have hemodynamically significant aortic stenosis. Uncorrected critical aortic stenosis carries a grave prognosis, but surgical aortic valve replacement or percutaneous aortic valvuloplasty can dramatically improve the long-term outlook, even in the very old. Although one should not overutilize diagnostic tests or subject patients with innocent murmurs to unnecessary evaluative procedures, it is important to identify correctly those patients with aortic stenosis who may significantly benefit from valvular surgery.

MEDICAL HISTORY

In a person over age 65 years, aortic stenosis most frequently involves a tricuspid (rather than a congenital bicuspid) valve in which progressive sclerosis and calcification have markedly restricted leaflet mobility and critically narrowed the valve orifice [1, 51]. Much less commonly, rheumatic and/or congenital valvular deformity may be the underlying pathology. A history of rheumatic or congenital heart disease or of a longstanding heart murmur may be helpful in establishing the diagnosis. The presence of exertional or postural syncope, progressive limitation of physical activity due to dyspnea on exertion, or angina pectoris is also important in the evaluation of need for surgical therapy [1]. The problem with using symptoms as indicators of severe aortic stenosis in elderly patients is that they are often the result of coronary artery disease and/or cerebrovascular disease and are not as specific for aortic stenosis as they are in a younger population. This problem is confounded by the coexistence in many elderly of both aortic stenosis and coronary artery disease [1, 52].

PHYSICAL FINDINGS

On physical examination, the "classic" signs of aortic stenosis may be less reliable and may be absent altogether in the elderly. For example, the location of the aortic ejection murmur may change so that instead of being most prominent at the base, it may be best heard at the apex [1, 51]. The duration or the time of onset of the murmur may not be as reliable an indicator of the severity of aortic stenosis in the elderly patient because left ventricular dysfunction may significantly alter these features [1, 51]. One of the most reliable physical findings of hemodynamically significant aortic stenosis in young adults—that of the delayed and diminished carotid upstroke—may be absent in the elderly because of noncompliant vasculature [1]. When the delayed carotid upstroke is present, however, it may be helpful in establishing the diagnosis of aortic stenosis, but it may also be confounded by the presence of severe carotid artery atherosclerosis. Although the aortic component of the second heart sound is frequently diminished in the presence of significant aortic stenosis, this is not a reliable sign either. Often with aortic stenosis there is a sustained apical impulse and an S_4 gallop. However, these findings are also often found in elderly patients who do not have aortic stenosis [1, 51]. A pale facial color is almost never helpful in diagnosing aortic stenosis in the elderly. When aortic stenosis becomes so severe that cardiac output is restricted, the systolic murmur may no longer be appreciated [1]. Thus, physical findings may be less reliable in the elderly.

ROUTINE LABORATORY EVALUATION

In routine laboratory testing the electrocardiogram may be helpful in supporting a suspicion of aortic stenosis. Findings compatible with left ventricular hypertrophy, especially in the absence of hypertension, suggest the possible presence of significant aortic stenosis. On the chest x-ray there may be evidence of left-sided cardiomegaly. However, because many elderly patients have a history of hypertension, these changes are less specific. In old kyphoscoliotic patients, chamber enlargement may be difficult to diagnose on the chest x-ray.

With all these limitations, one might ask whether the history, physical examination, and routine laboratory tests can ever reliably diagnose or exclude the presence of severe aortic stenosis in the elderly. The answer is that it is difficult but possible. As with any diagnostic tool, its strength increases with the user's knowledge of its weaknesses. A late-peaking systolic ejection murmur and a diminished or absent A_2 sound suggests aortic stenosis, especially in the presence of electrocardiographic evidence of left ventricular hypertrophy in a patient without a history of hypertension. If the systolic murmur is accentuated after a premature ventricular beat and decreases when the patient changes from a supine to a sitting or standing position and if aortic regurgitation is also audible, significant aortic stenosis is likely. The patient should be referred for noninvasive cardiovascular evaluation when aortic stenosis is suspected.

CARDIAC DIAGNOSIS AND CONFIRMATION

Echocardiography, Doppler studies, and phonocardiography can be very helpful in the noninvasive diagnosis of severe aortic stenosis [1, 53]. On the echocardiogram, thickening and diminished excursion of the aortic leaflets with left ventricular hypertrophy (usually concentric) suggest aortic stenosis. If in addition the left atrium is enlarged in the absence of mitral valve disease, the possibility of severe aortic stenosis is further enhanced [1]. In combination with these findings, if the phonocardiogram reveals a late-peaking systolic ejection murmur, a delayed carotid upstroke with a prolonged time to one-half peak level, a prolonged left ventricular ejection time, and a prolonged time interval from the Q wave to the peak of the murmur, it is likely that critical aortic stenosis is present [1]. If, on the other hand, echocardiography (M-mode or two-dimensional) demonstrates good systolic separation of the aortic leaflets (≥ 1.3 cm), especially in the absence of concentric left ventricular hypertrophy, it is unlikely that severe aortic stenosis is present [1]. In patients with thickened aortic leaflets with markedly diminished excursion, continuous-wave Doppler velocity estimation of the aortic valve gradient (both instantaneous and mean gradients) may be performed, and the aortic valve area can be estimated noninvasively [1, 53] to quantify the severity of the aortic stenosis. Cardiac catheterization is often performed to confirm the presence of critical aortic stenosis prior to valve replacement [53]. In addition, because older patients have a high prevalence of coronary artery disease, coronary arteriography should be performed prior to valvular surgery, so that coronary bypass grafts, if needed, may be inserted during the same operation [52].

AORTIC VALVE REPLACEMENT

If critical aortic stenosis has been diagnosed and the patient is a surgical candidate, aortic valve replacement should follow. Operative survival for aortic valve replacement is lower in the elderly (85 to 95 percent in those over 65 years versus 95 to 99 percent in younger patients). The choice of the valve—either a ball-cage, tilting disc, or biological tissue valve—depends on the circumstances of the specific case and the comparative merits of the durability of the valve, the hemodynamic characteristics, and the need for anticoagulation [1]. Because the porcine valve does not usually require long-term anticoagulation in the absence of atrial fibrillation, it is often the valve of choice for elderly patients, in whom anticoagulation may result in significant morbidity. On the other hand, physical size limitations may dictate the use of a ball-cage or a tilting disc prosthesis. A low-profile central-flow (St. Jude) prosthesis may be another alternative, but it does require anticoagulation.

A substantial proportion of elderly patients who undergo aortic valve replacement receive coincident coronary artery bypass grafts. These patients may have a slightly higher operative mortality and morbidity [1].

POSTOPERATIVE MANAGEMENT

Careful postoperative management of the elderly patient with aortic valve replacement includes frequent and thorough examination with treatment of problems, such as arrhythmias or heart failure, as they arise. Antibiotic prophylaxis for dental work and other procedures likely to result in bacteremia, and chronic anticoagulation with warfarin and dipyridamole if the prosthetic valve is not porcine or in the presence of atrial fibrillation even if it is porcine, are also required [1]. In addition, periodic evaluation of the patient's symptoms and physical examination findings should be performed to check for valvular dysfunction.

NONSURGICAL MANAGEMENT OF CRITICAL AORTIC STENOSIS

Recently, percutaneous balloon dilatation of calcific aortic stenosis (aortic valvuloplasty) has been successfully performed in elderly patients with aortic stenosis, achieving a reduction of the aortic gradient with increases in cardiac index and aortic valve area [1, 54]. This feasible, nonsurgical technique represents a major therapeutic advancement that should find wide application, especially in elderly patients with severe aortic stenosis for whom aortic valvular replacement is not an option (Fig. 14-8).

If neither surgery nor valvuloplasty is chosen, optimal medical management is directed at ameliorating the symptoms. Specifically, this includes (1) maintenance of the hematocrit within the normal range to optimize oxygen delivery; (2) control of atrial and ventricular arrhythmias to ensure adequate atrial transport and ventricular filling; (3) treatment of left ventricular heart failure with digitalis and/or diuretics; (4) enhancement of diastolic coronary perfusion with carefully titrated doses of nitrates; and (5) supplementation of inspiratory oxygen if clinically indicated. Without surgery or valvuloplasty, the average life expectancy after the development of symptoms, especially of congestive heart failure, may be less than two years.

FIGURE 14-8. *Aortic peak-to-peak gradient before and after valvuloplasty. Peak gradient decreased from 77 ± 27 to 39 ± 15 mm Hg. (From R. G. McKay, et al. Assessment of left ventricular and aortic valve function after aortic balloon valvuloplasty in adult patients with critical aortic stenosis.* Circulation *75: 192, 1987.)*

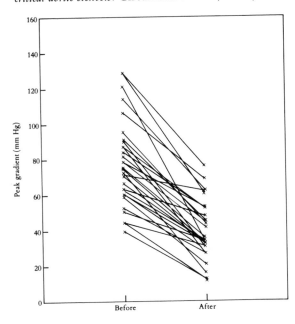

Although perioperative and long-term postoperative mortality rates for patients with aortic valve replacement are somewhat higher in elderly compared with younger patients with aortic stenosis [1, 52], the dismal prognosis on medical therapy alone as well as the potentially excellent surgical or valvuloplasty results justify an aggressive approach to the diagnosis and treatment of debilitating aortic stenosis in an otherwise intact and healthy elderly patient. Patients with isolated aortic stenosis complicated by left ventricular heart failure often have excellent operative survival and postoperative left ventricular functional improvement [1, 55]. It is important, therefore, to maintain a high degree of suspicion of aortic stenosis when appropriate and refer the patient for further evaluation if needed. In patients with cognitive impairment and/or serious multisystem problems, however, aortic valve replacement is not likely to improve cognitive function and/or long-term prognosis significantly [55].

Aortic Regurgitation
A major distinction between aortic stenosis and aortic regurgitation is that the stenotic lesion occurs only in the chronic form, whereas the regurgitant lesion may be either chronic or acute.

Chronic aortic regurgitation in the elderly develops as a result of hypertension, atherosclerosis, valvular deformity (e.g., due to sclerosis or congenital, rheumatic, or postendocarditic causes), or root dilatation (e.g., due to atherosclerosis, myxomatous degeneration, or aortitis). The regurgitant lesion can be very well tolerated and is often associated with a long asymptomatic period. Development of effort tolerance is usually the first symptom to appear and is followed by increasing symptoms of congestive heart failure. Diagnosis of chronic aortic regurgitation in the elderly is similar to that in the young (i.e., it is usually based on physical findings). Echocardiography and Doppler evaluation may be helpful in confirming the presence and estimating the severity of the lesion as well as in diagnosing the underlying disease mechanisms. Indications and timing for aortic valve replacement in patients with chronic aortic regurgitation have been somewhat controversial [1, 56]. In asymptomatic elderly persons, aortic valve replacement may not be necessary, whereas those who develop congestive heart failure secondary to aortic regurgitation should undergo prompt surgery.

The postoperative improvement after valve replacement for chronic aortic regurgitation (duration longer than 15 months) may not be as dramatic as that observed in patients with aortic stenosis. This difference may be due partly to irreversible muscle damage caused by left ventricular volume overload that occurred prior to the onset of severe clinical symptoms. Bonow et al. have indicated that surgery within 15 months of onset of left ventricular dysfunction may result in significant clinical improvement and reversal of ventricular dysfunction [56]. Our clinical impression is that postoperative improvement may not be as dramatic in the elderly, perhaps because of longer exposure time to the chronic regurgitant lesion.

Acute aortic regurgitation usually occurs as a result of either infective endocarditis (with valve perforation) or aortic dissection. In acute aortic regurgitation no time has been allowed for compensatory left ventricular hypertrophy or dilatation to develop, so that cardiac failure may occur following the abrupt increase in volume overload. In this case, a more aggressive approach should be taken toward valve replacement, even in elderly persons. Emergency operations may have to be considered during an active infection, particularly if it is fungal or if hemodynamic compromise or aortic valve ring abscess develops. If the acute regurgitation is due to aortic dissection, surgery requires both repair of the dissection and replacement of the valve and involves even higher operative risk. If indicated, it should be performed on an urgent or emergency basis.

MITRAL VALVE DISEASE

Mitral Stenosis

In elderly patients, mitral valve stenosis usually results from rheumatic heart disease, which is almost always acquired before the age of 20 years but which may not manifest clinical problems until several decades later [1, 57]. The diagnosis and management of mitral stenosis in elderly persons is usually not different from that in younger individuals, except that "silent" mitral stenosis may occur more commonly in the elderly and should be considered when dyspnea and/or atrial fibrillation are present. Occasionally, an elderly patient with no audible murmur may present with congestive heart failure and a small heart size on chest x-ray and will be found to have mitral stenosis on echocardiography.

The severity of mitral stenosis may be estimated by two-dimensional echocardiography and phonography, and the pressure gradient and mitral valve area may be determined by Doppler evaluation [1, 58]. The secondary effect of the mitral stenotic lesion on the pulmonary circulation and right heart should also be assessed noninvasively to optimize management of the patient [1, 57]. The natural history of mitral stenosis is related to several factors: severity of the lesion and its rate of progression, and the presence of pulmonary hypertension, atrial arrhythmias, and/or systemic embolism. Patients often adapt well for some time and may not become symptomatic until the onset of atrial fibrillation in the sixth or seventh decade. Management of atrial fibrillation should be directed at controlling the rapid ventricular rate followed by chemical and/or electrical attempts at conversion to sinus rhythm. Maintaining sinus rhythm may allow postponement of valve replacement or repair or balloon valvuloplasty and is associated with better long-term cognitive function.

Mitral Valve Prolapse

Mitral valve prolapse or mitral valve prolapse syndrome in the elderly has received substantial attention recently and continues to be defined and clarified [1, 59]. Certain elderly patients may present with problems that are similar to those of certain young patients, most commonly chest pain and arrhythmias, followed by progressive mitral regurgitation and congestive heart failure [1, 59, 60]. Severe congestive heart failure requiring valve replacement tends to be a more significant problem in certain elderly persons.

The management of elderly patients with mitral valve prolapse should consist of antibiotic prophylaxis against endocarditis for those with mitral regurgitation, symptomatic therapy including antiarrhythmic therapy for symptomatic arrhythmias, and antiplatelet therapy for those with prior cerebral emboli. Valve surgery should be considered only for severe mitral regurgitation.

Mitral Regurgitation
Mitral regurgitation may result from inadequate valve closure due to dysfunction of the left ventricle, papillary muscle(s), chordae tendinae, mitral valve leaflets, mitral annulus, or atrioventricular contractile sequence. In the elderly, the more common etiologies of mitral regurgitation include coronary artery disease and its complications, mitral valve prolapse, and mitral annular calcification. Diagnosing mitral regurgitation is usually not a problem and is similar for old and younger patients. Evaluation of severity of the regurgitation, however, may be more difficult.

Ruptured chordae tendinae may result from myxomatous degenerative and/or long-term mitral regurgitation in patients with mitral valve prolapse. Chordal rupture may also be due to infective endocarditis or trauma, or it may be idiopathic. The diagnosis of ruptured chordae tendinae may be made clinically and can be confirmed with Doppler echocardiography. Prognosis depends partly on the severity of the mechanical overload and partly on the cardiac reserve of the patient. Surgery may be necessary, occasionally on an emergency basis. In some cases, valvuloplasty may be performed without prosthetic valve replacement.

Postinfarction mitral regurgitation due to papillary muscle and/or ventricular wall dysfunction occurs commonly in the elderly and usually does not require aggressive therapy. When the infarcted papillary muscle is ruptured, however, catastrophic hemodynamic compromise may ensue [1, 37]. The development of cardiogenic shock may be abrupt and is sometimes unheralded by prior development of a murmur. Whereas conservative medical management may be associated with near certain mortality, prompt medical and surgical treatment may be lifesaving and may yield dramatic improvement, especially in patients in whom left ventricular wall motion is preserved [37–39]. The elderly, like younger patients, demonstrate excellent results, both short- and long-term, following prompt mitral valve surgery for postinfarction cardiogenic shock [39].

Infective endocarditis may cause abrupt mitral regurgitation by leaflet perforation or rupture of the chordae tendinae. These abrupt events dictate prompt medical and surgical therapy. Urgent surgery is indicated in the presence of hemodynamic compromise, fungal or *Staphylococcus aureus* infection, valve ring abscess, or new conduction block. If possible, surgery should be deferred until bacteriologic cure is attained or at least until bacteremia is no longer present. Elderly patients should receive the same considerations for surgery as younger individuals, but operative risk may be significantly higher in the aged.

Mitral Annular Calcification
Limited almost exclusively to the elderly population, mitral annular calcification is common and is usually benign. Most elderly patients are asymptomatic and demonstrate no significant hemodynamic changes. A diastolic murmur may be appreciated, but it seldom implies mitral stenosis. Although mitral valve replacement is generally not indicated, in rare instances the calcification is extensive, impeding mitral inflow and causing functional mitral stenosis [1, 61]. Antibiotic prophylaxis should be instituted if there is significant mitral regurgitation.

Infective Endocarditis
Aside from intravenous drug abusers, the elderly are becoming the most frequent victims of infective endocarditis [1, 62]. Diagnosis and management are similar to those practiced in younger patients, and emergency surgery is sometimes indicated [63]. Prophylaxis with appropriate antibiotic coverage for known bacteremic procedures is important for those with valvular deformity and regurgitant lesions. In the elderly person with a regurgitant valve lesion who presents with an undiagnosed fever, prompt wide spectrum antibiotic coverage during initial evaluation may be lifesaving in some cases.

Congestive Heart Failure
Congestive heart failure is a very common problem in clinical geriatrics. Its prevalence rises exponentially with increasing age, starting in the fifth decade [1]. Proper therapy can

probably benefit the patient more than treatment for any other condition of equal severity in old age. Congestive heart failure may result from compromise of either systolic or diastolic function or both, resulting in elevated ventricular end-diastolic pressures. Congestion of pulmonary or systemic veins and the organs they drain are the associated features. Although isolated left or right heart failure is not rare, combined left and right heart failure is more frequently observed. Recently, several studies have documented the high prevalence of diastolic dysfunction with impaired ventricular relaxation and filling with preserved systolic function in elderly patients with congestive heart failure [1, 64, 65]. Between 50 and 60 percent of old persons with congestive heart failure have normal or only slightly reduced ejection fractions [1, 64, 65], indicating adequate ventricular contraction. Elderly patients with impaired diastolic function are often erroneously treated for systolic heart failure with medications such as digitalis and vasodilators, which may exacerbate rather than improve their cardiac function. It is important, therefore, to be aware of this phenomenon and, as discussed below, tailor the therapy to the individual pathophysiology.

Although coronary artery disease is common in elderly patients with congestive heart failure, at autopsy approximately one-third to one-half of the hearts of elderly persons dying in congestive heart failure have been found to be without significant coronary disease [1, 10]. Therefore, congestive heart failure should not be equated with coronary heart disease.

PATHOPHYSIOLOGY

The heart adapts to an increased workload by one of the following mechanisms: (1) increased sympathetic nervous system stimulation, (2) myocardial hypertrophy, and (3) the Frank-Starling mechanism [1, 2, 66]. Responsiveness to beta-adrenergic stimulation is decreased with age, and there is greater dependence in elderly persons on the Frank-Starling mechanism [1, 22, 11]. Recent data in animals suggest that age blunts the hypertrophic response of the myocardium to a given increase in afterload [66]. The age-related prolongation in ventricular relaxation time together with the increased myocardial stiffness of the aged heart result in increases in the left ventricular end-diastolic pressures at rest and/or exercise such that pulmonary and systemic venous congestion may occur in the presence of preserved systolic function [1].

CLINICAL PRESENTATION

The usual symptoms and signs of congestive heart failure are similar for old and young patients, but atypical presentations are more frequent in the elderly. Nonspecific signs of illness such as somnolence, confusion, disorientation, weakness, and fatigue may be the presenting features, and dyspnea may be absent. Worsening of preexisting dementia is an important sign of congestive failure in many patients. Peripheral edema is not a reliable sign of heart failure, but jugular venous distention and hepatojugular reflux usually do indicate right heart failure. Although an S_4 gallop does not necessarily signify heart disease, an S_3, or early diastolic gallop, usually indicates heart failure. Inspiratory rales in the lower half of the lung fields may or may not indicate heart failure [1].

DIAGNOSIS

Although most attention has previously focused on systolic function, it is now more widely appreciated that diastolic function—i.e., ventricular stiffness and impaired left ventricular relaxation—may be more important than systolic dysfunction in the pathogenesis of heart failure in the elderly [1, 64, 65]. Noninvasive studies of left ventricular diastolic motion and ventricular diastolic filling using echocardiographic/Doppler and radionuclide scintigraphic techniques are very helpful in clarifying these points [1, 64, 65].

MANAGEMENT

In managing the patient with heart failure due to systolic dysfunction, allowances must be made for the specific circumstances of age. The mainstays of therapy are bed rest, digitalis, diuretics, and reduction of afterload and preload. Because prolonged bed rest is dangerous but necessary, an effective compromise is to have the patient sit in a chair with his/her legs elevated. Bed or chair rest enhances diuresis, as does oxygen supplementation insofar as it improves tissue oxygenation. Improved oxygenation of peripheral tissues increases renal perfusion, decreases venous tone, and consequently decreases preload [1].

The value of long-term digitalis therapy to elderly patients has recently been questioned [1, 67]. Digitalis is useful in managing acute and severe congestive heart failure in patients with sinus rhythm or atrial fibrillation. Although the inotropic response to cardiac glycosides may be diminished in senescent mammalian cardiac muscle, its toxic effects are not decreased in old age. Decreased renal clearance, combined with wide variability in extrarenal clearance reduces the predictability of serum digoxin levels in the elderly. In view of these age-related changes, including a possible decrease in inotropic response, the indications for digitalis should be considered in the context of its known toxicity.

Fortunately, we have access to efficacious diuretics, vasodilators, antihypertensive agents, and newer inotropic agents. Vasodilator therapy reduces afterload, thereby enhancing myocardial shortening and increasing stroke volume [1, 68]. The most frequently used vasodilators are the nitrates, which, alone or in combination with hydralazine, may be effective in reducing filling pressures, increasing cardiac output, increasing renal blood flow, and improving exercise tolerance [1, 68].

NEWER AGENTS

In some cases in which therapy with digitalis, diuretics, and vasodilators has not been sufficient, amrinone and its analog, milrinone, have been shown to be effective in producing a marked improvement in the stroke-work index and decreased pulmonary artery pressures [69]. Although milrinone has direct inotropic effects on cardiac muscle and, at high doses, a direct vasodilatory effect as well, another relatively new agent, captopril, an angiotensin-converting enzyme inhibitor, appears to work predominantly on the peripheral vasculature [70]. Captopril has also been shown to be very effective in patients who are refractory to digitalis, diuretics, and other vasodilators. Prazosin, an arterial and venous system vasodilator, reduces systemic and pulmonary venous pressure and may increase cardiac output [71], but its effectiveness in elderly patients with heart failure

has not been investigated. It is possible that a combination of these newer drugs with more conventional agents will result in additional synergistic effects. Which of these agents or combinations of them are best suited for the older patient with congestive heart failure remains to be established. Calcium antagonist therapy may prove beneficial for older patients with heart failure due to diastolic dysfunction [72].

Cardiomyopathy

The term *cardiomyopathy* refers to a diffuse or generalized myocardial disorder without underlying etiology [1]. Thus, by definition all patients so diagnosed have idiopathic or primary involvement of the myocardium. However, valvular, hypertensive, or coronary artery disease often coexists with primary cardiomyopathy. Three broad types of ventricular dysfunction (which may overlap) are described. Dilated or congestive cardiomyopathy is characterized by impaired systolic function with dilatation (sometimes mild) of chambers and increased muscle mass without significant increase in wall thickness. Hypertrophic cardiomyopathy is characterized by normal or small chamber size, increased wall thickness, hyperdynamic systolic ejection, and impaired diastolic filling. In restrictive or infiltrative cardiomyopathy, the myocardium shows increased stiffness secondary to infiltrative pathology; systolic function is impaired, and the atria are dilated in the late stages.

DILATED OR CONGESTIVE CARDIOMYOPATHY

Dilated cardiomyopathy may be misdiagnosed as heart failure secondary to coronary artery disease. Although thought to be uncommon in the elderly, approximately 10 percent of patients with this condition in several large studies are over the age of 65 [1]. It is possible that its low incidence in elderly patients may represent a selection process such that few people with susceptibility to myocardial damage of this type survive beyond the seventh decade. The diagnosis of dilated cardiomyopathy is based on exclusion of etiologic factors that may result in diffuse myocardial dysfunction (e.g., adriamycin toxicity, postradiation damage, and chronic alcoholism) and is generally confirmed by echocardiography, which reveals four-chamber dilatation with depressed systolic pump function. The increased tendency toward thrombus formation and subsequent systemic embolic events in these patients should be treated with anticoagulation therapy. Treatment for dilated cardiomyopathy is essentially the same as that for heart failure and arrhythmias, with emphasis on the use of vasodilator therapy in addition to diuretics and antiarrhythmic agents. Digitalis may be particularly effective in the presence of atrial fibrillation or other atrial arrhythmias. Its use in elderly patients with heart failure was discussed earlier in this chapter in the section on congestive heart failure. Dosages of vasodilator drugs should be adjusted with caution, since excessive hypotension may prove hazardous.

Acute myocarditis appears to be rare in the elderly and is difficult to diagnose clinically. Endomyocardial biopsy demonstrates conspicuous cellular infiltrates with cellular degeneration and necrosis. The common etiologic agents are viruses and rickettsia, with coxsackie infection being probably the most frequent cause in the western hemisphere. Although immunosuppressive therapy has been proposed for the treatment of subacute and chronic myocarditis, diagnostic criteria and therapeutic efficacy are uncertain, and it remains to be determined whether these agents are well tolerated by the elderly. Congestive heart failure with normal systolic function may represent hypertrophic cardiomyopathy or the early stages of restrictive cardiomyopathy, which may be seen at any age but is more frequently seen in the elderly.

HYPERTROPHIC CARDIOMYOPATHY
Diagnosis
Although it was previously thought that hypertrophic cardiomyopathy was rare in older patients, several studies have reported finding significant numbers of patients beyond the seventh decade [1, 73]. Echocardiography is helpful in identifying asymptomatic or mildly symptomatic elderly patients with idiopathic cardiac hypertrophy [1, 72–74]. The older patient often presents with symptoms similar to those of younger patients—dizziness, syncope, dyspnea, chest pain, and palpitations. Diagnosis is

often delayed because symptoms of dizziness and syncope are incorrectly attributed to cerebrovascular causes, coronary artery disease, or pulmonary disease; the proper diagnosis is considered in only one-third of cases prior to referral.

Left ventricular outflow tract "obstruction" in the form of intraventricular pressure gradients may be seen with the characteristic physical signs. The typical bifid carotid pulse, however, may be absent in many elderly hypertrophic patients [73]. Aortic regurgitation secondary to coexisting aortic valve calcification often coexists with hypertrophic "obstructive" cardiomyopathy.

The old hypertrophic heart does not appear dissimilar to that described in younger patients except that hypertrophy may be more pronounced and may be concentric with severe free wall hypertrophy. Natural history studies emphasize the rarity of sudden death in the elderly with this condition, which may indicate a different underlying mechanism for hypertrophic cardiomyopathy in old and young persons, or it may represent survival of a subgroup with a low propensity to sudden death. Fibrous endocardial thickening of the upper interventricular septum and of the anterior mitral leaflet is commonly observed. Associated abnormalities in the elderly commonly include mitral annular calcification and degenerative calcific aortic valves, with coexistence of valvular and myocardial diseases. The typical echocardiographic findings consist of asymmetrical left ventricular hypertrophy, hyperdynamic left ventricular systolic function, systolic anterior motion of the mitral valve, and left atrial dilatation [1, 73, 74]. Doppler findings include evidence of an impaired rate of diastolic filling and a left ventricular outflow tract gradient.

The syndrome of "hypertensive hypertrophic cardiomyopathy of the elderly" applies to patients with a history of hypertension who present with chest pain or dyspnea and on echocardiography are found to have severe concentric left ventricular hypertrophy with a small ventricular cavity and supernormal cardiac systolic function, with or without systolic anterior motion of the mitral valve and cavity obliteration [75]. The impaired diastolic function as manifest by a prolonged early diastolic filling period and a reduced peak rate of increase in diastolic dimension may be responsible for the presenting symptoms of pulmonary congestion [1, 72–75].

Management
Management of the elderly with hypertrophic cardiomyopathy is similar to that in the young. Symptomatic patients are managed with beta-adrenergic blocking agents and/or calcium channel-blocking agents; the elderly are less tolerant than younger patients of these drugs. Larger doses of calcium channel blockers may aggravate the clinical picture by causing significant hypotension and therefore should be avoided. Surgery, namely myotomy and myectomy, may be performed with an acceptable low operative mortality in symptomatic patients who have outflow gradients and who have failed medical therapy. Use of amiodarone may be less indicated in the elderly owing to decreased frequency of sudden death. Drugs such as digitalis, diuretics, and vasodilators may severely exacerbate the ventricular dysfunction in these patients and may be catastrophic in some cases [1].

RESTRICTIVE CARDIOMYOPATHY

Restrictive cardiomyopathy is characterized by small ventricles, large atria, elevated filling pressures, and thickened walls with a characteristic "sparkling" appearance on echocardiograms. The electrocardiogram shows low voltage with atrial fibrillation and conduction defects. Senile cardiac amyloidosis may be a separate pathologic condition that is usually observed in patients after the age of 70 years. The diagnosis is confirmed by rectal, gingival, or endomyocardial biopsy. The prevalence of amyloid deposition in the heart increases with age, reaching nearly 80 percent in the atria of persons over 90 years of age [10]. The macroscopic appearance, however, is often normal, and amyloid deposition may be largely limited to the atria [10]. Therefore, the term *restrictive cardiomyopathy* may not necessarily apply to all old hearts containing amyloid. Microscopically, the earliest deposits are seen in the atrial capillaries. In advanced cases, small deposits may be present in the atrioventricular valves, and conduction

tissue may be affected later, if at all. A restrictive type of physiology may occasionally result from radiation damage, which may not be observed until months or years after the radiation therapy. Restrictive cardiomyopathies are not commonly seen and rarely result in systolic heart failure. Treatment should be directed at optimizing filling and promoting diastolic function.

Arrhythmias
Atrial and ventricular arrythmias are common in the elderly, including those without clinically apparent heart disease. The incidence of frequent or complex arrhythmias is related to the presence and extent of underlying heart disease and reportedly ranges between 20 and 75 percent, with ventricular arrhythmias accounting for two-thirds and supraventricular arrhythmias for one-third of the cases [76, 77]. The clinical significance of supraventricular arrhythmias varies from trivial to life-threatening, and proper management depends on accurate diagnosis of the rhythm disturbance and knowledge of the clinical circumstances [1]. Both benign and potentially malignant ventricular arrhythmias are common in asymptomatic and other-wise healthy elderly individuals. Although minor ventricular arrhythmias also occur frequently in the symptomatic elderly, serious episodic arrhythmias are less common and often occur in relation to the onset of symptoms. Prognosis of a chronic arrhythmia is related to the severity of the underlying heart disease [1].

MANAGEMENT
Ventricular Arrhythmias
The management of ventricular arrhythmias in elderly patients is similar to that in younger patients [1, 77]. After a myocardial infarction, high-grade ectopic beats, especially in the presence of a low left ventricular ejection fraction, are associated with a poor prognosis and should be treated. However, whether antiarrhythmic therapy improves the prognosis in these patients is not yet established. A multicenter study is currently being conducted to address this issue. The long-term use of beta-blockade in elderly

infarct patients has been demonstrated to reduce significantly overall mortality, cardiac death, and reinfarction [1, 30, 32, 42].

The loading and maintenance doses of antiarrhythmic agents should be adjusted for age and body weight (see previous discussion on lidocaine in the section on acute myocardial infarction). Reduced clearance of quinidine and prolongation of its elimination half-life in elderly persons could predispose them to quinidine toxicity [1]. The high incidence of such side effects as diarrhea also limits the use of quinidine. A major disadvantage of using disopyramide in the elderly is its anticholinergic activity, which may result in urinary retention and visual blurring [1, 77]. Age-related decreases in renal clearance and excretion result in higher serum levels of procainamide and its active metabolite, N-acetyl procainamide (NAPA), in the elderly [77]. The development of procainamide-induced lupus is common and is a major disadvantage of this drug. It is clear that there is no ideal antiarrhythmic agent that is effective and has a long dosing interval and few side effects. The physician must therefore weigh the benefits and risks of antiarrhythmic therapy and select an appropriate agent carefully and empirically [1, 41, 77, 78].

Treatment of supraventricular arrhythmias is similar for all age groups. Atrial fibrillation may respond to drugs, electrocardioversion, or overdrive pacing. Although to date no definitive studies have been completed to address this issue, some authorities believe that in patients with atrial fibrillation, anticoagulation should be considered if no major contraindications exist. Atrial flutter may be treated with electrocardioversion if hemodynamic compromise warrants it. For those with sick sinus syndrome, a permanent pacemaker is indicated only if the patient is symptomatic, since pacemaker implantation does not alter the patient's life expectancy [1, 79].

Conduction System Disease

Although no single abnormality is confined to any age group, the sick sinus syndrome and trifascicular block can be regarded as predominantly geriatric diseases [1, 79, 80]. In symptomatic elderly patients with conduction defects or heart block, a pacemaker may alleviate the symptoms. Although pacemakers increase survival of the elderly who have complete heart block, they do not prolong life expectancy in cases of bifascicular or trifascicular block in the absence of symptoms [1, 79, 80]. Preservation of atrial transport, which may be vital to some patients, is accomplished by implanting an atrioventricular sequential pacemaker system. The prognosis of complete heart block—after permanent pacing is instituted—is related to the severity of the underlying heart disease [80]. Patients in their eighties who receive pacemakers for complete heart block can do very well with pacing and may survive as well as those without heart disease.

References

1. Wei, J. Y., and Gersh, B. J. Heart disease in the elderly. *Curr. Probl. Cardiol.* 12:1, 1987.
2. Wei, J. Y. Cardiovascular anatomic and physiologic changes with age. *Topics Geriatr. Rehab.* 2:10, 1986.
3. Yin, F. C. P. The Aging Vasculature and Its Effects on the Heart. In M. L. Weisfeldt (ed.), *The Aging Heart.* New York: Raven, 1980. Pp. 137–214.
4. Hutchins, G. M., Bulkley, B. H., and Miner, M. M. Correlation of age and heart weight with tortuosity and caliber of normal human coronary arteries. *Am. Heart J.* 94:196, 1977.
5. Goldberg, I. D., et al. Frequency of tetraploid nuclei in the rat increases with age. *Ann. N.Y. Acad. Sci.* 435:422, 1984.
6. Milch, R. A. Matrix properties of the aging arterial wall. *Monogr. Surg. Sci.* 2:261, 1965.
7. Potter, J. F., et al. The effect of age on the cardiothoracic ratio of man. *J. Am. Geriatr. Soc.* 30:404, 1982.
8. Gerstenblith, G., et al. Echocardiographic assessment of a normal adult aging population. *Circulation* 56:273, 1977.
9. Davies, M. J. Pathology of the conduction system. In F. L. Caird, J. L. C. Dalle, and R. D. Kennedy (eds.), *Cardiology in Old Age.* New York: Plenum, 1976. Pp. 57–59.
10. Pomerance, A. Pathology of the Myocardium and Valves. In F. L. Caird, J. L. C. Dalle, and R. D. Kennedy (eds.), *Cardiology in Old Age.* New York: Plenum, 1976. Pp. 11–53.
11. Rodeheffer, R. J., et al. Exercise cardiac output is maintained with advancing age in healthy human

subjects: Cardiac dilatation and increased stroke volume compensate for diminished heart rate. *Circulation* 69:203, 1984.

12. Shannon, R. P., et al. The effect of age and sodium depletion on cardiovascular response to orthostasis. *Hypertension* 5:438, 1986.

13. Wei, J. Y., et al. Post-cough heart rate response: Influence of age, sex and basal blood pressure. *Am. J. Physiol.* 245:R18, 1983.

14. Wei, J. Y., Spurgeon, H. A., and Lakatta, E. G. Excitation-contraction in rat myocardiums: Alterations with adult aging. *Am. J. Physiol.* 246:H784, 1984.

15. Shimada, K., et al. Age-related changes of baroreflex function, plasma norepinephrine, and blood pressure. *Hypertension* 7:113, 1985.

16. Maddens, M., et al. Does alpha-adrenergic responsiveness decrease with age? *Gerontologist* 26:154A, 1986.

17. Wei, J. Y., et al. Influence of age on cardiovascular reflex response in anesthetized rats. *Am. J. Physiol.* 249:R31, 1985.

18. Lipsitz, L. A., et al. Postprandial reduction in blood pressure in the elderly. *N. Engl. J. Med.* 309:81, 1983.

19. Ferguson, J. J., et al. Abnormalities in the arterial physical properties precede the development of hypertension in Dahl salt-sensitive rats. *Circulation* 72:255, 1985.

20. Tsunoda, K., et al. Effect of age on the renin-angiotensin-aldosterone system in normal subjects: Simultaneous measurement of active and inactive renin, renin substrate, and aldosterone in plasma. *J. Clin. Endocrinol. Metab.* 62:384, 1986.

21. Shannon, R. P., Minaker, K. L., and Rowe, J. W. Aging and water balance in humans. *Sem. Nephrol.* 4:346, 1984.

22. Raven, P. B., and Mitchell, J. The Effect of Aging on the Cardiovascular Response to Dynamic and Static Exercise. In M. L. Weisfeldt (ed.), *The Aging Heart.* New York: Raven, 1980. Pp. 269–295.

23. Nixon, J. V., et al. Ventricular performance in human hearts aged 61 to 73 years. *Am. J. Cardiol.* 56:932, 1985.

24. Kannell, W. B. Cardiovascular Risk Factors in the Aged. In *Second Conference on the Epidemiology of Aging.* Bethesda, MD: National Institute of Health, July, 1980.

25. Wei, J. Y., Ragland, J., and Li, Y. X. Effect of exercise training on resting blood pressure and heart rate in adult and aged rats. *J. Gerontol.* 42:11, 1987.

26. Li, Y. X., et al. Age-related differences in effect of exercise training on cardiac muscle function in rats. *Am. J. Physiol.* 251:H12, 1986.

27. Wei, J. Y., et al. Does chronic exercise training protect cardiac muscle against hypoxia? *Circulation* 70:235, 1984.

28. Larsson, B., et al. Health and aging characteristics of highly physically active 65 year old men. *Eur. Heart J.* 5:31, 1984.

29. Paffenbarger, R. S., Wing, A. L., and Hyde, R. T. Physical activity as an index of heart attack risk in college alumni. *Am. J. Epidemiol.* 108:161, 1978.

30. Wenger, N. K., Furberg, C. D. and Pitt, E. (eds.). *Coronary Heart Disease in the Elderly.* New York: Elsevier, 1986.

31. Mock, M. B., et al. Prognosis of Coronary Heart Disease in the Elderly Patient: The CASS Experience. In E. L. Coodley (ed.), *Geriatric Heart Disease.* Littleton, MA: PSG, 1983. Pp. 358–363.

32. Wei, J. Y. Cardiovascular drugs in the elderly: Antianginal agents. *Drug Ther.* 17:31, 1987.

33. Heller, G. V., Blaustein, A. S., and Wei, J. Y. Implications of elevated myocardial isoenzymes in the presence of normal serum creatinine kinase activity. *Am. J. Cardiol.* 85:24, 1983.

34. Hong, R. A., et al. Elevated MB with normal total CK in suspected myocardial infarction: Associated clinical findings and prognosis. *Am. Heart J.* 111:1041, 1986.

35. Wei, J. Y., et al. Time course of serum cardiac enzymes after intracoronary thrombolytic therapy. *Arch. Intern. Med.* 145:1596, 1985.

36. Fuentes, F., et al. Thrombolytic Therapy in Myocardial Infarction of the Elderly Patient. In E. L. Coodley (ed.), *Geriatric Heart Disease.* Littleton, MA: PSG, 1985. Pp. 404–410.

37. Wei, J. Y., Hutchins, G. M., and Bulkley, B. H. Papillary muscle rupture in fatal acute myocardial infarction: A potentially treatable form of cardiogenic shock. *Ann. Intern Med.* 90:149, 1979.

38. Weintraub, R. M., et al. Repair of post–infarction VSD in the elderly: Early and long-term results. *J. Thorac. Cardiovasc. Surg.* 85:191, 1983.

39. Weintraub, R. M., Wei, J. Y., and Thurer, R. L. Surgical repair of remediable post–infarction cardiogenic shock in the elderly: Early and long-term results. *J. Am. Geriatr. Soc.* 34:389, 1983.

40. Weiss, J. L., Wei, J. Y., and Kappelman, N. B. Ventricular septal defect complicating myocardial infarction. *Johns Hopkins Med. J.* 141:95, 1977.

41. Reidenberg, M. M., et al. Aging and renal clearance of procainamide and acetylprocainamide. *Clin. Pharmacol. Ther.* 28:732, 1980.

42. Gundersen, T., et al. Timolol-related reduction in mortality and reinfarction in patients aged

65–75 years surviving acute myocardial infarction. *Circulation* 66:1179, 1982.

43. Gersh, B. J., et al. Coronary Artery Surgery in Patients Over 65 Years of Age. In E. L. Coodley (ed.), *Geriatric Heart Disease.* Littleton, MA: PSG, 1985. Pp. 411–422.

44. Holmes, D. R., Jr. Percutaneous Transluminal Coronary Angioplasty. In E. L. Coodley (ed.), *Geriatric Heart Disease.* Littleton, MA: PSG, 1985. Pp. 439–449.

45. Hartzler, G. O., et al. Late results of multiple lesion coronary angioplasty in an aged population. *J. Am. Coll. Cardiol.* 7:21A, 1986.

46. Dorros, G., and Janke, L. Percutaneous transluminal coronary angioplasty in patients over the age of 70 years. *Cathet. Cardiovasc. Diagn.* 12:223, 1986.

47. St. John Sutton, M., Abdul, T. J., and McGoon, D. C. Atrial septal defect in patients ages 60 years or older: Operative results and long-term postoperative follow-up. *Circulation* 64:402, 1981.

48. Clarkson, P. M., et al. Results after repair of coarctation of the aorta beyond infancy: A 10- to 28-year follow-up with particular reference to late systemic hypertension. *Am. J. Cardiol.* 51:1481, 1983.

49. Liberthson, R. R., et al. Coarctation of the aorta: Review of 234 patients and clarification of management problems. *Am. J. Cardiol.* 43:835, 1979.

50. Stevenson, J. G., Kawabori, I., and Bailey, W. W. Noninvasive evaluation of Blalock-Taussig shunts: Determination of patency and differentiation from patent ductus arteriosus by Doppler echocardiography. *Am. Heart J.* 106:1121, 1983.

51. Roberts, W. C., Perloff, J. K., and Constantino, T. Severe valvular aortic stenosis in patients over 65 years of age. *Am. J. Cardiol.* 27:497, 1971.

52. Bonow, R. O., et al. Aortic valve replacement without myocardial revascularization in patients with combined aortic valvular and coronary artery disease. *Circulation* 63:243, 1981.

53. Currie, P. J., et al. Continuous-wave Doppler echocardiographic assessment of severity of calcific aortic stenosis: A simultaneous Doppler-catheter correlative study in 100 adult patients. *Circulation* 71:1162, 1985.

54. McKay, R. G., et al. Assessment of left ventricular and aortic valve function after aortic balloon valvuloplasty in adult patients with critical aortic stenosis. *Circulation* 75:192, 1987.

55. Henriksen, L. Evidence suggestive of diffuse brain damage following cardiac operations. *Lancet* 1:816, 1984.

56. Bonow, R. O., et al. Reversal of left ventricular dysfunction after aortic valve replacement for chronic aortic regurgitation: Influence of duration of preoperative left ventricular dysfunction. *Circulation* 70:570, 1984.

57. Selzer, A., and Cohn, K. Natural history of mitral stenosis in review. *Circulation* 45:878, 1972.

58. Smith, M. D., et al. Comparative accuracy of two-dimensional echocardiography and Doppler pressure half-time methods in assessing severity of mitral stenosis in patients with and without prior commissurotomy. *Circulation* 73:100, 1986.

59. Kolibash, A. J., et al. Mitral valve prolapse syndrome: Analysis of 62 patients aged 60 years and older. *Am. J. Cardiol.* 52:534, 1983.

60. Wei, J. Y., et al. Mitral valve prolapse syndrome and recurrent ventricular tacharrythmias: A malignant variant refractory to conventional drug therapy. *Ann. Intern. Med.* 88:6, 1978.

61. Osterberger, L. E., et al. Functional mitral stenosis in patients with massive mitral annular calcification. *Circulation* 64:472, 1981.

62. Robbins, N., Demaria, A., and Miller, M. H. Infective endocarditis in the elderly. *South Med. J.* 73:1335, 1980.

63. Reid, C. L., and Rahimtoola, S. H. Infective endocarditis. Role of echocardiography, cardiac catheterization, and surgical intervention. *Modern Concepts Cardiovasc. Dis.* 4:16, 1986.

64. Dougherty, A. H., et al. Congestive heart failure with normal systolic function. *Am. J. Cardiol.* 54:778, 1984.

65. Soufer, R., et al. Intact systolic left ventricular function in clinical congestive heart failure. *Am. J. Cardiol.* 55:1032, 1985.

66. Isoyama, S., et al. Does the capacity for left ventricular hypertrophy diminish with age? *Circ. Res.* 61:337, 1987.

67. Lee, D. C. S., et al. Heart failure in outpatients: A randomized trial of digoxin versus placebo. *N. Engl. J. Med.* 306:699, 1982.

68. Chatterjee, K., and Parmley, W. W. Vasodilator therapy for acute myocardial infarction and chronic congestive heart failure. *J. Am. Coll. Cardiol.* 1:133, 1983.

69. Baim, D. S., et al. Evaluation of a new bipyridine inotropic agent—milrinone—in patients with severe congestive heart failure. *N. Engl. J. Med.* 309:748, 1983.

70. Massie, B., et al. Hemodynamic and radionuclide effects of acute captopril therapy for heart failure: Changes in left and right ventricular volumes and function at rest and during exercise. *Circulation* 65:1374, 1982.

71. Parmley, W. W., et al. Hemodynamic effects of prazosin in chronic heart failure. *Am. Heart J.* 102:622, 1981.

72. Santinga, J. T., et al. Effect of age on left ventricular filling and hemodynamic response to a calcium antagonist. *Clin. Res.* 35:323A, 1987.

73. Shenoy, M. M., et al. Hypertrophic cardiomyopathy in the elderly. *Arch. Intern. Med.* 146:658, 1986.

74. Wei, J. Y., Weiss, J. L., and Bulkley, B. H. The heterogeneity of hypertrophic cardiomyopathy: An autopsy and one-dimensional echocardiographic study. *Am. J. Cardiol.* 45:24, 1980.

75. Topol, E. J., Traill, T. A., and Fortuin, N. J. Hypertensive hypertrophic cardiomyopathy of the elderly. *N. Engl. J. Med.* 312:277, 1985.

76. Martin, A., et al. Five-year follow-up of 101 elderly subjects by means of long-term ambulatory cardiac monitoring. *Eur. Heart J.* 5(7):592, 1984.

77. Dreifus, L. S. Cardiac arrhythmias in the elderly: Clinical aspects. *Cardiol. Clin.* 4(2):273, 1986.

78. Burk, M., and Peters, U. Disopyramide kinetics in renal impairment: Determinants of interindividual variability. *Clin. Pharmacol. Ther.* 34(3):331, 1983.

79. McAnulty, J. H., et al. Natural history of "high risk" bundle-branch block: Final report of a prospective study. *N. Engl. J. Med.* 307:137, 1983.

80. Ginks, W., Leatham, A., and Siddons, H. Prognosis of patients paced for chronic atrioventricular block. *Br. Heart J.* 41:633, 1979.

15

Altered Blood Pressure

JOHN W. ROWE
LEWIS A. LIPSITZ

High Blood Pressure

The prevalence of high blood pressure coupled with widespread recognition of its importance as a precedent for cardiovascular disease and the availability of effective, safe therapy has made management of hypertension a center-piece of the practice of modern medicine. It is surprising therefore, that despite these advances, generalized uncertainty persists regarding the proper management of high blood pressure in the elderly.

INFLUENCE OF AGE ON BLOOD PRESSURE

Numerous cross-sectional and longitudinal studies in Western countries have demonstrated similar trends for changes in blood pressure after adulthood (Fig. 15-1). The increase in systolic blood pressure is generally linear from age 30 to old age, whereas the increase in diastolic blood pressure is less prominent and peaks in the mid fifties in men and in the early sixties in women, declining slightly thereafter [1]. As a result of this pattern, pulse pressure increases in late life in both men and women. Although trends for blood pressure with age are similar in many Western societies, the well-documented lack of a rise of blood pressure with age in less developed countries [2] clearly indicates that the increases in blood pressure do not represent an inevitable consequence of normal human aging but rather are caused by some genetic or environmental factor common to developed countries.

PATHOPHYSIOLOGIC MECHANISMS UNDERLYING AGE-RELATED INCREASES IN BLOOD PRESSURE

The fact that systolic blood pressure rises despite the lack of increases in either cardiac output or stroke volume clearly points to changes in the peripheral vascular system as underlying the changes in blood pressure with age. Although peripheral vascular resistance clearly increases with age, this change alone would be expected to result in rises in both systolic and diastolic blood pressure. Age-related increases in pulse pressure and flattening of the dicrotic notch of the arterial pressure waves suggest that losses of vascular distensibility and elastic recoil [3] are important mechanisms underlying the rise in systolic blood pressure.

Although early studies suggested that differences in salt intake between primitive and developed countries might account for the changes in blood pressure with age, current evidence does not support this hypothesis [4]. Within Western societies longitudinal studies have shown that increases in blood pressure over time are more related to the initial blood pressure level and to subsequent weight gain than to age itself [5].

The relation of fatness to age-related increases in blood pressure has recently been examined

193

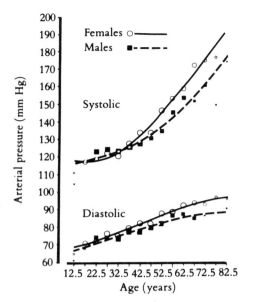

FIGURE 15-1. *Systolic and diastolic pressures for females and males for each 5-year age group of the population sample, together with the fitted curves. The area of each circle or square is proportional to the number of subjects in that age group.*

by Pan and co-workers in a cross-sectional study of over 30,000 white men and women. This study clearly indicated that systolic and diastolic blood pressure rises with age regardless of the presence or absence of obesity (Fig. 15-2) and confirmed prior studies that blood pressure levels are higher, at all ages, with progressive degrees of fatness [6].

DEFINITION AND PREVALENCE OF HYPERTENSION IN THE ELDERLY

Blood pressure is a continuous variable; increasing levels are associated with increasing cardiovascular risk, and there is no apparent threshold for the onset of the risk. The definition of any particular level as abnormal-pathologic must thus be empiric and varies from clinic to clinic and study to study. The definition of hyperten-

FIGURE 15-2. *Systolic and diastolic blood pressures for men and women by age and weight. (From W. H. Pan, et al. The role of weight in the positive association between age and blood pressure.* Am. J. Epidemiol. *124:612, 1986.)*

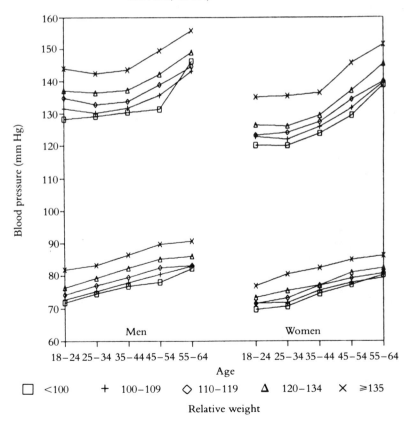

sion in the elderly can be approached in two general ways. One approach is to apply the same criteria for hypertension to all age groups. In this way one applies increasingly stringent criteria for high blood pressure in older age groups. Thus, if the definition of hypertension is systolic pressure over 160 or diastolic pressure over 95, as in the Framingham Study [7], one finds that 22 percent of men and 34 percent of women aged 65 to 74 can be considered hypertensive. Using the slightly lower cut-offs of 150 systolic and 95 diastolic, one finds that the prevalence of hypertension increases from 25 percent at age 50 to over 70 percent between ages 85 andf 95 [8]. A second approach views increasing blood pressure with age as normative and employs age-adjusted criteria for the definition of hypertension. Using such an approach the percentage of any given age cohort considered to be hypertensive will not change (for instance one-half of one standard deviation), but the level needed to reach this cut-off will increase with age. Although this approach takes into account the "normal" increase in blood pressure with aging, it overlooks the fact that

increases in blood pressure are associated with an increased risk of cardiovascular disease at any age. Therefore, the more appropriate definition of hypertension may be the establishment of some empiric but reasonable cutoff, such as 160 systolic and 95 diastolic, and application of these criteria regardless of age.

ISOLATED SYSTOLIC HYPERTENSION IN THE ELDERLY

The general age-related increase in systolic pressure and the fall in diastolic pressure after the middle years result in an increasing prevalence of isolated systolic hypertension (SBP > 160 mm Hg, DBP < 90 mm Hg) to 25 percent of men and women over the age of 75 (Fig. 15-3) [4]. There is general agreement that the major pathophysiologic factor underlying isolated systolic hypertension in the elderly is the age-related decrease in arterial compliance [9]. Although some systematic changes in circulating catecholamines and other endocrine factors have been shown to occur with age, to date these have not been shown to contribute importantly to the development of isolated systolic hypertension.

RISKS OF HIGH BLOOD PRESSURE

There is clear evidence from several large-scale epidemiologic studies that increasing levels of blood pressure are associated with increased

FIGURE 15-3. *Prevalence of isolated systolic hypertension (systolic blood pressure greater than 160 mm Hg, diastolic blood pressure less than 90 mm Hg) by age in men and women. (From W. B. Kannel, et al. Systolic blood pressure, arterial rigidity, and risk of stroke. J.A.M.A. 245:1228, 1981. Copyright 1981, American Medical Association.)*

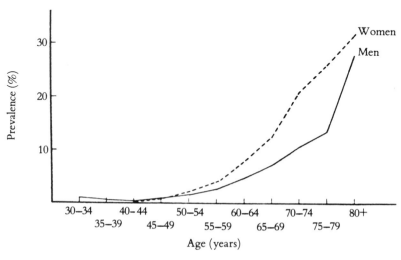

| Number of men | 591 | 1,628 | 2,539 | 3,282 | 3,975 | 3,617 | 2,817 | 1,795 | 985 | 350 | 22 |
| Number of women | 694 | 1,979 | 3,178 | 4,107 | 4,971 | 4,741 | 3,692 | 2,463 | 1,413 | 573 | 32 |

risk of morbidity and mortality from stroke, congestive heart failure, coronary heart disease, peripheral vascular disease, and maculopathy [10]. The bulk of the present evidence indicates that the "riskiness" of high blood pressure persists into old age, that systolic blood pressure, both current level and prior levels, are better predictors of risk than diastolic pressure, and that the risk associated with increasing levels of blood pressure is roughly equivalent for elderly men and women [11–13]. Although the risk of a stroke or other adverse cardiovascular event is greater in a hypertensive individual with already established end-organ damage such as left ventricular hypertrophy, the risks in individuals without end-organ damage are also considerable. These individuals deserve careful attention and appropriate treatment. Among the various cardiovascular events that have been studied, hypertension carries the greatest increase in risk for the development of stroke and seems to have the least impact on occlusive peripheral vascular disease. However, since the prevalence of coronary heart disease is so much greater than stroke, the absolute occurrence of death or related morbid events associated with coronary heart disease is much greater than that for stroke, even in hypertensive individuals.

RISK OF ISOLATED SYSTOLIC HYPERTENSION

The commonly held view that isolated systolic hypertension should not be treated is based on the misconceptions that since systolic hypertension accompanies "normal" aging it is harmless and that antihypertensive therapy is poorly tolerated by the elderly. Substantial information has now accumulated to indicate that neither of these views is correct.

The 1959 Build and Blood Pressure Study of the Society of Actuaries [14] reported on a 19-year follow-up of men and women aged 40 to 69 at entry in the study. For men whose diastolic pressure was 83 to 87 mm Hg, systolic blood pressures in the range of 158 to 167 mm Hg were associated with a 34 percent increase in mortality compared with those with systolic blood pressures in the range of 138 to 147 mm Hg. For women, similar increases in systolic blood pressure were associated with a doubling of mortality rate. The Chicago Stroke Study

[15] followed 2,100 lower socioeconomic class men and women aged 64 to 74 for three years. Of the group with diastolic blood pressures of less than 95 mm Hg those with systolic blood pressures of greater than 180 mm Hg suffered a mortality 59 percent higher than those with systolic blood pressures in the normal range. The Chicago Peoples' Gas Company Study [16] involved a 15-year follow-up of white men aged 40 to 59 at entry. Of the men whose diastolic blood pressures were less than 90 mm Hg, those with systolic blood pressures of over 140 mm Hg suffered a 70 percent greater mortality than those with lower systolic pressures. In a case-control study, Colandrea reported the findings of 72 patients with isolated systolic hypertension and 72 age-, sex-, and diastolic blood pressure-matched controls [17]. Mean age of entry was 69 years. Over a four-year follow-up, 10 of the hypertensive patients had fatal cardiovascular events, whereas only one member of the control group did.

In addition to the studies cited above reporting increased mortality, data are also available to indicate that substantial morbidity is associated with isolated systolic hypertension. Forette and colleagues [18] identified isolated systolic hypertension as a major risk factor for cerebrovascular events and acute myocardial infarction among elderly women (mean age 80 years) followed for 10 years. The Framingham Study [19] analyzed the probability of cerebrovascular or cardiovascular disease during prolonged follow-up of low-risk men and women according to their systolic blood pressure and age (Fig. 15-4). This study clearly demonstrated that at any systolic blood pressure level the risk of an adverse cardiovascular or cerebrovascular event increased dramatically with age. In addition, at any age the risk increased substantially with advancing systolic blood pressure. Finally, the relationship between elevated systolic blood pressure and increased risk was modified dramatically with age, the oldest age groups having the greatest relative risk for any given systolic pressure.

BENEFIT OF TREATMENT OF HYPERTENSION IN THE ELDERLY

A large body of data is accruing indicating the value of proper management of combined sys-

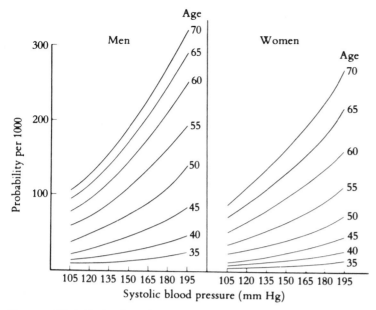

FIGURE 15-4. *Probability of cardiovascular disease in an 8-year period according to systolic blood pressure at specified ages in each sex. Low-risk subjects: those with serum cholesterol less than 185 mg/dl, non-smokers, no glucose intolerance, no electrocardiographic evidence of left ventricular hypertrophy. (From Framingham Heart Study— 18-year follow-up.)*

tolic and diastolic hypertension. The importance of strict control of blood pressure for the prevention of cerebral hemorrhage from intracerebral aneurysms, at any age, is unquestioned [20]. Although most studies of essential hypertension do not focus particularly on the elderly, the data available on geriatric patients suggest, but do not establish, that the benefits of treatment extend into old age. In the Veterans Administration Cooperative Trial [21] of blood pressure in men with diastolic pressure between 90 and 114, approximately 20 percent of the men were over 60 years old. In this older group, treatment was more than 50 percent effective in decreasing the likelihood of morbid cardiovascular events. The Hypertension Detection and Follow-up Program [22] has reported that long-term reduction of elevated diastolic blood pressure to levels below 90 mm Hg is associated with significant reductions in the incidence of fatal and nonfatal stroke in men and women aged 65 to 74 at initiation of treatment.

In 1985, an important multicenter international collaborative trial was reported that

will have a major impact on the management of hypertension in the elderly [23]. The European Working Party on High Blood Pressure in the Elderly [23] conducted a prospective randomized placebo-controlled study of 840 individuals over the age of 60 with well-established systolic (160 to 239 mm Hg) and diastolic (90 to 119 mm Hg) hypertension and no end-organ damage. Subjects were recruited from the community, hospital-based clinics, and long-term care facilities. The active treatment group received hydrochlorothiazide and triamterene as a first-line treatment, with methyldopa added if necessary to reach target blood pressure. Patient enrollment began in 1972, and patients remained in the study until its conclusion in 1984 unless they were lost to follow-up, had experienced an interruption of their study treatment for more than three months, died, or experienced one of several nonfatal cerebral or cardiovascular adverse effects of hypertension. Those removed from the double-blind portion of the trial continued to be followed until July 1984.

During the double-blind portion of the trial, blood pressure declined an average of 10 mm Hg systolic and 6 mm Hg diastolic in the placebo group and 32 mm Hg systolic and 13 mm Hg diastolic in the active treatment group. These blood pressure reductions were achieved in 65 percent of patients with administration of diuretic alone and in another 35 percent with the addition of methyldopa.

On overall intention-to-treat analysis, there was a statistically significant 27 percent reduction in cardiovascular mortality that primarily reflected a 38 percent reduction in cardiac mortality. There was a 43 percent reduction in cerebrovascular mortality that did not reach statistical significance (P = 0.15). Morbidity from severe congestive heart failure, accelerated hypertension, and cerebrovascular disease was significantly reduced in the treatment group.

In a follow-up [24] to the initial report from the European Working Party Trial, additional analysis has been presented regarding the relationships of age, sex, blood pressure, and previous cardiovascular disease to the study findings. This analysis clearly indicates that the beneficial effect of treatment on cardiovascular mortality and study-terminating events was evident in participants aged 60 to 79 years but could not be demonstrated beyond the age of 80. It should be noted, however, that most of the patients over age 80 were women (140 of 155) and that the majority (88 percent of the women and 81 percent of the men) were not community dwelling but were nursing home residents. Therefore, this finding may not be relevant to men or individuals living in the community. There was no effect of basal systolic or diastolic blood pressure or preexisting cardiovascular disease on the decrease in adverse cardiovascular or cerebrovascular outcomes in the treated group. This very large, lengthy trial provides direct substantive evidence for the first time of the benefit of treating hypertension in the elderly.

No data are yet available to indicate the benefit or lack of benefit of lowering *systolic* blood pressure in the elderly. However, a recent study, the Systolic Hypertension in the Elderly Program (SHEP) [25], has clearly documented that low doses of thiazide diuretics substantively lower systolic blood pressure in elderly individuals with isolated systolic hypertension without allowing development of excessive adverse effects. This important randomized blinded study included 551 men and women 60 years and older with documented systolic hypertension. Participants received either chlorthalidone (25 to 50 mg per day) or matching placebo. On one-year follow-up, 83 percent of the chlor-

thalidone group and 80 percent of the placebo group were still taking their medications, and of those taking chlorthalidone, 88 percent had reached their goal blood pressure without requiring additional medication. Analysis of the distribution of individual blood pressure responses to chlorthalidone showed that the response to treatment was rather uniform. Systolic blood pressure in the treatment group fell from 172 mm Hg to 146 mm Hg by the end of the first month of treatment with a slight continued decline through the first year. Diastolic blood pressure did not "bottom-out." Compliance with the medication regimen was excellent in both treatment and placebo groups. There was no significant increase in mild or severe side effects in the chlorthalidone group compared to placebo at one month or one year. Although chlorthalidone is commonly avoided in younger hypertensives because of its tendency to induce potassium depletion, this is not as serious a problem in the elderly, probably because of the lower glomerular filtration rate and renin and aldosterone levels that characterize normal aging. In the SHEP study, the mean decline in serum potassium was limited to 0.5 mEq per liter in the treatment group. There was no effect of chlorthalidone treatment on serum cholesterol or glucose levels. There was a very modest, clinically insignificant increase in serum creatinine levels from 1.05 ± 0.21 to 1.10 ± 0.32 and a modest increase in serum uric acid from 5.7 mg per dl to 6.8 mg per dl.

In summary, this important large randomized blinded study indicates that low-dose thiazide diuretic treatment is effective in lowering blood pressure and is safe in the management of elderly individuals with isolated systolic hypertension. An even larger multicentered randomized trial is currently underway to determine if lowering systolic blood pressure with antihypertensive medications in elderly individuals with isolated systolic hypertension is associated with a significant reduction in the risk of cerebrovascular or cardiovascular disease.

MANAGEMENT OF THE HYPERTENSIVE OLDER PATIENT

When faced with an elderly patient with hypertension, several important considerations deserve attention before a decision is made about whether to initiate therapy. In addition to the risks and benefits of therapy, one must consider the possible presence of secondary, or "curable," hypertension, the variability of blood pressure in the elderly, the presence of auscultatory gaps, and the possible presence of orthostatic hypertension, pseudohypertension, and end-organ damage.

The major cause of secondary hypertension that merits special attention in the elderly is renovascular disease. The ease of making this diagnosis is enhanced by the fact that the sensitivity and positive predictive value of saralasin infusion studies and stimulated renin measurements are increased in the elderly. These studies should be considered in elderly patients who are not responsive to first-line treatment of hypertension and who have recent significant reductions in renal function or evidence of severe aortic or large-vessel peripheral vascular disease. In elderly individuals with severe occlusive vascular disease that has led to major losses in renal function and subsequent hypertension, percutaneous transluminal angioplasty and, if necessary, operative vascular reconstruction in carefully selected individuals has met with surprising success, resulting in correction of blood pressure and return of renal function toward normal. The best candidates for this surgery are individuals with prominent collateral circulation on arteriography, which thus allows the nonfunctioning renal mass to maintain viability. Another major favorable prognostic finding is a proximal renal artery occlusion with a clear main renal artery distal to the occlusion. Some patients have undergone operative reconstruction months to years after loss of renal function and have recovered dramatically, often over long periods of time, to eventually become normotensive and gain considerable renal function [26, 27].

It is particularly important to measure blood pressure at least three times before instituting therapy, since blood pressure variability increases with age. Blood pressure should also be measured one hour after a meal to preclude significant postprandial hypotension (see later discussion). Auscultatory gaps are not uncommon among the elderly, and they can lead to underestimation of systolic blood pressure. Initially, it is best to measure blood pressure in both arms, selecting the arm with the highest reading for subsequent determinations and being certain that the blood pressure cuff is inflated to pressures over 230 mm Hg when determining the systolic pressure.

In addition to several baseline blood pressure measurements, it is important to obtain blood pressure with the patient both sitting and standing to detect orthostatic hypotension, which is common in the elderly and is discussed in detail later in this chapter.

Pseudohypertension is claimed to be more common among older persons. The elderly are more likely than the young to have a higher diastolic pressure reading on cuff measurement than on intraarterial measurements, the discrepancy often reaching 20 mm Hg or more. However, concordance between intraarterial and cuff measurements of systolic blood pressure is greater than that for diastolic pressure.

The presence of renal, hepatic, cardiac, and central nervous system dysfunction influences the choice of appropriate therapeutic agents. Evaluation of patients prior to initiation of therapy should include a detailed history and screening for diseases of these systems.

Goals of Therapy

There is substantial controversy about the level of blood pressure at which treatment is warranted as well as the blood pressure level that is a proper therapeutic goal. Since risk increases continuously with increases in systolic and, to a lesser extent, diastolic blood pressure, no clear cut-off points can be identified. Most clinicians accept a systolic blood pressure of 180 mm Hg as associated with markedly increased risk in older persons, and many feel that levels above 160 mm Hg should be treated. Similarly, elevations in diastolic blood pressure above 110 are generally agreed to be in the dangerous range, whereas levels between 90 and 110 are controversial.

One should not attempt to "normalize" pressure in an older patient to the level that one might find in healthy younger individuals. Reducing systolic blood pressures to 120 mm Hg in previously hypertensive older individuals is often associated with unwanted effects, possibly due to resetting of cerebral autoregulation at higher thresholds (see later discussion). A more reasonable therapeutic goal is a systolic blood pressure in the range of 140 to 160 mm Hg and a diastolic pressure less than 100 mm Hg. The general rule of thumb is to start with low doses of antihypertensive agents and then increase the doses to standard levels very slowly. Often there will be an initial reduction in systolic blood pressure of 10 to 15 mm Hg with further decreases requiring substantial increases in dosage. In some cases it is wise to accept a limited therapeutic goal, especially in the presence of isolated systolic hypertension for which the benefit of treatment has not yet been rigidly demonstrated, rather than to increase the chances of adverse reactions from aggressive dosing or the addition of multiple medications.

Specific Treatments
Both pharmacologic and nonpharmacologic therapy should be considered for managing hypertension in the elderly. At present, however, there is very little information about the efficacy of therapies such as weight loss, salt restriction, exercise, and various relaxation techniques. Since the physiologic basis of systolic blood pressure elevation among older persons is atherosclerosis rather than a hyperdynamic cardiovascular system as is found in younger individuals, one might expect that nonpharmacologic therapies, which are effective in young adults, may be ineffective in older patients. However, until this question is studied further, these therapies should certainly be considered for older patients who are highly motivated.

With regard to pharmacologic therapy, the approach to the management of fixed systolic and diastolic hypertension and isolated systolic hypertension is similar. As discussed in detail previously, the belief that the elderly are particularly susceptible to the adverse long-term effects of the usual antihypertensive agents is unfounded.

The first-line medications for older patients with hypertension are oral thiazide diuretics. In most cases, low doses of thiazides are appropriate, and a strong loop diuretic, such as furosemide or ethacrynic acid, is required only for those with significantly impaired renal function. Thiazide diuretics are well tolerated by the elderly, and the reductions in glomerular filtration rate and renin levels that are associated with normal aging often obviate the need for potassium supplementation. These age-related physiologic changes should make the physician wary of the administration of potassium-sparing diuretics to the elderly, especially to those whose serum creatinine levels are above 2 mg per dl. There does not appear to be a particular advantage of one thiazide diuretic over another, since both hydrochlorothiazide and chlorthalidone have been found to be effective in large trials. Thiazide diuretics are effective at low doses, from 12.5 to 50 mg. Doses above 50 mg offer no additional antihypertensive effect and increase the risk of hypokalemia.

There are a number of acceptable second-line drugs in the pharmacologic management of hypertension in the elderly. A clear understanding of the physiologic changes in the cardiovascular system with advancing age as well as knowledge of the patient's other diseases influence the proper choice of an antihypertensive. For instance, as discussed later in this chapter, age blunts baroreflexes, so that decreases in blood pressure are associated with smaller increases in heart rate in older persons than in their younger counterparts. Administration of peripheral vasodilators such as hydralazine is less likely to result in reflex tachycardia among the elderly than in younger individuals. Thus, low doses of peripheral vasodilators reduce blood pressure successfully in the elderly and can often be used alone.

Considerable controversy exists regarding the use of beta-adrenergic blocking agents for hypertension in the elderly. These drugs are often used, especially in elderly patients with other indications, such as recent myocardial infarction or angina. However, the high prevalence of clinical or subclinical congestive heart failure, chronic obstructive pulmonary disease, and peripheral vascular disease in older persons, all of which might be worsened with beta blockade, make these agents potentially dangerous. The combination of a peripheral vasodilator and a beta-blocking agent may be particularly dangerous for elderly persons with impaired baroreflexes and may result in an unacceptable incidence of orthostatic hypotension. Studies have shown that the sensitivity of the myocardium to beta-adrenergic stimulation and blockade is diminished in the elderly, thus casting further doubt on the effectiveness of beta blockers in this patient group. Beta blockers have also been associated with confusion and depression, particularly those agents, such as propranolol, that are lipid soluble and cross the blood-brain barrier.

A growing clinical experience would indicate that calcium channel-blocking agents are very effective and well tolerated in reducing elevations in blood pressure in older hypertensive patients. Although the current literature in this regard is very limited, it is highly likely that these agents will become the second line of therapy for most elderly patients with hypertension and the first-line therapy for patients with ischemic cardiac disease.

Substantial attention has been brought to the use of angiotensin-converting enzyme inhibitors, such as captopril and enalapril, in the treatment of hypertension in the elderly. Although these agents have been generally well tolerated, they carry an enhanced risk of side effects in the presence of impaired renal function that is particularly important in the elderly. In addition, these agents are at present much more expensive than some other effective antihypertensive agents such as thiazides. At present, they seem best reserved for use as second-line agents in patients not responsive to other medications.

A number of other agents have been found to be effective in lowering blood pressure in the elderly. At least two studies suggest that clonidine can be effective monotherapy in older patients with hypertension. In addition, as is shown in the European Working Party Study of Hypertension, methyldopa can effectively lower blood pressure in the elderly without substantially increasing adverse effects. Finally, an often overlooked effective agent for hypertension in the elderly is reserpine, which has the advantage of being effective in low doses given once daily.

As with pharmacotherapy of many disorders in old age, a sensible approach to the management of hypertension in the elderly employs a limited number of agents in as simple a regimen as possible in as low a dose as is effective. The elderly are at particular risk for the development of confusion and stroke from hypotension secondary to overenthusiastic antihypertensive

therapy [28–30]. Another major risk is the development of orthostatic hypotension and its adverse orthopedic sequelae from diuretic-induced volume depletion. Other important factors in the genesis of hypotension-induced central nervous system changes in this population are an age-related decrease in cerebral blood flow coupled with a hypertension-related increase in the threshold for cerebral autoregulation (see later discussion on cerebral blood flow).

Low Blood Pressure
PATHOPHYSIOLOGIC CHANGES UNDERLYING HYPOTENSIVE SYNDROMES IN THE ELDERLY
Baroreflexes

Baroreflex mechanisms play an important role in the regulation of systemic blood pressure by increasing heart rate and peripheral vascular resistance to resist transient decreases in arterial pressure and by decreasing heart rate and vascular tone to dampen transient increases in arterial pressure. With advancing age, there is a progressive decline in baroreflex sensitivity to both hypertensive and hypotensive stimuli such that the increase or decrease in heart rate in response to a physiologic stress is blunted in older persons compared with their younger counterparts [30,33,34]. Hyptertension, independent of age, also reduces baroreflex sensitivity [30]. Thus, elderly patients with hypertension often have doubly impaired baroreflex function, which is clinically manifest as an increase in blood pressure lability in response to the usual daily activities and a heightened sensitivity to hypotensive stimuli, particularly hypotensive medications.

Attenuation of baroreflex sensitivity is probably due in part to age-related arterial stiffening and a resultant damping of baroreceptor relaxation and stretch during changes in arterial pressure. Also, age clearly reduces cardiovascular responsiveness to adrenergic stimulation [35], an effect that diminishes baroreflex-mediated cardioacceleration and vasoconstriction during hypotensive stimuli.

Since age-related thickening of arterial intima and media is accelerated in the presence of hypertension, it is conceivable that control of hypertension might partially preserve barore-flex function [36]. This view is supported by the findings that sustained elevations or reductions in blood pressure can reset baroreflex sensitivity in healthy normotensive animals [37]. However, once pathologic vascular changes associated with aging and chronic hypertension become fixed lesions, this plasticity of baroreflex function may be lost. Whether long-term changes in baroreflex sensitivity can be prevented or reversed by the treatment of hypertension has not been established.

One possible physiologic consequence of diminished baroreflex sensitivity is an age-related increase in sympathetic nervous system activity. In healthy elderly subjects, "basal" plasma norepinephrine levels are elevated, and the norepinephrine response to posture change is heightened and prolonged [38]. Rowe and Troen [38] have speculated that a decrease in tonic inhibition of brainstem vasomotor centers due to diminished baroreceptor activity may enhance sympathetic nervous system activity. This increase in sympathetic activity may produce systolic hypertension, which becomes perpetuated by its own adverse effect on baroreflex function.

Cerebral Blood Flow
Age- and hypertension-related changes in baroreflex sensitivity become clinically significant when common hypotensive stressors, such as posture change, can no longer be offset by compensatory homeostatic mechanisms, and organ ischemia results. Age-related reductions in cerebral blood flow and hypertension-related alterations in cerebral autoregulation make the brain particularly vulnerable to underperfusion.

Cross-sectional and longitudinal studies in healthy subjects employing nitrous oxide and xenon inhalation techniques demonstrate a progressive age-related decline in cerebral blood flow with advancing age [39]. This decline is enhanced by the presence of risk factors (hypertension, heart disease, diabetes mellitus, and hyperlipidemia) for cerebrovascular disease [39]. Thus, many older persons (particularly those with hypertension or other risk factors for cerebrovascular disease) have resting cerebral blood flow that is so close to the threshold for cerebral ischemia that relatively small, acute reductions

in blood pressure may produce cerebral ischemic symptoms.

Ordinarily, cerebral autoregulatory mechanisms compensate for acute reductions in blood pressure. Autoregulation of cerebral blood flow in response to decreased perfusion pressure is generally preserved into old age, except in certain individuals with symptomatic postural hypotension [40]. However, since chronic hypertension raises the threshold for cerebral autoregulation [32], hypertensive older persons tolerate reductions in blood pressure less well than normotensive older persons.

Studies comparing treated and untreated groups of hypertensive rats or humans suggest that cerebral autoregulatory capacity can be improved with blood pressure reduction [41–43], and that elevated blood pressure can be gradually lowered to the normal range without risking cerebral ischemia.

ORTHOSTATIC HYPOTENSION
Orthostatic hypotension, defined as a systolic blood pressure reduction of 20 mm Hg or greater on standing upright, is a common clinical manifestation of impaired blood pressure homeostasis. Studies of community-dwelling elderly populations show a prevalence of orthostatic hypotension as high as 20 to 30 percent [44]. The prevalence has been reported to increase with advanced age and increased basal blood pressure [45]. In a study of normotensive older persons treated with diuretics to normalize blood pressure, a remarkably low prevalence of orthostatic hypotension (less than 5 percent) was found [46]. This prevalence did not increase with advancing age. These data suggest that hypertension rather than age may be the major determinant of orthostatic hypotension in old age.

Previous population-based studies of orthostatic hypotension have evaluated single postural blood pressure measurements for each subject, neglecting the large intraindividual variations in blood pressure often seen in the elderly. A recent study demonstrated a marked day-to-day intraindividual variability in postural blood pressure changes and a strong inverse relationship between each day's postural blood pressure change and basal supine blood pressure [47]. Thus, when first morning basal supine blood pressure is highest, the postural decline in blood pressure is greatest. The data lend further support to the notion that orthostatic hypotension in many elderly patients is related to blood pressure elevation rather than age.

Etiology

In view of the finding summarized above, orthostatic hypotension in the elderly may be viewed as two distinct clinical syndromes—one attributable to normal aging ("physiologic") and the other due to disease ("pathologic").

PHYSIOLOGIC ORTHOSTATIC HYPOTENSION

Physiologic orthostatic hypotension found in normal older persons varies dramatically from day to day, is related to blood pressure elevation, and is associated with the exaggerated norepinephrine response to posture change characteristic of normal aging. Although usually distinguished from a pathologic state by the lack of symptoms and lability, transient orthostatic hypotension may become clinically significant when complicated by stresses that reduce blood pressure further, such as volume depletion, hypotensive medications, or a Valsalva maneuver during voiding. Also, physiologic mechanisms may become further compromised during prolonged bed rest, resulting in severe postural hypotension. Although some degree of postural blood pressure reduction may be viewed as "normal" aging, it is certainly not harmless, since reductions of 20 mm Hg or more carry a significant risk for falls and syncope in otherwise well older persons.

PATHOLOGIC ORTHOSTATIC HYPOTENSION

Pathologic orthostatic hypotension is usually symptomatic (postural dizziness and syncope) and is associated with evidence of autonomic dysfunction such as a fixed heart rate, incontinence, constipation, inability to sweat, heat intolerance, impotence, and fatigability. Although the absence of cardioacceleration on standing has been used to distinguish orthostatic hypotension due to autonomic failure from hypovolemia, this sign may not be reliable in the elderly patient.

Symptomatic orthostatic hypotension may be secondary to a large number of diseases

TABLE 15-1. *Causes of orthostatic hypotension*

Drugs
  Phenothiazines and other neuroleptics
  Monoamine oxidase inhibitors
  Tricyclic antidepressants
  Antihypertensives
  Levodopa
  Vasodilators
  Beta blockers
  Calcium channel blockers
Central nervous system disorders
  Shy-Drager syndrome
  Brainstem lesions
  Parkinson's disease
  Myelopathy
  Multiple cerebral infarcts
Peripheral and autonomic neuropathies
  Diabetes
  Amyloidosis
  Tabes dorsalis
  Paraneoplastic syndromes
  Alcoholic and nutritional causes
Idiopathic

commonly found in elderly patients or to drugs used by elderly patients. In the absence of another cause, it may be primary or "idiopathic." Neuropathic causes of secondary orthostatic hypotension may be classified as central or peripheral (Table 15-1).

In contrast to physiologic orthostatic hypotension, elderly patients with the pathologic condition fail to increase plasma norepinephrine levels during posture change. The subset of patients with idiopathic orthostatic hypotension have lower basal plasma norepinephrine levels while supine, no increase in norepinephrine level with standing, a lower threshold for the pressor response to infused norepinephrine, and lower plasma norepinephrine levels in response to tyramine infusion despite a greater pressor response to the drug. These findings suggest that in idiopathic orthostatic hypotension there is a depletion of norepinephrine from sympathetic nerve endings with a resultant postsynaptic denervation supersensitivity. This is supported by the finding of Kontos et al. [48] in patients with idiopathic orthostatic hypotension that catechloamine-specific fluorescence is absent in sympathetic vasomotor nerves of deltoid muscle.

In patients with the Shy-Drager syndrome, circulating norepinephrine levels and the response to infused norepinephrine and tyramine are normal, but plasma norepinephrine levels also fail to increase with standing. This syndrome is associated with degeneration of neurons in several areas of the central nervous system including corticobulbar, corticospinal, extrapyramidal, and cerebellar systems of the brain as well as intermediolateral columns of the spinal cord. Thus, the Shy-Drager syndrome is a central disorder of sympathetic blood pressure control and is usually associated with extrapyramidal and cerebellar symptoms.

Another major category of causes of pathologic orthostatic hypotension includes disorders of the peripheral autonomic nervous system. This category includes insulin-dependent diabetes mellitus, in which severe peripheral neuropathy and other end-organ damage is evident, as well as less common entities such as amyloidosis, vitamin deficiencies, and the neuropathies associated with malignancies, particularly cancers of the lung and pancreas.

Perhaps the most commonly encountered cause of orthostatic hypotension is the adverse side effects of medications, including phenothiazines, tricyclic antidepressants, antianxiety agents, antihypertensive medications with central effects such as methyldopa and clonidine or peripheral actions such as prazosin, hydralazine, and guanethidine, and many other agents. Orthostatic hypotension may occur at doses within the usual therapeutic range and poses a difficult clinical dilemma when a positive therapeutic effect is achieved at the expense of this adverse side effect.

Management of Orthostatic Hypotension
The proper management of orthostatic hypotension begins with a clear definition of the presence of significant reductions in blood pressure on standing. The clinician should not assume that an elderly individual complaining of postural dizziness and lightheadedness is actually suffering from reductions in blood pressure but should measure blood pressure after the patient is recumbent for at least ten minutes and then after one and three minutes of quiet upright standing while carefully monitoring pulse rate. It is important to obtain these measurements on several occasions to confirm the con-

sistent reduction of blood pressure before the introduction of any therapy. The goal of therapy should be reduction or elimination of symptoms. This can often be achieved without complete correction of orthostatic reductions in blood pressure.

Initial therapeutic considerations include careful review of any prescribed and over-the-counter medications the patient is taking to identify a possible offending agent. In addition, it is important to train individuals to arise slowly from bed or a chair after a long period of recumbency or sitting. Dorsiflexion exercises of the feet prior to standing are often helpful in promoting venous return to the heart, accelerating the pulse, and increasing blood pressure. Initiation of a high salt intake program may result in modest weight gain and significant blunting of symptoms of orthostatic hypotension in many individuals. The use of elastic stockings is generally ineffective unless they cover the thigh as well as the calf, and in some cases abdominal binders may be useful. The head of the bed should be elevated by 5 to 20 degrees to prevent the nocturnal diuresis and supine hypertension that result from nocturnal shifts of interstitial fluid from the legs to the circulation.

A wide variety of pharmacologic maneuvers have been attempted in elderly individuals with orthostatic hypotension. Although most of these have either been found not to be effective or to require further study, one agent, fludrocortisone acetate, appears to be helpful. This mineralocorticoid, given in daily doses of 0.1 to 1.0 mg until mild peripheral edema develops, results in an increase in extracellular fluid volume and plasma volume and is accompanied by a modest increase in basal blood pressure. These physiologic changes appear to be adequate to circumvent the homeostatic defect on arising in many individuals with orthostatic hypotension, and a satisfactory response to this medication is seen in most individuals with mild or moderately severe symptoms. With the exception of occasional elevations of blood pressure beyond the acceptable range, complications of treatment are rare. The development of hypokalemia, a theoretical problem with large doses of mineralocorticoids, is rarely a practical problem. Other medications that are receiving increasing attention but are of unproved value in the management of orthostatic hypotension in the elderly include inhibitors of prostaglandin synthesis such as indomethacin and other nonsteroidal antiinflammatory agents, the peripheral α_2 agonist clonidine, the central α_2 antagonist yohimbine, and beta blockers that block β_2 vasodilator receptors or have intrinsic sympathomimetic activity such as pindolol. A variety of sympathomimetic agents have yielded inconsistent results. The administration of 250 mg of caffeine each morning can attenuate orthostatic hypotension. Ergot alkaloids including oral ergotamine tartrate or subcutaneous dihydroergotamine and caffeine have also been helpful in some patients. In very severe cases that are resistant to traditional therapeutic approaches, atrial pacing may be of value.

POSTPRANDIAL HYPOTENSION

It has recently been recognized that some elderly patients develop declines in blood pressure after meals. Studies of clinically stable, unmedicated institutionalized and community-dwelling elderly have demonstrated significant postprandial reductions in blood pressure after morning and noontime meals that do not occur in young subjects or in the absence of a meal [49,50] (Fig. 15-5). Approximately one-third of healthy elderly persons have postprandial blood pressure declines of 20 mm Hg or greater within one hour of eating a meal. This fall in blood pressure can be exaggerated by hypotensive medications given before a meal. As with orthostatic hypotension, postprandial hypotension is greatest in hypertensive elderly and in patients with postprandial syncope or autonomic dysfunction. This phenomenon is probably an important cause of falls and syncope in the elderly.

The mechanism of postprandial hypotension is unknown but presumably relates to impaired baroreflex compensation for splanchnic blood pooling during digestion. Like orthostatic hypotension, postprandial hypotension may have two clinical presentations: one, a physiologic, age-related phenomenon that is rarely symptomatic unless it is exacerbated by other hypotensive stresses, and two, a more severe pathologic syndrome related to autonomic insufficiency

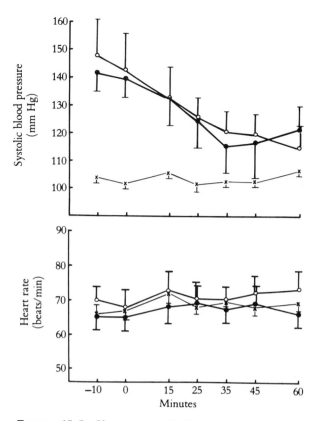

FIGURE 15-5. *Changes in systolic blood pressure and heart rate after a test meal in elderly patients with a history of syncope (○), elderly without history of syncope (●), and normal young controls. (From L. A. Lipsitz, et al. Postprandial reduction in blood pressure in the elderly. Reprinted by permission of* The New England Journal of Medicine *[309:81, 1983].)*

with more profound postprandial hypotension and syncope.

Health care providers for geratric patients should be alert for postprandial hypotension and carefully evaluate blood pressure before and after meals in patients with dizziness, falls, syncope, or other cerebral or cardiac ischemic symptoms that occur in the postprandial period.

Management

In the absence of clinical trials evaluating treatment approaches to postprandial hypotension, the management of this phenomenon relies on common sense. Symptomatic patients should avoid taking hypotensive medications before meals and should lie down after meals. Small, frequent feedings may be helpful.

Recent studies of patients with autonomic insufficiency suggest that indomethacin, caffeine with or without subcutaneous dihydroergotamine, or parenteral somatostatin given before a meal may ameliorate postprandial blood pressure reduction.

References

1. Gordon, T., and Shurtleff, D. Means at Each Examination and Inter-examination Variation of Specified Characteristics: The Framingham Study. In W. B. Kannel and T. Gordon (eds.), *The Framingham Study: An Epidemiologic Investigation of Cardiovascular Disease*. Department of Health, Education and Welfare Publication No. NIH 74478, Section 29. Washington, D.C.: U.S. Government Printing Office, 1974.
2. Page, L. P., and Sidd, J. J. Medical management of arterial hypertension. *N. Engl. J. Med.* 287: 960, 1972.
3. O'Rourke, M. F. Arterial hemodynamics in hypertension. *Circ. Res.* 6 (Suppl. 2): 123, 1970.
4. Tudge, C. The biggest risk factor of them all? *World Med.* 13:21, 1978.
5. Harlan, W. R., et al. A Thirty-Year Study of Blood Pressure in a White Male Cohort. In G. Onesti, K. E. Kim, and J. H. Moyer (eds.), *Hypertension: Mechanisms in Management*. New York: Grune & Stratton, 1973.
6. Pan, W. H., et al. The role of weight in the positive association between age and blood pressure. *Am. J. Epidemiol.* 124:612, 1986.
7. Shurtleff, D. Some Characteristics Related to the Incidence of Cardiovascular Disease and Death. In W. B. Kannel and T. Gordon (eds.), *The Framingham Study: An Epidemiologic Investigation of Cardiovascular Disease*. Department of Health, Education and Welfare Publication No. NIH 74-599. Section 30. Washington, D.C.: U.S. Government Printing Office, 1974.
8. Russek, H. I., and Zohman, B. L. Normal blood pressure in senescence. *Geriatrics* 1:113, 1946.
9. Rowe, J. W. Systolic hypertension in the elderly. *N. Engl. J. Med.* 309:1246, 1983.
10. Sperduto, R. D., and Hiller, R. Systemic hypertension and age-related maculopathy in the Framingham Study. *Arch. Ophthalmol.* 104:216, 1986.
11. Moore-Smith, B. The Management of Hypertension in the Elderly. In M. J. Denham (eds.), *The Treatment of Medical Problems in the Elderly*. Baltimore: University Park Press, 1980.
12. Whelton, P. K. Hypertension in the Elderly. In R. Andres, E. L. Biermon, and W. Hazzard (eds.), *Principles of Geriatric Medicine*. New York: McGraw-Hill, 1985. Pp. 536–551.
13. Kannel, W. B., et al. Epidemiologic assessment of the role of blood pressure in stroke—the Framingham Study. *J.A.M.A.* 214:301, 1970.
14. Morton, P. A. Ordinary insurance: The build and blood pressure study. *Trans. Soc. Actuar.* 11:987, 1959.
15. Shekelle, R., Ostfeld, A., and Kao, A. Hypertension and risk of stroke in an elderly population. *Stroke* 5:71, 1974.
16. Dyer, A. R., et al. Hypertension in the elderly. *Med. Clin. North Am.* 61:513, 1977.
17. Colandreci, M. A., et al. Systolic hypertension in the elderly: An epidemiologic assessment. *Circulation* 41:239, 1970.
18. Forette, F., et al. The proprostic significance of isolated systolic hypertension in the elderly: Results of a ten year longitudinal study. *Clin. Exp. Hypertens.* 174:1177, 1982.
19. Kannel, W. B., et al. Systolic blood pressure, arterial rigidity, and risk of stroke. *J.A.M.A.* 245:1229, 1981.
20. Pickering, G. Hypertension—definitions, natural history, and consequences. *Am. J. Med.* 52: 570, 1972.
21. Veterans Administration Cooperative Study Group on Anti-hypertensive Agents. Effects of treatment on morbidity and hypertension: III. Influence of age, diastolic pressure, and prior cardiovascular disease—further analysis of side effects. *Circulation* 45:995, 1972.
22. Hypertension Detection and Follow-up Program Cooperative Group. Five-year findings of the Hypertension Detection and Follow-up Program. *J.A.M.A.* 247:633, 1982.
23. Amery, A., et al. Efficacy of anti-hypertensive drug treatment according to age, sex, blood pressure, and previous cardiovascular disease in patients over the age of sixty. *Lancet.* 2:589, 1986.
24. Amery, A., et al. Mortality and morbidity results from the European Working Party on High Blood Pressure in the Elderly Trial. *Lancet* 1: 1349, 1985.
25. Hulley, S. B., et al. Systolic Hypertension in the Elderly Program (SHEP): Antihypertensive efficacy of chlorthalidone. *Am. J. Cardiol.* 56: 913, 1985.
26. Besarab, B., et al. Reversible renal failure following bilateral renal artery occlusive disease. *J.A.M.A.* 235:2838, 1976.
27. Libertino, J. A., et al. Renal artery revascularization. *J.A.M.A.* 244:1340, 1980.

28. Graham, D. I. Ischemic brain damage of cerebral profusion. Failure after treatment of severe hypertension. *Br. Med. J.* 4:739, 1975.
29. Jackson, J., et al. Inappropriate anti-hypertensive therapy in the elderly. *Lancet* 2:1317, 1976.
30. Gribbin, B., et al., Effect of age and high blood pressure on baroreflex sensitivity in man. *Circ. Res.* 29:424, 1971.
31. Skinhoj, E. Hemodynamic studies within the brain during migraine. *Arch. Neurol.* 29:95, 1973.
32. Stranguaard, S., et al. Autoregulation of brain circulation in severe arterial hypertension. *Br. Med. J.* 1:507, 1973.
33. McGarry, K., et al. Baroreflex function in elderly hypertensives. *Hypertension* 5:763, 1983.
34. Minaker, K. L., Rowe, J. W., and Sparrow, D. Impaired cardiovascular adaptation to vasodilation in the elderly (abstract). *Gerontologist* 20 (part II): 163, 1980.
35. Lakatta, E. G. Age-related alterations in the cardiovascular response to adrenergic mediated stress. *Fed. Proc.* 5:3173, 1980.
36. Haudenschild, C. C., and Chobanian, A. V. Blood pressure lowering diminishes age-related changes in the rat aortic intima. *Hypertension* 6:162, 1984.
37. Brown, A. M. Receptors under pressure: An update on baroreceptors. *Circ. Res.* 46:1, 1980.
38. Rowe, J. W., and Troen, B. R. Sympathetic nervous system and aging in man. *Endocrinal. Rev.* 1:167, 1980.
39. Meyer, J. S., and Shaw, T. G. Cerebral Blood Flow in Aging. In M. L. Albert (ed.), *Clinical Neurology of Aging*. New York: Oxford University Press, 1984.
40. Wollner, L., et al. Failure of cerebral autoregulation as a cause of brain dysfunction in the elderly. *Br. Med. J.* 1:1117, 1979.
41. Strandgaard, S. Autoregulation of cerebral blood flow in hypertensive patients. The modifying influence of prolonged antihypertensive treatment on the tolerance to acute, drug-induced hypertension. *Circulation* 53:720, 1976.
42. Vorstrup, S., et al. Chronic antihypertensive treatment in the rat reverses hypertension-induced changes in cerebral blood flow autoregulation. *Stroke* 15:312, 1984.
43. Hoffman, W. E., Miletich, D. J., and Albrecht, R. F. The influence of antihypertensive therapy on autoregulation in aged hypertensive rates. *Stroke* 13:701, 1982.
44. Caird, F. I., Andrews, G. R., and Kennedy, R. D. Effect of posture on blood pressure in the elderly. *Br. Heart J.* 35:527, 1973.
45. MacLennan, W. J., Hall, M. R. P., and Timothy, J. I. Postural hypertension in old age: Is it a disorder of the nervous system or of blood vessels? *Age Ageing* 9:25, 1980.
46. Myers, M. G., et al. Postural hypertension and diuretic therapy in the elderly. *Can. Med. Assoc. J.* 119:581, 1978.
47. Lipsitz, L. A., et al. Intraindividual variability in postural blood pressure in the elderly. *Clin. Sci.* 69:337, 1985.
48. Kontos, H. A., Richardson, D. W., and Norvell, J. E. Norepinephrine depletion in idiopathic orthostatic hypotension. *Ann. Intern. Med.* 82:336, 1975.
49. Lipsitz, L. A., et al. Postprandial reduction in blood pressure in the elderly. *N. Engl. J. Med.* 309:81, 1983.
50. Lipsitz, L. A., and Fullterton, K. J. Postprandial blood pressure reduction in healthy elderly. *J. Am. Geriatr. Soc.* 34:267, 1986.

16
Falls and Syncope

LEWIS A. LIPSITZ

FALLS AND SYNCOPE represent common, highly morbid syndromes in the elderly that may result in hip fracture, internal hemorrhage, aspiration pneumonia, soft tissue injuries, and loss of independent function. Both falls and syncope are due to a complex interaction between age-related physiologic changes, diseases that become more prevalent with advancing age, and environmental stresses. Although some falls are due to syncope or pathophysiologic processes that may also result in syncope, falls may be due to other disturbances in postural homeostasis that do not cause syncope, and episodes of syncope may not result in falls. Therefore, there are areas of overlap in the underlying pathology and diagnostic evaluation of these two important clinical syndromes as well as features unique to each syndrome.

This chapter reviews the age-related, disease-related, and environmental factors underlying each of these clinical problems. The diagnostic evaluation of both falls and syncope will be discussed together to avoid redundancies, but information specific for each syndrome will be highlighted. The reader should recognize the importance of distinguishing falls from syncope in order to narrow the spectrum of diagnostic possibilities and focus the clinical evaluation in the most cost-effective manner.

Falls

A pathologic fall can be defined as an unintentional change in position, occurring under circumstances in which normal, homeostatic mechanisms would preserve postural stability. Falling is a symptom, not a diagnosis, that may result from common, age-related changes that impair homeostatic capacity and may also be a manifestation of any disease process in the elderly.

EPIDEMIOLOGY OF FALLS

Approximately 35 to 40 percent of community-dwelling people over the age of 65 and up to 45 percent of institutionalized elderly fall at least once each year. The incidence is highest in women and the very old [1,2].

Despite this high prevalence of falls in the geriatric population, relatively few episodes are associated with injury. Over half of all falls result in no injury, 28 percent are associated with trivial soft tissue injury, 11 percent produce severe soft tissue injury, and 6 percent result in fractures [1]. However, there is an age-related increase in death rate due to falls, as high as 525 deaths per 100,000 population in white females over the age of 85 [3].

Falling episodes in elderly persons are often recurrent. Up to one-third of elderly patients with falls have recurrent episodes, possibly due to an underlying physiologic substrate that makes them vulnerable to postural instability or transient loss of consciousness. In some patients falls may cluster several weeks or months before death. Falling episodes are often observed to precede a period of gradual functional decline and the development of acute confusional states in elderly patients [1].

FACTORS CONTRIBUTING TO FALLS IN THE ELDERLY

Age-Related Physiologic Changes

The process of aging is associated with several important physiologic changes that predispose to falling. These changes can be classified into two categories: those responsible for postural instability and those that affect blood pressure homeostatic mechanisms and result in transient dizziness or syncope.

POSTURAL INSTABILITY

Age-related changes in postural stability are manifest as an increase in body sway. Body sway can be measured simply with a marking pencil projecting anteriorly from the mid-pelvis and inscribing a line on a piece of graph paper. Recently, computerized forceplates have been developed to measure body sway in anterior-posterior and lateral directions. With any of these techniques, body sway has been shown to increase with advancing age, particularly in women and with the eyes closed. Some studies have correlated an increase in body sway with falling episodes [4]. Although this may not be a clinically useful tool in predicting falls, body sway does represent the combined effects of physiologic changes that perturb postural stability.

Wyke demonstrated the presence of cervical articular mechanoreceptors, located on cervical apophyseal joints with afferent fibers to the brain stem, cerebellum, and cortex, which provide information about where the head and neck are located in space [5]. With progressive degeneration of the mechanoreceptors due to aging and/or degenerative arthritis, knowledge of one's position in space can be severely impaired. This may lead to a sensation of dizziness or instability and may result in falling when the patient is confronted with an environmental hazard.

Other age-related changes that affect gait and postural stability include degeneration of afferent proprioceptive fibers and sensory receptors and a reduction in nerve conduction velocity. As a result, many elderly individuals lose Achilles reflexes and position and vibration senses in their lower extremities.

Basal ganglion atrophy, loss of dopaminergic neurons in the substantia nigra, and diminution in dopamine levels in the caudate nucleus are also associated with the aging process [6]. These changes produce parkinsonian features such as a slow gait and an increase in motor tone and increase susceptibility to medications such as haloperidol that further block dopaminergic nerve transmission in the central nervous system.

In addition to attrition of dopaminergic neurons in the basal ganglia, Betz cells in the motor cortex undergo age-related changes. These cells lose dendritic spines in the fourth to fifth decades of life, and more than one-third of these cells disappear by the sixth or seventh decades. The axons of Betz cells innervate the large proximal antigravity muscles of the arm, trunk, back, and lower extremities. They are responsible for diminishing antigravity tone in the extensors prior to a motor act. Their attrition may, therefore, contribute to increased motor tone and the slow, stiff muscle activity that is often seen in elderly patients [7].

BLOOD PRESSURE HOMEOSTASIS

Impaired regulation of systemic blood pressure is another important age-related change that may result in transient hypotension, underperfusion of the brain, and a fall, usually in association with syncope [8]. Age-related changes in blood pressure homeostasis that produce syncope are discussed later in this chapter.

Disease-Related Factors

The elderly patient is at risk of falling not only from numerous age-related changes in homeostatic mechanisms but also from the large burden of disease that is often present. Surveys of community-dwelling elderly reveal that each has an average of three to four chronic coexisting diseases.

Several recent studies have demonstrated that

falls in elderly patients are more likely due to combinations of multiple disorders than to single diseases. Tinetti et al. [9] have demonstrated that the risk of falling increases as the number of chronic disabilities increases. Risk factors that cumulatively increase the risk of falling include impaired mobility, a low morale score (Philadelphia Geriatric Morale Scale), a low mental status score (Set Test), distant corrected vision worse than 20/30 in both eyes, moderate or severe hearing loss, a mean orthostatic blood pressure drop of 20 mm Hg or more at three minutes standing, inability to extend the back or perform activities of daily living, and drugs such as antidepressants, phenothiazines, or sleeping medications.

Drachman and Hart [10] also emphasized the importance of multiple impairments in their investigations of the dizzy patient. Of 125 patients evaluated for dizziness, 13 percent had multiple sensory deficits. Patients with this syndrome were typically elderly and suffered from such conditions as peripheral neuropathy, cervical spondylosis, vestibular abnormalities, visual impairments, and orthopedic problems.

Environmental Factors
The combination of multiple pathologic conditions is likely to result in falls owing to an inability to compensate for common environmental hazards. Such falls account for nearly 50 percent of falls in the elderly and are often called "accidental." However, normal reflex mechanisms in healthy individuals are usually able to prevent these episodes, suggesting that they result from underlying pathologic abnormalities and are not truly accidental.

Examples of environmental hazards precipitating falls include poor lighting, slippery floors, loose rugs, assistive devices, unexpected objects, stairs, poor fitting shoes, bed siderails, and medications. Stair accidents are quite common due to dimensional irregularities in broken-down flights of stairs or visual distractions that make it difficult to perceive the end of a tread. Such visual distractions include patterned carpeting or shadows that fall across a flight of stairs, creating visual illusions such as stripes running parallel to the tread edge. Stairs should be designed to allow proper detection of

the edge, to eliminate shadows and glare, and to provide handrails over the entire length of stair [11].

SPECIFIC SYNDROMES PRODUCING FALLS
Drop Attacks
The drop attack is a descriptive term found primarily in the British literature that refers to the sudden loss of postural tone without loss of consciousness that sometimes occurs while the person is walking and turning the neck to look to the side or up at an object. The victim of a drop attack often claims that the knees buckled under him or her and vigorously denies loss of consciousness. Sometimes the victim cannot resume an upright posture until he or she places the soles of the feet on a firm surface. Although it is thought that the drop attack may represent vertebral basilar artery insufficiency, the term *drop attack* is merely a description of a syndrome that is associated with a variety of medical conditions, including cardiac and cerebrovascular diseases, seizure disorders, vestibular disease, carotid sinus hypersensitivity, or subclavian steal syndrome. The prognosis following a drop attack is determined by the underlying medical condition [12].

Locomotor Falls
Locomotor problems include any condition that causes a chronic impairment in neuromuscular function or postural stability and manifests as a gait disorder. Locomotor falls may present as accidents because of a patient's inability to compensate for environmental hazards.

Neurologic diseases with motor system involvement are common causes of locomotor falls in the elderly. These diseases include stroke, transient ischemic attacks, multiple sclerosis, Parkinson's disease, amyotrophic lateral sclerosis, hydrocephalus, cerebral palsy, and myopathy. Brain stem ischemia, Parkinson's disease, or cervical cord compressions may manifest as drop attacks. Each of these conditions is associated with focal neurologic abnormalities that point to the anatomic location of the lesion.

Many of the neurologic diseases responsible for falls are diagnosable by a careful examination of the gait. For example, the parkinsonian patient has difficulty with axial movement, starting, stopping, and turning. These patients are characteristically slow with a shuffling gait, absent arm swing, and stiff posture. Some elderly patients have a frontal lobe gait apraxia (Brun's apraxia), the "march-a-petit-pas." This is a small, stepped shuffle or magnetic gait, which appears as though the feet are glued to the floor. The patient can often walk quite well if holding on to another person. These patients have substantially larger ventricles than other patients of the same age, possibly representing hydrocephalus due to impaired absorption of cerebral spinal fluid from the subarachnoid space [13]. Expansion of the lateral ventricles is thought to compress the descending motor fibers innervating the lower extremities. The more severe syndrome, normal pressure hydrocephalus, is associated with the development of dementia and urinary incontinence. Some of these patients seem to improve their gait after a spinal tap that removes small amounts of cerebral spinal fluid.

Acute orthopedic injuries as well as chronic skeletal deformities, kyphoscoliosis, arthritis, tendonitis, Paget's disease, and the myopathies also impair gait and postural stability. Although many elderly people adapt quite well to these problems, an acute exacerbation of any of them, or the addition of a second condition, may impair one's precarious compensation and result in a fall.

Other Conditions Producing Falls
Other common conditions that predispose to falls include perceptual deficits due to cataracts, macular degeneration, hearing loss, peripheral neuropathies, and labyrinthine disorders. Each of these impair spatial orientation and judgment of the environment. Since many of these changes occur quite gradually with advancing age, patients are usually able to adapt to perceptual deficits. When cataracts or hearing impairments are suddenly treated with cataract extraction or a hearing aid, the new sensory input may disorient the patient even further and result in a paradoxical fall at a time when improvement in the underlying perceptual deficit is expected. The patient may take months to a year to adapt to new lenses or a hearing aid. Cataract glasses produce a visual image that is 25 percent

larger than usual; objects appear nearer, straight lines look curved, and a ring scotoma appears. For this reason, a lens implant is preferable to improve vision in the aphakic eye.

Drugs and alcohol are very common contributors to gait abnormalities and falls in the elderly. Their sedative or hypotensive effects produce perceptual impairments, instability, and dizziness. Deficiencies of acetylcholine and dopamine in the aging brain make elderly patients particularly vulnerable to the confusional and parkinsonian effects of anticholinergic and antidopaminergic drugs, respectively.

In addition to the above-mentioned diseases and related factors, any acute process can precipitate a fall in an elderly patient. Due to age-related physiologic changes that impair postural stability and blood pressure homeostasis, falling may occur as the first manifestation of heart failure, sepsis, a viral syndrome, metabolic disorder, or gastrointestinal bleed.

The combination of multiple physical impairments and recurrent falls may result in loss of confidence in walking, a fear of falling, and recurrent falls. Walking is an automatic activity that becomes difficult if it is de-automatized, easily demonstrated by trying to walk across a room holding a cup of coffee. This task is easy when one does not try to be careful but becomes almost impossible once attention is paid to it.

Syncope

Syncope, one of many causes of falling, is a sudden, transient loss of consciousness characterized by unresponsiveness and loss of postural control, with spontaneous recovery not requiring specific resuscitation procedures. It occurs as a result of inadequate delivery of oxygen or metabolic substrate to the brain or, in a seizure, as a result of disorganized electrical activity in the brain. Syncope also is not a disease but a symptom of numerous disease processes [14].

EPIDEMIOLOGY
Although the prevalence and incidence of syncope have not been studied in the general population of elders, approximately 25 percent of institutionalized elderly have histories of syncope

within the past 10 years of their lives, and 6 to 7 percent experience syncope each year. In approximately one-third of cases, syncope is recurrent [15].

Syncope in institutionalized elderly is *not* an independent risk factor for mortality but is associated with physical disability and subsequently functional decline [15]. Both falls and syncope may be markers of serious underlying disease with an associated high morbidity and mortality.

PATHOPHYSIOLOGY

Syncope is due to the inadequate delivery of oxygen or metabolic substrate to the brain. The accumulation of multiple age- and disease-related conditions that threaten cerebral blood flow or reduce oxygen content in the blood may bring cerebral oxygen delivery dangerously close to the threshold needed to maintain consciousness. Any additional stress that further reduces cerebral blood flow or blood oxygen content may precipitate syncope (Fig. 16-1).

For example, aging is associated with a progressive reduction in cerebral blood flow. Cerebral oxygen delivery may fall close to the threshold for cerebral ischemia when common conditions that reduce blood oxygen content are present, such as chronic obstructive lung disease or anemia. The addition of congestive heart failure with dyspnea and hyperventilation can decrease cerebral blood flow by 40 percent, thus bringing cerebral oxygen delivery below the threshold for the maintenance of consciousness and resulting in syncope. The sudden superimposition of any condition that reduces blood pressure such as pneumonia, a hypotensive drug, a cardiac arrhythmia, or even a situational stress may also result in syncope [14].

Elderly patients often develop syncope in response to situational stresses such as taking medication, eating a meal, defecating, or changing posture [16]. Therefore, syncope is due to the interaction of multiple coexisting clinical abnormalities that impair cardiovascular compensation for these common hypotensive stresses.

Numerous cardiovascular and neuroendocrine homeostatic mechanisms normally maintain a blood pressure adequate for cerebral perfusion. However, with advancing age there is a progressive decline in homeostatic capacity such that elderly individuals have a blunted ability to adapt to hypotensive stress. The su-

FIGURE 16-1. *Accumulation of age- and disease-related conditions in some elderly may reduce brain oxygen delivery close to the level needed to maintain consciousness. In such an individual, an added stress—for example, dyspnea with hyperventilation—can cause syncope. (From L. A. Lipsitz. Syncope in the elderly patient.* Hosp. Pract. [Off.] *21:33, 1986. Illustration by Albert Miller.)*

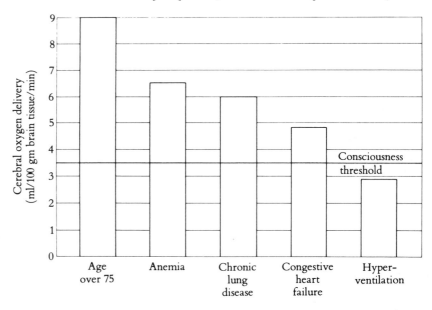

perimposition of drugs and diseases that are highly prevalent in the elderly population further impairs blood pressure regulation. Therefore, seemingly minor everyday stresses such as change in posture, eating, acute illness, or a new drug may threaten blood pressure homeostasis and precipitate a syncopal episode.

As discussed in detail in Chapter 15, baroreflex mechanisms play an important role in the regulation of systemic blood pressure. With advancing age there is a progressive decline in baroreflex sensitivity to both hypertensive and hypotensive stimuli [17,18]. This decline is readily apparent in the blunted heart rate response to posture change found in many elderly patients. Similarly, elderly patients are less able to cardioaccelerate to compensate for the hypotensive effect of many medications.

Other important age-related physiologic changes are the progressive decrease in basal and stimulated renin levels and the decreases in aldosterone production that impair renal sodium conservation and maintenance of intravascular volume [19]. The older person is more likely to become dehydrated with consequent hypotension in response to a diuretic, an acute febrile illness, or a situation in which access to salt and water is limited. Recent studies have also shown that healthy elderly are less likely to experience thirst when exposed to hypertonic dehydration [20]. This dehydration can lead to rapid volume depletion, orthostatic hypotension, and syncope.

DISEASE-RELATED CAUSES OF SYNCOPE

The causes of syncope are listed in Table 16-1, divided into hypotensive syndromes, abnormalities in blood composition, cardiac diseases, and primary cerebral disorders.

Hypotensive syndromes that are particularly important in the elderly include orthostatic and postprandial hypotension (see Chap. 15).

Orthostatic hypotension occurs in 20 to 30 percent of community-dwelling elderly and accounts for about 4 percent of falls. Postural hypotension is defined as a 20-mm Hg or greater drop in systolic blood pressure on standing. Although it is usually asymptomatic, it is an important risk factor for falls and syncope. It may be due to the age-related physiologic changes mentioned above and/or to conditions found

TABLE 16-1. *Causes of syncope*

I. Hypotension
   A. Vasomotor instability
      1. Orthostatic hypotension
      2. Carotid sinus syndrome
      3. Micturition, defecation, cough, swallow syncope
      4. Vasovagal syncope
   B. Volume depletion
   C. Drugs
II. Abnormal blood composition
   A. Hypoxemia
   B. Hypoglycemia
III. Cardiac disease
   A. Anatomic
      1. Aortic stenosis
      2. Mitral prolapse and regurgitation
      3. Hypertrophic cardiomyopathy
      4. Myxoma
   B. Myocardial
      1. Ischemia and infarct
      2. Cardiomyopathy
      3. Pulmonary embolism
   C. Electrical
      1. Tachyarrhythmia
      2. Bradyarrhythmia
      3. Heart block
      4. Sick sinus syndrome
IV. Cerebral disorders
   A. Vascular insufficiency
   B. Seizures

in many elderly, including volume depletion, drugs, and autonomic insufficiency syndromes such as idiopathic orthostatic hypotension, the Shy-Drager syndrome, or multiple cerebral infarctions. Elderly individuals are usually able to maintain postural blood pressure homeostasis, but when exposed to mild volume depletion (e.g., during diuretic therapy), they may develop a profound postural blood pressure decline [21].

Another recently identified abnormality in blood pressure homeostasis is postprandial hypotension [22]. Institutionalized and healthy community-dwelling elderly have an average 11-mm Hg decline in blood pressure by one hour after a meal. Although in most elders this is an asymptomatic age-related abnormality, individuals with postprandial syncope have more profound declines in blood pressure that are probably responsible for their fainting episodes [23]. Postprandial hypotension may be related to an inability to compensate for splanchnic blood pooling after a meal.

Anemia may also threaten oxygen delivery to

the brain. When transient hypotension due to any condition occurs, the anemic patient may not have sufficient oxygen content in the blood to maintain cerebral function.

Any cardiac illness that abruptly and momentarily diminishes cardiac output can result in syncope. Cardiac output may be transiently compromised by the anatomic, myocardial, or rhythm abnormalities listed in Table 16-1.

Primary cerebral disorders such as vascular insufficiency or seizures are important causes of syncope. Syncope can be attributed to cerebrovascular disease only if transient, focal neurologic deficits are associated with the episode. Although a seizure disorder may present as syncope, syncope from other causes may be associated with seizure activity. Clinical features such as occurrence of syncope in the horizontal position, an olfactory or gustatory aura, tongue biting, fecal incontinence, and postictal confusion all support a diagnosis of epilepsy.

Studies of syncope in institutionalized elderly have shown that syncope (like falls in general) is more likely to occur in patients with two or more coexisting abnormalities, such as coronary artery disease, postural blood pressure reduction, aortic stenosis, insulin therapy, or overall functional impairment [16].

Diagnostic Evaluation of Falls and Syncope

The diagnostic approaches to falls and syncope are similar and will be discussed together. Since both symptoms are usually due to multiple interacting abnormalities rather than to a single disease entity, it is difficult to establish an algorithm that leads the clinician to a specific diagnosis. Instead, the clinician must search for age- and disease-related abnormalities and environmental precipitants that threaten postural homeostasis.

The evaluation of falls and syncope in the elderly patient begins with a careful history and physical examination, which is sufficient to identify underlying precipitants in a majority of cases. It is important to ask individuals who have witnessed a fall what activities preceded it. Also, family members or caretakers can often identify recent changes in a patient's function that may point to the underlying pathophysiol-

ogy. If the fall was associated with syncope or near syncope, the evaluation should pay particular attention to hypotensive stresses and cardiovascular conditions that compromise delivery of oxygen and glucose to the brain.

The history should include a careful search for predisposing diseases, including visual and hearing impairments and previous orthopedic disabilities, fractures, and deformities in the case of the fall, or hypotensive syndromes, cardiac arrhythmias, valvular heart disease, or seizure disorders in the case of syncope or near-syncope. Equally important are prescribed drugs as well as over-the-counter and eye medications. Many over-the-counter medications have anticholinergic properties that cause confusion or tachyarrhythmias and precipitate falls. Similarly, eye medications have autonomic effects, and topical ophthalmic beta blockers have systemic effects such as bronchospasm and heart failure that may be associated with falls or syncope. The onset and nature of recovery from a fall can give important clues to its etiology. Falls due to vasovagal syncope will be preceded by hunger, fatigue, emotional stress, and a typical autonomic prodrome. The recovery is usually rapid. In contrast, a seizure may have a sudden onset and a slow recovery. Precipitants such as taking a medication, eating a meal, or straining at stool are important clues.

Evaluation of a fall or faint also relies on a careful physical examination, focused particularly on the following areas. Postural vital signs are essential to rule out orthostatic hypotension. The blood pressure and heart rate should be taken supine after a 10-minute rest period and then again after one and three minutes of standing if the patient is able to do so. Although a standing position is most sensitive in detecting immediate and delayed postural blood pressure reduction, vital signs while sitting are helpful if the patient is unable to stand. A diminished heart rate response to upright posture may be a clue to baroreflex impairment.

The carotid arteries should be examined for evidence of flow abnormalities or bruits (to exclude conditions contraindicating carotid sinus massage—see later discussion) as well as the quality of the carotid upstroke. Although aortic stenosis typically produces a slow and low amplitude upstroke in younger individuals, the upstroke may be deceptively brisk in elderly patients with significant aortic stenosis [24]. This is due to the increase in vascular rigidity that accompanies aging such that when aortic stenosis intervenes, the upstroke may diminish in intensity to that which is normal for a younger person.

The heart should be examined for murmurs of aortic stenosis, mitral regurgitation, or hypertrophic cardiomyopathy, all of which are relatively common in elderly patients. An apical heave, a loud, late-peaking, systolic murmur, and a diminished second aortic sound suggest significant aortic stenosis. Classically, mitral regurgitation creates a holosystolic murmur at the cardiac base, but this murmur may also be present in elderly patients with aortic stenosis or hypertrophic cardiomyopathy. If the patient is able to perform a valsalva maneuver, hypertrophic cardiomyopathy may be distinguishable from aortic stenosis and mitral regurgitation by accentuation of its systolic murmur.

The stool should be examined for blood to rule out the possibility of gastrointestinal bleeding and associated anemia.

A careful neurologic examination is essential to evaluate gait, motor function, coordination, balance, and sensation. All of the neurologic diseases mentioned above can be diagnosed from the neurologic evaluation. Bedside evaluations of hearing and vision are essential to identify abnormalities in these senses, since visual and hearing impairments are important risk factors for falls.

One of the most important parts of the physical examination for the evaluation of a fall is an observation of gait and balance, particularly during the activity that caused the fall. It is very useful to observe the patient getting up from a chair (with arms folded in front, if possible), walking 20 feet, making a 180-degree turn, and standing still for the Romberg maneuver with eyes closed and then with eyes opened and a slight sternal push. Difficulty arising from a chair or the need to push off with the arm suggests significant quadriceps weakness. Instability or difficulty in performing any of the other procedures suggests postural incompetence and a predisposition toward falling.

More specialized studies are necessary only if the history and physical examination fail to reveal a cause of falling or if they point to a particular abnormality that requires laboratory evaluation. Since disease can present atypically in elderly patients, some screening tests are often useful. These include a white blood cell count to look for evidence of occult sepsis and hematocrit to diagnose anemia, which can threaten oxygen delivery to the brain. Electrolytes, blood urea nitrogen (BUN), and creatinine values are helpful in assessing hydration status and ruling out electrolyte disorders. A serum glucose concentration is useful to rule out hypoglycemia or hyperglycemia. Hyperosmolar dehydration with hyperglycemia may first present as falling or syncope.

If the patient is taking antiarrhythmic, anticonvulsant, or bronchodilator drugs or lithium, drug levels are useful to determine whether the patient is in the therapeutic or toxic range. If the drug level is in the subtherapeutic range, the fall may be due to inadequate treatment of a known predisposing condition, such as a seizure disorder.

The electrocardiogram is another important test that should be included in the evaluation of most falls. If there are ischemic changes and/or a history of chest pain associated with a fall or, more commonly, a syncopal episode, cardiac enzymes and isoenzymes should be obtained to rule out myocardial infarction. Although arrhythmias are common and often asymptomatic in elderly patients, rhythm disturbances and conduction disease are occasional causes of falls.

There is considerable controversy about other tests for the evaluation of falls or syncope that remain unexplained after the above evaluation. The 24-hour ambulatory cardiac monitor is often used to evaluate falls and syncope but is difficult to interpret because of the high prevalence of asymptomatic arrhythmias, which are rarely coincident with the event. In one study a higher prevalence of serious arrhythmias during ambulatory cardiac monitoring was found in elderly institutionalized fallers than in nonfallers [25]. Two-thirds of fallers with arrhythmias ceased falling after treatment of their arrhythmia. However, the medications used to treat these arrhythmias often have toxic side effects, and many fallers stop falling spontaneously without treatment. Therefore, it is best to obtain the ambulatory electrocardiographic recording only in patients whose arrhythmias would be treated despite the risk of toxicity. These include syncopal or near-syncopal patients with underlying cardiovascular disease or recent myocardial infarction who are at highest risk of sudden death [26].

Carotid sinus massage should be performed on those fallers with no evidence of cerebrovascular disease (a carotid bruit, previous stroke, or transient ischemic attack) or cardiac conduction abnormalities. Although there are case reports of serious complications from carotid sinus massage, these reports include only a few very sick individuals. There are numerous reports of hundreds of elderly patients undergoing carotid sinus massage without complication. Since this procedure can identify a treatable cause of a fall in elderly patients, it is indicated when no other apparent cause of falling and none of the above contraindications are present [27]. The carotid sinus syndrome, defined as greater than a three-second sinus pause or more than a 50-mm Hg drop in systolic blood pressure during carotid sinus stimulation, increases in prevalence with advancing age and cardiovascular disease. It is detected by gentle circular massage of each carotid sinus, one at a time for five seconds, while observing the electrocardiogram. A blood pressure reading is taken before and immediately after the procedure. Patients with carotid sinus syndrome can often be helped by eliminating cardioinhibitory or hypotensive medications. If this is not effective, patients with the cardioinhibitory variety can be treated with cardiac pacing, and those with associated hypotension may benefit from pressors such as ephedrine.

The electroencephalogram and brain computed tomography scan are often ordered for the evaluation of falls and syncope. However, recent studies suggest that these are of little value unless there are underlying focal abnormalities on neurologic examination. Recently, magnetic resonance imaging (MRI) has gained popularity for the more sensitive diagnosis of lacunar infarctions, brain stem abnormalities, and cervical myelopathy.

In a patient with a cardiac murmur, the echocardiogram, phonocardiogram, and cardiac Doppler examination are often used in increasing or decreasing one's suspicion of hemodynamically significant valvular heart disease. These studies may also identify hypertrophic cardiomyopathy, which is relatively common and often unsuspected in elderly patients.

The patient with true vertigo, or a sensation of movement associated with a fall, should be referred to an otorhinolaryngologist for a careful auditory and vestibular assessment. True vertigo is a useful symptom for identifying the patient who is likely to have labyrinthine disease.

Cervical spine films are useful in selected patients with gait disorders and lower extremity spasticity and hyperreflexia, which suggest cervical spondylosis. It is important to obtain lateral neck films in both flexion and extension to evaluate the dimensions of the spinal canal. A dimension of less than 12 mm suggests a significant encroachment on the cervical cord and can be confirmed with MRI or myelography. These patients may require neurosurgical consultation.

Finally, fallers who experience pain with walking may have an orthopedic or rheumatologic problem. A careful bone and joint examination should be performed, and radiographs of painful areas should be obtained. The gait observation often reveals that the patient favors one side. Orthopedic or rheumatologic consultation may be helpful.

Therapeutic Approach

The first step in the treatment of an elderly faller is to identify and treat all predisposing pathologic conditions that might contribute to a fall or faint. For example, the anemic patient might benefit from vitamin supplementation, iron, or a transfusion, depending on the cause of the anemia. The patient with postural hypotension might benefit from liberalized salt intake, support hose, and elevation of the head of the bed at night. Adjusting the time of hypotensive medication administration to avoid a peak effect after a meal may help ameliorate postprandial hypotension. The patient with ischemic heart disease and angina should be given antianginal therapy if it does not result in severe blood pressure reduction. The patient with carotid sinus hypersensitivity should have a careful drug evaluation to be sure that cardioinhibitory drugs such as digoxin, beta blockers, methyldopa, or calcium channel blockers are not contributing to this condition. A similar approach should be applied to the patient with cardiac conduction disease. The patient with arthritis and mobility impairment due to pain may benefit from analgesics, nonsteroidal anti-inflammatory agents, or local measures to relieve discomfort. By treating each of these predisposing factors, falls and syncope can often be prevented.

Environmental hazards should also be eliminated. If possible, a home visit should be arranged to identify such common hazards as excessive furniture, doorstops, slippery floors, throw rugs, poor lighting, or unsafe stairways. The institution of handrails, bath mats, raised toilet seats, and sliding doors in bathrooms may help reduce the risk of falling. Changes in ground topology should be marked with contrasting colors. Due to age-related losses of green and blue perceptions, red and yellow are better seen.

A physical therapy consultation should be requested to evaluate the patient for assistive devices and to institute gait training. Physical therapists can also reduce the fear of falling by repeatedly helping patients through a frightening activity until they become accustomed to it.

It is important to identify and teach the patient to avoid common precipitants of falls, such as arising quickly from bed, particularly in the middle of the night. Patients should be taught to sit at the side of the bed and flex the feet prior to standing. In patients with postprandial hypotension, small frequent feedings and lying down after a meal may prevent falls or syncope. Also, the Valsalva maneuver, associated with straining at stool, can be avoided through patient education, bowel softeners, and dietary alterations.

References

1. Gryfe, C. I., Amies, A., and Ashley, M. J. A longitudinal study of falls in an elderly population: I. Incidence and morbidity. *Age Aging* 6:201, 1977.
2. Nickens, H. Intrinsic factors in falling among the elderly. *Arch. Intern. Med.* 145:1089, 1985.
3. Iskrant, A. P. The etiology of fractured hips in females. *Am. J. Publ. Health* 58:485, 1968.
4. Overstall, W., et al. Falls in the elderly related to postural imbalance. *Br. Med. J.* 1:261, 1977.
5. Wyke, B. Cervical articular contributions to posture and gait: Their relation to senile disequilibrium. *Age Aging* 8:251, 1979.
6. Finch, C. E., Randall, P. K., and Marshall, J. F. Aging and basal gangliar functions. *Ann. Rev. Gerontol. Geriatr.* 2:49, 1981.
7. Scheibel, A. B. Falls, motor dysfunction, and correlative neurohistologic changes in the elderly. *Clin. Geriatr. Med.* 1:671, 1985.
8. Lipsitz, L. A. Abnormalities in blood pressure homeostasis that contribute to falls in the elderly. *Clin. Geriatr. Med.* 1:637, 1985.
9. Tinetti, M. E., William, T. F., and Mayewski, R. Fall risk index for elderly patients based on number of chronic disabilities. *Am. J. Med.* 80:429, 1986.
10. Drachman, D. A., and Hart, C. W. An approach to the dizzy patient. *Neurology* 22:323, 1972.
11. Archea, J. C. Environmental factors associated with stair accidents by the elderly. *Clin. Med.* 1:555, 1985.
12. Meissner, I., et al. The natural history of drop attacks. *Neurology* 36:1029, 1986.
13. Sudarsky, L., and Ronthal, M. Gait disorders among elderly patients: A survey study of 50 patients. *Arch. Neurol.* 40:740, 1983.
14. Lipsitz, L. A. Syncope in the elderly. *Ann. Intern. Med.* 99:92, 1983.
15. Lipsitz, L. A., Wei, J. Y., and Rowe, J. W. Syncope in an elderly, institutionalized population: Prevalence, incidence, and associated risk. *Q. J. Med.* 55:45, 1985.
16. Lipsitz, L. A., et al. Syncope in institutionalized elderly: The impact of multiple pathological conditions and situation stress. *J. Chron. Dis.* 39:619, 1986.
17. Gribbin, B., et al. Effect of age and high blood pressure on baroreflex sensitivity in man. *Circ. Res.* 29:424, 1971.
18. McGarry, K., et al. Baroreflex function in elderly hypertensives. *Hypertension* 5:763, 1983.
19. Rowe, J. W. Aging and renal function. *Ann. Rev. Gerontol. Geriatr.* 1:161, 1980.
20. Fish, L. C., Minaker, K. L., and Rowe, J. W. Altered thirst threshold during hypertonic stress in aging man. *Gerontologist* 25:118, 1985.
21. Shannon, R. P., et al. The effect of age and sodium depletion on cardiovascular response to orthostasis. *Hypertension* 8:438, 1986.
22. Lipsitz, L. A., et al. Postprandial reduction in blood pressure in the elderly. *N. Engl. J. Med.* 309:81, 1983.
23. Lipsitz, L. A., et al. Cardiovascular and nor-

epinephrine responses after meal consumption in elderly (older than 75 years) persons with post-prandial hypotension and syncope. *Am. J. Cardiol.* 58:810, 1986.

24. Flohr, K. H., Weir, E. K., and Chesler, E. Diagnosis of aortic stenosis in older age groups using external carotid pulse recording and phonocardiography. *Br. Heart J.* 45:577, 1981.

25. Gordon, M., Huang, M., and Gryfe, C. I. An evaluation of falls, syncope, and dizziness by prolonged ambulatory cardiographic monitoring in a geriatric institutional setting. *J. Am. Geriatr. Soc.* 30:6, 1982.

26. Kapoor, W. N., et al. Syncope in the elderly. *Am. J. Med.* 80:419, 1986.

27. Murphy, A. L., et al. Carotid sinus hypersensitivity in elderly nursing home patients. *Aust. N.Z. J. Med.* 16:24, 1986.

17

Peripheral Vascular Disease

Burt Adelman

As the number of elderly persons in our society continues to grow, those conditions that result from advanced atherosclerosis will have an increasing impact on the national health. Although stroke, myocardial infarction, and peripheral vascular disease all too often leave a surviving individual unable to continue an independent life-style, recent medical and surgical advances permit many affected patients to continue to lead productive lives. Advances in the prevention and management of peripheral vascular disease will depend on an increased understanding of the process of atherosclerosis and its consequences. As complex treatment modalities are developed that aim at both prevention of the disease and amelioration of the secondary effects of diseased arteries, the practicing physician will be required to have a broad understanding of the pathobiology of atherosclerosis and its related complications.

This chapter focuses on the pathobiology of atherosclerosis, especially peripheral vascular disease, and its management in the elderly; cerebrovascular disease and coronary artery disease are discussed elsewhere in this book (see Chaps. 25 and 14, respectively).

Normal Vascular Anatomy

Atherosclerosis is primarily a disease of the elastic arteries—the aorta and its major branches (subclavian, innominate, and proximal common carotid) and the muscular (distributing) arteries (renal, internal carotid, femoral, mesenteric). The wall of both elastic and muscular arteries consists of three concentric tunics: (1) the tunica intima, (2) the tunica media, and (3) the tunica adventitia.

The boundaries of the intima are formed by a single layer of endothelial cells on the luminal side and the internal elastic lamina on the vessel wall side (Fig. 17-1). In all arteries the endothelial cells lie on a thin, extracellular matrix called the *subendothelium*. In arteries free of vascular disease the intima is a thin layer, and the media contains the bulk of the vessel wall. In muscular arteries the media is composed of a thick band of smooth muscle cells and an extracellular matrix that contains collagen and elastin. In elastic arteries the media is composed of circumferential bands of elastin between which are dispersed smooth muscle cells. In all arteries the media provides the necessary strength to allow the vessel to withstand systolic pressure. The adventitia in both vessel types is composed primarily of fibroblasts and contains no smooth muscle cells. In both elastic and large muscular arteries this coat of fibroblasts provides support for the nerve fibers that penetrate the vessels and the vaso vasorum (vessels of the vessel) that provide nourishment to the outer portion of the media. The adventitia cannot provide adequate

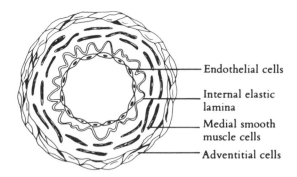

FIGURE 17-1. *Anatomy of the blood vessel wall.*

- Endothelial cells
- Internal elastic lamina
- Medial smooth muscle cells
- Adventitial cells

physical support to the vessel if the media is weakened.

Cell Biology of Vessel Wall
THE ENDOTHELIAL CELL

Both endothelial and smooth muscle cells are critical to the normal function of the vascular system. The endothelial cell, an important regulator of vascular function and integrity, provides a nonthrombogenic surface to passing blood, synthesizes von Willebrand's factor (an important constitutent of the coagulation protein factor VIII), and secretes collagen into the underlying subendothelial basement membrane (contributing to the hemostatic and thrombogenic potential of the vessel wall) [1]. Endothelial cells contribute to the nonthrombogenic quality of the vessel surface by producing prostaglandin I_2 and heparin–like compounds [2]. In addition, endothelial cells maintain a tight barrier that prevents plasma constituents, notably lipid, from passing randomly into the vessel wall. After a fibrin clot forms within a vessel lumen, the endothelial cells are thought to initiate activation of plasminogen to plasmin, thereby facilitating fibrinolysis and clot removal. Clearly, disruption of this important cell will result in major alterations in vessel homeostasis.

Smooth Muscle Cells

Smooth muscle cells have a significant function in the vessel beyond that of establishing vascular tone. They produce many components of the extracellular matrix, including collagen, elastin, and a number of proteoglycans. Smooth

muscle cells respond to vascular injury by migrating from the media into the intima, where they proliferate and at the same time produce extracellular matrix. Smooth muscle cell proliferation can also be initiated by low-density lipoproteins and by a platelet-derived mitogenic factor (platelet-derived growth factor). For these reasons, smooth muscle cell activity plays an important role in the development of the atherosclerotic lesion [3–5].

Arteriosclerosis

Atherosclerosis is only one form of arteriosclerosis; arteriosclerosis includes all processes that result in loss of elasticity and "hardening" of the arteries. Other entities that are considered arteriosclerotic processes include thromboangiitis obliterans (Buerger's disease), Monckeberg's medical calcinosis, and those changes strictly associated with aging. The word *atherosclerosis* is derived from the Greek word *athera* meaning "gruel" and an apt description for the grumous, gruel-like, material that is commonly found in the central portion of an atherosclerotic plaque.

AGE-RELATED CHANGES IN THE ARTERIAL WALL

Although atherosclerosis is commonly considered a disease of aging, it is not merely an age-related process. Only those biologic changes that affect all individuals in a progressive, irreversible fashion can be considered secondary to the aging process. Age-related vascular changes may predispose the individual to the development of atherosclerosis, but they are not specifically atherogenic.

Study of animal and human vascular tissue has identified specific histologic changes that occur with aging in the aorta and arteries. As aging progresses, most major vessels develop changes in mineral and protein content. The intima, a thin layer at birth, becomes thickened owing to cellular proliferation and fibrosis. Elastin fibers, the extracellular material that gives arteries elasticity, become calcified, thinned, and fragmented. Collagen content increases in both the intima and the media, and with time, this collagen becomes progressively more rigid and insoluble due to nonenzymatic cross-linking. In addition, as the structural composition of the vessel wall changes, lipid accumulation increases. Although the mechanism underlying these changes is not understood, one prominent hypothesis holds that they are a response to constant stress [6].

From a functional standpoint these age-related changes result in a progressive stiffening of vessels, which raises peripheral resistance and limits the capacity of the vascular system to increase organ blood flow. Furthermore, baroreceptor function is impaired because stiff vessel walls dampen the transmission of the systolic pressure wave.

The Atherosclerotic Plaque
HISTOLOGY
The characteristic atherosclerotic lesion is a thickening of the intima that extends into the lumen. In extensive lesions the media is also involved. Within the plaque a number of distinct regions are seen. The roof of the plaque is composed of fibrous connective tissue containing collagen, smooth muscle cells, and amorphous extracellular material. Underlying the fibrous cap is the lipid-containing region, in which cholesterol crystals may be seen along with calcium deposits and fat-filled cells. Some plaques are predominantly fibrotic, and others contain large amounts of grumous lipid material. The advanced plaque can further progress to a "complicated plaque" following any of a number of possible events: rupture of the fibrous cap, necrosis of the underlying media, or hemorrhage into the lesion. Such a lesion is highly thrombogenic and liable to promote embolization of its lipid contents or of adherent thrombus.

From this description of the atherosclerotic lesion, it becomes clear how this slowly progressing process can suddenly cause dramatic clinical events. Progressive encroachment on the vascular lumen by plaque formation causes the syndromes of angina pectoris and intermittent claudication. Transient ischemic attacks may be due to embolization of plaque contents, thrombus material, or intermittent vascular obstruction promoted by advanced lesions. In patients with amaurosis fugax, it is possible to visualize cholesterol emboli passing through the retinal vessels by direct ophthalmoscopy. These emboli are characteristically refractile in appearance. Stroke, myocardial infarction, gangrene of the extremities, and ischemic bowel syndromes may be due to any single or combined process. In the aorta the associated surface is highly thrombogenic and can promote the development of secondary thrombotic events, including obstruction of the distal aorta and embolization to the extremities.

MECHANISM OF PLAQUE FORMATION
The leading hypothesis of the development of atherosclerosis is called the "response to injury" theory; it holds that the initiating event in the early development of the atherosclerotic lesion is endothelial cell injury, either desquamation of endothelial cells or alterations in their functional integrity [7–9]. Desquamation would allow for platelet adhesion and secretion of platelet-derived growth factor into the media, where it would stimulate smooth muscle cell proliferation and migration into the intima. Entry of low-density lipoprotein into the media would also be facilitated by endothelial cell damage and would also cause smooth muscle cell proliferation.

The continuous repetition of these initiating events in the appropriate setting of hypertension, cigarette smoking, diabetes, and hypercholesterolemia would allow for the development of full-fledged atherosclerotic lesions. Experimental evidence from animal studies suggests that regrowth of endothelial cells over these early lesions in the presence of elevated serum cholesterol levels can actually contribute to the trapping and concentration of lipid within the arterial wall [10]. In humans the factors that cause the initial endothelial cell injury have not been identified specifically, but evidence from animal experiments supports the possible role of cigarettes, hypertension, antibody-antigen complexes, and cholesterol [11,12]. Finally, there are numerous hereditary factors, all of which are poorly understood, that determine an individual's overall response to any and all of these factors.

Epidemiology of Atherosclerotic Vascular Disease
Extensive epidemiologic study has identified several risk factors for the development of ath-

TABLE 17-1. *Incidence of cardiovascular events according to age and sex*

	AVERAGE ANNUAL INCIDENCE PER 1,000							
	CORONARY HEART DISEASE		CEREBROVASCULAR ACCIDENT		PERIPHERAL ARTERIAL DISEASE		CONGESTIVE HEART FAILURE	
AGE	MEN	WOMEN	MEN	WOMEN	MEN	WOMEN	MEN	WOMEN
45 to 54	9.9	3.1	2.0	0.9	1.8	0.6	1.8	0.8
55 to 64	20.8	9.5	3.2	2.9	5.1	1.9	4.3	2.7
65 to 74	20.4	14.5	8.4	8.6	6.3	3.8	8.2	6.8

SOURCE: Modified from W. B. Kannel and T. Gordon. Cardiovascular Risk Factors in the Aged: The Framingham Study. In S. G. Haynes and M. Feinleb (eds.), *Epidemiology of Aging.* NIH Publication No. 80-969. Washington, D.C.: U.S. Government Printing Office, 1980.

erosclerosis. Atherosclerotic vascular disease is most prevalent in Western industrialized areas and is closely associated with dietary habits that contribute to elevated levels of serum cholesterol. Other important risk factors include cigarette smoking, hypertension, type A personality traits, diabetes, male sex, and hereditary influences [13]. Table 17-1, from the Framingham Study 20-year follow-up, shows the incidence of specific cardiovascular events according to age and sex.

While the incidence of cardiovascular disease continues to increase with age, the impact of some specific risk factors, including serum cholesterol levels, cigarette smoking, and diabetes, declines after age 65. Hypertension, however, remains a significant factor even in the elderly (see Chap. 15). Since no level of elevated blood pressure is without a discernible effect on risk, careful attention must be given to treatment of high blood pressure in the elderly (Table 17-2). Interestingly, high-density lipoprotein (HDL) in both men and women up to the age of 80 continues to play an important role in inhibiting atherosclerosis.

Epidemiology of Peripheral Vascular Disease

Because the main clinical focus of this chapter is on peripheral vascular disease, some specific comments on its epidemiology are indicated. The incidence of intermittent claudication continues to rise with age in both sexes (Table 17-3). In addition, there is a high correlation between the presence of peripheral vascular disease, as indicated by claudication, and the sub-

TABLE 17-2. *Attributable risk for hypertension according to age**

AGE	OVERALL MORTALITY	CARDIO-VASCULAR MORTALITY	CARDIO-VASCULAR MORBIDITY
Men			
45 to 54	17.9	29.3	16.4
55 to 64	16.1	21.4	17.9
65 to 74	8.4	12.9	18.8
Women			
45 to 54	12.0	28.6	17.4
55 to 64	8.5	17.5	26.5
65 to 74	14.9	34.5	26.9

*Attributable risk = total population rate − nonhypertensive population rate/total population rate × 100.
SOURCE: Modified from W. B. Kannel and T. Gordon. Cardiovascular Risk Factors in the Aged: The Framingham Study. In S. G. Haynes and M. Feinleb (eds.), *Epidemiology of Aging.* NIH Publication No. 80-969. Washington, D.C.: U.S. Government Printing Office, 1980.

TABLE 17-3. *Average annual incidence of intermittent claudication according to age and sex per 10,000*

AGE GROUP (YEARS)	NUMBER OF MEN	NUMBER OF WOMEN
45 to 54	18	5
55 to 64	51	19
65 to 74	59	40

SOURCE: From N. C. Peabody, W. B. Kannel, and P. M. McNamara. Intermittent claudication: Surgical significance. *Arch. Surg.* 109:693, 1974. Copyright 1974, American Medical Association.

sequent occurrence of a major cardiovascular event (Table 17-4).

All major studies of the epidemiology of peripheral vascular disease have identified cigarette smoking and diabetes as the most signifi-

TABLE 17-4. *Subsequent occurrence of major cardiovascular events in persons aged 50 to 76 years with claudication*

YEARS AFTER ONSET OF INTERMITTENT CLAUDICATION	CUMULATIVE % WITH WITH CARDIOVASCULAR DISEASE	
	MEN	WOMEN
2	7	20
4	25	34
6	43	39
8	47	45
10	56	66

SOURCE: From N. C. Peabody, W. B. Kannel, and P. M. McNamara. Intermittent claudication: Surgical significance. *Arch. Surg.* 109:693, 1974. Copyright 1974, American Medical Association.

cant risk factors. In the Framingham Study a strong association was found between peripheral vascular disease and cigarette smoking in men of all ages and in women over 60. Between the ages of 60 and 69 the incidence of intermittent claudication in cigarette smokers is twice that of nonsmokers [14]. Diabetes imparts an even greater risk. The cumulative incidence of peripheral vascular disease following the diagnosis of diabetes is estimated to be 15 percent at 10 years and 45 percent at 20 years. In addition, among persistent smokers and diabetics, progression from stable claudication to advanced ischemia requiring amputation is quite high [15,16].

Clinical Manifestations of Peripheral Vascular Disease

The primary cause of obstructive arterial disease affecting the lower extremities is atherosclerosis. When obstructed vessels cannot supply muscle, skin, and nerves adequately, ischemic complications develop. Although affected individuals commonly have diffuse vascular disease in both limbs at the time of presentation, clinical symptoms are usually a result of a critical narrowing in one particular part of the arterial tree [17,18].

CLINICAL PRESENTATION

The most characteristic clinical sign of atherosclerotic disease in the legs is pain on exertion that is relieved by rest, known as intermittent claudication. Although cramping pain is the most common complaint, individuals can also report fatigue and weakness in affected legs. An important characteristic of intermittent claudication is the consistency of the precipitating event; the amount of exertion that produces symptoms in any one individual is constant—for example, cramping pain always occurs after walking the same number of city blocks.

Location of the critical stenosis often determines the specific symptoms. High aortic obstruction is associated with buttock and low back pain. Aortoiliac disease may cause thigh and calf pain. Iliofemoral disease usually causes calf pain, while popliteal and calf artery obstruction affects the foot.

The spectrum of clinical symptoms associated with occlusive vascular disease is determined by the relative adequacy of collateral flow around areas of critical stenosis, the presence of multiple segmental occlusions or stenosing lesions, the degree of exertion required by the patient to function satisfactorily, and a host of systemic factors such as cardiac output, presence of anemia, blood viscosity, and recurrent embolization.

Rest Pain, Ulcers, and Gangrene

Pain at rest results from advanced obstructive disease complicated by poor collateral flow. Affected individuals complain of pain that first begins in the toes and may progress to involve the entire lower leg. Painful ulcerations of the foot and ankle may also develop in these individuals. Ischemic neuropathy may accompany rest pain, causing patients to suffer various disturbing sensations, including numbness and burning. In advanced diabetes, however, neuropathic changes may actually result in loss of pain sensation in the foot or lower leg. Gangrene is the most severe complication of ischemic vascular disease; its presence signifies total loss of blood flow to the affected area.

PHYSICAL EXAMINATION

A careful physical examination will help to identify arterial insufficiency as the cause of leg pain. Loss of normal or previously present pulses is helpful in localizing the distal side of a stenotic lesion. Bruits are also indicative of stenosis. Careful examination of the abdomen and popliteal vessels is performed to detect aneurysm.

Skin color may suggest vascular insufficiency. Pallor on elevation and rubor on dependency are characteristic of arterial insufficiency in the legs. In normal individuals the plantar surfaces of the feet remain pink during elevation; in patients with vascular insufficiency and poor collateralization, the plantar surface develops pallor during this maneuver. Venous filling time can be estimated by asking the patient to place his or her feet in a dependent position following elevation. In normal individuals venous filling occurs within 20 seconds; in the presence of severe arterial insufficiency, filling time may exceed 30 seconds.

Characteristic trophic changes include thinning of the skin, loss of hair, and thickening of the nails. The thinned skin is susceptible to fissure formation, which often results in infection and ulceration. Muscle mass may decrease in ischemic areas, further contributing to patient complaints of weakness.

Additional diagnostic procedures may be undertaken to better define the extent and severity of disease or to assist in making a diagnosis in an unusual situation. Many medical centers are equipped with a noninvasive vascular diagnostic laboratory [19]. Using ultrasonic flow (Doppler) detectors, systolic pressure can be measured along the arterial supply of the leg, and significant obstructing lesions can be localized. By measuring systolic pressure at the ankle before and after exercise the functional significance of an identified lesion can be assessed.

Angiography is rarely indicated as a diagnostic tool; its main usefulness is in evaluating patients before arterial reconstruction and in detecting emboli. Caution must be exercised when using angiography because elderly patients are particularly susceptible to the toxic effects of contrast media on the kidney.

Differential Diagnosis

In general, differentiation of occlusive atherosclerotic vascular disease from other entities causing leg pain or affecting blood flow in the extremities is not difficult. Vascular syndromes in the elderly that affect the legs include advanced atherosclerosis, arterial embolism, and venous disease.

ARTERIAL EMBOLUS

Symptoms associated with arterial embolus may vary from pain at rest to intermittent claudication; however, the onset of symptoms is almost always sudden. The acute loss of a pulse in a patient with no other evidence of severe vascular disease should make the examiner suspicious of an embolic event, but a specific source for emboli must be identified before the diagnosis can be confirmed. The most common source of peripheral emboli is the heart, particularly in the setting of atrial fibrillation, recent myocardial infarction, or infective endocarditis. Less commonly, embolli may dislodge from a complicated atherosclerotic plaque in the aorta or iliac or femoral arteries. Such embolic events often result in infarction of a toe. A popliteal aneurysm can also suddenly become occluded or release embolic material, resulting in acute ischemia below the knee.

VENOUS DISEASE

Pain is commonly associated with both deep venous thrombosis and chronic venous insufficiency. Differentiating venous from arterial disease can usually be accomplished by obtaining a careful history and performing a physical examination. Patients with acute or chronic venous disease complain of leg swelling, especially in the evening after ambulating during the day. This swelling is commonly relieved by elevation. Pain associated with acute phlebitis is localized over the affected vein, which may be palpable as a cord. Chronic venous disease is characterized by increased pigmentation of the medial aspect of the calf with ulcer formation over the medial malleolar area; arterial insufficiency ulcers are more commonly located over the lateral malleolus. In difficult situations noninvasive studies performed in the vascular laboratory can help determine the correct diagnosis.

MUSCULOSKELETAL DISORDERS

Patients with degenerative joint disease involving the hip or knee experience pain on exertion, particularly in association with weight bearing. Physical examination reveals pain elicited by the movement of the affected joint. In inflammatory arthritis, synovial effusion or thickening is found.

NEUROLOGIC DISORDERS

Lumbar disk disease is commonly associated with pain on exertion. However, because pain is related to pressure on nerves and is not affected by metabolic demand, bedside examination can reproduce the pain syndrome. Sciatic and femoral nerve syndromes have characteristic pain patterns and are often accompanied by specific defects noted on neurologic examination, such as muscle group weakness and loss of reflexes. The presence of intact pulses helps to rule out arterial disease.

Spinal stenosis resulting from hypertrophic bony growth or disk herniation can cause a "pseudoclaudication" syndrome in which compressions of the cauda equina or its vascular supply causes lower back and leg pain during activity. Spinal stenosis may be differentiated from aortoiliac occlusion by a careful history, which may reveal that the specific events leading to the production of pain are not as precisely reproducible as one would expect in atherosclerotic vascular disease. Often patients with spinal stenosis report that they obtain relief from pain by assuming unusual positions. Noninvasive laboratory testing will help to differentiate pseudoclaudication from true vascular insufficiency. Confirmation of the diagnosis may require computerized axial tomography or myelography.

Neuropathic pains and paresthesias are associated with both vascular and nonvascular disease. A careful history and physical examination will help sort out the diagnosis. However, particularly in diabetic patients, primary neuropathic and vascular problems may be present together. In these patients the physician must use his or her clinical judgment to determine if extensive evaluation is needed to establish whether correctable vascular or neurologic disease is present.

Clinical Course and Prognosis

The clinical course of atherosclerosis of the lower extremities is surprisingly benign [15,17, 20]. Progressive disease requiring arterial reconstruction or amputation develops in less

TABLE 17-5. *Cardiovascular comorbidity in Framingham study subjects developing intermittent claudication**

CARDIOVASCULAR DISEASE	101 MEN		61 WOMEN	
	No.	%	No.	%
None	51	52	39	64
Coronary heart disease	44	44	21	34
Atheromatous brain infarction	4	4	2	3
Congestive heart failure	11	11	4	7

*Subjects aged 35 to 76 years. Cardiovascular events not mutually exclusive.
SOURCE: From N. C. Peabody, W. B. Kannel, and P. M. McNamara. Intermittent claudication: Surgical significance. *Arch. Surg.* 109:693, 1974. Copyright 1974, American Medical Association.

than 10 percent of patients who have intermittent claudication. However, in diabetics or in patients who continue to smoke cigarettes after the onset of symptoms, progression of the disease is more common, and the amputation rate is higher.

It is important to recognize that intermittent claudication is usually associated with generalized atherosclerotic vascular disease. As seen in Table 17-5, individuals in whom intermittent claudication develops have a high incidence of generalized cardiovascular morbidity and mortality. Any individual who has intermittent claudication deserves a careful cardiovascular assessment and continued follow-up study.

General Principles of Therapy

The intention of either medical or surgical therapy in patients with atherosclerotic vascular disease of the lower extremities is to relieve pain, preserve tissue, and maintain as high a level of physical function as possible [21]. Medical therapy necessitates a common sense approach that recognizes that most affected individuals have advanced generalized atherosclerosis. Because hypertension is associated with an increased risk of accelerated vascular impairment, it should always be treated adequately. In addition, hyperlipidemia should be treated, and diabetes, if present, should be controlled. It is unlikely, however, that control of diabetes will prevent progression of vascular disease.

All patients who are obese should be encouraged to lose weight. Exercise is currently included in the rehabilitation of patients with coronary artery disease and should also be part of the treatment plan for patients with intermittent claudication. By routinely exercising, half to two-thirds of patients can extend the distance that they can walk before the onset of pain. All patients who smoke must be encouraged to stop. Although this will not improve the symptoms, it may prevent progression of atherosclerosis and some secondary features, particularly the development of skin ulcers, since nicotine decreases blood flow to the skin.

The use of vasodilator drugs is without proven merit and cannot be recommended. Whatever beneficial effects vasodilation can have on blood flow can be achieved by advising patients to keep their legs warm.

Recently the methylxanthine derivative pentoxifylline has been shown to be of some benefit in the pharmacologic management of peripheral vascular disease. This agent appears to reduce blood viscosity by increasing the deformability of the red cell membrane. In a number of clinical trials patients treated with pentoxifylline have shown improved blood flow in ischemic areas. In a multicenter controlled trial patients receiving this agent were able to increase their walking distance significantly as measured on a treadmill [22]. In general, the side effects of pentoxifylline are minimal.

All patients with ischemic leg disease need careful instruction regarding care of skin and nails. The skin should be kept lubricated with lanolin or other mild emollients, and nails should be kept trimmed. Fungal infections should be treated immediately, and any other infection given close attention. Foot care is often best administered by a podiatrist or surgeon who is particularly sensitive to the complications of vascular insufficiency. Patients should be informed that any break in the skin that does not heal rapidly should be brought to the attention of their physician.

SURGICAL TREATMENT

Surgical treatment of peripheral vascular disease includes sympathectomy, arterial bypass, or amputation. Sympathectomy results in vasodilatation of cutaneous blood vessels and thus may be helpful in the treatment of patients with rest pain and ischemic ulcers. The effect of sympathectomy on skeletal muscle is minimal; therefore, no improvement will be noted by patients with intermittent claudication. The procedure can be performed via local instillation of alcohol or by direct surgical section. Before considering sympathectomy in any patient, it is important to demonstrate that sympathetic activity is intact and that interruption of sympathetic innervation will result in improved blood flow in the affected area.

Bypass Surgery

Arterial bypass surgery in a patient with advanced peripheral vascular disease can result in improved functional capacity and salvage of dangerously ischemic tissue. However, because more than two-thirds of affected individuals have stable disease, careful selection of patients for operation is essential. The primary reason for surgical intervention is the presence of significant ischemic symptoms at rest, especially pain and ulceration. Rapid progression of symptoms or intermittent claudication of such severity that the patient suffers intolerable changes in life-style are adequate reasons for surgery. Because patients generally have diffuse disease, the operative procedure is aimed at alleviating the most significant lesions.

Careful arteriographic examination of the circulation in the affected extremity and aoritic bifurcation is usually necessary to help plan the procedure and evaluate the extent of collateral flow. Furthermore, the general condition of the patient is also an important consideration; in particular, the location and extent of other sites of atherosclerotic disease must be determined. Severe carotid or coronary artery disease may require prior surgical or medical treatment to improve operative morbidity for intended peripheral vascular surgery. In addition, most surgeons believe that continued cigarette smoking will adversely affect the patency of grafts and therefore insist that persons considered for surgery stop smoking.

Aortoiliac Disease

The favored surgical technique for the amelioration of aortoiliac disease is replacement of the bifurcation with a prosthetic graft. This necessitates an intraabdominal approach that can be quite stressful to the patient. Overall mortality for this procedure is between 2.5 and 9.3 percent, and five-year patency rates are between 70 and 90 percent [17,23,24]. Complications include groin infection and aneurysm formation at the site of anastomosis. Return of symptoms is usually the result of progression of disease distal to surgical repair.

In patients too ill to undergo extensive abdominal surgery, an axillofemoral bypass procedure may be attempted. In this procedure a synthetic graft is tunnelled subcutaneously between the axillary artery and the femoral artery. The operative mortality is less than 2 percent, and although the thrombosis rate at one year is as high as 40 percent, the graft can be easily thrombectomized so that patency rates of 76 percent have been reported at five years [17,20]. Femoral-femoral bypass procedures can also be utilized in high-risk patients.

Femoropopliteal Disease and Distal Disease

Surgical repair of disease in the femoropopliteal region usually necessitates the placement of an autogenous saphenous vein graft. If a vein suitable for grafting is not available, synthetic materials can be used. It is difficult to evaluate the published results of these procedures because indications for surgery as well as extent of disease vary. In general, operative mortality ranges from 2 to 7 percent; five-year patency rates vary from 58 to 72 percent [26].

Obstructed vessels of the calf can also be bypassed surgically. Such procedures also involve the use of autogenous vein grafts. A successful outcome can prevent the loss of a foot or toes through gangrene.

Amputation

Amputation remains a necessary form of treatment in some patients with advanced atherosclerosis. Gangrene involving the foot or leg or intractable pain are the usual indications for amputation. Arteriography should be performed to ensure that a bypass procedure cannot be attempted. Amputations should involve the least amount of tissue necessary but should be at a level at which an adequate vascular supply will ensure satisfactory healing.

Percutaneous Transluminal Angioplasty

Direct dilation of obstructed peripheral arteries by a balloon catheter became possible after de-velopment of the flexible balloon catheter by Gruntzig and Hopff in 1974. Although many patients with peripheral vascular disease have been treated by balloon dilation there remains no clear consensus to support its general application. Recent studies have helped to define the patient population most likely to benefit from percutaneous angioplasty and have indicated that it is important to distinguish clinical success (improved patient status) from technical success (a dilated vascular lumen) when evaluating outcome [27]. Patients most likely to benefit from this procedure have claudication rather than limb-threatening ischemia, focal rather than diffuse lesions, immediate return of peripheral pulses after dilation, good blood flow distal to the obstruction, and no diabetes [27,28]. Currently, percutaneous angioplasty should be considered an adjunct to surgery rather than a replacement for it.

Abdominal Aortic Aneurysm

In general, the greatest incidence of abdominal aneurysm appears to be during the seventh decade. Men are affected six times as often as women. The same risk factors associated with other forms of atherosclerosis apply to the development of aortic aneurysms. The majority of patients with atherosclerotic aneurysms have associated cardiovascular disease.

Dilatation of the abdominal aorta beyond 3 cm is considered aneurysmal. Once the media is sufficiently weakened to allow expansion of the vessel, progressive widening becomes inevitable because wall tension increases as the radius increases (LaPlace's law). The majority of aneurysms are fusiform in shape, although some may be saccular. All are filled with laminated thrombus, which only rarely obstructs the lumen. Over 97 percent of abdominal aneurysms begin below the renal arteries; distal extension commonly includes the aortic bifurcation and can involve the iliac arteries.

Approximately 40 percent of patients with an abdominal aneurysm have symptoms at the time of discovery. The most common symptoms include abdominal pain, groin pain, back pain, pulsation in the abdomen, and discovery of an abdominal mass. On physical examination the most important finding is a pulsatile abdominal mass. Aneurysms less than 4.5 cm in diameter may be difficult to feel. Because ultrasound examination can provide definitive diagnostic information in almost every instance, any suspicious lesion should be examined by this technique. Angiography is not generally indicated for diagnosis and can actually provide misleading information; the actual size of the aneurysm is difficult to assess by angiography because clot is present in the lumen of the aorta [29].

The natural history of untreated abdominal aneurysms is dismal. The five-year survival of affected patients approximates 30 percent, with over half of the patients dying of rupture. In general, the risk of rupture is directly related to the size of the aneurysm. The five-year risk of rupture of a 4-cm aneurysm is less than 15 percent, however, it is more than 75 percent for an 8-cm aneurysm.

In light of the high risk of fatal rupture, elective surgical reapir of an abdominal aneurysm is usually indicated. All patients with an aneurysm of over 6 cm should be considered for elective surgery. An aneurysm measuring between 4 and 5 cm should be carefully followed by serial abdominal echo examination, and surgery should be recommended if the growth rate exceeds 1 cm in a year [29]. Others recommend repair of all aneurysms in patients who appear able to tolerate surgery [30].

Operative mortality appears to depend on the general status of the patient; the most important factor is whether or not the aneurysm has ruptured or is leaking. Currently, operative mortality in good-risk patients should approximate 3 to 5 percent, with many centers reporting mortality rates of less than 2 percent. Five-year survival following surgery ranges between 50 and 78 percent. Operative mortality in patients with an expanding aneurysm rises to between 5 and 15 percent, and in patients with a ruptured aneurysm, operative mortality is approximately 50 to 60 percent [29]. Age alone is not a significant risk factor; a number of studies have indicated that immediate surgical mortality in the elderly can be kept to 5 percent by applying the same guidelines for patient selection as are used for the general population [30,31].

Acute complications of aneurysm surgery in-clude myocardial infarction, peripheral arterial occlusion, acute renal insufficiency, colonic arterial insufficiency, aortoenteric fistula with gastrointestinal bleeding, and wound infection. Late complications include graft occlusion or stenosis, false aneurysm formation, enteric fistula, and infection.

Anticoagulants and Antiplatelet Agents

Although drugs that inhibit thrombus formation are commonly used in patients with coronary artery disease or cerebrovascular disease, their general value in the treatment of peripheral vascular disease has not been established. However, their use in specific situations may be indicated, such as after percutaneous angioplasty, in patients with recurrent embolic events, or following repeated thrombosis at a site of revascularization. For these reasons and to supplement the information presented in the chapter on cerebrovascular disease (see Chap. 25), a brief discussion of these agents follows.

Drugs that affect blood clotting are divided into two classes. Agents that affect the fluid phase coagulant proteins are commonly referred to as anticoagulants; agents that inhibit platelet function are called antiplatelet agents. The major anticoagulants are heparin, bishydroxycoumarin (Dicumarol), warfarin (Coumadin, Panwarfarin), and the indanedione derivatives.

Heparin inhibits clotting by accelerating the activity of antithrombin III, a naturally occurring protein inhibitor of activated coagulation factors. It is commonly used for therapy in acute deep venous thrombosis, pulmonary embolization, and in some cases, arterial thrombosis or embolization. Because it must be administered parenterally, its chronic use is awkward.

The other anticoagulants are administered orally and thus are suitable for long-term use. All have the same pharmacologic action—interference with synthesis of the vitamin K-dependent coagulant proteins, factors II, VII, IX, and X. As is the case with heparin, this effect ultimately prevents fibrinogen conversion to fibrin and interrupts clot formation. Elderly individuals placed on oral anticoagulants should be closely followed because a number of studies have demonstrated an age-related increase in the pharmocodynamic effect of these agents despite stable pharmacokinetics [32].

References

1. Gimbrone, M. A., Jr. Culture of Vascular Endothelium. In T. H. Spaet (ed.), *Progress in Hemostasis and Thombosis*. Vol. III. New York: Grune & Stratton, 1976.
2. Moncada, S., and Amezcua, J. L. Prostacyclin, thromboxane A_2 interactions in hemostasis and thrombosis. *Haemostasis* 8:252, 1979.
3. Ross, R., and Glomset, J. S. Atherosclerosis: A problem in the biology of the arterial smooth muscle cell. *Science* 180:1332, 1973.
4. Scher, C. D., et al. The Initiation of Cell Replication by Cationic Polypeptide Hormones. In F. E. Bloom (ed.), *Peptides: Integrators of Cell and Tissue Function*. New York: Raven, 1980.
5. Fischer-Dzoga, K., and Wissler, R. W. Stimulation of proliferation in stationary primary cultures of monkey aortic smooth muscle cells: II. Effect of varying concentrations of hyperlipemic serum and low density lipoproteins of varying dietary fat origins. *Atherosclerosis* 24:515, 1976.
6. Kohn, R. R. Heart and Cardiovascular System. In C. E. Finch and L. Hayflick (eds.), *Handbook of the Biology of Aging*. New York: Van Nostrand Reinhold, 1977.
7. Harker, L. A., Ross, R., and Glomset, J. A. The role of endothelial cell injury and platelet response in atherogenesis. *Thromb. Haemost.* 39:312, 1978.
8. Wissler, R. W. Principles of the Pathogenesis of Atherosclerosis. In E. Braunwald (ed.), *Heart Disease: A Textbook of Cardiovascular Medicine*. Philadelphia: Saunders, 1980.
9. Ross, R., and Glomset, J. A. The pathogenesis of atherosclerosis. *N. Engl. J. Med.* 295:369, 1976.
10. Minick, C. R., Stemerman, M. B., and Insull, W., Jr. Role of endothelium and hypercholesterolemia in intimal thickening and lipid accumulation. *Am. J. Pathol.* 95:131, 1979.
11. Kottke, B. A., and Sobbiah, M. T. R. Pathogenesis of atherosclerosis concepts based on animal models. *Mayo Clin. Proc.* 53:35, 1978.
12. McGill, H. C., Jr. Atherosclerosis: Problems in Pathogenesis. In R. Paoletti and A. M. Gotto (eds.), *Atherosclerosis Reviews*. Vol. 7. New York: Raven, 1979.
13. Dawber, T. R. *The Framingham Study: The Epidemiology of Atherosclerotic Disease*. Cambridge: Harvard University Press, 1980.
14. Kannel, W. B., and Shurtleff, D. Cigarettes and the development of intermittent claudication. *Geriatrics* 28:61, 1973.
15. Juergens, J. L., Barker, N. W., and Hines, E. A., Jr. Atherosclerosis obliterans: Review of 520 cases with special reference to pathogenic and prognostic factors. *Circulation* 21:188, 1960.
16. Melton, L. J., III, et al. Incidence and prevalence of clinical peripheral vascular disease in a population-based cohort of diabetic patients. *Diabetes Care* 3:650, 1980.
17. Coffman, J. D. Intermittent claudication and rest pain: Physiologic concepts and therapeutic approaches. *Progr. Cardiovasc. Dis.* 22:53, 1979.
18. Juergens, J. L., and Bernatz, P. E. Atherosclerosis of the Extremities. In J. L. Juergens, J. A. Spittell, and J. F. Fairbairn II (eds.), *Peripheral Vascular Diseases*. Philadelphia: Saunders, 1980.
19. Sobel, M., and Skillman, J. J. Noninvasive Evaluation of the Lower Extremity and Carotid Circulation. In M. Aronson and T. Delbanco (eds.), *Manual of Clinical Evaluation: Strategies for Cost-Effective Care*. Boston: Little, Brown, (in press, 1988).
20. Imparato, A. M., et al. Intermittent claudication: Its natural course. *Surgery* 78:795, 1975.
21. Fairbairn, J. F. II, and Juergens, J. L. Principles of Medical Management. In J. L. Juergens, J. A. Spittell, and J. F. Fairbairn II (eds.), *Peripheral Vascular Diseases*. Philadelphia: Saunders, 1980.
22. Porter, J. M., Cutler, B. S., and Lee, B. Y. Pentoxifylline therapy in intermittent claudication. *Am. Heart J.* 104:66, 1982.
23. Mulcane, R. S., Royster, T. S., and Lynn, R. A. Long-term results of operative therapy for aortoiliac disease. *Arch. Surg.* 113:601, 1978.
24. Malone, J. M., Moore, W. S., and Goldstone, J. The natural history of bilateral femoral bypass grafts for ischemia of the lower extremities. *Arch. Surg.* 110:1300, 1975.
25. Johnson, W. C., Logrefo, F. W., and Vollman, R. W. Is axillo-bilateral femoral graft an effective substitute for aortic-bilateral iliac/femoral graft? An analysis of ten years' experience. *Ann. Surg.* 186:123, 1977.
26. Hansteen, V., et al. Long-term follow-up of patients with peripheral arterial obliterans treated with arterial surgery. *Acta Chir. Scand.* 141:725, 1975.
27. Cambria, R. P., et al. Percutaneous angioplasty for peripheral arterial occlusive disease. *Arch. Surg.* 122:283, 1987.
28. Morin, J. F., Johnston, K. W., and Rae, M. Improvement after successful percutaneous transluminal dilation treatment of occlusive peripheral

arterial disease. *Surg. Gynecol. Obstet.* 163:453, 1986.

29. Weintraub, A. M., and Gomes, M. N. Clinical Manifestations of Abdominal Aortic Aneurysm and Thoracoabdominal Aneurysm. In J. Lindsay, Jr. and J. W. Hurst (eds.), *The Aorta.* New York: Grune & Stratton, 1979.
30. Rutherford, J. D. Infrarenal Aortic Aneurysms. In R. R. Rutherford (ed.), *Vascular Surgery.* Philadelphia: Saunders, 1984.
31. Baker, W. H., and Munns, J. R. Aneurysmectomy in the aged. *Arch. Surg.* 110:513, 1975.
32. Smith, T., Viverette, F., and Adelman, B. The use of antithrombotic therapy in the elderly. *Geriatr. Clin.* 1:887, 1985.

18

Renal System

JOHN W. ROWE

Renal Anatomy

Advancing age is associated with progressive loss of renal mass in humans, with renal weight decreasing from 250 to 270 gm in young adulthood to 180 to 200 gm by the eighth decade. In the absence of hypertension or marked vascular disease, the senescent kidney maintains its relatively smooth contour. The loss of renal mass is primarily cortical, with relative sparing of the renal medulla. The total number of identifiable glomeruli decreases with age, roughly in accordance with the changes in renal weight. The number of hyalinized or sclerotic glomeruli identified on light microscopy increases from 1 to 2 percent during the third to fifth decade, to as high as 30 percent in some apparently healthy 80-year-olds; the mean prevalence after age 70 is approximately 10 to 12 percent [1,2].

Aging is associated with a loss of lobulation of the glomerular tuft, thus decreasing the effective filtering surface. Although the total number of nuclei per glomerulus is unchanged with age, the filtering surface is further diminished by a progressive increase in the number of mesangial cells and a reciprocal decrease in the number and percentage of epithelial cells. The glomerular filtration characteristics, as estimated by dextran clearance, indicate no change in permeability with age [3].

Several changes have been documented in the renal tubule with age. Of particular interest is the observation by Darmady and coworkers [4] that diverticuli of the distal nephron, which are essentially absent in kidneys from young individuals, become increasingly prevalent with advancing age, reaching a frequency of three diverticuli per tubule at the age of 90 years. It has been suggested that these diverticuli represent the origin of the simple retention cysts commonly seen in the elderly.

It is generally agreed from histologic studies that normal aging, independent of hypertension or renal disease, is associated with variable sclerotic changes in the walls of the larger renal vessels. These sclerotic changes do not encroach on the lumen and are augmented in the presence of hypertension. Smaller vessels appear to be spared, and only 15 percent of senescent kidneys from nonhypertensive individuals display arteriolar changes [2,5,6].

Radiographic studies in normotensive individuals demonstrate an increasing prevalence after the seventh decade of abnormalities similar to those seen in persons with hypertension, including abnormal tapering of interlobar arteries, abnormal arcuate arteries, increased tortuosity of intralobular arteries, and a predilection for age-related vascular abnormalities in the polar region.

Combined microangiographic and histologic studies have identified two very distinctive patterns of change in arteriolar-glomerular units

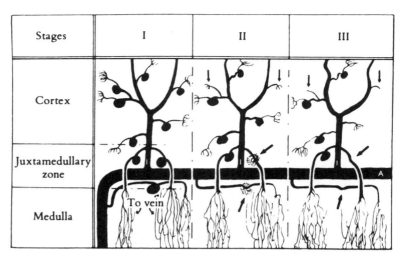

Stages	I	II	III
Cortex			
Juxtamedullary zone	To vein		A
Medulla			

FIGURE 18-1. *Changes in the intrarenal arterial pattern with age. Stage I: Basic adult pattern shows glomerular arterioles. Stage II: Partial degeneration of some glomeruli. Two cortical afferent arterioles ramify into remnants of glomerular tufts (small arrows). Two juxtamedullary arterioles pass through partially degenerated glomeruli (large arrows). There is a slight spiraling of interlobular arteries and afferent arterioles. Stage III: Two cortical afferent arterioles now end blindly (small arrows), and two juxtamedullary arterioles are a glomeruli (large arrows). The corresponding glomerular tufts have degenerated completely. The spiraling of interlobular arteries and afferent arterioles is now more pronounced. (A = arcuate artery; I = interlobular artery.) (From A. Ljungqvist and C. Lagergren. Normal intrarenal arterial pattern in adult and aging human kidney. J. Anat. 96:285, 1962. By permission of Cambridge University Press.)*

with senescence [7,8] (Figs. 18-1, 18-2). In one type (see Fig. 18-1), hyalinization and collapse of the glomerular tuft is associated with obliteration of the lumen of the preglomerular arteriole and a resultant loss in blood flow. This type of change is seen primarily in the cortical area. The second pattern (see Fig. 18-2), seen primarily in the juxtamedullary area, is characterized by the development of anatomic continuity between the afferent and efferent arterioles during glomerular sclerosis. The end point is thus loss of the glomerulus and shunting of blood flow from afferent to efferent arterioles. Blood flow is maintained to the arteriolar rectae verae, the primary vascular supply of the medulla, which are not decreased in number with age.

Renal Physiology
RENAL BLOOD FLOW
A progressive reduction in renal plasma flow from 600 ml per minute in young adulthood to 300 ml per minute by 80 years of age is well established. Factors contributing to this decrease include an age-related decline in cardiac output and the reduction in the renovascular bed already outlined. Xenon washout studies in healthy potential renal donors ranging in age from 17 to 76 years indicate that the age-related decrease in flow is not purely a reflection of decreased renal mass, but that flow per gram of tissue falls progressively after the fourth decade

	Forms of communication between the arterioles and the glomeruli at the vascular pole			
	I	II	III	IV
Cortical type				
Juxtamedullary type				

(left axis label: Forms of efferent arterioles)

FIGURE 18-2. *The degenerative process in the cortical and juxtamedullary nephrons. (From E. Takazakura, et al. Intrarenal vascular changes with age and disease. Reprinted from* Kidney International *2:224, 1972.)*

[9]. There is a highly significant decrease with advancing age in the cortical component of blood flow with preservation of medullary flow—a finding consistent with histologic studies showing selective loss of cortical vasculature. These cortical vascular changes probably account for the patchy cortical defects commonly seen on renal scans in healthy elderly adults [10]. This histologic and functional demonstration of selective decrease in cortical flow may explain the observation that filtration fraction (the fraction of renal plasma flow that is filtered at the glomerulus) actually increases with advancing age, since outer cortical nephrons have a lower filtration fraction than juxtamedullary nephrons.

To clarify the relative contributions of functional "spasm" to the observed change in blood flow, Hollenberg and associates [9] studied young and old subjects before and during intra-arterial administration of acetylcholine and angiotensin. If age-related functional spasm was present, maximal renal blood flow after acetycholine-induced vasodilation might be expected to be independent of age. Renal blood flow was increased in all age groups by acetylcholine, but the relation between flow and age was similar after acetylcholine administration to that in the control studies, indicating a fixed or structural etiology for the observed decrease in flow with age. Consistent with these findings, vasoconstrictor response to angiotensin was not influenced by age.

GLOMERULAR FILTRATION RATE

The major clinically relevant functional defect arising from these histologic and physiologic changes is a progressive decline after maturity in the glomerular filtration rate (GFR). Age-adjusted normative standards for creatinine clearance have recently been established (Fig. 18-3). Creatinine clearance is stable until the middle of the fourth decade, when a linear decrease of about 8.0 ml/minute/1.73 m² per decade beings [11,12] (Fig. 18-4).

Long-term longitudinal studies indicate substantial variability in the effect of age on creatinine clearance; as many as one-third of individuals show no decline in GFR with age [13]. This variability suggests that factors other than aging per se may be responsible for the apparent

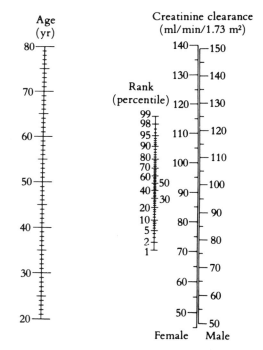

FIGURE 18-3. *Nomogram for ascertaining age-adjusted percentile rank in creatinine clearance. Nomogram is constructed for use with creatinine clearance and with creatinine determinations done by automated "total chromogen" method. A line through the subject's age and creatinine clearance intersects the percentile rank line at a point indicating the subject's age-adjusted percentile rank. (From J. W. Rowe, et al. Age-adjusted normal standards for creatinine clearance in man. Ann. Intern. Med. 84:567, 1976.)*

effect of age on renal function. This view is supported by the finding in longitudinal studies that increasing blood pressure levels are associated with accelerated loss of renal function [14] (Fig. 18-5).

The argument that entire nephrons drop out with advancing age is supported by the rather striking parallel declines with age in GFR and several proximal tubular functions, including maximum excretion of paraaminohippurate and Diodrast and maximal absorption of glucose. Additional observations regarding glucose absorption indicate that the renal threshold for glycosuria, which relates inversely to the degree of "splay" in reabsorptive capacity of individual nephrons, increases with age. A healthy older individual is less likely than his or her younger counterpart to show a false-positive

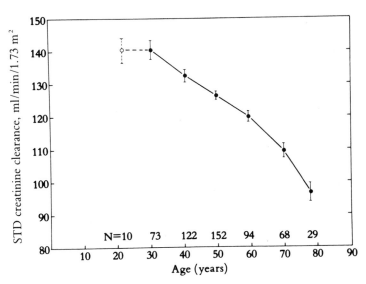

FIGURE 18-4. *Cross-sectional differences in standard creatinine clearance with age. The number of subjects in each age group is indicated above the abscissa. Values plotted indicate mean ± SEM. (From J. W. Rowe, et al. The effect of age on creatinine clearance in man: A cross-sectional and longitudinal study. J. Gerontol. 31:155, 1976.)*

urinary glucose test in postprandial screening for diabetes. Likewise, glucose will appear in the urine of a young diabetic patient at a lower blood glucose level than that seen in an elderly diabetic.

SERUM CREATININE CONCENTRATION

Since muscle mass, from which creatinine is derived, falls with age at roughly the same rate as GFR, the rather drastic age-related loss of GFR is not reflected in an elevation of serum creatinine (Table 18-1). Thus, the serum creatinine concentration overestimates GFR in the elderly. A healthy 80-year-old man with a creatinine clearance of 32 ml per minute less than his 30-year-old counterpart will have the same serum creatinine concentration. Depressions of GFR severe enough to result in an elevation of serum creatinine above 1.5 mg/dl are rarely due to normal aging and so indicate the presence of a disease state. In clinical practice the doses of many drugs excreted primarily to the kidneys are routinely adjusted to compensate for alterations in renal function (Table 18-2), especially digoxin preparations and aminoglycoside antibiotics. Unfortunately, these adjustments are usually based on serum creatinine values, with the resultant predictable overdose in elderly patients. Dose adjustments should ideally be based on creatinine clearances; when only serum creatinine is available, the influence of age must be

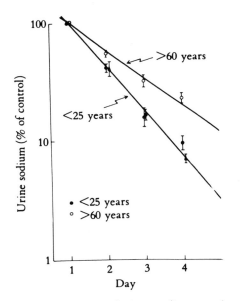

FIGURE 18-5. *Response of urinary sodium excretion to restriction of sodium intake in normal humans. The mean half-time for eight subjects over 60 years of age was 30.9 ± 2.8 hours, exceeding the mean half-time of 17.6 ± 0.7 hours for subjects under 25 years of age. (P = 0.01.) (Reprinted from M. Epstein. Effects of aging on the kidney. Federation Proceedings 38:168, 1979.)*

TABLE 18-1. *Cross-sectional age differences in creatinine clearance, serum creatinine, and 24-hour creatinine excretion*

AGE (YEARS)	NO. OF SUBJECTS	CREATININE CLEARANCE (ML/MIN/1.73 M^2)*	SERUM CREATININE CONCENTRATION (MG/DL)	CREATININE EXCRETION (MG/24 HR)
17–24	10	140.2 ± 3.7	0.808 ± 0.026	1,790 ± 52
25–34	73	140.1 ± 2.5	0.808 ± 0.010	1,862 ± 31
35–44	122	132.6 ± 1.8	0.813 ± 0.009	1,746 ± 24
45–54	152	126.8 1.4	0.829 ± 0.008	1,689 ± 18
55–64	94	119.9 ± 1.7	0.837 ± 0.012	1,580 ± 22
65–74	68	109.5 ± 2.0	0.825 ± 0.012	1,409 ± 25
75–84	29	96.9 ± 2.9	0.843 ± 0.019	1,259 ± 45

*Values indicate mean ± 1 SEM

TABLE 18-2. *Common renally excreted drugs for which dose adjustment in normal elderly persons may be required*

Aminoglycoside antibiotics
  Gentamicin
  Kanamycin
  Tobramycin
  Amikacin
Vancomycin
Nitrofurantoin
Tetracycline
Digoxin
Hypoglycemic agents
  Acetohexamide
  Chlorpropamide
Procainamide
Cephaloridine

considered and can be accomplished by use of this formula [15]:

$$\text{creatinine clearance (ml/minute)} = \frac{(140 - \text{age}) \times \text{weight (kg)}}{72 \times \text{serum creatinine (mg/dl)}}$$

(15 percent less in females)

Fluid and Electrolyte Balance

In normal circumstances age has no effect on plasma sodium or potassium concentration, plasma pH, or the ability to maintain normal extracellular fluid volume. However, adaptive mechanisms responsible for maintaining constancy of the volume and composition of the extracellular fluid are impaired in the elderly.

Because of these physiologic changes, acute illness in geriatric patients is often complicated by development of derangements in fluid and electrolyte balance that delay recovery and prolong hospitalization. These changes in homeostasis are best understood in terms of renal sodium and water excretion after acute alterations in salt and fluid intake.

SODIUM BALANCE
Sodium Deficiency
The aged kidney's response to sodium deficiency is blunted. Studies of the renal response to acute reductions in salt intake (100-mEq to 10-mEq sodium intake per day) have shown that although aged patients are capable of sodium conservation and attainment of salt balance on this markedly restricted intake, their response is sluggish compared to that in younger adults. In the studies of Epstein and Hollenberg [16], the half-time for reduction of urinary sodium after salt restriction was 17.6 hours in young and 30.9 hours in old subjects (see Fig. 18-5). The cumulative sodium deficit before daily renal losses equal intake is thus greater in the elderly. Since old patients are more likely to experience confusion, loss of sense of thirst, and disorientation when acutely ill, this "salt-losing" tendency is aggravated by failure of adequate salt intake, leading to further depletion of the extracellular fluid volume and impaired cardiac, renal, and mental function. This vicious

cycle is too often continued in the hospital when physicians, dreading pulmonary edema, are reluctant to administer substantial amounts of sodium-containing fluids intravenously to acutely ill, volume-depleted geriatric patients.

This salt-losing tendency of the senescent kidney is due both to nephron loss, which leads to increased osmotic load per nephron and resultant mild osmotic diuresis, and to important age-related alterations that occur in the renin-aldosterone system. Basal renin, whether estimated by plasma renin concentration or renin activity, is diminished by 30 to 50 percent in the elderly in the face of normal levels of renin substrate. This basal difference between young and old is magnified by maneuvers designed to augment renin secretion, such as salt restriction, diuretic administration, and upright posture [17,18].

Lowered renin levels are associated with 30 to 50 percent reductions in plasma concentrations of aldosterone as well as significant reductions in the secretion and clearance rates of aldosterone [19]. That aldosterone deficiency of old age is a function of the coexisting renin deficiency and not secondary to intrinsic adrenal changes is suggested by studies showing that plasma aldosterone and cortisol responses after adrenocorticotropic hormone (ACTH) stimulation are not impaired with advancing age [18]. The functional significance of the aldosterone deficiency in the elderly is evident in studies indicating that significant enhancement of distal tubular sodium reabsorption occurs after aldosterone administration [20].

The impact of normal aging on plasma renin levels must be considered when assigning hypertensive patients to specific pathophysiologic groups based on renin levels. A geriatric hypertensive patient, and occasionally a normotensive patient with the normal elevation of systolic blood pressure that occurs with advancing age, may be labeled as having "low renin hypertension" when actually the renin level is not low but normal for the patient's age.

An additional factor that may play an important role in age-related alterations in sodium balance is atrial natriuretic factor (ANF). Although only a few preliminary studies have appeared, these uniformly indicate that ANF levels, while very variable in the elderly, are, on

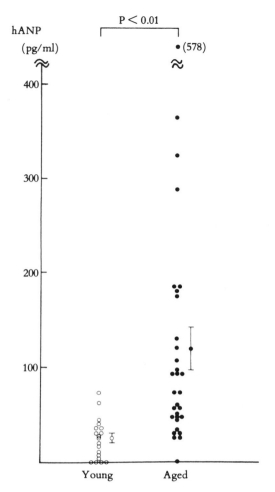

FIGURE 18-6. *Circulating atrial natriuretic factor levels in healthy young and old individuals. (From M. Ohaski, et al. High plasma concentration of human atrial natriuretic polypeptide in aged men. J. Clin. Endocrinol. Metab. 64:81. © 1987 by The Endocrine Society.)*

average, substantially higher than those seen in healthy younger adults [21] (Fig. 18-6). These elevated levels may play a role in the salt-losing tendency of the aged kidney.

The management of sodium depletion and its resultant deleterious effects on cardiac, central nervous system, renal, and intestinal function includes the prompt administration of sodium chloride. If extracellular depletion is mild, oral administration of fluids and foods with a high sodium content for several days is often sufficient. If volume depletion is more marked, as reflected by decreased blood pressure, tissue turgor, or orthostatic hypotension, intravenous administration of isotonic saline is indicated. The administration of hypotonic fluids, such as 5% glucose in water, will lead to hyponatremia while failing to correct the salt depletion and may aggravate the patient's overall condition.

Sodium Excess

Just as volume depletion is more likely to develop in old patients who are salt- and water-deprived, volume expansion is a commonly encountered problem. Primarily because of its lower glomerular filtration rate, the senescent kidney is less able to excrete an acute salt load than the younger kidney. Geriatric patients, with or without preexisting myocardial disease, are thus at risk for expansion of the extracellular fluid volume in the presence of an acute salt load (from inappropriate intravenous fluids, dietary indiscretions, or, as commonly happens, after the administration of sodium-rich radiographic contrast agents such as those used in intravenous pyelography).

The mainstay of management of acute volume expansion with pulmonary congestion remains the intravenous administration of potent diuretics such as furosemide or ethacrynic acid. However, in the absence of preexisting cardiomegaly, administration of excess fluid generally does not result in precipitation of acute congestive heart failure but rather in modest weight gain and the appearance of mild peripheral edema. Over the course of several days, this excess salt is generally excreted. The administration of oral diuretics can be helpful if the volume expansion aggravates preexisting heart failure or hypertension.

POTASSIUM BALANCE

Hyperkalemia

The age-related decreases in renin and aldosterone mentioned earlier contribute to an increased incidence of type 4 renal tubular acidosis (hyporeninemic hypoaldosteronism) in the elderly and to an increased risk of developing hyperkalemia in a variety of clinical settings. Through its action on the distal renal tubule, aldosterone increases sodium reabsorption and facilitates the renal excretion of potassium. Aldosterone represents one of the major protective mechanisms that prevent hyperkalemia during periods of potassium challenge. Since the glomerular filtra-

tion rate (another major determinant of potassium excretion) is also impaired in old patients, serious elevations of plasma potassium are likely to develop, especially in the presence of gastrointestinal bleeding (a major source of potassium) or when potassium salts are given intravenously. This tendency toward hyperkalemia is further aggravated in any clinical setting associated with acidosis, since the senescent kidney is sluggish in its response to acid loading, resulting in prolonged depression of pH and concomitant potassium elevation. Potent antagonists of renal potassium excretion, such as spironolactone or triamterene, which impair renal potassium excretion, as well as indomethacin, beta-adrenergic blockers, and converting enzyme inhibitors, which also inhibit potassium disposal, should be administered with caution to the elderly, and the concomitant administration of these agents and potassium should be avoided.

The initial management of hyperkalemia includes discontinuation of any sources of potassium in the diet, discontinuation of potassium-sparing diuretics, and prompt optimization of renal function in patients with volume depletion or heart failure. Severe hyperkalemia, which is reflected in electrocardiographic abnormalities, including symmetrically peaked T waves and widened QRS complexes, requires prompt treatment with intravenous calcium salts (calcium chloride or calcium gluconate), which directly antagonize the effect of hyperkalemia on the myocardium and often normalize the electrocardiogram. Also indicated are sodium bicarbonate, glucose, and insulin. Because such emergency treatment is of temporary benefit in controlling serum potassium and has no effect on total body potassium, these emergency efforts should be accompanied by initiation of efforts to deplete total-body potassium. These include oral or rectal administration of sodium-potassium exchange resin (Kayexalate) and potent intravenous diuretics such as furosemide or ethacrynic acid.

WATER BALANCE

Dehydration

The clinical impact of the aged kidney's inability to regulate salt balance properly under stress is compounded by similar abnormalities in water metabolism. The capacity of elderly individuals to conserve water and elaborate a concentrated urine under conditions of either water deprivation or infusion of antidiuretic hormones is impaired [22,23]. The cause of the decreased concentrating capacity of the aged kidney is unclear but probably is related to the concomitant decline in GFR and an age-related decrease in renal response to antidiuretic hormone (ADH).

Although the decline in water-conserving capacity is not severe enough to be clinically significant under conditions of free access to water, it may become important when fluid intake is limited because of the decreased thirst sensation that occurs in old age or in the presence of exaggerated insensible losses such as occur with fever. Regarding thirst, Phillips and colleagues have clearly demonstrated [24] that subjective measures of thirst and objective measures of water-drinking behavior following water deprivation were increased in the elderly and were associated with impaired recovery from hyperosmolality. Studies employing hypertonic saline infusions have also shown that healthy individuals over age 75 have markedly blunted thirst sensation [25]. Elevations of the serum sodium concentration to levels that impair mental function (greater than 160 mEq/L) are commonly seen in the geriatric age group. Both the salt and water-losing tendencies of the senescent kidneys and the thirst deficit contribute to the common clinical presentation of acutely or subacutely ill elderly patients with hypertonic volume depletion. The incidence of hypernatremia among the elderly exceeds one case per hospital per month [26]. The insidious onset of volume depletion, coupled with the fact that common presentations are nonspecific and include a preponderance of neurologic and psychiatric symptoms, often delays diagnosis and worsens morbidity.

In the initial management of the patient with severe hypertonic volume depletion it is important to focus on volume repletion as potentially life-saving and to treat such patients with rapid intravenous infusion of isotonic saline until cardiovascular stability is attained. In the presence of marked hypernatremia, these isotonic fluids are actually "hypotonic" relative to the patient's plasma, and serum sodium will begin to fall as volume is expanded. Once blood pressure and intravascular volume are corrected, hypotonic fluids should be administered until the serum sodium level is below 150 mEq/L. Severe hypertonic dehydration in the elderly is uniformly associated with marked alterations in consciousness. Although the volume and the composition of the extracellular fluid may be normalized within 72 hours of admission, mental state alterations commonly persist for some time, and slow recovery over two weeks is not infrequent. This persisting confusion, despite normal electrolyte values, should not necessarily precipitate invasive clinical evaluation. Patience is often rewarded in such cases, and the complications of lumbar punctures and the costs of sophisticated noninvasive radiologic procedures are avoided.

Water Intoxication

Perhaps the most serious and least well-recognized electrolyte disorder in geriatric patients is their tendency to develop water intoxication. One survey in a geriatric unit demonstrated that over 10 percent of patients had hyponatremia (serum sodium levels below 130 mEq/L); administration of thiazide diuretics and intravenous hyptonic solutions were the most commonly identified causes [27]. A similar survey in another long-term care facility found an incidence of hyponatremia of 23 percent. Three of every four hyponatremic patients had symptoms that were felt to be secondary to water intoxication [28].

The clinical presentation of hyponatremia is nonspecific, with depression, confusion, lethargy, anorexia, and weakness the most common findings. When hyponatremia is severe (serum sodium concentrations below 110 mEq/L), seizures and stupor may be seen, and central nervous system damage may be irreversible. It is not unusual for geriatric patients to become hyponatremic in the presence of any stress, including surgery, fever, or acute viral illness.

Clinical evaluation of the elderly hyponatremic patient usually reveals one of three general causes. One is decreased renal capacity to excrete water as a consequence of acute or chronic reduction in renal blood flow. This occurs in patients with extracellular volume depletion, congestive heart failure, hypoalbuminemia associated with cirrhosis or nephrosis, or drug-induced hypotension. In addition to the evidence on history and physical examination of the possible presence of any of these disorders, a laboratory examination is often helpful. In this category of patients laboratory examination reveals prerenal azotemia, with blood urea nitrogen (BUN) elevations out of proportion to elevations in serum creatinine.

The second group of elderly hyponatremic patients comprises those on diuretics, especially thiazide diuretics. Although the precise pathophysiology remains unclear, the well-known effect of diuretics on decreasing renal diluting capacity certainly is an important component, especially when combined with the decreased diluting capacity of the aged kidney. However, this fails to explain the tremendous variability between apparently well elders in the tendency to develop hyponatremia on diuretics or the very rapid rate at which the serum sodium concentration falls in some patients.

The third group of patients with hyponatremia shows a constellation of findings consistent with oversecretion of ADH as a cause of the water retention. These findings include low serum sodium, evidence of good renal function (low BUN), mild extracellular fluid expansion (normal to slightly full neck veins, trace edema), and evidence of inappropriate renal water retention (urine osmolality greater than maximally dilute and in many cases more concentrated than serum). In addition, excess ADH secretion, because of the slight extracellular fluid expansion and subsequent reduction in aldosterone secretion and elevation of glomerular filtration rate, is associated with the presence of modest to large amounts of sodium in the urine (greater than 20 mEq/L).

Excess ADH secretion is commonly associated with pneumonia, tuberculosis, stroke, meningitis, subdural hematoma, and a variety of other pulmonary and central nervous system disorders. As discussed in Chapter 9, the elderly seem particularly prone to this complication. This special vulnerability of the elderly may also hold true for drug-induced ADH excess. In one study, elderly patients accounted for most cases of hyponatremia developing from use of chlorpropamide [29]. Elderly patients may develop hyponatremia in a variety of clinical set-

TABLE 18-3. *Drugs known to impair water excretion and induce hyponatremia*

Vasopressin	Amitriptyline
Oxytocin	Thiothixene
Chlorpropamide	Aspirin
Vincristine	Acetaminophen
Cyclophosphamide	Narcotics
Fluphenazine	Barbiturates
Clofibrate	Haloperidol
Carbamazepine	

tings, including fever, psychological stress, general anesthesia, and acute viral illness [30]. Although hyponatremic, these patients are unable to excrete a water load, but after resolution of the acute illness water metabolism is normal. In many cases the same patient returns several weeks or months later with another acute illness and again develops hyponatremia.

One must maintain a high degree of suspicion for hyponatremia in geriatric patients, particularly in view of the slow, insidious nature of the development of water intoxication and its nonspecific clinical presentation. Physicians caring for the elderly should be cautious when prescribing medications known to increase ADH secretion, such as chlorpropamide and barbiturates (Table 18-3), as well as when administering hypotonic fluids in the presence of recent surgery or any acute illness.

Management of water intoxication is dictated by the level and rate of fall of the serum sodium level, the clinical manifestations, and the cause. In all cases, strict water restriction is appropriate. Medications possibly associated with water intoxication, such as diuretics or agents that increase ADH (see Table 18-3), should be withheld promptly. In patients in whom hyponatremia is associated with reduced renal blood flow, therapy should be aimed at maximizing renal function by either correction of congestive heart failure, volume repletion of patients with extracellular fluid depletion, or restoration of blood pressure to normal in hypotensive patients.

In cases of excess ADH secretion, fluid restriction alone generally results in a slow return of plasma osmolality toward normal levels. In resistant cases or when fluid restriction is impractical, the water-retaining effects of ADH can be inhibited by oral administration of dimethyl chlorotetracycline in doses of 300 mg two or three times a day. This nephrotoxic agent induces a state of partial nephrogenic diabetes insipidus and predictably results in correction of hyponatremia over the course of several days. Since it is a nephrotoxic agent, the serum creatinine and BUN levels should be followed closely.

Severe hyponatremia (serum sodium concentrations of less than 115 mEq/L) that is associated with seizures or major central nervous system abnormalities requires prompt correction. The most effective approach is the administration of hypertonic saline; 500 ml of 3% sodium chloride can safely be administered intravenously to most patients over a period of 12 hours and will generally increase the serum sodium concentration 8 to 10 mEq/L, placing the patient out of immediate danger while other therapeutic modalities are initiated.

Renal Vascular Disorders

RENAL EMBOLI

Occlusive arterial disease is an important cause of both acute and chronic renal failure in the elderly. Renal arterial emboli occur in any setting associated with peripheral embolization, such as acute myocardial infarction, chronic atrial fibrillation, subacute bacterial endocarditis, and aortic surgery or aortography. The manifestations of renal emboli in the elderly may vary from an essentially clinical silent event to a full-bown syndrome of severe flank pain and tenderness, hematuria, hypertension, spiking fevers, marked reduction in renal function, and elevations of serum lactate dehydrogenase. Small emboli are very difficult to detect because renal scans may show focal perfusion defects in many apparently normal elderly patients. Major emboli may be suggested by the finding of differential contrast excretion on pyelography and confirmed by renal scanning and aortography. Surgery is generally not indicated, and anticoagulant therapy may be of major benefit. In many cases when renal function is discernibly impaired, improvement may occur over a period of several days to weeks.

Renal cholesterol embolization is a specific geriatric syndrome that may occur spontaneously or in association with aortic surgery or angiography in patients with diffuse atherosclerosis. Diagnosis may be difficult because a definitive diagnosis requires visualization of cholesterol crystals on renal biopsy, and a presumptive diagnosis is frequently clouded by other concomitant potential causes of reduced renal function, such as hypotension or administration of angiographic contrast material. The clinical course is highly variable. Although most patients go on to progressive renal failure, some develop only moderate renal impairment and may regain renal function over time [31]. No specific treatment is available.

RENAL ARTERY THROMBOSIS

Thrombotic occlusive renal arterial disease frequently complicates severe aortic and renal arterial atherosclerosis, especially in the setting of decreased renal blood flow caused by congestive heart failure or volume depletion. Renal artery stenosis secondary to dysplastic changes in the arterial walls is essentially limited to young age groups and is not an important disorder in the geriatric population. Symptoms of renal arterial occlusion may be remarkably absent. In patients in whom renal function was previously good, the only manifestation of unilateral thrombosis may be an increase in serum BUN, creatinine, and perhaps a modest increase in blood pressure. In cases with preexisting renal impairment and azotemia, renal arterial occlusion may precipitate congestive heart failure, marked hypertension, and emergence of the uremic syndrome.

The value of currently available diagnostic tests for detection of renovascular hypertension is influenced by age. Recent studies indicate that the number of falsely positive results on either stimulated plasma renin study or saralasin infusion study decreases markedly with age. Similarly, the older the patient, the more likely a high stimulated renin or positive saralasin infusion study indicates significant renovascular hypertension [32]. Thus, either or both of these studies are useful tests in identifying elderly patients for further study, including timed intravenous pyelography, renal vein renin determinations, and, ultimately, angiography. There should be a careful evaluation for a coexisting abdominal aortic aneurysm, which may lead to renal arterial occlusion by extension of atheromata or dissection. Angiography should involve the least amount of contrast possible in order to minimize the likelihood of a nephrotoxic reaction, which, while generally limited to several days of oliguria and mild azotemia, may take the form of severe acute oliguric renal failure. When technically feasible, surgical revascularization should be carefully considered. Substantial return of renal function can be obtained after prompt revascularization, and in some cases recovery occurs even if surgery is delayed until several months after the vascular occlusion.

ACUTE RENAL FAILURE

Age influences renal disease either by altering the prevalence of specific diseases or by affecting the presentation, course, and response to treatment of conditions seen in both early and late adult life. Acute renal failure is seen more frequently in old patients simply because the common inciting events, including hypotension associated with marked volume depletion, major surgery, sepsis, major angiographic procedures, or the injudicious use of antibiotics, are more common in multiply impaired elderly, who are often at increased risk because of pre-existing moderate renal insufficiency.

The management of acute renal failure in the elderly is a complex and demanding task worthy of the effort. The aged kidney retains the capacity to recover from acute ischemic or toxic insults over the course of several weeks. Although the usual acute tubular necrosis (ATN), comprising 2 to 10 days of oliguria followed by a diuretic phase preceding recovery of function, is seen in the elderly, "nonoliguric" acute renal failure is being recognized with increasing frequency. In these cases, renal function, as reflected in serum BUN and creatinine levels, is impaired for several days after a brief hypotensive episode associated with surgery, sepsis, overmedication, or volume depletion, or after the administration of nephrotoxic radiographic contrast agents. After this brief period of azotemia, renal function gradually returns to its previous level. Despite this transient and reversible loss of renal function, oliguria is not a prominent component of the clinical picture. Since the clinical hallmark of renal failure is generally thought to be a dramatic reduction in urine output, cases of nonoliguric acute renal failure may go unrecognized. This lack of recognition of suppressed renal function may result in an inadvertent overdose of medications excreted predominantly via renal mechanisms, including digitalis preparations and aminoglycoside antibiotics such as gentamicin.

The management of elderly patients with full-blown acute renal failure complicated by oliguria is guided by the same general principles employed in younger patients. The most important principle is the careful exclusion of urinary obstruction as a cause of the renal failure, particularly in men with prostatic hypertrophy or prostatic carcinoma and in women with gynecologic malignancy.

The major causes of death during acute renal failure are volume overload precipitating acute pulmonary edema, hypertensive crisis, hyperkalemia, and infection. Dialysis, whether it be hemodialysis or peritoneal dialysis, is effective in the elderly, and the complication rate seems to be dictated more by coincident cardiovascular disease than by the patient's age. Dialysis often substantially simplifies management; thus, one should not wait until an emergency situation is present before initiating dialysis in a patient with acute renal failure. It is more prudent to initiate dialysis early in patients in whom it is very likely that renal function will not return before the dialysis will be needed. The immediate indications for emergency dialysis include pulmonary edema unresponsive to diuretics, hyperkalemia, uremic pericarditis, and seizures, or uncontrolled bleeding on a uremic basis. The use of intravenous catheters placed in the femoral vein for dialysis has been a recent major advance in the management of elderly patients with acute renal failure. These catheters are easily placed, may be left in for several days to a week with a very low incidence of infection or thrombosis, and circumvent the need for implantation of arteriovenous shunts for dialysis access in acute renal failure.

Aside from initiation of dialysis, careful attention to the balance of several factors is necessary. Water and salt balance must be monitored carefully. Due to catabolism, the usual patient with acute renal failure will lose about one pound of body weight mass per day. Attempts to keep body weight constant will result in gradual expansion of the extracellular fluid volume and a consequent increase in blood pressure and risk of precipitation of cardiac failure. Similarly, overzealous fluid restriction will impair the patient's general condition and central nervous system function and may delay the recovery of renal function. In general, the administration of approximately 600 ml of fluid a day, in addition to insensible losses, provides adequate fluid balance.

Potassium balance is crucial, and hyperkalemia must be avoided if possible and treated promptly if present. Acidosis progresses with the length and degree of renal failure, and sodium bicarbonate should be administered in an effort to maintain circulating bicarbonate levels in the range of 15 to 19 mEq/L. Administration of sodium bicarbonate may expand extracellular fluid volume, and thus patients should be watched carefully for the presence of congestive heart failure.

Infection is a common and lethal complication of acute renal failure. Urinary infection secondary to unnecessary urinary catheterization is particularly common. Little is gained from placing a urinary catheter in an oliguric patient in whom volume status and serum levels of BUN, creatinine, and potassium are better guides to progress and treatment than urinary output. Infection of intravenous lines is also common, and these should be scrupulously monitored and discontinued when possible.

Additionally, routine measures include administration of oral phosphate-binding agents in an effort to minimize the elevation of serum phosphorus levels associated with acute renal failure and administration of a diet limited in protein content to blunt the rise in BUN. It is of major importance to pay careful attention to the alteration in dose-interval of medications excreted via the kidney and to recognize the enhanced sensitivity of elderly uremic patients to psychotropic medications such as hypnotics and major tranquilizers.

CHRONIC RENAL FAILURE

Many forms of chronic renal failure are seen more commonly late in life because the renal disease is secondary to other age-dependent diseases. Examples include prostatic hypertrophy or cancer leading to hydronephrosis, reno-vascular hypertension or renal failure secondary to atherosclerosis, multiple myeloma, drug-related causes of renal insufficiency, and, perhaps most common, prerenal azotemia from congestive heart failure or volume depletion.

Recognition

Although the general principles of management of renal failure are similar in young and old adults, the geriatric patient with chronic renal insufficiency presents several special considerations. With regard to diagnosis, the serum creatinine level generally fails to rise as high in the elderly as in the young despite equivalent levels of residual renal function because muscle mass, the ultimate source of creatinine, falls with age, particularly in the presence of nutritional deficits such as those seen in uremia. Since serum creatinine underestimates the degree of renal failure, many debilitated, uremic elderly patients will not be recognized as uremic since their creatinine levels may be less than 10 mg/dl, whereas substantially higher levels are common in younger uremic patients.

Another factor that often delays recognition of chronic renal failure in the elderly is the presentation of renal failure as decompensation of a previously impaired organ system before the emergence of specific symptoms of uremia. Examples include worsening of preexisting heart failure due to inability to excrete salt and water, gastrointestinal bleeding in the presence of previous gastrointestinal malignancy or ulcer, or mental confusion in a borderline demented patient who becomes increasingly azotemic.

Diagnosis

Once the presence of chronic renal failure is established, the definitive cause should be identified. Most chronic renal failure in the elderly is due to chronic glomerulonephritis, hypertensive and atherosclerotic vascular disease, diabetes, or, in some cases, late-presenting polycystic kidney disease. The most important diagnostic consideration is strict exclusion of potentially reversible causes, such as urinary tract obstruction, particularly in men with symptoms of prostatism; renal arterial occlusion that may be reparable; hypercalcemia; or administration of nephrotoxic agents.

Management

If no reversible component is identified, the patient should be followed closely so that the rate of loss of renal function can be judged accurately. Appropriate adjustments to account for the renal failure should be made in the doses and dose schedules of all medications, especially digoxin. Hypertension should be controlled carefully. As serum phosphate rises, phosphate-binding antacids should be given with meals to suppress parathyroid hormone and its resultant adverse effects on bone. As serum phosphate falls in response to treatment, serum calcium will generally rise toward the normal range. If hypocalcemia persists after normalization of phosphate levels, it should be treated with preparations of vitamin D or its congeners (vitamin D_1, 50,000-unit tablets two or three times a day; dihydrotachysterol, 0.2 to 0.4 mg twice a day; 1,25-dihydroxyvitamin D_3, 0.25 to 0.5 mg twice a day) in order to increase intestinal calcium absorption.

Anemia associated with chronic renal failure often requires more aggressive management in elderly patients because of coexisting cardiac disease. Red cell indices are not a reliable estimate of iron deficiency in uremia. Iron deficiency should be excluded by evaluation of serum iron and ferritin, and oral or parenteral iron supplements should be administered if indicated. In the absence of iron deficiency, the anemia of chronic renal failure was managed until recently with monthly injections of androgens (nandrolone decanlate, 200 mg intramuscularly). Preparations of erythropoietins developed through genetic engineering have become available and promise to be very effective in controlling the anemia of chronic renal failure.

Dietary management of elderly patients with chronic renal failure is often overdone, compounding the nutritional impact of the disease. Protein and salt restriction is often needed in young individuals to suppress the volume expansion and BUN elevations. Many elderly patients ingest only 60 to 70 gm of protein daily and 4 to 5 gm of salt under normal conditions, and strict limitations of these dietary constituents is often unnecessary. Similarly, hyperkalemia should be avoided and dietary potassium controlled, but the reductions required in the el-

derly are often moderate. Acidosis should be controlled with oral sodium bicarbonate tablets with the aim of keeping serum bicarbonate levels near 18 to 20 mEq/L. The best approach to these modifications is careful alteration of the diet to the proved needs of the individual patient.

Pruritus is a major problem in elderly uremic patients, especially in the presence of coexisting xerosis. In addition to skin moisteners, ultraviolet treatments have been found effective and safe for elderly uremic patients. Administration of so-called antipruritic agents, such as antihistamines, and ataractics are rarely helpful because they act primarily by causing sedation and may produce adverse nervous system effects in the elderly.

Dialysis in the Elderly

Chronic maintenance dialysis—generally hemodialysis but occasionally chronic ambulatory peritoneal dialysis—remains the mainstay of treatment of elderly uremic patients. Elderly patients often do very well on dialysis, and the frequency of complications seems to be related more to the coexisting extrarenal disease than to age itself. Psychologically, elderly patients often are more able to adapt to chronic dialysis than are their younger counterparts. Once it is clear that a patient will need dialysis at some time in the near future, early creation of an arteriovenous fistula for access to hemodialysis is important, particularly in the elderly patient, since such fistulas often mature rather slowly. At present, renal transplantation is generally not considered in individuals over the age of 60.

Nephrotic Syndrome

Nephrologists have traditionally taught that age plays an important role in the etiology of nephrotic syndrome, with the likelihood of lipoid nephrosis decreasing and amyloidosis increasing with advancing age. Several series have now been reported that include biopsy and clinical data on large numbers of elderly nephrotics [33–35]. In general, age has no impact on the frequency of any specific histologic type of glomerular change. In particular, the most common cause of nephrosis in old age is membranous glomerulonephritis, and minimal-change disease and amyloidosis are seen with equal frequency in young and old patients. There is no impact of age on the generally excellent response of patients with minimal-change disease to corticosteroids and immuno-suppressants. In addition, some elderly with membranous disease respond to steroid or cy-clophosphamide therapy. In many cases, cyclo-phosphamide may be the treatment of choice to avoid the steroid-associated worsening of common preexisting conditions in the elderly, such as glucose intolerance, hypertension, os-teoporosis, and cataracts. It is clear from the available literature that renal biopsy remains a critically important procedure in the proper evaluation of an elderly patient with nephrotic syndrome.

Acute Glomerulonephritis

Acute glomerulonephritis is receiving increas-ing attention as a disease in which presentation and prognosis are clearly age-related. In chil-dren and young adults, acute glomerulonephri-tis is frequently associated with recent strep-tococcal infection and, less commonly, with one of a wide variety of conditions, including Schönlein-Henoch purpura, crescentic nephritis with or without pulmonary hemorrhage, he-molytic uremic syndrome, or generalized vas-culitis. The presentation, regardless of etiology, is fairly uniform, with hematuria, heavy pro-teinuria, edema, hypertension, and the develop-ment in many cases of pulmonary congestion. The prognosis is generally good in poststrepto-coccal disease in young patients, and there is a variable outcome in nonpoststreptococcal cases.

In old patients, acute glomerulonephritis is manifestly different [36,37]. The presentation is nonspecific, with nausea, malaise, arthralgias, and a rather striking predilection for pulmo-nary infiltrates initially. Commonly, the clinical picture is believed to represent worsening of a preexisting illness, especially congestive heart failure. Proteinuria is generally moderate. Hy-pertension or edema, although unusual, usually indicates a poststreptococcal etiology and a fa-vorable prognosis; otherwise, the prognosis is poor, with crescentic glomerulonephritis char-acterized by focal, segmental necrotizing, and fibrosing glomerulitis the most frequent histo-logic finding [38]. Management is presently controversial, and the value of treatment with corticosteroids, immunosuppressive agents, anticoagulants, and plasmapheresis is hotly debated.

References

1. McLachlan, M. S. F., et al. Vascular and glo-merular changes in the aging kidney. *J. Pathol.* 121:65, 1977.
2. Tauchi, H., Tsuboi, K., and Okutomi, J. Age changes in the human kidney of the different races. *Gerontologie* 17:87, 1971.
3. Artursen, G., Groth, T., and Grotte, G. Human glomerular membrane porosity and filtration pressure: Dextran clearance data analyzed by theoretical models. *Clin. Sci.* 40:137, 1971.
4. Darmady, E. M., Offer, J., and Woodhouse, M. S. The parameters of the aging kidney. *J. Pathol.* 109:195, 1973.
5. McLachlan, M. S. F. The aging kidney. *Lancet* 2:143, 1978.
6. Griffiths, G. J., Cartwright, G. O., and McLach-lan, M. S. F. Loss of renal tissue in the elderly. *Clin. Radiol.* 26:249, 1975.
7. Takazura, E., et al. Intrarenal vascular changes with age and disease. *Kidney Int.* 2:224, 1972.
8. Ljungqvist, A., and Lagergren, C. Normal intra-renal arterial pattern in adult and aging human kidney. *J. Anat.* 96:285, 1962.
9. Hollenberg, N. K., et al. Senescence and the renal vasculature in normal man. *Circ. Res.* 34:309, 1974.
10. Friedman, S. A., et al. Functional defects in the aging kidney. *Ann. Intern. Med.* 76:41, 1972.
11. Rowe, J. W., et al. Age-adjusted normal stan-dards for creatinine clearance in man. *Ann. Intern. Med.* 84:567, 1976.
12. Rowe, J. W., et al. The effect of age on creatinine clearance in man: A cross-sectional and longitu-dinal study. *J. Gerontol.* 31:155, 1976.
13. Lindeman, R. D., Tobin, J. D., and Shock, N. W. Longitudinal studies on the rate of decline in renal function with age. *J. Am. Geriat. Soc.* 33:278, 1985.
14. Lindeman, R. D., Tobin, J. D., and Shock, N. W. Association between blood pressure and the rate of decline in renal function with age. *Kidney Int.* 26:861, 1984.
15. Cockcroft, D. W., and Gault, M. H. Prediction of creatinine clearance from serum creatinine. *Nephron* 16:31, 1976.
16. Epstein, M., and Hollenberg, N. K. Age as a de-

terminant of renal sodium conservation in normal men. *J. Lab. Clin. Med.* 87:411, 1976.

17. Crane, M. G., and Harris, J. J. Effect of aging on renin activity and aldosterone excretion. *J. Lab. Clin. Med.* 87:947, 1976.

18. Weidmann, P., et al. Effect of aging on plasma serum and aldosterone in normal man. *Kidney Int.* 8:325, 1975.

19. Flood, C., et al. The metabolism and secretion of aldosterone in elderly subjects. *J. Clin. Invest.* 46:960, 1967.

20. Nunez, M., et al. Renal management of sodium under indomethacin and aldosterone in the elderly. *Age Aging* 9:165, 1980.

21. Ohaski, M., et al. High plasma concentration of human atrial natriuretic polypeptide in aged men. *J. Clin. Endocrinol. Metab.* 64:81, 1987.

22. Rowe, J. W., Shock, N. W., and DeFronzo, R. The influence of age on urine concentrating ability in man. *Nephron* 17:279, 1976.

23. Lindeman, R. D., et al. Influence of age, renal disease, hypertension, diuretics and calcium on the anti-diuretic response to suboptimal infusion of vasopressin. *J. Lab. Clin. Med.* 68:206, 1966.

24. Phillips, P. A., et al. Reduced thirst after water deprivation in healthy elderly men. *N. Engl. J. Med.* 12:753, 1984.

25. Minaker, K. L., et al. Altered thirst threshold during hypertonic stress in aging man. *Clin. Invest. Med.* 8:2, 1985.

26. Mahowald, J. W., and Himmelstein, D. U. Hypernatremia in the elderly: Relation to infection and mortality. *J. Am. Geriat. Soc.* 20:177, 1981.

27. Sunderam, S. G., and Mankiker, G. D. Hyponatremia in the elderly. *Age Aging* 12:77, 1983.

28. Kleinfeld, J., Casimir, M., and Bona, S. Hyponatremia as observed in a chronic disease facility. *J. Am. Geriat. Soc.* 27:156, 1979.

29. Weissman, P. N., Shenkman, L., and Gregerman, R. I. Chlorpropamide hyponatremia. *N. Engl. J. Med.* 284:65, 1971.

30. Deutsch, S., Goldberg, M., and Dripps, R. D. Postoperative hyponatremia with the inappropriate release of antidiuretic hormone. *Anesthesiology* 27:250, 1966.

31. Smith, M., et al. The clinical spectrum of renal cholesterol embolization. *Am. J. Med.* 71:174, 1981.

32. Andersen, G. H., et al. Effect of age on diagnostic usefulness of stimulated plasma renal activity and saralasin test in detection of renovascular hypertension. *Lancet* II:821, 1980.

33. Fawcett, I. W., et al. Nephrotic syndrome in the elderly. *Br. Med. J.* 2:387, 1971.

34. Lustig, S., et al. Nephrotic syndrome in the elderly. *Israel J. Med. Sci.* 18:1010, 1982.

35. Moorthy, A. V., and Zimmerman, S. W. Renal disease in the elderly: Clinopathologic analysis of renal disease in 115 elderly patients. *Clin. Nephrol.* 14:233, 1980.

36. Arieff, A., et al. Acute glomerulonephritis in the elderly. *Mod. Geriatr.* 3:77, 1973.

37. Boswell, D. C., and Eknoyan, G. Acute glomerulonephritis in the aged. *Geriatrics* 23:73, 1968.

38. Potvliege, P. R., DeRoy, G., and Dupuis, F. Necropsy study on glomerulonephritis in the elderly. *J. Clin. Pathol.* 28:891, 1975.

19

Urinary Incontinence—
A Treatable Disorder

Neil M. Resnick

URINARY INCONTINENCE IN THE ELDERLY is clearly a major problem—it is prevalent, morbid, costly, and neglected. The prevalence of incontinence depends on which segment of the elderly population one examines. At least one-third of community-dwelling American elderly have difficulty controlling their urine until they can get to a toilet, and nearly 10 percent soak their clothes or the floor weekly or more frequently [1,2]. In acute care settings, about one-third of individuals are afflicted [3,4], half of whom become so with the onset of acute illness [3]. Among institutionalized elderly, the prevalence of incontinence is approximately 50 percent [5]. Factors associated with incontinence include female sex, neurologic disease, and immobility, but surprisingly, neither age nor bacteriuria are independent risk factors [6].

The burden of incontinence is substantial and must be measured in medical, psychosocial, and economic terms. Medically, incontinent individuals are predisposed to perineal rashes, pressure sores, urinary tract infections, urosepsis, falls, and fractures. Another unappreciated complication is recurrent lower limb cellulitis, which occurs when incontinent individuals' shoes are chronically soaked by urine, become hardened, and abrade their feet; it is especially apt to occur in individuals with impaired peripheral sensation.

The psychosocial aspects of incontinence are also significant. Individuals are frequently embarrassed, isolated, stigmatized, depressed, and regressed; they are also predisposed to institutionalization, although to what extent remains undefined [7]. Economically, the costs of incontinence are startling. In America, over $8 billion was spent on incontinence in 1984 [8]. This figure exceeds the annual amount devoted to dialysis and coronary artery bypass surgery combined [6].

Despite its considerable prevalence, morbidity, and expense, however, incontinence remains a largely neglected problem. Only 20 percent of incontinent individuals consult a health care provider or agency. Sadly, when they do, only one physician in three will initiate even the most rudimentary evaluation [6]. This fact is unfortunate because incontinence is no more a part of normal aging than is chest pain, and, like chest pain, it is a symptom of a variety of underlying conditions. Moreover, several studies have documented that, regardless of the context in which it is found, incontinence is a highly treatable disorder: It is curable or virtually curable in two-thirds of patients and manageable in most of the rest [9–14].

This chapter reviews the basic aspects of urinary incontinence in the elderly. This review entails a brief discussion of the anatomy and physiology of the lower urinary tract, an examination of the impact that normal aging has on the urinary system, a theoretical consideration of what can go wrong, and a review of what does go wrong. This knowledge is used to formulate a targeted clinical evaluation of the incontinent individual and to propose a logical diagnostic and therapeutic approach.

Anatomy and Physiology

Details of the anatomy and physiology of normal micturition remain controversial [15]. For our purposes, however, we can simplify both. The anatomy of the lower urinary tract is easiest to conceptualize if it is considered in three sections: the bladder and its outlet, the local innervation, and the connections to the central nervous system.

The lower urinary tract comprises the urethral outlet and a muscular storage and contractile portion known as the detrusor. The proximal portion of the urethra is surrounded by a sphincter, known as the internal urethal sphincter. It is located in the region of the bladder neck, is predominantly smooth muscle, and is autonomically innervated. A few centimeters distal to this sphincter lies the external sphincter, which is composed of striated muscle and lies primarily in the mural portion of the urethra, at the level of the urogenital diaphragm.

The innervation of the lower urinary tract is derived from three sources: the parasympathetic (from S_2-S_4), the sympathetic (from $T_{10}-L_2$), and the somatic (voluntary) nervous systems (from S_2-S_4). The parasympathetic nervous system innervates the detrusor; increased cholinergic activity increases the force and frequency of detrusor contraction, while reduced activity has the opposite effect. The sympathetic nervous system innervates both the bladder and the urethra, with its effect determined by local receptors. Although adrenergic receptors are sparse in the bladder body, those normally present are beta receptors; their stimulation relaxes the bladder. Receptors at the base of the bladder and in the proximal urethra, on the other hand, are alpha receptors; their stimulation contracts the internal sphincter. Thus, activation of the sympathetic nervous system facilitates storage of urine in a coordinated manner. The somatic nervous system innervates the urogenital diaphragm and the ex-

ternal sphincter, although the external sphincter probably receives other innervation as well [16].

Storage of urine is mediated by detrusor relaxation and closure of the sphincters. Detrusor relaxation is accomplished by central nervous system inhibition of parasympathetic tone, while sphincter closure is mediated by a reflex increase in alpha-adrenergic and somatic activity. Voiding occurs when detrusor contraction, mediated by the parasympathetic nervous system, is coordinated with sphincter relaxation.

The Impact of Age on the Lower Urinary Tract

Normal aging affects the lower urinary tract in a variety of ways, but incontinence is not one of them. Although there is still a dearth of data and no longitudinal studies, several points emerge from cross-sectional studies. Bladder capacity, the ability to postpone voiding, bladder compliance, and urinary flow rate probably decline in both sexes, while maximum urethral closure pressure and urethral length probably decline in women [17]. The prevalence of uninhibited contractions probably increases with age, but there are few studies of younger individuals available for comparison [17]. Postvoiding residual volume may increase but probably to no more than 25 to 50 ml [17]. Another important age-related change is an alteration in the pattern of fluid excretion. Although younger individuals excrete the bulk of their daily ingested fluid before bedtime, many healthy elderly excrete the bulk of theirs during the night, even those individuals without peripheral venous insufficiency, renal disease, heart failure, or prostatism. Thus, one to two episodes of nocturia per night may be normal, especially if the pattern is long-standing and unchanged and other conditions have been excluded [17].

None of these age-related changes causes incontinence, however, since all are derived from studies of either asymptomatic or continent individuals. Nonetheless, each of these changes *predisposes* to incontinence. This predisposition, coupled with the increased likelihood that an older person will be subjected to additional pathologic, physiologic, or pharmacologic insults, underlies the higher incidence of inconti-

TABLE 19-1. *Common causes of transient incontinence*

D elirium/confusional state
I nfection—urinary (symptomatic)
A trophic urethritis/vaginitis
P harmaceuticals
   Sedative/hypnotics, especially long-acting agents
   "Loop" diuretics
   Anticholinergic agents (antipsychotic agents,
     antidepressants, antihistamines, anti-Parkinsonian
     agents, antiarrhythmics (disopyramide),
     antispasmodics, opiates, antidiarrheal agents)
   Alpha-adrenoceptor agonists and antagonists
   Calcium channel entry blockers
   Vincristine
P sychological, especially depression
E ndocrine (hypercalcemia, hyperglycemia)
R estricted mobility
S tool impaction

nence in the elderly. The corollary is equally important. The new onset or exacerbation of incontinence in an older person is likely to be due to a precipitant outside the lower urinary tract that is amenable to medical intervention. Treatment of the precipitant alone may be sufficient to restore continence. These principles provide a rationale for dividing the causes of incontinence in the elderly into transient and established categories.

Transient Incontinence

Transient incontinence is common in the elderly, affecting up to one-third of community-dwelling incontinent individuals [10] and up to half of hospitalized incontinent patients [3,9]. The causes can be recalled easily using the mnemonic DIAPPERS (misspelled with an extra P; Table 19-1) [18].

D is for delirium, a state of confusion characterized by acute or subacute onset as opposed to the insidious onset and slow progression of dementia. Delirium can result from virtually any drug or medical illness—including pneumonia, thrombophlebitis, or heart failure—or the pain associated with a fracture. Each of these underlying causes may present atypically and, if unrecognized, is associated with significant mortality. Incontinence in this setting is merely an associated symptom that will abate once the underlying cause of confusion is identified and treated. Thus, the patient needs medical rather than bladder management.

Symptomatic urinary tract *infection* causes transient incontinence when dysuria and urgency defeat the older person's ability to reach a nearby toilet. Asymptomatic infection, on the other hand, which is extraordinarily common in the elderly, is not a cause of incontinence [17,19].

Atrophic vaginitis is a common cause of transient incontinence [20]. It can present as urethral "scalding," dysuria, dyspareunia, urinary urgency, or urge or stress urinary incontinence. In demented individuals it may present as agitation. The symptoms are readily responsive to treatment with a low dose of estrogen, administered either orally (0.3 mg conjugated estrogen per day) or topically. The optimal route is unclear. Orally administered, estrogen has adverse hepatic-mediated effects but beneficial effects on blood lipids [21] and costs less than 10 cents per day. Applied intravaginally, estrogen is considerably more expensive and inconvenient; additionally, systemic levels equivalent to orally administered estrogen are attained, and the hepatic effect is not eliminated. More recently, estrogen has been given transcutaneously, but studies of its impact on atrophic vaginitis are not yet available. The transcutaneous route seems promising, however, because it requires application only twice weekly, and preliminary data suggest that it has beneficial effects on lipids without adverse hepatic effects [22]. Whichever route is chosen, symptoms may respond in as short a period as a few days or as long as six weeks. Although the duration of therapy has not been well established, we administer a low dose of estrogen on a daily basis for one to two months and then start to taper it. Eventually, most patients can probably be weaned to a dose as infrequent as two to four times per month; after six months, estrogen can be discontinued entirely in some patients, although recrudescence is common. Since the estrogen dose is low and is given briefly, its carcinogenic effect is probably slight, if present at all. In fact, the only adverse effect we have seen is mild and irregular vaginal bleeding in a small percentage of patients. However, if long-term treatment with estrogen is required, it probably should be cyclic and accompanied by a progestin if the patient still has a uterus. Mammography should probably be performed prior to its initiation. Of note, the dose of estrogen employed for treatment of atrophic vaginitis is substantially lower than that recommended by the National Institutes of Health for treatment of osteoporosis.

Pharmaceuticals are one of the most common causes of voiding dysfunction. Long-acting sedative hypnotics, such as diazepam and flurazepam, have longer half-lives in the elderly and thus may accumulate, inducing confusion and secondary incontinence [17]. Another sedative used by patients is alcohol, which both induces a diuresis and clouds the sensorium. "Loop" diuretics induce a brisk diuresis, which may overwhelm bladder capacity and result in incontinence. Vincristine can cause a partially reversible neuropathy associated with urinary retention [23].

Drugs with anticholinergic properties are in common use. Older patients often take several nonprescribed preparations for insomnia, coryza, pruritus, vertigo, and so on. Because three-quarters of the elderly use nonprescription agents [24], and because many do not regard them as "medicines" worth mentioning to their physicians, it is worth inquiring about such drugs directly. If the agents taken have anticholinergic effects, urinary retention and overflow incontinence may result.

Adrenergic agents also affect the lower urinary tract. Because the proximal urethra contains primarily alpha-adrenoreceptors, its tone can be decreased by alpha antagonists and increased by alpha agonists. Alpha antagonists make up much of modern medicine's antihypertensive armamentarium. When taken by an older woman, whose urethra has shortened and weakened with age, these drugs may precipitate stress incontinence. On the other hand, nonprescribed preparations containing alpha agonists (such as decongestants) may provoke acute retention in a man with otherwise asymptomatic prostatic enlargement, especially if the preparation additionally contains an antihistamine (anticholinergic). It is apparent that many nonprescription cold remedies are effectively, albeit inadvertently, formulated to cause lower urinary tract dysfunction in older men. In fact, a not uncommon cause of urinary retention occurs when an older man gets a cold and medicates himself with a multicomponent "cold" capsule, long-acting nosedrops, and a hypnotic (usually an antihistamine). How commonly this scenario results in an unnecessary or premature prostatectomy is unknown.

Calcium channel blockers reduce smooth muscle contractility throughout the body, and the bladder is no exception; they not infrequently induce urinary retention that is occasionally significant [17].

Psychologic causes of incontinence have not been well studied in the elderly but are probably much less common than in younger individuals. Intervention is properly directed at the psychologic disturbance, usually depression or lifelong neurosis. However, once the psychologic disturbance has been treated, persistent incontinence warrants further evaluation.

Endocrine causes of incontinence include those conditions that both cloud the sensorium and induce a diuresis, primarily hypercalcemia and hyperglycemia. Diabetes insipidus may also cause incontinence, albeit rarely.

Reduced mobility is a common characteristic contributing to incontinence in the elderly. It can result from arthritis, hip deformity, poor eyesight, inability to ambulate, or simply being tied to a bed or a chair. A careful search will often identify correctable causes of the impaired mobility. If not, a urinal or bedside commode may still improve or resolve the incontinence.

Stool impaction has been implicated as a cause of urinary incontinence in up to 10 percent of patients referred to incontinence clinics [17]. The mechanism is unknown, but patients usually present with either urge or overflow incontinence and typically have associated fecal incontinence as well. Disimpaction restores continence.

These eight reversible causes of incontinence should be assiduously sought in every elderly patient. In our series of hospitalized patients, most of those in whom incontinence developed in the context of acute illness became continent by the time of their discharge—invariably because one of these eight conditions was reversed [3]. Regardless of their frequency, however, their identification is important in all settings because they are easily treatable.

A case presentation may illustrate these points more effectively. An 80-year-old man was referred for evaluation of urinary incontinence.

He had been healthy until a year ago, when he noted progressive generalized stiffness and trouble in walking. He then fell, was hospitalized for a hip fracture, and subsequently developed pneumonia and confusion. The confusion was treated with haloperidol and the pneumonia with antibiotics. He was noted to be newly incontinent, and the incontinence persisted even after the pneumonia cleared. A urologist thought the prostate was palpably enlarged and suggested a prostatectomy, but the family refused. Awaiting placement in a nursing home, the patient remained on haloperidol. Physical examination revealed confusion, congestive heart failure, parkinsonism, a distended bladder, an enlarged prostate, and fecal impaction.

The etiology of his incontinence was multifactorial. During the prior year he had developed Parkinson's disease, which limited his mobility, was the cause of his fall, and was exacerbated by haloperidol. The anticholinergic effect of haloperidol also contributed to fecal impaction and urinary retention. Congestive heart failure, as well as the discomfort of urinary retention and fecal impaction, and the anticholinergic effect of haloperidol, all led to his becoming confused. Obviously, the role played by his prostate could not yet be determined, especially since the size of the prostate as palpated rectally correlates poorly with the presence of outlet obstruction [18,25].

Therefore, he was disimpacted and diuresed, haloperidol was discontinued, the bladder was drained, physical therapy was begun, and fiber was added to his diet. L-Dopa/carbidopa (Sinemet) was initiated because moderately severe Parkinson's disease had preceded treatment with haloperidol. Within two weeks, the stigmata of Parkinson's disease subsided, bowel movements became regular, exercise tolerance increased, ambulation improved, and incontinence resolved; the postvoiding residual was 10 ml, and prostatectomy was deferred. He remains dry and asymptomatic a year later.

Established Incontinence

If leakage persists after transient causes of incontinence have been addressed, the more established causes (Table 19-2) must be consid-

TABLE 19-2. *Common causes of established incontinence*

Detrusor overactivity
  Neurogenic causes (stroke, Parkinson's disease, Alzheimer's disease)
  Nonneurogenic causes (bladder carcinoma/carcinoma in situ, cystitis, urethral obstruction/incompetence)
Detrusor underactivity
  Neurogenic (disk compression, plexopathy, surgical damage [anteroposterior resection], autonomic neuropathy [e.g., diabetes mellitus])
  Nonneurogenic (sequelae of outlet obstruction, idiopathic)
Outlet incompetence
  Neurogenic (surgical lesion—rare)
  Nonneurogenic (urethral hypermobility due to pelvic floor laxity, sphincter damage [type 3 stress incontinence] due to fibrosis from prior "suspension" operations)
Outlet obstruction
  Neurogenic (detrusor-sphincter dyssynergia in spinal cord disease)
  Nonneurogenic (prostatic enlargement/urethral stricture in men; large cystourethrocele/distal urethral stenosis in women [uncommon])

ered. These causes comprise dysfunction of the bladder, the outlet, or both.

The lower urinary tract can malfunction in only four ways, two of which involve the bladder and two of which involve the outlet: The bladder either contracts when it should not (detrusor overactivity) or fails to contract when or as well as it should (detrusor underactivity), or the outlet resistance is high when it should be low (obstruction) or low when it should be high (outlet incompetence). Since incontinence in older individuals is frequently due to a cause other than the classic types of "neurogenic bladder" [26] it is probably better to think of the causes of incontinence in terms of the four pathophysiologic mechanisms just mentioned and to realize that each mechanism has a set of "neurogenic" as well as "nonneurogenic" causes (Table 19-2). This section provides an overview of the four basic mechanisms and their causes; a later section provides more clinical details and treatment strategies for each.

Detrusor overactivity is a condition in which the bladder contracts precipitously, with little warning, and usually empties itself completely. Recently, detrusor overactivity has been shown to exist as two physiologic subsets: one in which contractile function is preserved and one in which it is impaired. The latter condition has been termed *detrusor hyperactivity* with impaired contractile function (DHIC) [27] and is discussed below under Cystometry.

Detrusor overactivity presents clinically as urge incontinence. It may result from damage to the central nervous system inhibitory centers due to a stroke, Alzheimer's disease, or Parkinson's disease. Alternatively, the cause may be in the urinary tract itself, where a source of irritation—such as cystitis (interstitial, radiation- or chemotherapy induced), a bladder tumor, or a stone—overwhelms the ability of even a normal brain to inhibit bladder contraction. Two other important local causes are outlet obstruction and outlet incompetence, both of which may lead to secondary detrusor overactivity [28,29].

Detrusor underactivity may be caused by damage to the nerves supplying the bladder, which may be due to disk compression or tumor involvement, or to the autonomic neuropathy of diabetes, pernicious anemia, alcoholism, or tabes dorsalis. Alternatively, the bladder muscle may be replaced by fibrosis and connective tissue, as occurs in men who have chronic outlet obstruction, so that even when the obstruction

is removed, the bladder fails to empty normally. Detrusor replacement by fibrosis may also occur in women, but the cause is unknown.

Outlet incompetence is caused most often by pelvic floor laxity, which results in "urethral hypermobility" and allows the proximal urethra and bladder neck to "herniate" through the urogenital diaphragm when abdominal pressure increases. Such herniation results in unequal transmission of abdominal pressure to the bladder and urethra and consequent stress incontinence (Fig. 19-1). A less common cause of outlet incontinence is "sphincter incompetence," in which the sphincter is so weak that merely the hydrostatic weight of a full bladder overcomes outlet resistance. This condition is known as type 3 stress incontinence [31]. In the elderly it generally results from diabetes or surgically induced periurethral fibrosis, but occasionally no precipitant is identified.

Outlet obstruction is the final established cause of incontinence. If due to neurologic disease, it is invariably associated with spinal cord damage. In this situation, pathways that normally coordinate outlet opening with bladder contraction are interrupted. As a result, rather than relaxing when the bladder contracts, the outlet actually contracts simultaneously, leading to severe outlet obstruction, hydronephrosis, and renal failure—a condition termed detrusor-sphincter dyssynergia. Alternatively, and much more commonly, obstruction results from prostatic enlargement or urethal stricture in men; anatomic obstruction is uncommon in

FIGURE 19-1. *Pathophysiology of stress incontinence (SUI) due to urethral hypermobility. Normally, resting urethral pressure is greater than bladder pressure; with a stress maneuver (such as coughing, straining, laughing, or bending over), the increase in abdominal pressure is transmitted equally to the bladder and the outlet, and the individual remains dry. In the woman with urethral hypermobility, however, the proximal urethra "herniates" through the urogenital diaphragm (UGD) into the pelvis with a stress maneuver. Since abdominal pressure is no longer transmitted equally, instantaneous leakage occurs.*

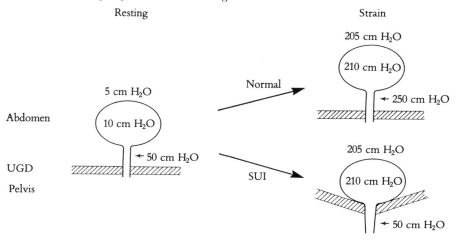

women in the absence of a large cystocele, which can prolapse and kink the urethra if the patient augments voiding by the use of abdominal straining.

Clinically, it is useful to rearrange these four basic pathophysiologic mechanisms into two categories: disorders of storage (detrusor overactivity or outlet incompetence), in which the bladder empties at inappropriate times, and disorders of evacuation (detrusor underactivity or outlet obstruction), in which the bladder empties incompletely, leading to progressive urine accumulation and overflow. In the first category, the bladder is normal in size; in the second, it is distended.

Clinical Evaluation

HISTORY

The first step in clinical evaluation (Table 19-3) is to characterize the patient's usual voiding pattern and determine if symptoms of abnormal voiding, such as straining to void or a sense of incomplete emptying, are present. One must be

TABLE 19-3. *Clinical evaluation of the incontinent patient*

History
    Type (urge, reflex, stress, overflow, mixed)
    Frequency, severity, duration
    Pattern (diurnal, nocturnal, or both; following
        medications, etc.)
    Associated symptoms (straining to void, incomplete
        emptying, dysuria)
    Other relevant factors (cancer, diabetes, acute illness,
        neurologic disease, pelvic or lower urinary tract
        surgery)
    Medications, including non-prescription agents
Physical examination
    Test for stress-induced leakage with bladder full
    Observe/listen to void
    Palpate for bladder distention after voiding
    Pelvic examination (atrophic vaginitis/urethritis; pelvic
        floor laxity; pelvic mass)
    Rectal examination (resting tone and voluntary control
        of anal sphincter; prostate nodules; fecal impaction)
    Neurologic examination (mental status and elemental
        examination, including sacral reflexes and perineal
        sensation)
Initial investigation
    Metabolic survey (electrolytes, calcium, glucose, urea
        nitrogen)
    Urinalysis and culture
    Incontinence chart
    Postvoid residual volume

careful in eliciting these symptoms, however, since many elderly people strain at the end of voiding to empty the last few drops; these individuals often report incomplete bladder emptying because the final few drops are passed after voiding has ceased. On the other hand, many patients have been straining for so long that they fail to acknowledge it. Thus, additional observations by the physician and family members are extremely useful.

One then elicits a detailed description of the incontinence, focusing on its onset, frequency, severity, pattern, precipitants, palliating features, and associated symptoms and conditions [32]. It is also helpful to know if the patient leaks at night. Generally, individuals with detrusor overactivity gush intermittently both day and night. Individuals with pure stress incontinence, on the other hand, are usually dry at night because they are in the supine position and are not straining. However, individuals with type 3 stress incontinence, especially those who also have a poorly compliant bladder, may leak only at night if they allow their bladder to fill to a volume greater than their weakened outlet can withstand. These individuals may admit to postural-related dribbling as well, leaking continually while sitting or standing.

Prostatism is another symptom complex worth additional comment. Regardless of whether the patient has "irritative" or "obstructive" symptoms, the physician can easily be misled. Several investigators have found that about one-third of patients referred for operative treatment of prostatism actually have an abnormality other than obstruction that is the cause of the incontinence [33,34]. Usually the abnormality is an overactive detrusor, which, if unaccompanied by outlet obstruction, may be exacerbated by operative intervention [35]. Thus, symptoms are a clue to the diagnosis of obstruction but alone are insufficiently specific to confirm it.

VOIDING RECORD

One of the most helpful parts of the history is the voiding record kept by the patient, family, or nursing staff. These charts note the time of each void or leakage at two-hour intervals for a 48-hour period. Although many incontinence records have been proposed, few have been ade-

Time ?	Wet or dry?	How wet? (mild, moderate, severe?)	Amount voided?	Comments
8 AM	W	Severe	10 oz	On way to bathroom
10 AM	D	—	6 oz	Voided before going out
12 noon	D	—	—	
2 PM	W	Moderate	9 oz	Choked and coughed

FIGURE 19-2. *Sample voiding record. Instructions for filling it out should be given to the responsible person. The record should be reviewed by the physician with the patient (see text).*

quately tested. A sample of our record is shown in Figure 19-2.

To record the volume voided, an individual at home can use a measuring cup, coffee can, pickle jar, or other large container. Information regarding the volume voided provides an index of an individual's functional bladder capacity and, together with the pattern of voiding and leakage, can be quite helpful in pointing to the cause of the leakage. For example, incontinence that occurs only between 8 A.M. and noon may be caused by a morning diuretic. If a chairfast man with congestive heart failure wets himself each half hour at night but remains dry during a four-hour daytime nap in his wheelchair, the problem is probably not prostatic enlargement but rather the postural diuresis associated with his heart failure [18]. One woman's chart showed a single episode of leakage each day, always at 1 A.M. Closer questioning revealed her regular use of a "nightcap" to induce sleep!

The information gathered from the history and voiding record permits characterization of the incontinence as *urge,* in which precipitant leakage of a large volume is preceded by a brief warning of seconds to minutes; *reflex,* in which precipitant leakage is not preceded by a warning; *stress,* in which leakage occurs coincident with, and only in association with, increases in abdominal pressure; *overflow,* in which continual dribbling occurs; and *mixed,* which is usually a combination of urge and stress [30]. Each of these types correlates fairly well with the pathophysiologic mechanisms already mentioned: urge and reflex with detrusor overactivity, stress with an incompetent outlet, overflow with outlet obstruction or detrusor underac-

tivity, and mixed with both an overactive detrusor and an incompetent outlet.

PHYSICAL EXAMINATION

The examination should check for signs of neurologic disease—such as delirium, dementia, stroke, Parkinson's disease, cord compression, and neuropathy (autonomic or peripheral)—as well as for general medical illnesses such as heart failure and peripheral edema. Additionally, one should check for bladder distention (pointing to an evacuation disorder) and stress leakage. The latter is assessed by asking the patient, whose bladder should be full, to assume a position as close to upright as possible, to relax, spread her legs, and cough. The diagnosis of stress incontinence can be missed if any of these maneuvers is omitted. If leakage occurs, it is also important to note whether it occurs coincident with the stress maneuver or is delayed for more than 5 to 10 seconds. If delayed, such leakage suggests detrusor overactivity (triggered by coughing) rather than outlet incompetence.

The rectal examination checks for fecal impaction and masses. It is less important to assess the size of the prostate because, as determined by palpation, it correlates poorly with the presence or absence of outlet obstruction [18,25]. The remainder of the rectal examination is actually a detailed neurologic examination because the same sacral roots (S_2-S_4) innervate both the external urethral and the anal sphincters. One assesses the afferent supply by testing perineal sensation. To assess motor innervation, one asks the patient to contract and relax the anal sphincter volitionally. Many neurologically unimpaired elderly patients are unable to do so; if they can, however, it is strong evidence against a cord lesion. One can assess motor innervation further by testing the anal wink and bulbocavernosus reflexes (Fig. 19-3). Although ab-

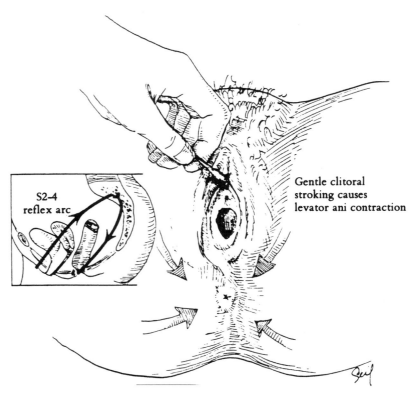

S2–4
reflex arc

Gentle clitoral
stroking causes
levator ani contraction

FIGURE 19-3. *Bulbocavernosus reflex. Determination of integrity of the sacral cord reflex arc (S_1–S_4). (From J. A. Fantl. Clinical Investigation of the Lower Urinary Tract—Urodynamic Studies. In W. G. Slate (ed.), Disorders of the Female Urethra and Urinary Incontinence [2nd ed.]. © 1982 The Williams & Wilkins Co., Baltimore.)*

normal, the absence of these reflexes is not necessarily pathologic, however, nor does their presence exclude an underactive detrusor (due to a diabetic neuropathy, for example).

In women one should check for pelvic floor laxity (cystocele, rectocele, enterocele, uterine prolapse) and pelvic masses. After removing one blade of the vaginal speculum (or using a Sims speculum), one checks for laxity by sequentially applying the remaining blade to the anterior and posterior vaginal walls and asking the patient to cough. If bulging of the anterior wall is detected when the posterior wall is stabilized, a cystocele is present; conversely, if bulging of the posterior wall is detected, a rectocele is present. Although the extent of pelvic floor laxity may be underestimated if the patient is checked in only the supine position, the presence of laxity can usually be determined in any position. It is important to realize, however, that the presence or absence of pelvic floor laxity reveals little about the cause of an individual's leakage. Detrusor overactivity may exist in addition to a cystocele, and stress incontinence may exist in the absence of a cystocele.

Thus, knowledge of pelvic floor muscle strength is useful primarily in informing the surgeon's choice of operation. The one exception to this statement occurs in the woman with a large cystocele: Descent of the cystocele may kink the urethra and cause outlet obstruction.

Atrophic vaginitis must also be sought. It is characterized by mucosal friability, petechiae, telangiectasia, and vaginal erosions [20]; loss of rugal folds and the presence of a thin, shiny-appearing mucosa are signs of vaginal atrophy rather than atrophic vaginitis. The bimanual examination excludes pelvic masses.

Two other tests should be mentioned. The first is the Q-tip test, in which a lubricated, sterile cotton swab is inserted into the urethra, and the patient is then asked to strain abdominally. The change in Q-tip angle is measured and used as an index of pelvic floor laxity [36].

As pointed out earlier, however, pelvic floor laxity is of little value in determining the cause of a patient's leakage, and hence the utility of this test is limited. The second test is the Bonney (or Marshall) test. If stress leakage coincident with abdominal straining is detected, the Bonney test can determine whether such leakage can be prevented by stabilizing the bladder base, thereby preventing its herniation through the urogenital diaphragm [37]. This stabilization is accomplished by placing two fingers in the lateral vaginal fornices and asking the patient to cough again. Urethral hypermobility is considered present if leakage is prevented. However, the value of this test is also limited in the elderly. Vaginal stenosis is common in the elderly and may lead to a false-positive result by precluding accurate finger placement; if one's fingers are not placed far enough laterally, they may occlude the bladder outlet rather than stabilizing it, preventing leakage even in a patient with detrusor instability. Furthermore, even if the test is correctly performed, a false-positive result may occur if the first episode of leakage was due to a cough-induced detrusor contraction, which, having emptied the bladder, does not recur during the Bonney test. A final caveat: The patient should not be asked to strain if she has a strong urge to void because the urge may be due to an uninhibited contraction. If the contraction is accompanied by physiologic sphincter relaxation and the patient then coughs, leakage will occur instantaneously, prompting the physician to misdiagnose a detrusor abnormality as outlet incompetence. Finally, if stress testing provokes delayed leakage of a large amount, suggesting detrusor overactivity, the patient should be asked to interrupt the stream. If she is able to do so, it probably augurs well for bladder retraining.

The examination concludes when the patient voids into a toilet (equipped with a receptacle) and is catheterized for a postvoiding residual volume (PVR) test. Adding the PVR to the voided volume provides an estimate of total bladder capacity and a crude assessment of bladder proprioception. A PVR of more than 50 to 100 ml suggests either bladder weakness or outlet obstruction, but smaller values do not exclude either diagnosis, especially if the patient

strained during the void. Thus, it is important to observe or listen to the voided stream. If straining is observed, one must ask the patient whether she is using her usual voiding technique and must take this fact into account when interpreting the PVR. A urine sample is then sent for urinalysis and culture.

Although the literature is replete with statements and uncontrolled studies asserting that "the bladder is an unreliable witness" and that the history is an unreliable guide to the cause of incontinence, our experience differs. In a prospective and blinded study, we recently found that the clinical evaluation correctly predicted the urodynamically determined cause of leakage in over 90 percent of cases [38]. The discrepancy between our experience and that of others may arise because we do not rely on any single symptom or sign. Rather, we dissect each symptom for its full diagnostic significance, and we integrate information from the history with that from the voiding record, physical examination, the observed void, and the PVR determination. Furthermore, even in nursing home patients, an algorithmic approach—relying only on information obtainable at the bedside by a nurse—has yielded the correct diagnosis in 83 percent of cases and correctly guided treatment in 93 percent [39]. Therefore, although the specificity of a given symptom may be low, we believe that an informed, carefully performed, and comprehensive clinical evaluation can determine the cause of incontinence most of the time.

URODYNAMIC EVALUATION

If the cause of the patient's incontinence still cannot be determined, urodynamic evaluation is the next step. Although some investigators have proposed "bedside testing" [40,41], no data are yet available to evaluate its performance in the 10 to 20 percent of patients whose diagnosis has eluded clinical evaluation. Since these "bedside tests" require additional time, expertise, equipment, and cost, and since they have not been evaluated in debilitated elderly, their role remains unclear at present.

Urodynamic testing, on the other hand, has been used in debilitated elderly and has proved feasible, safe, and reproducible [42]. It is probably warranted when diagnostic uncertainty may affect therapy; when the morbidity associated with potentially misdirected empiric therapy is high; when empiric therapy has failed; when surgical intervention is planned; and when the patient has overflow incontinence, to exclude obstruction [6].

Urodynamic testing consists of a battery of tests. It is difficult to know in advance what to include in the battery, however, and therefore only a physician conversant with the pathophysiology of incontinence should perform the evaluation. Generally, the evaluation includes simultaneous measurement of bladder, urethral, and rectal pressures during the filling and emptying phases of the micturition cycle. Optimally, the study is fluoroscopically monitored, and periurethral electromyography may occasionally be required. Some of the more commonly used tests are described below.

Cystometry

Cystometry (CMG) evaluates bladder proprioception, compliance, capacity, and stability (in regard to detrusor overactivity). It assesses only the bladder—not the outlet—and only during filling, not voiding. Therefore, it yields only one-fourth of the information needed to establish a diagnosis. It is performed by inserting a catheter into the bladder, filling it with gas or fluid, and plotting the bladder's pressure response to increasing volume. Artifacts are common, especially in the elderly, but they can be minimized by having the test performed by a knowledgeable physician (not a technician), by infusing fluid rather than gas, by using moderate infusion rates rather than rapid ones (100 ml per minute), by using fluoroscopy, and by measuring abdominal and bladder pressures simultaneously to differentiate rises in bladder pressure from rises in abdominal pressure.

Uninhibited contractions are phasic bladder contractions and are usually seen easily. They may be missed, however, especially in patients in whom detrusor hyperactivity coexists with detrusor weakness (DHIC) [27]. In these patients, detrusor contraction pressure may rise only 2 to 6 cm H_2O. Because DHIC is the most common cause of incontinence in nursing home patients and because it is easily missed, it can be a great mimic, masquerading variously as "re-flex urethral instability," stress incontinence, and outlet obstruction [26]. For instance, if the low-pressure uninhibited contraction is missed cystometrically, physiologic relaxation of the urethral sphincter may be misdiagnosed as "urethral instability." If the low-pressure contraction coincides with a stress maneuver, co-incident leakage may be misdiagnosed as stress incontinence. And since the symptoms, flow rate, and postvoid residual of DHIC are all similar to those seen in prostatism, a man with DHIC may easily be misdiagnosed as having a prostatic obstruction. The first two mistakes can be avoided by fluoroscopically monitoring the urodynamic evaluation, since a bladder contraction will be seen to coincide with leakage. DHIC can be distinguished from obstruction by the use of pressure/flow studies and micturitional urethral pressure profilometry (MUPP), as described below. If these tools are unavailable, however, the distinction can be quite difficult. We are currently devising ways to simplify the diagnosis of DHIC, examining the importance of the distinction, and exploring whether DHIC will exacerbate or simplify our ability to treat detrusor hyperreflexia.

Urethral Profilometry (Resting and Dynamic)

There are two types of profilometry, depending on whether urethral pressure is measured during bladder filling or bladder contraction. The first is called urethral closure pressure profilometry (UCPP), and the second is known as micturitional urethral pressure profilometry (MUPP). UCPP is performed by inserting a catheter into the bladder, slowly withdrawing it through the urethra, and plotting urethral pressure at each point [43]. Using this trace one measures urethral anatomic length, functional length, maximum urethral pressure, maximum urethral closure pressure (urethral pressure minus bladder pressure), and (in males) the length and height of the prostatic area. Although there is a correlation between the presence of stress incontinence and both the strength of the urethral sphincter and the length of the urethra, the values overlap substantially, reducing the utility of these parameters in the individual patient. Similarly, values obtained for prostatic length and area are of limited value. Nonetheless, UCPP is occasionally useful for testing the bulbocavernosus reflex and for fluid bridge testing; the latter is an extremely sensitive test for stress incontinence [44,45]. Additionally, UCPP will help differentiate stress incontinence due to urethral sphincter weakness from that due to urethral hypermobility; in the former the urethral pressure is low, whereas in the latter it is normal [31].

Urethral profilometry is also used to exclude detrusor-sphincter dyssynergia. Generally, only the distal urethral sphincter is evaluated; normally it should relax just prior to or coincident with detrusor contraction. The response of the smooth muscle sphincter is more complex and is reviewed elsewhere [46].

MUPP is quite useful for evaluating incontinent men [47]. It is performed by withdrawing the catheter through the urethra as the patient voids. Its interpretation is based on the principle that urethral pressure proximal to the membranous urethra should equal bladder pressure during voiding. In the setting of a urethral obstruction, however, the pressure distal to the obstruction will be much lower than bladder pressure. If an obstruction is detected, fluoroscopy will allow one to localize the site. MUPP is more accurate than cystoscopy for determining the presence of an obstruction and judging its severity.

Uroflowmetry

Uroflowmetry is used as a screening test for obstruction, although when used in this manner it is probably analogous to relying on a blood pressure measurement to determine the presence of critical aortic stenosis. The flow rate depends not only on the presence of an outlet obstruction but also on the strength of detrusor contractions. To interpret the test, one must know the voided volume, the residual volume, whether the void was augmented by abdominal straining, the peak and mean flow rates, and the configuration of the accompanying trace. Interrupted and oscillatory patterns suggest abdominal straining or outlet obstruction. Although age-related norms have been devised to aid interpretation of the test, one should realize that the studies on which they are based are significantly flawed and include few patients over age 70 [17]. Thus, the ability of isolated uroflowmetric test to differentiate obstructed from unobstructed elderly males remains undefined. One can, however, derive some information from it. In the older man with symptoms of prostatism, a normal flow rate—in the absence of a Valsalva maneuver and with a PVR of less than 50 ml—probably allows exclusion of clinically significant outlet obstruction. On the other hand, when performed in conjunction with a full urodynamic evaluation, uroflowmetry is quite helpful in assessing detrusor contractility and detecting the presence of obstruction.

Electromyography

Electromyography (EMG) [48] is used to evaluate the distal urethral sphincter by determining the integrity of its innervation; testing its response to reflex stimuli (such as bladder filling [guarding reflex] and bulbocavernosus stimulation), and characterizing its behavior during voiding. A variety of techniques are available for performing EMG, including employment of surface or needle electrodes, recording the response of single or multiple nerve fibers, and evaluating the nerve supply to the urethral sphincter or the pelvic floor musculature (through vaginal, anal, or perineal probes). In the most accurate approach a needle electrode is inserted directly into the distal urethral sphincter. Although most elderly patients can tolerate EMG performed in this fashion, the results can be difficult to interpret (e.g., a few polyphasic potentials in a 90-year-old may or may not be really abnormal), the equipment is expensive, and, if urodynamic evaluation is performed as already detailed, EMG adds little new information. If fluoroscopically monitored multichannel urodynamic capability is not available, however, EMG is useful. Unfortunately, in these situations only surface or anal EMG is usually performed. Since these techniques yield results fraught with artifact, they should be interpreted with caution.

Radiographic Evaluation

Optimally, radiographic and urodynamic evaluations are performed simultaneously, allowing correlation of visual and manometric information. If this is not feasible, substantial information can still be gleaned from cystography. A full evaluation includes posterior-anterior and oblique (or lateral) views of the bladder, at rest and during straining and voiding. These films will reveal bladder trabeculation, diverticula, masses, bladder neck competence, and ureteral reflux. Although the urethrovesical angle and axis are also generally measured, the reliability and relevance of these measurements are controversial [49]. The voiding films allow one to check for outlet obstruction. Postvoiding residual volume can also be assessed radiographically, but there are pitfalls. Elderly patients are frequently rushed through busy radiography departments and may feel too inhibited to void to completion; the radiologist, who may have been absent during the examination, may then erroneously conclude that the residual volume is elevated. Conversely, a low volume does not exclude a weak bladder if the patient augmented the void using the Valsalva maneuver. Therefore, the radiographer should be viewed as a partner in the evaluation rather than being asked to read films blindly after the examination is completed.

The precise role of urodynamic testing in the evaluation of the incontinent elderly individual remains to be determined. Although it pinpoints pathologic abnormalities, it may not identify which of the abnormalities actually causes the patient's incontinence unless it is performed by a trained urodynamicist and incorporated into the overall clinical evaluation.

Whatever its role, however, urodynamic evaluation of elderly patients is reproducible, safe, and feasible to perform, even in frail and debilitated individuals. In our series of over 100 consecutively evaluated nursing home patients, whose mean age was 88 and all of whom received prophylactic antibiotics, we induced only three cases of asymptomatic bacteriuria; no cases of urosepsis, pyelonephritis, endocarditis, or cardiac ischemia were observed. All but two patients were able to complete the examination at one sitting, and the original diagnosis was confirmed in all 21 cases in which the examination was repeated. It must be emphasized, however, that an extra person was employed whose sole job was to explain the procedure and comfort the patient during the test. Several modifications in the urodynamic suite were made as well [38, 42].

Treatment

DETRUSOR OVERACTIVITY

Detrusor overactivity is characterized by frequent periodic voiding; the patient is generally dry between voids. Leakage is moderate to large in volume, nocturnal frequency and incontinence are common, sacral sensation and reflexes are preserved, voluntary control of the anal sphincter is intact, and the postvoiding residual volume is generally low. A residual volume in excess of 50 ml in a patient with detrusor overactivity suggests outlet obstruction (although the residual may be nil in early obstruction), DHIC, or puddling of urine in a cystocele. It is also found in patients with Parkinson's disease or spinal cord injury [27].

Initial management involves identification and treatment of reversible causes. Suspicion of a spinal cord disorder (an appropriate history and/or the finding of a dermatomal sensory "level") warrants a complete neurourologic evaluation. Sterile hematuria, if present, must be evaluated to exclude bladder stone, carcinoma in situ, or carcinoma. Uroflowmetry, if available, can detect important outlet obstruction, as described above.

It cannot be overemphasized that obstruction and stress incontinence may cause *secondary* detrusor overactivity that will remit with correction of the outlet abnormality [28,29]. Failure to evaluate the outlet may not only cause the patient harm (e.g., by prescribing an anticholinergic agent to an obstructed patient) but will also lead to overlooking easily correctable incontinence. Obstruction and stress incontinence are common in the elderly, including frail and cognitively impaired individuals [26]. With recent advances in surgical technique, correction of outlet abnormalities is now potentially feasible even in these patients [17,26]. Thus, evaluation of the outlet is critically important.

Unfortunately, however, many of the causes of detrusor overactivity are not amenable to specific therapy, or a cause may not be found. Treatment must then be symptomatic. Simple measures such as providing a bedside commode or urinal and asking the patient to void more frequently are often successful. Toileting regimens, based on analysis of the incontinence chart, are also beneficial, even in patients with advanced cognitive impairment [50,51]. For the demented patient, the technique known as prompted voiding is used. One uses the incontinence chart to predict when leakage is likely to occur and escorts the patient to the bathroom in advance. Positive reinforcement is also used, but negative reinforcement is not employed. A blinded controlled study conducted in two nursing homes found nearly a 50 percent decrease in incontinence in the first day of using the technique in this manner, a decrease that persisted as long as the technique was utilized [12]. Techniques such as behavior modification in less mentally impaired patients permit the interval between voidings to be progressively lengthened. For instance, if the incontinence chart reveals that the patient is wet every three hours, one then asks the patient to void every two hours. If the patient is able to remain dry for three consecutive days using this regime, the interval is lengthened by ½ hour, and the process is repeated. One need not ask patients to get up to void at night; once they are dry during the day, they are generally dry at night as well. Biofeedback may be added to this regimen, but its marginal benefit is unclear.

Pharmacologic intervention can be added, although there is a dearth of data regarding efficacy and toxicity in this population, and comparative or controlled trials are rare [17]. Smooth muscle relaxants, such as flavoxate (300 to 800 mg per day) and calcium channel blockers have been used, as have anticholinergic agents such as propantheline (15 to 120 mg per day). Oxybutynin (5 to 20 mg per day), combining both smooth muscle relaxant and anticholinergic properties, and imipramine (50 to 150 mg per day), whose mechanism of action is more complex, are also frequently successful. All these drugs are given in divided doses. The decision regarding which drug to employ is often based on factors unrelated to bladder function [17]. In the incontinent patient with dementia or the patient taking other anticholinergic agents, propantheline is best avoided. In the patient with associated hypertension, angina pectoris, or abnormalities of cardiac diastolic relaxation, a calcium channel-blocking agent may be preferred. Orthostatic hypotension, common in the elderly, often precludes the use of imipramine and nifedipine and should be watched for if these agents are used. Occasionally, combining low doses of two agents with complementary actions, such as oxybutynin and imipramine, will maximize benefit and minimize side effects. Medications with a rapid onset of action (such as oxybutynin) can be employed prophylactically if incontinence occurs at predictable times. But regardless of which medication is used, postvoiding residual volume and common indexes of renal function (blood urea nitrogen, serum creatinine, and urine output) should be monitored, since urinary retention may develop. On the other hand, inducing urinary retention and using intermittent catheterization may be a viable approach for patients whose incontinence defies other remedies (such as those with DHIC) and for whom intermittent catheterization is feasible.

Other remedies for urge incontinence, including electrical stimulation, bladder distention, and selective nerve blocks, are less widely used, although some are quite successful in selected situations. For instance, McGuire et al. developed an innovative approach using intermittent bilateral transcutaneous stimulation of the peroneal or posterior tibial nerve, with promising preliminary results [52].

Adjunctive measures, such as pads and special undergarments, are invaluable if incontinence proves refractory, and a wide variety of these are now available, allowing the recommendation to be tailored to the individual's problem. For instance, for bedridden individuals a launderable bedpad may be preferable [53], whereas for those with a stroke, a diaper or pant that can be opened using the good hand may be preferred. For ambulatory patients with large gushes of incontinence, a wood pulp-containing product is generally preferable to those containing a polymer gel, since the polymer gel generally cannot absorb the large amount of rapid flow these individuals produce, whereas the wood pulp product can easily be doubled up if necessary. Optimal products for men and women also differ because of the location of the "target zone." Finally, one must know whether the patient has fecal incontinence as well in order to choose the most appropriate product [9,53].

Condom catheters are helpful for men, although they are associated with skin breakdown and often a decreased motivation to become dry. A satisfactory external collecting device has not yet been devised for women, especially for elderly women in whom the problem is further complicated by the high prevalence of atrophic vaginitis and vaginal stenosis. In-dwelling urethral catheters are not recommended for this condition because they usually exacerbate detrusor overactivity. If they must be used (e.g., to allow healing of a pressure sore in a patient with refractory detrusor overactivity), a small catheter with a small balloon is preferable to minimize irritability and consequent "leakage around the catheter." Such leakage almost invariably results from bladder "spasm," not a catheter that is too small. Increasing the size of the catheter and balloon only aggravates the problem, and, over time, may result in progressive urethral erosion and sphincter incompetence. If "bladder spasm" persists, agents such as oxybutynin can be employed. Especially in the elderly, alternative agents with more potent anticholinergic side effects (e.g., belladonna suppositories) should be avoided.

Stress Incontinence

Involuntary leakage that occurs only during stress is common in elderly women but is uncommon in men unless the sphincter has been damaged during surgery. The definition excludes overflow incontinence, which, although exacerbated by stress, occurs at other times as well and is associated with bladder distention. Typical stress incontinence is characterized by daytime loss of small to moderate amounts of urine, infrequent nocturnal incontinence, and a low postvoiding residual volume in the absence of urine puddling in a large cystocele. The sine qua non of the diagnosis is leakage that, in the absence of bladder distention, occurs *simultaneously* with the stress maneuver. The usual cause is "urethral hypermobility" due to pelvic floor laxity (Fig. 19-1), but other conditions must be considered. These include intrinsic "sphincter incompetence" (type 3 stress incontinence) [31], stress–induced detrusor overactivity, and urethral instability [54].

Sphincter incompetence (type 3 stress incontinence) was described above. One should realize that the term is actually a misnomer because if the weight of urine in the bladder exceeds the

ability of the sphincter to retain it leakage can occur even when the patient sits quietly, which is a helpful diagnostic point.

Stress-induced detrusor instability is merely an uninhibited bladder contraction triggered by stress maneuvers. These uninhibited contractions usually occur at other times as well, giving rise to urgency, frequency, nocturia, urge incontinence, and nocturnal incontinence. The key point is to assess the integrity of the outlet as described earlier. If it is competent, then the problem is detrusor-mediated and should be treated as detrusor overactivity. If the outlet is incompetent, then the patient has either stress incontinence or mixed incontinence (see below) and should be treated as such.

Urethral instability occurs when the sphincter abruptly and paradoxically relaxes in the absence of a detrusor contraction [54]. In our experience this condition is rare in the elderly. In fact, it may be less common than believed in younger individuals as well, since most investigators have failed to use fluoroscopic monitoring. This omission may lead one to miss an uninhibited contraction (DHIC) and mistakenly identify the accompanying physiologic sphincter relaxation as a pathologic sphincter abnormality [26].

The most common cause of stress incontinence, however, is urethral hypermobility, which is improved by weight loss if the patient is obese, by therapy of precipitating conditions such as coughing or atrophic vaginitis, and occasionally by insertion of a pessary [55]. Pelvic floor muscle exercises are time-honored and frequently effective [17,51,56], especially if they are combined with orally or topically administered estrogen. The patient is instructed to sit on the toilet and begin voiding. Once voiding has started, the patient is asked to interrupt the stream by contracting the sphincter for as long as possible. Initially, most elderly women are able to do so for no more than a second or two, but after a few weeks, many can prolong the duration of the contraction. Once the patient recognizes which muscle to contract, she can do the exercises at any time and during any activity. The optimal regimen remains to be determined. We advise patients to increase the duration of muscle contraction to about ten seconds, to contract the muscle as many as 25 times per set, and to complete four to five sets per day. When the patient is able to comply, the exercises are extremely efficacious. However, many older women are unable or unmotivated to follow this regimen. If so, we contact them more frequently or add biofeedback, if available. If not contraindicated by other medical conditions, treatment with an alpha-adrenergic agonist such as phenylpropanolamine (50 to 100 mg per day in divided doses) may be added and is often beneficial for women, especially when administered with estrogen. In fact, these two agents work for women with sphincter incompetence as well. Phenylpropanolamine is inexpensive, is available without a prescription, and is contained in many "diet pills." However, the physician should prescribe the dose and guide the choice of preparation, since some capsules contain additional agents such as chlorpheniramine in doses that can be troublesome for elderly patients. Imipramine, with beneficial effects on the bladder and the outlet, is a reasonable alternative for patients with evidence of both stress and urge incontinence if postural hypotension has been excluded.

If these methods fail, further evaluation of the lower urinary tract is warranted. If urethral hypermobility is confirmed, surgical correction may be performed and is successful in the majority of elderly patients [17]. If sphincter incompetence is diagnosed instead, it too can be corrected, but a different surgical approach is generally required, morbidity is higher, and precipitation of chronic urinary retention is more likely than with correction of urethral hypermobility [17]. Other treatments for sphincter incompetence include periurethral injection of Teflon and insertion of an artificial sphincter, both of which are effective in selected cases [17].

If all other interventions fail, prostheses such as condom catheters or penile clamps may be useful for men, but most such prostheses require substantial manual dexterity and are often poorly tolerated. An alternative product for men is a penile sheath, such as the McGuire prosthesis (similar to an athletic supporter) or the self-adhesive sheath produced by several manufacturers, especially if it is lined with a polymer gel or cellulose. Unfortunately, no similar satisfactory prostheses are available for elderly women. Pads and undergarments are employed as adjunctive measures as discussed above, but in these cases, thin, superabsorbent polymer gel pads are frequently successful because the gel can more readily absorb the smaller amount of leakage. Some products, e.g., Tranquility, consist of pads that can actually be flushed down the toilet, which is quite convenient for ambulatory women. Electrical stimulation is promising, whether applied rectally or vaginally, but is still investigational [17].

OUTLET OBSTRUCTION

Outlet obstruction is the cause of incontinence in up to 5 percent of elderly women [17,26]. The etiology, as noted earlier, is usually a large cystocele that distorts or even kinks the urethra, especially if the patient strains when she voids. Other causes of outlet obstruction in women include bladder neck obstruction, which is rare, and distal urethral stenosis, which may afflict as many as 2 to 3 percent of incontinent women. If a large cystocele is the problem, surgical correction is usually required and should include an outlet suspension if urethral hypermobility is also present. Prior urodynamic evaluation is helpful as well: If incompetence of the bladder neck or low urethral closure pressure (< 20 cm H_2O) is observed, a different surgical approach will be required to avoid converting incontinence due to obstruction into incontinence due to sphincteric incompetence. Bladder neck obstruction is also corrected easily, using local anesthesia, and is thus feasible for even the most frail elderly patient. Distal urethral stenosis can be dilated and treated with estrogen. If meatal stenosis is present, more extensive intervention may be necessary; alternatively, dilation can be repeated at fairly frequent intervals. It should be noted that many women who undergo dilation at present do not have urethral stenosis but rather an underactive detrusor; for these women, dilation is usually unhelpful and may be harmful.

In men, the cause of obstruction is usually a stricture or prostatic enlargement. As noted above, neither the size of the prostate nor a past history of prostatectomy correlates well with obstruction. Estimates of prostatic size are unreliable, and following a prostatectomy the patient may have a bladder neck contracture or stricture; regrowth of the prostate following a prostatectomy is uncommon. Although transurethral resection prostatectomy (TURP), or even suprapubic or retropubic prostatectomy, is optimal and feasible for the elderly, newer approaches have made surgical decompression feasible for even the frailest and most debilitated individuals. These procedures include transurethral incision of the prostate and bladder neck as well as bladder neck incision with bilateral prostatotomy [17,57]. These procedures, as well as the TURP in some instances [58], can be done with local anesthetic and can be completed in less than 30 minutes of operating time. Unlike the TURP and open resections, these newer procedures do not fully resolve the problem, but in frail elderly individuals recrudescence of obstruction two to three years later may not be an issue.

Another new approach to the obstructed individual involves administration of alpha-adrenergic antagonists, such as prazosin or phenoxybenzamine. Numerous double-blind placebo-controlled trials have documented the symptomatic efficacy of these agents, and in some trials postvoiding residual volume, outlet resistance, and urinary flow rate have improved as well; in only two controlled studies has a benefit in urodynamic parameters failed to appear [59]. Phenoxybenzamine in adequate doses (5 to 20 mg per day) is probably superior to prazosin (1 to 2 mg four times a day), but concern about its carcinogenic potential in mice has mitigated against its use. Neither agent is a panacea for outlet obstruction. Rather, each allows the physician to treat the problem symptomatically until more definitive therapy is necessary and feasible.

UNDERACTIVE DETRUSOR

Incontinence due to an underactive detrusor is associated with a large postvoiding residual volume and overflow incontinence. Leakage of small amounts of urine occurs frequently throughout the day and night. The patient may also notice hesitancy, diminished and interrupted flow, a need to strain to void, and a sense of incomplete emptying. If the problem is neurologically mediated, perineal sensation, sacral reflexes, and control of the anal sphincter are frequently impaired. Before this entity can be diagnosed, one must first exclude outlet obstruction.

Management of detrusor underactivity is directed at reducing the postvoiding residual volume and preventing urosepsis. The first step is to use in-dwelling or intermittent catheterization to decompress the bladder for at least 10 to 14 days while reversing potential contributors to impaired detrusor function (fecal impaction and medications). If this does not restore bladder function, then augmented voiding techniques (such as double voiding and implementation of the Credé or Valsalva maneuver) may help if the patient is able to initiate a detrusor contraction. An alpha blocker such as prazosin may further facilitate emptying by reducing outlet resistance. Bethanechol (40 to 200 mg per day in divided doses) is occasionally useful in a patient whose bladder contracts poorly because of treatment with anticholinergic agents that cannot be discontinued (e.g., neuroleptic agents). In other patients, bethanechol may decrease the postvoiding residual volume if sphincter function and local innervation are normal, but evidence for its efficacy is equivocal [60,61], and residual volume should be monitored to assess its effect.

On the other hand, if the detrusor is acontractile, these interventions are apt to be fruitless, and the patient should be started on intermittent catheterization or an in-dwelling urethral catheter. Intermittent self-catheterization is preferable and requires only clean, rather than sterile, catheter insertion. The individual can purchase two or three of these catheters inexpensively. One or two are used during the day and another is kept at home. Men can carry their catheter in a coat pocket, and women can carry theirs in a purse, because the catheter used for females is only a few inches long. The catheters are cleaned daily, allowed to air dry at night, and sterilized periodically, and may be reused repeatedly. Prophylaxis against urinary tract infection is probably warranted if the individual gets more than an occasional infection or has an abnormal heart valve. Intermittent catheterization is painless, safe, inexpensive, and effective, and allows individuals to carry on with their usual daily activities.

Unfortunately, despite the benefits and proven feasibility of intermittent catheterization, most elderly individuals choose indwelling catheterization instead. Complications of chronic in-dwelling catheterization include bladder and urethral erosions, bladder stones, and bladder cancer, as well as urosepsis. There is still no consensus regarding the optimal composition of the catheter or the best time to change it, but several points should be mentioned. First, asymptomatic bacteriuria is ubiquitous in the chronically catheterized individual [62]. It is pointless to treat these asymptomatic infections, since all one does is replace one organism with a more virulent one. Symptomatic infections, on the other hand, should be treated. Second, recent studies have revealed that organisms colonizing catheter encrustations may be unrelated to the organism causing a given bladder infection [63]. For this reason, before treating a symptomatic infection, one should pull the old catheter and obtain a culture from a newly inserted one. Third, the use of mandelamine for the chronically catheterized patient is useless, both theoretically and in practice [64]. Mandelamine is inert unless activated, a process that takes at least 60 to 90 minutes in acidic urine. Because urine in the catheterized patient remains in the bladder for only a few minutes, mandelamine will do nothing to sterilize it.

When indicated, in-dwelling catheters can be extremely effective, but their use should be restricted. They are indicated in the acutely ill patient to monitor fluid balance, in the patient with a nonhealing pressure sore, and in the patient with overflow incontinence refractory to other measures. Even in long-term care facilities, they probably should not be used in more than 1 or 2 percent of patients [17].

MIXED INCONTINENCE

Especially in the elderly, more than one type of incontinence may be present. For example, urge incontinence may develop in a woman with a history of stress incontinence. Such mixed incontinence differs from stress-induced detrusor overactivity; in the latter only detrusor overactivity is present, whereas in the former both detrusor overactivity and impaired outlet integrity are present. Urodynamic evaluation is fre-

quently helpful in such cases because it can help the physician decide which is the predominant lesion and target therapy more effectively.

References

1. Resnick, N. M., et al. Urinary incontinence in community-dwelling elderly: Prevalence and correlates. Proceedings of the 16th Annual Meeting, International Continence Society, Boston, 1986. Pp. 76–78.
2. Diokno, A. C., et al. Prevalence of urinary incontinence and other urological symptoms in the non-institutionalized elderly. J. Urol. 136:1022, 1986.
3. Resnick, N. M., and Paillard, M. Natural history of nosocomial incontinence. Proceedings of the 14th Annual Meeting, International Continence Society, Innsbruck, 1984. Pp. 471–472.
4. Sier, H., Ouslander, J., and Orzeck, S. Urinary incontinence among geriatric patients in an acute-care hospital. J.A.M.A. 257:1767, 1987.
5. Ouslander, J. G., Kane, R. L., and Abrass, I. B. Urinary incontinence in elderly nursing home patients. J.A.M.A. 248:1194, 1982.
6. Resnick, N. M., and Yalla, S. V. Management of urinary incontinence in the elderly. N. Engl. J. Med. 313:800, 1985.
7. Ory, M. G., Wyman, J. F., and Yu, L. Psychosocial factors in urinary incontinence. Clin. Geriatr. Med. 2(4):657, 1986.
8. Hu, T. The economic impact of urinary incontinence. Clin. Geriatr. Med. 2(4):673, 1986.
9. Willington, F. L. Problems in urinary incontinence in the aged. Geront. Clin. 11:330, 1969.
10. Yarnell, J. W. G., and St. Leger, A. S. The prevalence, severity, and factors associated with urinary incontinence in a random sample of the elderly. Age Aging 8:81, 1979.
11. Fossberg, E., Sander, S., and Beisland, H. O. Urinary incontinence in the elderly: A pilot study. Scand. J. Urol. Nephrol. (Suppl.) 60:51, 1981.
12. Schnelle, J. F., et al. Management of geriatric incontinence in nursing homes. J. Appl. Behav. Anal. 16:235, 1983.
13. Castleden, C. M., et al. Factors influencing outcome in elderly patients with urinary incontinence and detrusor instability. Age Aging 14:303, 1985.
14. Overstall, P. W., Rounce, K., and Palmer, J. H. Experience with an incontinence clinic. J. Am. Geriatr. Soc. 28:535, 1980.
15. Torrens, M., and Morrison, J. F. B. Neuro-

morphology. Introduction and Terminology. In M. Torrens and J. F. B. Morrison (eds.), *The Physiology of the Lower Urinary Tract*. New York: Springer-Verlag, 1987. Pp. 1–2.

16. Dixon, J., and Gosling, J. Structure and Innervation in the Human. In M. Torrens and J. F. B. Morrison (eds.), *The Physiology of the Lower Urinary Tract*. New York: Springer-Verlag, 1987. Pp. 3–22.

17. Resnick, N. M. Voiding dysfunction in the elderly. In S. V. Yalla, et al. (eds.), *Neurology and Urodynamics: Principles and Practice*. New York: Macmillan, 1988. Pp. 303–330.

18. Resnick, N. M. Urinary incontinence in the elderly. *Med. Grand Rounds* 3:281, 1984.

19. Boscia, J. A., et al. Lack of association between bacteriuria and symptoms in the elderly. *Am. J. Med.* 81:979, 1986.

20. Robinson, J. M. Evaluation of Methods for Assessment of Bladder and Urethral Function. In J. C. Brocklehurst (ed.), *Urology in the Elderly*. New York: Churchill Livingstone, 1984. Pp. 19–54.

21. Chetkowski, R. J., et al. Biologic effects of transdermal estradiol. *N. Engl. J. Med.* 314:1615, 1986.

22. Jensen, J., et al. Long-term effects of percutaneous estrogens and oral progesterone on serum lipoproteins in postmenopausal women. *Am. J. Obstet. Gynecol.* 156:66, 1987.

23. Wheeler, J. S., et al. Vincristine-induced bladder neuropathy. *J. Urol.* 130:342, 1983.

24. Goldsmith, M. F. Research on aging burgeons as more Americans grow older. *J.A.M.A.* 253:1369, 1985.

25. Meyhoff, H. H., et al. Accuracy in preoperative estimation of prostatic size. *Scand. J. Urol. Nephrol.* 15:45, 1981.

26. Resnick, N. M., Yalla, S. V., and Laurino, E. The pathophysiology and clinical correlates of established urinary incontinence in frail elderly. *N. Engl. J. Med.* (in press).

27. Resnick, N. M., and Yalla, S. V. Detrusor hyperactivity with impaired contractile function. An unrecognized but common cause of incontinence in elderly patients. *J.A.M.A.* 257:3076, 1987.

28. McGuire, E. J., and Savastano, J. A. Stress incontinence and detrusor instability/urge incontinence. *Neurourol. Urodynam.* 4:313, 1985.

29. Abrams, P. Detrusor instability and bladder outlet obstruction. *Neurourol. Urodynam.* 4:317, 1985.

30. Hald, T., et al. *The Standardisation of Terminology of Lower Urinary Tract Function*. Glasgow: International Continence Society, 1984. Pp. 1–34.

31. McGuire, E. J., et al. Stress urinary incontinence. *Obstet. Gynecol.* 47:255, 1976.

32. Resnick, N. M. Urinary incontinence in the elderly. *Hosp. Pract. [Off.]* 21(11):80C, 1986.

33. Eastwood, H. D. H. Urodynamic studies in the management of urinary incontinence in the elderly. *Age Aging* 8:41, 1979.

34. Abrams, P. H., and Feneley, R. C. L. The significance of the symptoms associated with bladder outflow obstruction. *Urol. Internat.* 33:171, 1978.

35. Abrams, P. H. Prostatism and prostatectomy: The Role of urine flow rate measurement in the preoperative assessment for operation. *J. Urol.* 117:70, 1977.

36. Chrystle, C. D., Charmel, S., and Copeland, W. E. Q-tip test for stress urinary incontinence. *Obstet. Gynecol.* 38:313, 1971.

37. Marshall, V. F., Marchetti, A. A., and Krantz, K. E. Correction of stress incontinence by simple vesicourethral suspension. *Surg. Gynecol. Obstet.* 88:509, 1949.

38. Resnick, N. M., and Yalla, S. V. A prospective, blinded trial of clinical vs. urodynamic evaluation of the incontinent patient. *J. Urol.* 137:188A, 1987.

39. Resnick, N. M., et al. Evaluation of a clinical algorithm to identify the cause of incontinence in the elderly. *J. Urol.* 135:168A, 1986.

40. Sutherst, J. R., and Brown, M. C. Comparison of single and multichannel cystometry in diagnosing bladder instability. *Br. Med. J.* 288:1720, 1984.

41. Ouslander, J. G., et al. Diagnostic tests for geriatric incontinence. *World J. Urol.* 4:16, 1986.

42. Resnick, N. M., Yalla, S. V., and Laurino, E. Feasibility, safety, and reproducibility of urodynamics in the elderly. *J. Urol.* 137(4/2):189A, 1987.

43. Schmidst, R. R., Witherow, R., and Tanagho, E. Recording urethral pressure profile. Comparison of methods and clinical implications. *Urology* 10:390, 1977.

44. Sutherst, J. R., and Brown, M. C. Detection of urethral incompetence in women using the fluid bridge test. *Br. J. Urol.* 52:138, 1980.

45. Yalla, S. V., Finn, D., and DeFelippo, N. Fluid bridge test in the evaluation of male urinary continence. *J. Urol.* 128:1241, 1982.

46. Resnick, N. M., and Yalla, S. V. Initiation of voiding in human subjects: The temporal relationship and nature of urethral sphincter responses. Submitted for publication.

47. Yalla, S. V., and Resnick, N. M. Vesicourethral static pressure profile during voiding: Meth-

odology and clinical utility. *World J. Urol.* 2:196, 1984.

48. Blaivas, J. G. Sphincter electromyography. *Neurourol. Urodynam.* 2:269, 1983.

49. Fantl, J. A., et al. Bead-chain cytourethrogram: An evaluation. *Obstet. Gyncecol.* 58:237, 1981.

50. Hadley, E. Bladder training and related therapies for urinary incontinence in elderly people. *J.A.M.A.* 256:372, 1986.

51. Burgio, K. L., and Burgio, L. D. Behavior therapies for urinary incontinence in the elderly. *Clin. Geriatr. Med.* 2(4):809, 1986.

52. McGuire, E. J., et al. Treatment of motor and sensory detrusor instability by electrical stimulation. *J. Urol.* 129:78, 1983.

53. Brink, C. A., and Wells, T. J. Environmental support for incontinence: Toilets, toilet supplements, and external equipment. *Clin. Geriatr. Med.* 2(4):829, 1986.

54. McGuire, E. J. Reflex urethral instability. *Br. J. Urol.* 50:200, 1978.

55. Bhatia, N. N., Bergman, A., and Gunning, J. E. Urodynamic effects of a vaginal pessary in women with stress during urinary incontinence. *Am. J. Obstet. Gynceol.* 147:876, 1983.

56. Mohr, J. A., et al. Stress urinary incontinence: A simple and practical approach to diagnosis and treatment. *J. Am. Geriatr. Soc.* 31:476, 1983.

57. Orandi, A. Transurethral incision of prostrate (TUIP): 646 cases in 15 years—a chronological appraisal. *Br. J. Urol.* 57:703, 1985.

58. Sinha, B., et al. Transurethral resection of the prostate with local anesthesia in 100 patients. *J. Urol.* 135:719, 1986.

59. Caine, M. The present role of alpha-adrenergic blockers in the treatment of benign prostatic hypertrophy. *J. Urol.* 136:1, 1986.

60. Downie, J. W. Bethanechol chloride in urology—a discussion of issues. *Neurourol. Urodynam.* 3:211, 1984.

61. Finkbeiner, A. Is bethanechol chloride clinically effective in promoting bladder emptying? A literature review. *J. Urol.* 134:443, 1985.

62. Warren, J. W., et al. Sequelae and management of urinary infection in the patient requiring chronic catheterization. *J. Urol.* 125:1, 1981.

63. Grahn, D., et al. Validity of urinary catheter specimen for diagnosis of urinary tract infection in the elderly. *Arch. Intern. Med.* 145:1858, 1985.

20

Pulmonary System

DAVID SPARROW
SCOTT T. WEISS

GROWTH AND DEVELOPMENT of the human lung continues until about age 20. Following a variable period of stability, many parameters of pulmonary function decline steadily with advancing age. Knowledge of the normal growth and decline of pulmonary function facilitates an understanding of the effects of genetic and environmental factors, particularly cigarette smoking, that can modify normal function.

The influence of normal physiologic changes and epidemiologic risk factors on the decline of pulmonary function and the development of chronic obstructive lung disease are described in this chapter. Discussion focuses on important physiologic changes that occur in the areas of pulmonary mechanics, alveolar gas exchange, control of respiration, and pulmonary defense mechanisms. These physiologic data are integrated with epidemiologic risk factors such as cigarette smoking, atopy, and airways responsiveness to describe aging of the respiratory system.

Physiologic Age Changes
COMPLIANCE

The lungs and chest wall are bound together by the potential pleural space and function like a bellows. At the end of quiet expiration, the tendency of the lungs to recoil inward is just balanced by the tendency of the chest wall to recoil outward. The entire system is at its resting volume, the functional residual capacity.

Cross-sectional studies have shown that there is a progressive age-related loss of lung elastic recoil after ages 20 to 25 that results in increased lung compliance [1,2]. This loss of elastic forces cannot be accounted for by loss of collagen or elastin in pulmonary parenchyma [3] or a decrease in the total length and diameter of elastic fibers [4]. Instead, alterations in the location and orientation of individual elastic fibers may provide some explanation for the decline in lung elasticity. Other as yet undescribed factors may also be important, such as changes in the composition and turnover of pulmonary surfactant with age and the release of oxidant and antioxidant enzymes.

With advancing age, the compliance of the chest wall also changes. The chest wall begins to stiffen after about age 20, and hence its natural tendency to expand outward is inhibited [5,6]. This stiffening has been attributed to age-related changes in the rib cage, particularly the calcification of its articulations [7].

LUNG VOLUMES

Decreasing elastic recoil and stiffening of the chest wall with age explain age-related changes in several standard lung volumes and capacities defined below. Total lung capacity (TLC) is the total amount of air in the lungs following a

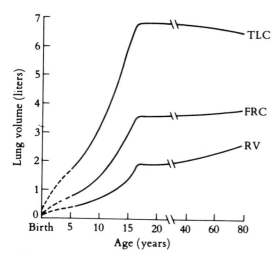

FIGURE 20-1. *Total lung capacity (TLC), functional residual capacity (FRC), and residual volume (RV) as a function of age from birth to 80 years for an "average" body build. (From J. F. Murray. The Normal Lung. Philadelphia: Saunders, 1976.)*

maximum inspiration. Residual volume (RV) is the amount of air in the lungs at the end of a maximum expiration. Vital capacity is the maximum amount of air one can expire after a maximum inspiration. The amount of air in the lungs at the end of a quiet expiration is called functional residual capacity (FRC).

The relationships between lung volumes and age are depicted in Figure 20-1. The TLC remains essentially constant with age after adulthood is attained. In contrast, the RV increases during the adult years due to airways collapse at higher lung volumes secondary to the loss of elastic recoil [8]. Vital capacity, therefore, declines slightly, since vital capacity is equal to TLC minus RV. The FRC represents the point at which the inward elastic recoil of the lungs is balanced by the outward elastic recoil of the chest wall. As lung recoil forces decrease with advancing age, FRC increases slightly.

AIRFLOW

Muscular strength and elastic recoil have an important influence on the rate of flow achieved in the lungs, but these effects on flow rates depend on lung volume [9]. When lung volumes are large, both muscular strength and the pressure supplied by lung elastic recoil have a significant impact on the flow rate. When lung volumes

are small, the elastic recoil of the lungs is probably the major determinant of air flow [10].

Various indexes of airflow have been shown to decline with age including the forced vital capacity (FVC), the forced expiratory volume in 1 second (FEV_1), and the forced expiratory $flow_{25-75}$, or the flow between 25 and 75 percent of the vital capacity (FEF_{25-75}). The greatest decline is seen in FEF_{25-75}, reflecting reduced flow at low lung volumes and the primacy of a decrease in elastic recoil. FEV_1 and FVC reflect flows at high lung volumes and thus depend on muscular strength more than on elastic recoil.

The most important clinical variables that determine flow rates and lung volumes are age, height, and sex. As a result, patients' measured values are routinely compared with predicted values that are based on healthy individuals of the same age, height, and sex [11,12]. After accounting for these clinical variables, there is still considerable interindividual variability in level of pulmonary function, which is reflected in the wide range of levels considered within the normal range (e.g., 80 to 120 percent predicted FEV_1 is considered normal). Other factors that may explain interindividual variation are discussed later in the section on development of respiratory symptoms and disease.

GAS EXCHANGE

The exchange of oxygen and carbon dioxide is the main function of the respiratory system. Adequate exchange of gas depends on the close matching of ventilation (the amount of air taken into the lungs) to perfusion (the amount of blood flow into the lungs). In the normal young lung, ventilation and perfusion are matched very closely, although there are regional variations [13]. Because ventilation and, to greater extent, perfusion increase proceeding from top to bottom in the upright lung, the ratio of ventilation to perfusion ($\dot{V}_A/\dot{Q}$) is greater than one at the apex and less than one at the base. The overall $\dot{V}_A/\dot{Q}$ ratio is close to one.

With advancing age, loss of elastic recoil causes closure of small airways in the lower regions of the lung during the normal respiratory cycle. Inspired gas appears to be preferentially distributed to the upper regions without decreasing blood flow to the lower regions [14]. A ventilation-to-perfusion mismatch results that

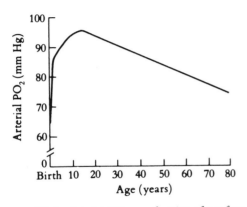

FIGURE 20-2. *Arterial PO$_2$ as a function of age from birth to 80 years. (From J. F. Murray.* The Normal Lung. *Philadelphia: Saunders, 1976.)*

may have an adverse effect on arterial oxygenation in the elderly.

The influence of age on arterial PO$_2$ has been examined in several studies [15–17], and results are summarized in Figure 20-2. Among adults there is a small but steady decrease in arterial PO$_2$ of approximately 4 mm Hg for each decade of age. In contrast, alveolar PO$_2$ stays constant or increases slightly with age. The most likely explanation for this age-dependent widening of the alveolar-arterial oxygen difference is the functional alteration in ventilation-perfusion dynamics described above. In addition, the pulmonary diffusing capacity declines progressively with age [18,19], perhaps as a result of loss of alveolar capillary units, and may contribute a small amount to age-related hypoxia.

CONTROL OF RESPIRATION

Respiration is controlled by a complex system of sensors, effectors, and a central controller in the brain stem. The central controller coordinates the information it receives from sensors and adjusts the activity of the respiratory muscles. The central chemoreceptor, located in the medulla, is responsible for most of the ventilatory response to hypercapnia. The peripheral chemoreceptors, located in the carotid and aortic bodies in the neck, are responsible for all of the increase in ventilation that accompanies hypoxemia.

Presently available data indicate that the ventilatory response to hypercapnia decreases with increasing age [20–23]. This decrease may re-

flect diminished neural output to the respiratory muscles [22] or altered mechanics of the respiratory system in the elderly [6,24]. However, the response to hypoxia in the elderly is less clear-cut. Some reports have found that the ventilatory response to hypoxia is blunted as well [20,22]. However, Chapman and Cherniack failed to confirm these reports [23]. The reasons for these study differences are unclear and may reflect population selection, biologic heterogeneity, differences in test procedure, or variables that are unknown or uncontrolled.

DEFENSE MECHANISMS

The lung has a variety of defenses against inhaled chemicals, toxic dusts, and microorganisms. Defense mechanisms involve the epiglottis and upper airway, which prevent aspiration, and the cough reflex, which expels mucus or unwanted material from the lung. In addition to these local mechanisms, cellular and humoral immunity play an important role in defending the lung from microorganisms.

There is a paucity of data on the relationship of age to humoral immunity. Secretory immunoglobulin (IgA) of the nasal and respiratory mucosal surfaces, a major deterrent to viruses, may fall with age [25]. Serum IgG levels increase with age, although this increase may reflect antibody to intrinsic antigens (or self) rather than foreign antigens. Weksler has speculated that this ineffective increase in antibody may reflect defective helper T-cell function [26].

FIGURE 20-3. *Frequency histogram (percent of total number of analyzed disks) of individual disk velocities in young (broken line) and elderly (solid line) nonsmokers. (From R. M. Goodman, et al. Relationship of smoking history and pulmonary function tests to tracheal mucous velocity in nonsmokers, young smokers, ex-smokers, and patients with chronic bronchitis.* Am. Rev. Respir. Dis. *117:205, 1978.)*

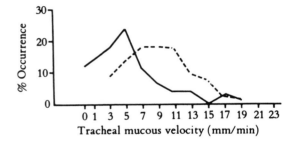

Further investigation in this area is required. Cellular immune function as measured by skin test declines with age [27,28]. Increased suppressor T-cell activity appears to contribute to this impaired cellular response [26], and the resulting anergy is associated with an increased mortality [29]. However, the relationship of impaired cellular response to pulmonary disease in the elderly is unclear.

Local airway protection, including both cough and laryngeal reflexes, also declines with age. There is a marked age-related reduction in sensitivity to inhaled ammonia as a cough stimulus, with older individuals tending to cough less than younger individuals [30]. The relationship of decrease in cough and laryngeal reflexes to increased aspiration is still unclear. Other factors besides attenuation of reflexes may also be important. It has been observed (using radiopaque disks) that mean tracheal mucus velocity is slower in nonsmoking elderly subjects [31], although, as seen in Figure 20-3,

there is considerable overlap between young and older subjects. In view of the seriousness of pneumonia in elderly populations, further effort needs to be directed toward the definition and investigation of the above changes in local defenses.

Development of Respiratory Symptoms and Disease

Figure 20-4 presents a model of pulmonary function in relation to normal growth and disease that is modified from work done by Fletcher et al. [32]. As shown in this figure, pulmonary function tends to reach a maximal level by the early twenties. After a variable period of stability, loss of pulmonary function begins. This loss appears to be relatively linear but may accelerate with increase in age. An early life exposure (such as respiratory illness) could conceivably inhibit the maximally attained pulmonary function (curve B) and thus increase the individual's risk of developing adult symptoms.

Patients generally do not develop dyspnea until their pulmonary function is roughly half of the normal maximally attained value, which, for an average-sized man, corresponds to an FEV_1 of approximately 2 liters. The higher the initial level (see Fig. 20-4, curve A) and the slower the decline in adult life, the longer the time needed to develop symptoms.

FIGURE 20-4. *Theoretical curves representing varying rates of change in FEV_1 by age. Curve A depicts normal decline in FEV_1 without cigarette smoking, curve B with smoking. Curve D depicts the effect of smoking cessation also seen in disabled individuals (curve E). Often, the disability-related decline continues as a variable rate (curves C and F). (From F. E. Speizer and I. B. Tager. Epidemiology of mucus hypersecretion and obstructive airways disease. Epidemiol. Rev. 1:124, 1979.)*

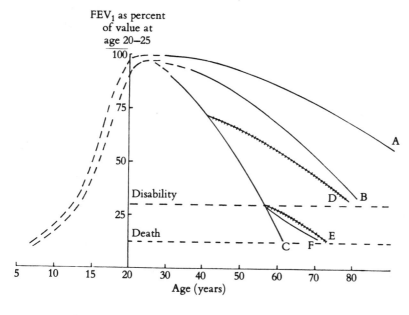

Chronic obstructive lung disease (COLD) generally refers to patients who have chronic bronchitis, emphysema, or a mixture of the two. Chronic bronchitis is defined as cough and phlegm production on most days for three consecutive months for two consecutive years. The prevalence of chronic bronchitis increases with advancing age. Emphysema is a pathologic term referring to dilatation and destruction of air spaces distal to the terminal bronchioles. The clinical term reflecting the pathologic entity of emphysema is chronic airflow obstruction. Chronic airflow obstruction generally refers to decreased flow rates (an FEV_1 usually less than 65 percent of predicted for age, sex, and height and often less than 50 percent of predicted) and increased lung volumes (TLC, RV, FRC), signifying loss of elastic recoil. Risk factors for the development of chronic bronchitis and chronic airflow obstruction to be discussed below are cigarette smoking, atopy, and airways responsiveness.

CIGARETTE SMOKING

Cigarette smoking is the single most important factor in the development of chronic bronchitis and chronic airflow obstruction [32]. During childhood, smoking ("active" or "passive") may act to inhibit the maximally attained level of pulmonary function [33] and in turn increase a subject's risk of developing clinically significant airflow obstruction in adult life (see Fig. 20-4, curve B). During adulthood, the normal decline in FEV_1 of approximately 20 to 30 ml per year is doubled or tripled in the smoker (see Fig. 20-4, curves B and C). This accelerated loss of pulmonary function markedly increases disease risk in individuals with low maximally attained levels or those who smoke a greater amount (assuming a dose response). Cigarette smoking leads to cough symptoms by increasing mucus secretion and irritating nerves. The impact of smoking on cough and phlegm production is particularly evident from the population attributable risks (amount of chronic cough and phlegm in a population attributable to smoking) reported in several studies (Table 20-1).

ATOPY

Atopy is defined as an altered state of reactivity of the host to foreign antigens. Atopy is usually

TABLE 20-1. *Attributable risk for smoking in chronic bronchitis from various population-based studies*[a]

REFERENCE	POPULATION	POPULATION-ATTRIBUTABLE RISK PERCENTAGE,[b] BASED ON GROUP STUDY
Anderson and Ferris (1962)	Random sample, 25 years of age	46
Anderson and Ferris (1965)	Random sample, 25 years of age	52
Higgins (1957)	Random sample, 25 years of age	50
Colley (1974)	Cohort of men and women followed from birth to 20 years of age	46
Huhti (1965)	Total population	70
Tager and Speizer (1976)	Random sample 15 years of age	66

SOURCE: I. B. Tager and F. E. Speizer. Risk estimates for chronic bronchitis in smokers: A study of male-female differences. *Am. Rev. Resp. Dis.* 113:619, 1976.
[a] No female participant smoked more than half a pack per day; therefore, data on women were not calculated.
[b] Population-attributable risk = rate in population − rate in nonsmokers; population-attributable risk percentage = (population-attributable risk/rate in population) × 100.

assessed with allergen skin tests and levels of immunoglobulin E (IgE) and, less frequently, with the number of peripheral blood eosinophils. Figure 20-5 shows the relationship of age to allergen skin test reactivity and total serum IgE in a population sample of white subjects in Tucson, Arizona [28]. In adulthood, both skin test reactivity and IgE level decline with advancing age.

Cross-sectional studies have related various measures of atopy to pulmonary function, but these relationships are limited to specific subgroups. Higher IgE levels are associated with decreased levels of FEV_1 but only among subjects reporting respiratory symptoms [34]. Eosinophilia is associated with decreased levels of FEV_1 among never smokers older than 54 years of age [35]; among younger subjects, the association is confined to never smokers with positive skin tests [35,36]. There is also an association between skin test reactivity and reduced pulmonary function but only among current and former cigarette smokers [37]. Longitudinal studies have revealed only a weak connec-

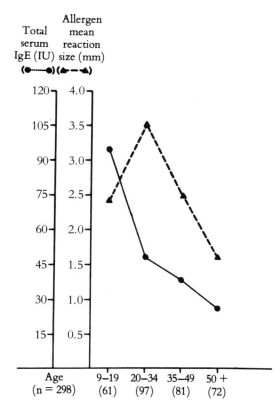

Total serum IgE (IU) (●----●)	Allergen mean reaction size (mm) (▲--▲)
120	4.0
105	3.5
90	3.0
75	2.5
60	2.0
45	1.5
30	1.0
15	0.5

Age (n = 298)	9–19 (61)	20–34 (97)	35–49 (81)	50 + (72)

FIGURE 20-5. *Relationship of allergen skin-test reactivity (mean reaction size in millimeters) and total serum IgE (geometric mean of natural log) to age. (Adapted from R. A. Barbee, et al. Allergen skin-test reactivity in a community population sample: Correlation with age, histamine skin reactions and total serum immunoglobulin E. J. Allergy Clin. Immunol. 68:15, 1981.)*

tion between atopy and pulmonary function. Higher absolute eosinophil counts are associated with a faster rate of decline of FEV_1 but only among never smokers [38]. Other measures of atopy including serum IgE and skin test are unrelated to rate of decline of pulmonary function [38,39].

AIRWAYS RESPONSIVENESS
Increased levels of airways responsiveness to nonspecific stimuli (e.g., methacholine, histamine) are present in the majority of active asthmatics and in some healthy individuals [40,41]. In population samples, nonspecific airways responsiveness is unimodally distributed [42] and is of similar magnitude in males and females [43,44]. Children and older adults have rela-

tively greater responsiveness (Fig. 20-6). In Figure 20-6 this responsiveness is depicted as subjects responding at small methacholine areas. Responsiveness decreases gradually up until the late thirties and then gradually increases in later life [44,45]. Chronic cigarette smoking is associated with increased nonspecific responsiveness in most studies [41,46–49].

Currently available data from population studies suggest an association between increased airways responsiveness and more rapid rates of decline in pulmonary function. In most of the longitudinal studies [38,50,51], airways responsiveness was only measured toward the end of follow-up, making it unclear whether accelerated decline in function follows or precedes airways hyperresponsiveness. One longitudinal study assessed airways responsiveness at baseline and found that decline in FEV_1 was significantly greater among hyperresponders than in less responsive subjects [52]. Hyperresponsiveness was also associated with the subsequent development of occasional cough, sputum, and chronic bronchitis.

Although the role of increased airways responsiveness as a risk factor for the development of COLD remains unsettled, in patients with established disease the presence of this trait clearly implies a poor prognosis with an accelerated decline in pulmonary function.

COLD is an insidious process that only develops over many years. Current research is directed at understanding why only a minority of cigarette smokers develop this illness. Current theories suggest that those subjects with allergies and increased levels of airways responsiveness may be at greater risk. In addition, cigarette smoking may interact to increase the effect of these risk factors. Because of the complexity of these research questions longitudinal studies will be necessary to answer them.

Therapy for Chronic Airflow Obstruction
The basic principles of therapy for airflow obstruction do not change simply because the patient is elderly. However, recognition of age-related physiologic changes leads to some important modifications. For example, hypoxemia caused by functional alterations in ventilation-

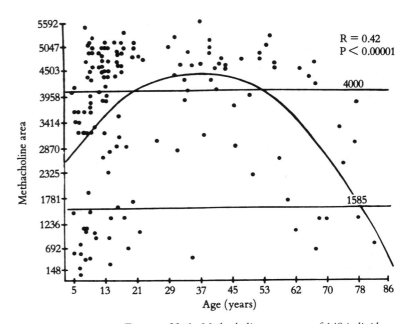

R = 0.42
P < 0.00001

4000

1585

Methacholine area

5592
5047
4503
3958
3414
2870
2325
1781
1236
692
148

Age (years)

5   13   21   29   37   45   53   62   70   78   86

FIGURE 20-6. *Methacholine responses of 148 individuals from a selected American population. Methacholine areas > 4000 indicate a normal response, areas > 1535 indicate moderately increased responsiveness, and areas < 1535 indicate markedly increased responsiveness (From R. J. Hopp, et al. The effect of age on methacholine response.* J. Allergy Clin. Immunol. *76:609, 1985.)*

perfusion dynamics is important because it could worsen congestive heart failure, arrhythmias, or delirium, all common problems in the elderly.

For the patient with chronic symptoms of dyspnea secondary to bronchospasm, bronchodilators (sympathomimetics, methylxanthines) are the mainstay of a therapeutic regimen. However, since loss of elastic recoil may play a major role in a decrease in airflow and because this is not amenable to bronchodilator therapy, recognition of the limits of bronchodilators is necessary [53].

In addition, the frequent association of occult heart failure in the elderly with airflow obstruction may be important, although it is difficult to detect. Home oxygen therapy is necessary in any patient who has a persistent PaO_2 of less than 55 mm Hg. In addition, the presence of polycythemia (hematocrit greater than 50) or cor pulmonale is also a clear-cut indicator for oxygen therapy. Oxygen must be used for a minimum of 12 to 15 hours a day to effectively decrease pulmonary artery pressure [54]. Finally, for the stable outpatient, it is sometimes noted that cessation of smoking will revert the rate of loss of pulmonary function to normal in two to three years.

Acute exacerbations of chronic airflow obstruction are common and are the most frequent cause of hospitalization for patients with chronic airflow obstruction. The common causes of acute exacerbations of chronic airflow obstruction are (1) respiratory infection, (2) myocardial infarction, (3) sedative drugs (narcotics, sleep medications), (4) air pollution, and (5) systemic illness (sepsis or other organ failure).

Although respiratory infection is the most common cause for acute exacerbations in any age group, in the elderly, "silent" myocardial infarction presenting as respiratory failure and respiratory failure secondary to sepsis or other organ system failure are of increased importance. Because of the decrease in respiratory drive noted with increased age, the prescription of hypnotic, psychotropic, and sedative drugs can precipitate respiratory failure in the elderly. The coexistence of other diseases such as heart failure can increase the work of breathing or predispose to infection, and the use of drugs such as diuretics may exacerbate respiratory failure by inducing chloride depletion and metabolic alkalosis, with further respiratory depression. Finally, although respiratory infections will not permanently decrease pulmonary function, the transient effect in a patient with severe airflow obstruction can be life-threatening. The elderly patient is more susceptible for the following reasons. First, the decrease in pulmonary function associated with aging implies a decrease in pulmonary reserve, and, in addition, the depression of respiratory drive implies a diminished ability to respond to stress. Finally, the mechanical work of moving the chest is greater in an older person. For example, Turner and coworkers [1] estimate that the work of breathing is 20 percent greater in a 60-year-old than in a 20-year-old.

Treatment for the acute exacerbation involves the use of oxygen, bronchodilators, and antibiotics, if appropriate. Bronchodilator dosage must be adjusted carefully in the elderly. Lower doses of sympathomimetics, 0.2 to 0.3 ml of 1:1,000 epinephrine and 0.25 mg of terbutaline subcutaneously or 2.5 mg of terbutaline by mouth should be used in the elderly patient because of the risk of cardiac arrhythmias. Similarly, the effect of aminophylline directly depends on liver function and hepatic blood flow. Silent loss of hepatic function in many elderly patients makes a downward adjustment in dose mandatory. Therapeutic levels (10–20 μg/ml) of aminophylline can be achieved with a standard loading dose (5 mg/kg), given only if the patient has not received the drug before. A maintenance infusion of from 0.2 to 0.4 mg/kg per hour should be used, as opposed to the rate of 0.8 to 1.2 mg/kg per hour used in young adults.

If conservative therapy (e.g., O_2, bronchodilators, and antibiotics) for an acute exacerbation of COLD is not successful, then mechanical ventilation must be considered. Age per se is not a contraindication to intubation. A variety of studies have shown that the level of pulmonary function rather than age is the primary determinant of mortality in patients with COLD. Because of their decreased ventilatory drive and decreased pulmonary reserve, elderly patients are more likely to require mechanical ventilation than younger patients. Obviously, the decision to use mechanical support must be based on all aspects of the patient's clinical condition and with the patient's active participation.

Medical Intensive Care for the Elderly

One of the most frequently encountered clinical issues in pulmonary medicine is the role of medical intensive care for elderly patients. Coronary artery disease, congestive heart failure, chronic obstructive lung disease, pneumonia, and gastrointestinal bleeding are the most common reasons for admission to an intensive care unit (ICU) for elderly patients. Selection factors will limit, to some extent, which elderly patients are considered ICU candidates. Given that the elderly who were in the best health before the onset of acute illness are more likely to enter the ICU, most studies find no increase in ICU [55] or total hospital costs [56] related to age. Most studies do find that ICU mortality is age related [55,56]. Campion and coworkers studied 2,693 admissions to an ICU/cardiac care unit (CCU) over a two-year period. Hospital mortality was 16 percent for subjects over 75 years of age, 14 percent for subjects 65 to 74 years of age, and 8 percent for subjects 55 to 64 years of age. Major life support interventions such as mechanical ventilation were more common in elderly patients. Elderly patients were just as likely as younger patients to return to their preadmission living situation but were less likely to regain their preadmission activity level [56].

These data suggest that elderly patients do not in general fare as well as younger patients in the ICU setting. Most ICU physicians would be very loath to deny an individual patient ICU care on the basis of age alone because the prognoses of ICU patients are poorly predicted by any variable or combination of variables, and age alone is an insufficient basis for any clinical decision. Better predictive models are clearly needed for ICU medicine.

Lung Cancer

Lung cancer represents the number one cause of cancer death in men. The disease has a dismal 5-year survival, with an overall survival rate of 5 percent. Survival is modified by cell type, anatomic extent of disease (e.g., stage), clinical staging (fever, weight loss), and age. This disease is almost uniformly fatal, and surgery is the only reasonable chance for cure. However, thoracotomy for unresectable disease carries an increased mortality, and both mortality and morbidity of thoracotomy increase with increasing age. These factors make careful clinical assessment of the elderly patient a necessity.

Careful staging is the only answer to this clinical dilemma. In general, it is rare in clinical practice to find patients who meet the criteria of resectability and are over age 70. However, age alone is a poor criterion for clinical decision making, and bronchoscopy, computed tomographic scanning, pulmonary function testing and, if necessary, mediastinoscopy allow more accurate clinical assessment.

References

1. Turner, J. M., Mead, J., and Wohl, M. E. Elasticity of human lungs in relation to age. *J. Appl. Physiol.* 25:664, 1968.
2. Knudson, R. J., et al. Effect of aging alone on mechanical properties of the normal adult human lung. *J. Appl. Physiol.* 43:1054, 1977.
3. Hance, A. J., and Crystal, R. G. The connective tissue of lung. *Am. Rev. Respir. Dis.* 112:675, 1975.
4. Niewoehner, D. E., and Kleinerman, J. Morphometric study of elastic fibers in normal and emphysematous human lungs. *Am. Rev. Respir. Dis.* 115:15, 1977.
5. Frank, N. R., Mead, J., and Ferris, B. G., Jr. The mechanical behavior of the lungs in healthy elderly persons. *J. Clin. Invest.* 36:1680, 1957.
6. Mittman, C., et al. Relationship between chest wall and pulmonary compliance and age. *J. Appl. Physiol.* 20:1211, 1965.
7. Rizzato, G., and Marazzini, L. Thoracoabdominal mechanics in elderly men. *J. Appl. Physiol.* 28:457, 1970.
8. Jones, R. L., et al. Effects of age on residual volume. *J. Appl. Physiol.* 44:195, 1978.
9. Fry, D. L., and Hyatt, R. E. Pulmonary mechanics. A unified analysis of the relationship between pressure, volume and gas flow in the lungs of normal and diseased human subjects. *Am. J. Med.* 29:672, 1960.
10. Mead, J., et al. Significance of the relationship between lung recoil and maximum expiratory flow. *J. Appl. Physiol.* 22:95, 1967.
11. Morris, J. F., Koski, A., and Johnson, L. C. Spirometric standards for healthy nonsmoking adults. *Am. Rev. Respir. Dis.* 103:57, 1971.
12. Dockery, D. W., et al. Distribution of forced expiratory volume in one second and forced vital capacity in healthy, white, adult never-smokers in six U.S. cities. *Am. Rev. Respir. Dis.* 131:511, 1985.
13. West, J. B. *Ventilation/Blood Flow and Gas Exchange.* Oxford: Blackwell, 1977. Pp. 28–29.
14. Holland, J., et al. Regional distribution of pulmonary ventilation and perfusion in elderly subjects. *J. Clin. Invest.* 47:81, 1968.
15. Nelson, N. M. Neonatal pulmonary function. *Pediatr. Clin. North Amer.* 13:769, 1966.
16. Sorbini, C. A., et al. Arterial oxygen tension in relation to age in healthy subjects. *Respiration* 25:3, 1968.
17. Mansell, A., Bryan, C., and Levison, H. Airway closure in children. *J. Appl. Physiol.* 33:711, 1972.
18. Hamer, N. A. J. The effect of age on the components of the pulmonary diffusing capacity. *Clin. Sci.* 23:85, 1962.
19. Muieson, G., Sorbini, C. A., and Grassi, V. Respiratory function in the aged. *Bull. Eur. Physiopathol. Resp.* 7:973, 1971.
20. Kronenberg, R. S., and Drage, C. W. Attenuation of the ventilatory and heart rate responses to hypoxia and hypercapnia with aging in normal men. *J. Clin. Invest.* 52:1812, 1973.
21. Altose, M. D., et al. Effects of hypercapnia and inspiratory flow—resistive loading on respiratory activity in chronic airways obstruction. *J. Clin. Invest.* 59:500, 1977.
22. Peterson, D. D., et al. Effects of aging on ventilatory and occlusion pressure responses to hypoxia and hypercapnia. *Am. Rev. Respir. Dis.* 124:387, 1981.
23. Chapman, K. R., and Cherniack, N. S. Aging effects on the interaction of hypercapnia and hypoxia as ventilatory stimuli. *J. Gerontol.* 42:202, 1987.
24. Rebuck, A. S., et al. Control of tidal volume during rebreathing. *J. Appl. Physiol.* 37:475, 1974.
25. Alford, R. H. Effect of chronic bronchopulmonary disease and aging on human nasal secretion IgA concentrations. *J. Immunol.* 101:984, 1968.
26. Weksler, M. E. Senescence of the immune system. *Med. Clin. North Am.* 19:73, 1983.
27. Barbee, R. A., et al. Immediate skin-test reactivity in a general population sample. *Ann. Intern. Med.* 84:129, 1976.
28. Barbee, R. A., et al. Allergen skin-test reactivity in a community population sample: Correlation with age, histamine skin reactions and total serum immunoglobulin E. *J. Allergy Clin. Immunol.* 68:15, 1981.
29. Roberts-Thomson, I. C., et al. Ageing, immune response and mortality. *Lancet* 2:368, 1974.
30. Pontoppidan, H., and Beecher, H. K. Progres-

sive loss of protective reflexes in the airway with the advance of age. *J.A.M.A.* 174:2209, 1960.

31. Goodman, R. M., et al. Relationship of smoking history and pulmonary function tests to tracheal mucous velocity in nonsmokers, young smokers, ex-smokers, and patients with chronic bronchitis. *Am. Rev. Respir. Dis.* 117:205, 1978.

32. Fletcher, C. M., et al. *The Natural History of Chronic Bronchitis and Emphysema.* London: Oxford University Press, 1976.

33. Tager, I. B., et al. Longitudinal study of the effects of maternal smoking on pulmonary function in children. *N. Engl. J. Med.* 309:699, 1983.

34. Burrows, B., et al. Interactions of smoking and immunologic factors in relation to airways obstruction. *Chest* 84:657, 1983.

35. Burrows, B., et al. Epidemiologic observations on eosinophilia and its relation to respiratory disorders. *Am. Rev. Respir. Dis.* 122:709, 1980.

36. Kauffman, F., et al. Eosinophils, smoking, and lung function. An epidemiologic survey among 912 working men. *Am. Rev. Respir. Dis.* 134:1172, 1986.

37. Burrows, B., Lebowitz, M. D., and Barbee, R. A. Respiratory disorders and allergy skin-test reactions. *Ann. Intern. Med.* 84:134, 1976.

38. Taylor, R. G., et al. Bronchial reactivity to inhaled histamine and annual rate of decline in FEV_1 in male smokers and ex-smokers. *Thorax* 40:9, 1985.

39. Vollmer, W. M., et al. Relationship between serum IgE and cross-sectional and longitudinal FEV_1 in two cohort studies. *Chest* 90:416, 1986.

40. Chatham, M., et al. A comparison of histamine, methacholine, and exercise airways reactivity in normal and asthmatic subjects. *Am. Rev. Respir. Dis.* 126:235, 1982.

41. Sparrow, D., et al. The relationship of non-specific bronchial responsiveness to the occurrence of respiratory symptoms and decreased levels of pulmonary function. The Normative Aging Study. *Am. Rev. Respir. Dis.* 35:1255, 1987.

42. Cockcroft, D. W., Berscheid, B. A., and Murdock, K. Y. Unimodal distribution of bronchial responsiveness to inhaled histamine in a random human population. *Chest* 83:751, 1983.

43. Weiss, S. T., et al. The epidemiology of airways responsiveness in a population sample of adults and children. *Am. Rev. Respir. Dis.* 129:898, 1984.

44. Hopp, R. J., et al. The effect of age on methacholine response. *J. Allergy Clin. Immunol.* 76:609, 1985.

45. Malo, J., et al. Reference values of the provocative concentration of methacholine that cause 6% and 20% changes in forced expiratory volume in one second in a normal population. *Am. Rev. Respir. Dis.* 128:8, 1983.

46. Welty, C., et al. The relationship of airways responsiveness to cold air, cigarette smoking, and atopy to respiratory symptoms and pulmonary function in adults. *Am. Rev. Respir. Dis.* 130:198, 1984.

47. Buczko, G. B., et al. Effects of cigarette smoking and short-term smoking cessation on airway responsiveness to inhaled methacholine. *Am. Rev. Respir. Dis.* 129:12, 1984.

48. Kabiraj, M. U., et al. Bronchial reactivity, smoking, and alpha$_1$-antitrypsin. A population-based study of middle-aged men. *Am. Rev. Respir. Dis.* 126:864, 1982.

49. Enarson, D. A., et al. Predictors of bronchial hyperexcitability in grainhandlers. *Chest* 87:452, 1985.

50. Vollmer, W. M., Johnson, L. R., and Buist, A. S. Relationship of response to a bronchodilator and decline in forced expiratory volume in one second in population studies. *Am. Rev. Respir. Dis.* 132:1186, 1985.

51. Tabona, M., et al. Host factors affecting longitudinal decline in lung spirometry among grain elevator workers. *Chest* 85:782, 1984.

52. Pham, Q. T., et al. Prognostic value of acetylcholine challenge test: A prospective study. *Br. J. Ind. Med.* 41:267, 1984.

53. Lertzman, M. M., and Cherniack, R. M. Rehabilitation of patients with chronic obstructive pulmonary disease. *Am. Rev. Respir. Dis.* 114:1145, 1976.

54. Nocturnal Oxygen Therapy Trial Group. Continuous or nocturnal oxygen therapy in hypoxemic chronic obstructive lung disease: A clinical trial. *Ann. Intern. Med.* 93:391, 1980.

55. Fedullo, A. J., and Swinburn, A. J. Relationship of patient age to cost and survival in a medical ICU. *Crit. Care Med.* 11:155, 1983.

56. Campion, E. W., et al. Medical intensive care for the elderly: A study of current use, costs, and outcomes. *J.A.M.A.* 246:2052, 1981.

21

Immune System and Immunoproliferative Disorders

Donald A. Jurivich
Harvey J. Cohen

THE IMPORTANCE OF AGE-RELATED CHANGES in the immune system has been underscored by numerous clinical observations of common diseases in the elderly. Taken collectively, these observations recapitulate a theme of age as an immunodeficient state. That age-related diseases have, in part, an immunologic basis is supported by epidemiologic studies that show an increased incidence of morbidity and mortality in the elderly due to infectious diseases and cancer [1,2]. Because the immune system has such a large role in the containment of microbial infections and neoplastic events, it follows that a decline in this system could ultimately account for a large proportion of illness and suffering in the aged population. Since current understanding of normal immune function, while quite extensive, is far from complete, age-related processes are difficult to establish. Furthermore, the task of distinguishing normal aging of the immune system from disease within it may be formidable. This latter point is particularly relevant if it is kept in mind that not all age-dependent changes in the immune system are deleterious. Some changes over time may represent an appropriately orchestrated readjustment to a different and age-related venue. Thus, the premise that immunosenescence can be either avoided or reversed must take into account that correction of one part of the immune system, such as autoanti-

body production, may have a negative impact on another part of the system, such as immune clearance of decaying cells [3].

The goal of reconstituting the immune system in old age raises some critical questions about establishing the cornerstone of normal aging. For instance, does failure in the immune system arise from precursor immunocytes or does it stem from more differentiated cells [4]? The immune system is a heterogeneous collection of cells that vary in their capacity for replication and differentiation. Consequently, what is observed in one component of the immune system may not necessarily be generalized to other components. Indeed, the various parts of the immune system may age differently and at different rates. Are these changes inevitable, and, more critically, are they irreversible [5]? To answer these last questions, the geriatrician/gerontologist must move the study of immunosenescence from simple observation to definitive intervention in age-dependent events.

In addition to diminishing the effects of age-dependent diseases, it is thought that reconstitution of the immune system in old age may either maximize or prolong human longevity. The shortened life spans of immunodeficient strains of mice compared to wild-type strains lend support to an "immunologic theory of aging" [6]. This theory suggests that senescence of the organism is due to an age-related decline in the immune system [7]. The crux of this theory rests on the observation of the predictable and progressive attrition of the thymus. As such, the steady atrophy of the thymus resembles the unwinding of a biologic clock. Detractors of the immunologic theory of aging point out that early thymectomy, which may occur in surgical cases, does not portend a shortened life span. Furthermore, pathologic evaluation of thymus tissue from various age groups suggests that the demise of this gland occurs much before any discernible change in the function of the immune system.

Nevertheless, efforts to link immunologic problems to abbreviated life expectancy have given some credibility to the immunologic theory of aging [8]. In one prospective longitudinal study the presence of autoantibody was statistically associated with a higher probability of death due to cancer or vascular disease than its absence [9]. Similarly, elderly patients who failed to mount a delayed-hypersensitivity skin reaction to common antigens were more likely to die during a two-year period than their skin-reactive cohorts [10]. Whether other decrements in immune function can be measured and assessed as predictors of the human life span is a possibility that needs further investigation. It is intriguing to consider that indicators of immune function may serve as biomarkers of physiologic aging—i.e., preservation of immunologic function into old age may predict those individuals who will become the oldest of the old. What remains to be seen is whether the promise of intact immune function throughout old age is matched with sustained mental and physical vigor.

To fully understand immunosenescence, normal immunologic function needs to be examined. The following section provides a review of basic immunologic processes and currently available data from human studies concerning age-dependent changes in the immune system. This review will provide the basis for discussion of clinical disorders associated with the immune system.

Normal Immune System

The immune system can be considered in terms of a peripheral part and a central part [11]. The former is represented by immunocytes in the peripheral blood, whereas the latter is composed of spleen, bone marrow, encapsulated lymph nodes, thymus, and organized lymphoid tissue such as Peyer's patches. Categorization of the immune system in this somewhat anatomic fashion is helpful because it reminds us that much of our knowledge of immune function in old age is based on studies of the peripheral immune branch and not necessarily of the central branch. To understand the protective nature of the immune system one must understand its cellular components and their function.

B-CELL SYSTEM

One of the essential components, the B-lymphocyte group, is responsible for the maintenance of the immunoglobulin profile found in serum, body secretions, and tissue. These cells are characterized by surface membrane or cytoplasmic immunoglobulin. Typically, the peripheral blood lymphocytic population is made up of 10 to 25 percent B-cells.

Activation of B-lymphocytes is a critical event in the production of antibodies. Assessment of B-cell activation can be achieved in vitro with a wide range of substances such as anti-immunoglobulins, lipopolysaccharides, lectins, calcium ionophores, and a variety of other agents, especially those capable of cross-linking B-cell receptors. Cross-linkage of a few B-cell receptors is not itself sufficient to drive this cell into an antibody-secreting cell. Both the quantity and quality of receptor cross-linkage determine whether a B-cell progresses from the G_1 phase to the S phase. Furthermore, other signals are needed to regulate B-cell function, and substances such as interleukin-2 (IL-2) and macrophage-activating factor appear to be necessary requirements for full B-cell activation [12]. Once B-cells become activated, they expand clonally and differentiate into antibody-secreting plasma cells. Some of these cells acquire an immunologic memory and generate a secondary humoral response when the body is rechallenged with antigen. The persistent capacity to respond and replicate and the ability to maintain fidelity of secreted products are important factors in the assessment of immunosenescence [13].

T-Cell System

T-lymphocytes are a heterogeneous collection of cells. Identified by agglutination with sheep red blood cells, 60 to 80 percent of circulating lymphoid cells are T-cells. By correlating the function of T-cells with their respective monoclonal antibody markers, T-lymphocytes can be categorized as helper, suppressor, or cytotoxic cells. This categorization is not a robust account of T-lymphocytes, however, and it is clear that subsets of T-cells occur even within the previously identified subpopulations. Evaluation of T-cell subsets and the assessment of T-helper to T-suppressor ratios have recently become a general measure of immune dysfunction.

T-helper cells perform a variety of duties. They secrete products that affect the activation and differentiation of fellow T-cells, B-cells, monocytes, and other hematopoietic cells. In addition to secretion of immunomodulating substances, T-helper function is based on cell-to-cell interactions. In this regard, some T-helper cells recognize class II antigens (HLA DR), which may play an important role in the up or down regulation of other immunocytes. Interestingly, some of the helper cells that lack the IL-2 receptor appear to have the ability to convert to suppressor cell function. Thus, it appears that T-helper cells have a varied potential for influencing immunologic events.

T-suppressor cells work toward inhibitory activity, insurance of self-tolerance, and controlled immune responses. T-cytotoxic cells can kill foreign or allogenic cells. They have the means to recognize class I surface antigens (HLA A, HLA B) and to lyse their targets. Another cellular immune response has been investigated in cells that appear as lymphocytes and are designated natural killer (NK) cells. These cells destroy foreign cells without any apparent cooperation or dependency on other immunocytes.

Monocyte-Macrophage System

In addition to lymphoid cells, immune function decidedly depends on the activity of the monocyte-macrophage system [14]. These cells, which make up 2 to 7 percent of circulating white blood cells, produce immunoregulatory substances and participate in cell-to-cell interactions. They also serve as scavengers. Like the T-cell system, the monocyte-macrophage system is composed of subpopulations. Perhaps the best known secretogogue of the monocyte-macrophage system is interleukin-1 (IL-1). This substance has an important role in stimulating other cells and contributing toward the febrile response. Other substances such as complement, superoxide, and interferon are produced by macrophages. Furthermore, these cells have been found to either activate or inhibit cellular responses. Like the T-lymphocyte, the monocyte-macrophage can either up-regulate or down-regulate immunologic activity (Fig. 21-1). These cells also act as antigen presenters. Their surface membrane recognizes particular cell types and offers the antigen to them for further reaction.

Cell-to-Cell Interactions

The crux of immune function lies in the interrelationship between immunocytes. This network of cells may have a distant relationship when immunoregulatory substances such as interleukin-2 are secreted, or it may be direct in nature, as seen in cell-to-cell interactions [15]. The affinity of one immunocyte for another is a critical determinant of immunologic activation and down-regulation.

One clear example of cell-to-cell interaction occurs during antigen processing. As part of the process, antigen-presenting cells such as the monocyte-macrophage contact helper T-lymphocytes. The contact is initiated after antigen is internalized and then processed onto the macrophage membranes in association with major histocompatibility complex II molecules. Helper T-lymphocyte recognition of activated macrophages subsequently leads to a cascade of lymphokine production and perhaps other cell-to-cell interactions [12]. Antigen processing by B-cells and presentation to T-cells has also been documented.

Finally, immunocyte-to-nonimmunocyte interactions are important in tumor surveillance [16], and because they are salient to the normal aging process they are discussed further below.

Immunosenescence

In reviewing immunosenescence it is clear that appropriate interpretation of the data is fraught with problems. First, because of the difficulties

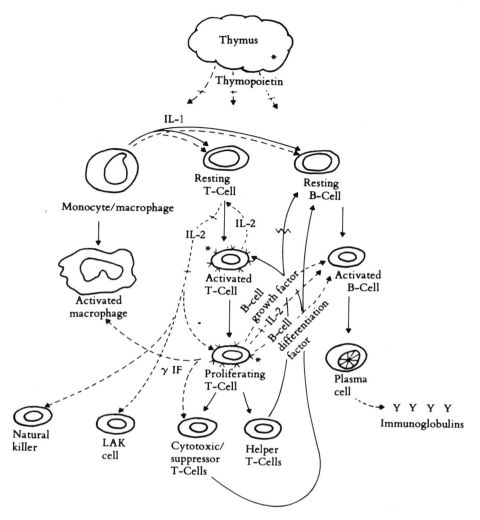

FIGURE 21-1. *Diagrammatic representation of several important cellular events and interactions that occur in the normal and aging immune system. Abbreviations: (-----) represents lymphokines and cellular products; (_____) represents intercellular events; (-) represents definite age-related alterations; (∨∨∨) represents possible age-related alterations; (*) represents functional changes with age; (∨) indicates cell receptor; IL-1 = interleukin 1; IL-2 = interleukin 2; IF = interferon; LAK = lymphokine-activated killer cell. (Adapted from A. S. Fauci, et al. Immunomodulators in clinical medicine. Ann. Intern. Med. 106:422, 1987.)*

intrinsic to the study of processes that encompass the human life span, animal models have been used heavily in the study of the immune system. Information gained from animal studies can provide valuable leads to understanding the human system, but such data cannot always be reproduced in humans. Second, data generated from human subjects comes mainly from cross-sectional studies and contain the weaknesses implicit in such studies (see Chap. 34). Third, examination of extremely old subjects, whose survival may be based on atypical immunologic vigor, may lead to a misrepresentation of normal aging. Finally, the complexity of immune responses creates a situation in which the elucidation of normal aging effects is offset by an incomplete understanding of what constitutes maximal or appropriate immune function. An important lesson to be gained from the study of immunosenescence is that age-related changes in this system are multifactorial [17]. As such, the immune system may exhibit heterogeneity in the expression of senescent change [18]. Thus, not all observed changes in the immune system over time may be experienced by all elderly, and different organs age at different rates—for example, the thymus versus the spleen. Despite the variability of the aging process, it is the search for common trends that helps to distinguish normal aging from age-related disease.

QUANTITATIVE CHANGES

The most impressive morphologic change in the aging immune system is thymic involution. The aging thymus has been portrayed as an essential link to the aging phenomenon and perhaps the critical determinant of human longevity. Cross-sectional autopsy studies have shown a linear decline in the thymic epithelial space commencing at birth as well as a similar decline in perivascular lymphoid tissue starting around puberty [19]. Curiously, extrapolation of these data indicates that functional thymic tissue should become extinct within 120 years—a period thought possibly to represent the absolute life span of man. While total loss of thymic tissue in extreme old age remains to be proved, it is clear that the aging thymus gland accumulates adipose tissue while lymphoid and epithelial tissue decrease. Although there is a relative decrease in the content of thymic macrophages, cell marker studies have verified a full spectrum of immature and mature lymphocytes that persist in the wisps of aging thymic tissue.

Morphologic studies of the peripheral elements of the immune system do not provide evidence of impressive age-related changes. The appearance of circulating white blood cells does not change with old age. Likewise, the constituents of the white blood cell population maintain their overall profile with old age [20]. Data from the Duke and Baltimore longitudinal studies have verified that both the white blood cell count and its differential are preserved in old age. Additionally, when ill or debilitated individuals are excluded, it is apparent that healthy elderly men longitudinally maintain their absolute number of peripheral blood lymphocytes [21–23]. Curiously, one study detected a decline in the lymphocyte count three years prior to death [24]. However, a premortem decline in the lymphocyte count may not represent an aging phenomenon. Physiologic stress has a profound influence on lymphocyte counts, and it is interesting to note that in one instance ambulatory male patients with health problems had elevated lymphocyte counts, whereas other groups had reduced counts. Thus, deviation of lymphocyte counts in old age may best be considered a barometer of illness and debilitation.

Because cell counts and morphologies do not change with age, attention has been given to the assessment of immunocytes by cell surface markers. Monoclonal antibody markers to cell surface antigens permit examination of subpopulations of immunocytes in old age. Such studies indicate that the numbers of circulating B- and T-cells do not change. Observations about age-related changes in subpopulations of T-lymphocytes have been marked by controversy and conflicting reports. Overall, there seems to be agreement with the finding that the number of mature T-lymphocytes, as detected by OKT3 monoclonal antibody, is preserved with old age [25]. By contrast, quantitation of helper and suppressor/cytotoxic T-lymphocytes in the elderly does not lend itself to a clear-cut consensus. Helper T-lymphocytes appear to remain unchanged with age; however, illness may lead to a reduction in their number. The number of suppressor/cytotoxic T-lymphocytes variably has been found to stay the same in the aged or decline. Likewise, the ratio of helper to suppressor/cytotoxic T-lymphocytes (T_4/T_8 ratio) has been shown to either increase with aging or remain unchanged. It is likely that claims of increased or decreased helper or suppressor cells in old age arise from studies that do not fully account for debilitated or ill elderly. Furthermore, circadian rhythms in the proportions of T-helper and T-suppressor cells would confound many of the claims that normal aging is accompanied by variances in the helper and suppressor T-cell populations [76]. The data certainly are not clear on the issue of age-related changes in the T-cell subpopulations, and while mouse studies do show a change in these cell types with senescence, it would not be prudent to assume that a parallel situation occurs in man. Quantification of T-lymphocyte subsets by more specific cell markers may eventually help resolve the issue of whether some of these cells undergo age-related diminution.

BIOCHEMICAL CHANGES

As part of the general phenomenon of cellular aging, immunocytes undergo biophysical and biochemical alterations over time [27]. Several intracellular defects have been found in lymphocytes from the aged. Many of these defects have been implicated in the age-associated impairment of mitogenesis [28]. For instance, stimulated lymphocytes from elderly persons manifest delays in enzyme activation as well as diminished glycolytic enzyme activity compared to that in young adults [9]. In addition to depressed energy-related events, these cells may have age-dependent fluxes in the activity of adenylate and guanylate cyclases [30]. Imbalances in the intracellular pool of nucleotide second messengers could further account for altered activation of resting lymphocytes into functional cells [31]. Thus, the overall impression is that aging significantly affects the metabolic and regulatory activities of lymphocytes.

In addition to altered intracellular activities with age, it appears that lymphocytic membranes undergo time-dependent change [32]. Membrane fluidity as detected by lipid probes is decreased in the aged [7,33]. By contrast, membrane protein organization in resting lymphocytes does not appear to change with age [34]. Thus, a dichotomy in age-related effects in lymphocytic membranes may exist where the lipid domain is more susceptible to senescent change than the protein domain. Furthermore, the cytoskeleton of lymphocytes from the elderly has been found to undergo subtle changes compared to that in lymphocytes from young adults [35]. One critical step toward lymphocyte activation is the capping of membrane components, and this too is altered with age [36–38].

Part of the reason that lymphocytes undergo change with age lies in their reduced ability to adjust to external stressors and internal errors. For instance, it is known that lymphocytes sustain increasing chromosomal damage with increasing age [39]. Lymphocytes from the elderly are also more susceptible to irradiating damage than lymphocytes from young adults [40]. The net effect of age on lymphocytes is to make these cells less capable of responding to physiologic and stressful stimuli in a timely and proficient manner.

FUNCTIONAL CHANGES

In contrast to morphologic studies of the aging immune system, functional studies provide the most insight about important age-related changes [41]. Results from these studies must be interpreted cautiously, however, for several reasons. First, many of the studies are in vitro phenomena and may not reflect in vivo situations. Second, most functional studies are performed on peripheral immunocytes and not on centrally located cells. Third, current knowledge of immune dysfunction with age is limited to observations of altered outcomes, such as the increase in autoantibodies, rather than to findings of altered mechanisms, such as how B-cells produce these autoantibodies. Given these caveats, we can critically examine both humoral and cellular immunity in old age.

Peripheral blood lymphocytes have been examined more frequently than any other immunocytes in the elderly because of the general inaccessibility of central lymphoid tissue from healthy elderly. Consequently, the information about normal immunologic aging in humans has been based on a population of cells that are thought to be rapid responders to external stimuli. These "front-line" cells may not necessarily reflect the functional ability of central lymphoid cells, in which immunologic memory and regulation have a prominent role. Peripheral blood lymphocytes in the aged have been studied in essentially two ways. In the first method, the cellular characteristics of resting or unstimulated lymphocytes in culture from young adult donors have been compared to those from aged donors. These studies have found inconsistent and, at best, subtle differences between resting young and old cells. The general impression has been that age-dependent differences in lymphocytes are made manifest on stimulation of these cells. Thus, the second and more telling method of detecting age-related changes in lymphocytes has been to examine their behavior when challenged antigenically or provocatively [42].

T-Lymphocytes

The preponderance of immunosenescent changes seems to reside in the T-lymphocyte [43]. As a very gross measure of functional change in T-lymphocytes with age, the cutaneous delayed hypersensitivity reaction is less vigorous in certain elderly [44]. Evidence that reactivity to tuberculin antigens diminishes with age has been suggestive of waning memory T-cell function, but studies that have elucidated this phenomenon have not clearly separated sick from healthy elderly [45]. Analysis of in vivo T-cell function, regardless of immunologic memory, has been undertaken by skin testing with a novel antigen, dinitrochlorobenzene [46]. Patients over the age of 70 have been found to respond to the skin test less well than young adults. Animal studies that have examined graft-versus-host reactivity have verified an age-dependent loss of T-lymphocyte function and add further credence to human in vivo findings [47].

In vitro studies of T-lymphocyte function have also shown an age-dependent decrement. In general, cultured lymphocytes respond to plant lectins such as concanavalin A and phytohemagglutinin by transforming into lymphoblasts. The response is markedly reduced in lymphocytes from healthy elderly, with the impairment greater in T-lymphocytes than in B-lymphocytes [25,48]. An undefined subpopulation of lymphocytes seems to retain its proliferative capacity in old age when a certain mitogen is utilized [49], suggesting that loss of mitogenic responsiveness in old age is selective. Loss of T-cell proliferative ability does not seem to be due to lack of mitogenic receptors in lymphocytes from the aged; thus, an intracellular defect must prevent uniform activation [46]. Lymphocytes from the elderly appear to divide well initially, but after the first division, their T-lymphocytes do not replicate as vigorously as those from young adults [50].

In addition to their in vitro ability to proliferate, T-lymphocyte function can be assessed by their ability to synthesize and secrete cellular products such as lymphokines [38,51]. Production of interleukin-2, an important stimulator in the immune response, is substantially reduced in the aged [52,53] and this decrease is accompanied by an altered ability of cells to respond to this lymphokine [54,55]. By contrast, production of another lymphokine, interferon, does not decrease with age [56], suggesting that some responses are preserved in senescent lymphocytes.

Although not produced by T-lymphocytes, thymosin is thought to be critical to the maturation of these cells, and reduced levels of this growth and differentiation substance have been found in the aged [57,58]. Whether reduced thymosin levels reflect an appropriate response to decreased turnover of this immunoregulatory substance or an immunodeficient situation is not clear [59].

B-Lymphocytes

Although a clearly demonstrable decline in T-lymphocyte function occurs with age, a parallel situation with B-lymphocyte function is not quite as apparent [60]. If anything, B-lymphocyte function decline may be related more to declines in requisite T-cell activity. For instance, overactivity of T-suppressor cells or underactivity by T-helper cells could downgrade B-cell function. Nevertheless, some data suggest that B-lymphocytes undergo intrinsic changes quite separate from T-lymphocyte dysfunction [61]. Pokeweed mitogen, a polyclonal activator thought to stimulate B-cells especially, has been found in one instance to activate cultured lymphocytes from elderly less well than those from young adults when radioactively labeled thymidine incorporation was measured [62]. In addition to promoting DNA synthesis, pokeweed mitogen can stimulate antibody synthesis in cultured lymphocytes, and in aged subjects a reduced ability to produce IgM was found [63]. Because pokeweed mitogen has T-lymphocyte dependency, loss of in vitro immunoglobulin synthesis after stimulation with this lectin does not indicate an intrinsic B-cell defect with age. Exposure to an antigen derived from salmonella purportedly activates B-cells independently from T-cells, and by this method both IgG and IgM production in vitro were found to be reduced in the aged [63].

Because B-lymphocyte studies in humans are limited to peripheral blood constituents, it is helpful to examine rodent studies in assessing the behavior of these cells in central lymphoid tissue. Here again, B-lymphocytes from splenic samples demonstrate an age-related decline in function that cannot be completely remedied by enrichment of cell cultures with accessory immunocytes or lymphokines [64]. A particularly interesting finding has been that certain clones of cultured B-lymphocytes from aged mice show a youthful ability to synthesize immunoglobulin, whereas up to 50 percent of other clones were unable to synthesize appropriate amounts of immunoglobulin [65]. This finding suggests that subpopulations of B-lymphocytes succumb to age-dependent events instead of the entire cell population. This apparent heterogeneity of aging in murine B-lymphocytes suggests that a particular component of the human immune system such as the bone marrow or spleen may be the nidus of B-lymphocyte senescence.

Other methods of assessing B-lymphocyte function have centered on evaluation of serum immunoglobulins. Serum determination of immunoglobulin concentration with age has revealed intact levels of IgG and IgA, whereas IgM levels appear to diminish by about 50 percent in the very old (Fig. 21-2) [66]. An interesting footnote in one longitudinal study was that a premorbid peak in IgG concentration occurred almost within a year of an elderly individual's demise [67]. Other studies have suggested that falling IgG levels are associated with a reduced life expectancy [68].

Naturally occurring antibodies such as isohemagglutinins have been found to decrease with increasing age [69]. Provocative studies that test for immunoglobulin production after challenge with an antigen or vaccine have also shown an age-related loss. Investigations of immunoglobulin response to influenza and pneumococcal vaccinations in the elderly have demonstrated diminished peak antibody responses compared to vaccinated young adults [70]. Furthermore, postvaccination maintenance of antibody levels is reduced in older individuals. Whether the primary humoral response is affected any differently from the secondary humoral response in aged humans is not clearly established, but murine studies have shown a substantial decrement in the primary immune response with age. Likewise, avidity of antibodies produced in the elderly have not been well delineated. Animal studies suggest that the

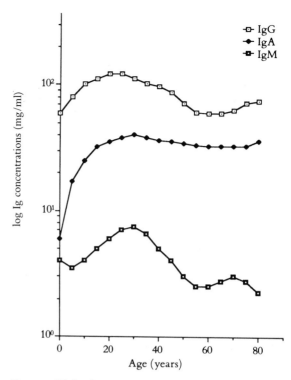

FIGURE 21-2. *Serum immunoglobulin levels in the elderly. (Adapted from C. E. Buckley, et al. Longitudinal changes in serum immunoglobulins in older humans.* Fed. Proc. *33:2037, 1974.)*

fidelity of the variable portion of the immunoglobulin to its antigenic target may decline in old age [71].

Monocytes
Monocyte function in old age has not been extensively studied despite the view that increased susceptibility to infections in the elderly is possible due to phagocytic dysfunction. One study of peripheral blood monocytes from hospitalized elderly found no measurable decrement in chemotactic responsiveness and phagocytosis [72]. The ability to migrate in response to a chemoattractant and the ability to kill *Candida* yeast both were comparable to the action of monocytes from young adults. Other functions of monocytes in old age, such as antigen presentation or cell-to-cell interaction, have not yet been examined. With current information, it appears that monocyte function, unlike that of T-lymphocytes, is preserved with aging. Why aging should have a preferential effect on one

cell type of the immune system is an interesting and incompletely understood phenomenon. Because immunocytes so freqently depend on growth factors and regulatory substances from autosecretion or from other cells, the apparent functional preservation of monocytes in old age suggests that these cells may hold the key to understanding maintenance of immunologic vigor over time.

Local Immune Function
Various organs such as the lungs, skin, and gut are laden with immunocytes that are responsible for local protection. Maintenance of local immune function in old age is poorly understood, mainly due to a paucity of studies in this area. Nevertheless, loss of fidelity in local immune function may be an important aspect of the aging process. For instance, the increased incidence of pulmonary infections in the elderly could be explained by altered immunologic function in the respiratory tree. Bronchoalveolar lavage of normal and sick elderly has shown fluctuations in pulmonary immunocyte composition [73,74]. These data, coupled with the recently reported finding of reduced phagocytosis by neutrophils in old age [75], suggest one mechanism in the loss of local immune responsiveness in the aged lung.

Age-related changes in cutaneous immune function have been suggested by the increased incidence of cutaneous neoplasia and shingles in the elderly [76]. The search for cutaneous immunosenescence has led to two observations. First, the density of Langerhans' cells in the epidermis decreases with age. Because these cells appear to have an immunoregulatory role by virtue of their ability to secrete interleukin-1-like substances and to present antigens to T-lymphocytes, it has been proposed that loss of these cells increases the susceptibility of the aged to cutaneous infections and neoplasms [77]. Second, there appears to be a loss of production of epidermal thymocyte-activating factor in elderly keratinocytes as well as a decreased responsiveness of lymphocytes to this substance. Furthermore, it has been observed that contact sensitivity to a neoantigen such as dinitrochlorobenzene is reduced in the elderly [77]. Thus, there is emerging evidence that

within the epidermis significant age-dependent events lead to immune dysfunction.

Mucosal immunity may also decline with age. Despite a 45 to 60 percent increase in basal levels of salivary IgA from elderly patients, secretion of this antibody under stress, such as occurs with influenza infection, may decline with age. The gut-associated lymphoid tissue (GALT) also undergoes age-dependent change [78]. In particular, Peyer's patches are reduced by 50 percent in the elderly. The actual impact of diminished GALT is not certain, but Japanese statistics [79] suggest that elderly patients experience a marked increase in gastrointestinal infections. Thus, local immune function associated with the gut must be altered. Studies in aged mice show reduced helper lymphocytes in Peyer's patches, but the net changes with age in humans are not clear. The limited information on gut-associated immunity in old age suggests that alterations in secretory function and changes in lymphoid composition of the gut may lead to an age-related increase in gut neoplasms and infections.

Clinical Manifestations
Clinical immunologic problems usually relate to cell proliferation. For example, lymphomas represent proliferation of immunocytes, and multiple myeloma represents proliferation of plasma cells and their secreted product, immunoglobulins. Hypoproliferative immune disorders, other than of the thymus, are less commonly encountered in the elderly than in the pediatric population. Additional age-related deficiencies in immune regulation may allow the emergence of other problems such as neoplasia, autoimmunity, immunocytopenias, and immune complex disorders. These disorders will be discussed first, followed by review of intrinsic immunocyte problems that lead to a spectrum of disorders ranging from monoclonal gammopathies to chronic leukemias.

DISORDERS OF ALTERED REGULATION
Neoplastic Disease
Over one-half of all cancers occur in people aged 65 and above [80]. The incidence of can-

cer rises continuously throughout life in both sexes, although the rise slows somewhat in the oldest old [81]. One of the factors frequently cited as important in this relationship is immunosenescence. Although there is evidence for this relationship in animal models, the link remains largely circumstantial in humans [82].

The major attraction to this theory is its logic—i.e., the immune system appears to be important in controlling tumor growth; its function diminishes with age—therefore, cancer may arise more frequently. Unfortunately, the relationship is far from this simple. As is obvious from Figure 21-1, there are many competing factors at work in immune system regulation. The immune response to a tumor is highly dependent on many factors including tumor antigenicity, factors produced by the tumor that influence the host, and the host's ability to respond [16,83]. The host responses include T-cell-mediated cytotoxicity, natural killer cells, macrophage-mediated cytotoxicity, antibody-dependent cell killing, and others [16].

As shown predominantly in animal models, some of these responses may be influenced by age. For example, decreased responsiveness of tumor-specific cytotoxic T-cells has been noted during the age-related decrease in the ability of mice to reject a transplanted fibrosarcoma [84]. Similarly, the increasing susceptibility of certain mouse species to a spontaneous lymphoma appears to be related to the decline in T-cell function [85]. Since many of the animal studies, such as tumor transplantation, are artificial and contrived, they must be interpreted carefully. In man, among the aspects of the immune system noted above to be putatively involved in tumor control, only T-cell function declines appreciably with age.

The control of the malignancy growth rate is another possible function of the immune system and has become a controversial issue because it is not clear whether the rate of growth of tumors in elderly people is different from that in the young. Anecdotal reports have suggested that tumor growth might actually be slower in the elderly [86], but other epidemiologic evidence does not support this contention and suggests a much more complex relationship [81,87,88]. Regardless, studies of immune function (again in animals) in this connection are interesting because they indicate the care that must be taken before fully accepting attempts at immunomodulation for cancer treatment. Thus, it appears that in some instances the immune system response to a tumor stimulates rather than inhibits the growth of the tumor [83,89]. This response may depend on type, stage, and antigenicity and may involve a highly complex immunoregulatory interaction [83]. How the changes in immune function with age relate to this phenomenon is not certain, but in some situations the potential exists for these changes to be advantageous as well as detrimental [89]. Thus, the use of immunomodulatory agents in the elderly will have to be carefully monitored.

Autoimmune Disorders

Because the incidence of autoantibodies increases with increasing age, it is important for the geriatrician to understand the relationship between autoantibody presence and the expression of autoimmune disease. Autoantibodies in the elderly do not always indicate autoimmune disease nor do they necessarily represent a proclivity to develop autoimmune disease. Furthermore, there is an emerging hypothesis that suggests that the occurrence of autoantibodies in old age may be in part an appropriate response in the down-regulation of some immune responses that had previously been under some other type of control [90]. A complementary view might be that the emergence of autoantibodies represents the aged immune system's way of readjusting to self-recognition and self-tolerance.

Some autoantibodies postulated to represent regulatory idiotypes may have a functional role in the immune system. A variety of data have been cited to support the hypothesis of an idiotypic network, and a review of the subject has been published [91]. The observation of a transient rise in rheumatoid factor after vaccination of normal subjects indirectly supports the idea that antibodies directed against immunoglobulins serve a physiologic purpose [69]. Until further information is available it is best to recognize that idiotypy may be part of a regulatory network that possibly may have additional importance in the aging process.

In examining the spectrum of autoantibodies in old age it is clear that these immunoglobulins can occur spontaneously as well as in response to induction [92]. There is some evidence that the presence of autoantibodies is associated with a higher incidence of mortality [9]. Commonly found autoantibodies in the elderly include rheumatoid factor, antinuclear antibodies, and antithyroglobulin. Of course, many other autoantibodies can be found in the elderly and may be associated with disease. Antibodies against cell receptors have been detected in Graves' disease (TSH receptor), type II diabetes mellitus (insulin receptor), and myasthenia gravis (acetylcholine receptor). Other antibodies may occur that may be more systemic in nature. These autoantibodies can be found in autohemolytic anemia, immune thrombocytopenia, and idiopathic neutropenia. The prevalence of antibodies increases with age and may involve 30 to 40 percent of all men and women above the age of 80 years. The general rule is that multiple autoantibodies can be found in the elderly, and there may be great variation in the titers of autoantibodies. A recent study found that the B-cell pool from elderly bone marrow was more likely to produce IgM rheumatoid factor on stimulation with the polyclonal B-cell activator, Epstein-Barr virus, than the B-cell pool from peripheral blood [69]. The size of the B-cell pool producing rheumatoid factor increased with increasing age. Interestingly, the B-cells that produced rheumatoid factor in the elderly seemed to be a less mature cell type than the B-cells that were associated with rheumatoid arthritis. The conclusions of the study were that the bone marrow was the primary respository of autoreactive B-cells in humans, and that IgM rheumatoid factor produced by these cells might serve a physiologic rather than a destructive purpose.

Perhaps one of the more important autoimmune phenomena in the elderly is drug-induced lupus erythematosus. Although drug-induced lupus is discussed in Chapter 31, it needs to be reiterated that certain features of this iatrogenic disease differ from the idiopathic condition. One key difference is that drug-induced lupus is more likely than idiopathic lupus to lead to polyserositis. Thus, pleural effusion and pericarditis could be one of the most serious side effects of lupus-inducing drugs. Although the suggestion has been made that slow hepatic acetylators have a greater likelihood of developing a lupus-like reaction from some drugs [93], it is not clinically possible to predict with certainty which elderly patients will experience a drug-related autoimmune effect. The astute geriatrician will maintain close follow-up in elderly patients who necessarily need to take drugs associated with lupus such as procainamide, isoniazid, and hydralazine.

Immune Cytopenias

Disturbances in the immune system that lead to an autoimmune basis for neutrophil, erythrocyte, or platelet destruction appear to increase with increasing age. Autoimmune hemolysis, although a rare event, occurs more frequently in the elderly than in younger adults [94,95]. Many of the cases are idiopathic or drug-related. With increasing age there seems to be a higher incidence of warm autoantibodies to erythrocytes than cold autoantibodies. The basis for this discrepancy in old age is not clear other than perhaps the higher incidence of drug use in the elderly population than in other adult groups. In fact, almost all of the drug-induced cases of autoimmune hemolysis are due to alpha-methyldopa, which has been associated with warm-type autoantibodies. It should be stressed that alpha-methyldopa can cause autoantibodies to emerge without clear evidence of hemolysis or reduced red blood cell life span.

The diagnosis of autoimmune hemolytic anemia is based on several laboratory features. The Coombs' test and reticulocyte count are the mainstay of investigation into hemolytic anemias, and further inquiry can be made by testing for cold-reacting antibodies and Donath-Landsteiner antibodies. Treatment of autoimmune hemolytic anemias depends on removing the underlying cause. Steroid therapy is usually warranted in idiopathic cases, and it will be effective in most of the cases. Refractory cases may require higher doses of steroid therapy; alternatively, the use of danazol, azathioprine, or cyclophosphamide may be necessary. Occasionally, splenectomy is performed after failure to obtain remission with drugs and plasmapheresis.

Neutrophils and platelets are also subject to destruction by an immunologic mechanism. Drugs that have provoked immunologic destruction of hematopoietic elements do so primarily through aberrant antibody formation. The antibodies may bind with the drug and form an immune complex, which in turn binds to the cell membrane. Alternatively, the drug may bind to the cell membrane and act as a hapten. Antibodies develop against this membrane-hapten complex. Finally, a drug may alter the surface membrane in such a way that de novo antibodies are formed against native membrane. Table 21-1 lists many of the drugs that have been implicated in immunologic destruction of red blood cells, platelets, and neutrophils.

Immune Complex Disorders
The formation of antigen-antibody complexes in the elderly can lead to immune complex disease. Nonspecific clinical findings such as weakness and low-grade temperature may be the only clues indicative of immune complex dis-

TABLE 21-1. *Drugs associated with autoimmune hemolytic anemia, autoimmune thrombocytopenia, and autoimmune neutropenia*

AUTOIMMUNE HEMOLYTIC ANEMIA		
Acetaminophen	Cephalothin	Chlordiazepoxide
Chlorpromazine	Chlorpropamide	Cyclophosphamide
Erythromycin	Ibuprofen	Indomethacin
Insulin	Isoniazid	L-Dopa
Mefenamic acid	Melphalan	Mephenytoin
Methadone	Methyldopa	Nalidixic acid
p-Aminosalicylic acid	Penicillin	Phenytoin
	Quinidine	Quinine
Procainamide	Streptomycin	Tetracycline
Rifampin	Triamterene	Phenylbutazone
Tolbutamide		

AUTOIMMUNE THROMBOCYTOPENIA		
Acetazolamide	Carbamazepine	Chlorothiazide
Chlorpropamide	Desipramine	Gold salts
Hydroxy-chloroquin	Methyldopa	p-Aminosalicylic acid
	Quinidine	
Phenytoin	Sulfa compounds	Quinine
Rifampin		

IMMUNE MEDIATED NEUTROPENIA	
Phenothiazine derivatives	Sulfonamides

SOURCE: Data for autoimmune hemolytic anemia adapted from J. Javid. Immune hemolytic anemia in the aged. *Clin. Geriatr. Med.* 1(4): 757, 1985.
 Data for autoimmune thrombocytopenia adapted from A. J. Marcus. Hemorrhagic Disorders: Abnormalities of Platelet and Vascular Function. In J. B. Wyngaarden, and L. H. Smith, (eds.), *Cecil Textbook of Medicine*. Philadelphia: Saunders, 1985. P. 1032.

ease in the elderly. These complexes deposit in tissue and lead to inflammatory reactions, which may not be as fulminant in the elderly as in younger adults. Detection of immune complex disease in the elderly can be done through a Clq-binding assay or a RAJI cell assay. The ability of these tests to detect immune complexes is such that they are complementary. Immune complexes not detected by Clq may be found by the RAJI cell assay and vice versa. Some of the more common immune complex diseases in the elderly include subacute bacterial endocarditis, drug reactions, and glomerulonephritis. In old patients the incidence of immune complex disease may be superimposed on preexisting illness and as such may appear as an indolent worsening of a chronic condition.

INTRINSIC IMMUNE DISORDERS
B-Cell Disorders
Foremost on the list of intrinsic immune system disorders during senescence are the B-cell disorders. It seems paradoxical that B-cells are able for the most part to maintain their ability to produce antibodies with age, yet are increasingly likely with age to go awry in their proliferative or maturational status. For instance, why does the incidence of monoclonal gammopathies increase with increasing age? Part of the explanation may be found in the age-related disruption of maturational events that are a necessary process in the progression of pre–B-cells to lymphoblasts. Other reasons for the development of B-cell disorders in old age surely exist and need to be elucidated, but clearly a range of B-cell disorders can be found in the elderly. Most important, each B-cell disorder has different clinical ramifications. For instance, the monoclonal gammopathies may be, on one hand, a laboratory phenomenon without apparent clinical repercussions, but on the other hand they may contribute to a clinically significant problem such as hyperviscosity syndrome. The same could be said for chronic lymphocytic leukemia, which may be either "smoldering" or fulminant in nature. In a broader sense, we can examine the clinical aspects of B-cell disorders according to whether they should contribute primarily to paraproteinemias or to proliferative problems.

 The B-cell disorders characterized by elevated serum protein levels include the mono-clonal gammopathy of unknown significance (MGUS), Waldenström's macroglobulinemia, and multiple myeloma. One of the key questions in geriatrics is whether a condition such as MGUS is a precursor to multiple myeloma. Treatment of B-cell disorders is briefly indicated in each of the following sections, but a more complete review is offered elsewhere [96].

MONOCLONAL GAMMOPATHY OF UNKNOWN SIGNIFICANCE

The prevalence of MGUS increases with increasing age. One study documented the range to be 1 percent at age 65 to 5 percent at age 80 [97]. A more recent study, utilizing different methodology, identified the prevalence of MGUS in retirement home residents as 7.4 percent in the age group of 70 to 79 years and 14.2 percent in elderly over the age of 90 years [28].

The importance of identifying MGUS in the aged lies in the association of this disorder with development of plasma cell or lymphoproliferative disorders. Twenty to twenty-eight percent of longitudinally followed patients with MGUS go on to develop some type of lymphoproliferative disorder. Although it is not known which of the patients with MGUS will develop a malignancy, a heightened clinical suspicion may allow early detection and treatment of this latter possibility.

Detection of MGUS has few clinical clues, and protein electrophoresis is the only certain means of identifying the presence of a monoclonal gammopathy. Agarose gel electrophoresis is more sensitive in detecting monoclonal proteins than cellulose acetate electrophoresis. Whether improved methodology in the detection of MGUS has clinical relevance with regard to the risk of progressing to malignancy has not yet been established. Ancillary clues to the presence of MGUS in the elderly include elevation of the erythrocyte sedimentation rate, red blood cell rouleaux formation, and elevated serum protein levels. The plasma viscosity may also be elevated, and urinary light chains may be detected.

The presence of MGUS, unlike multiple myeloma, does not usually result in the suppression of other immunoglobulin levels. The level of monoclonal immunoglobulin is generally

TABLE 21-2. *Clinical features of myoclonal gammopathy of unknown significance and multiple myeloma*

FEATURE	MONOCLONAL GAMMOPATHY OF UNKNOWN SIGNIFICANCE	MULTIPLE MYELOMA
Monoclonal immunoglobulin level	Usually <3.0 g/dl with stable concentration over time	>3.0 gm/dl with increasing concentration over time
Urine light chains	Possible, but infrequent	Present
Quantitative immunoglobulins	No change	Decrease
Albumin	No change	Decrease
Hemoglobin	No change	Decrease
Neutrophils	No change	Decrease
Platelets	No change	Decrease
Skeletal x-ray	No change	(+) Lytic lesions
Bone marrow	<10% plasmacytosis	>30% plasmacytosis
Plasma cell morphology	No change	Nucleolar size increase

under 3.0 gm/dl, and serial determinations of the protein concentration over a period of years commonly show little fluctuation. In fact, a precipitous rise in the immunoglobulin level is a probable indication that the monoclonal gammopathy has progressed to multiple myeloma. Distinguishing features between MGUS and myeloma are outlined in Table 21-2. Bone marrow examination is an important part of this workup.

Once an active disease process is ruled out, the patient can be followed without specific treatment. Patients with monoclonal gammopathies of unknown significance usually remain stable. Occasionally the gammopathy will resolve spontaneously, but at least 10 percent of patients eventually develop myeloma. Utilizing the serum protein levels as a major index, the initial diagnosis of MGUS must be confirmed by followup studies that show no progression in a three- to six-month period. Less frequent but continued followup should be maintained thereafter.

MULTIPLE MYELOMA

Multiple myeloma (MM) is one of the most striking age-related phenomena among the neoplastic disorders in humans [99] (Fig. 21-3). It is

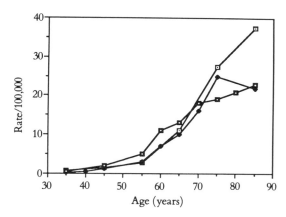

FIGURE 21-3. *Incidence of multiple myeloma from three different studies. (Adapted from H. J. Cohen. Multiple myeloma. Clin. Geriatr. Med. 1(4):829, 1985.)*

interesting to note that the relative prevalence of monoclonal gammopathies is 100 to 1 when compared to the frequency of multiple myeloma. Thus, it has been postulated that the etiology of multiple myeloma may be associated with a low incidence of genetic alteration in monoclonal-producing clones, which in turn leads to uncontrolled proliferation. This oncogenic event is probably a random occurrence rather than an age-related phenomenon because the ratio of monoclonal gammopathies to multiple myeloma does not change with time.

The primary clinical manifestations of multiple myeloma occur in bone and blood. Bone pain is common and is frequently located in the back. Osteoporosis with or without lytic lesions also occurs. This bone loss seems to be due to the direct absorptive effect of plasma cells and the indirect effect of osteoclastic-activating factors. Due to the insidious and fluctuating nature of bone pain from multiple myeloma it is possible to mistake this symptom for arthritic or degenerative bone and joint changes. In the elderly, lower extremity weakness with neurologic findings consistent with a spinal cord lesion could herald an oncologic emergency secondary to a spinal plasmacytoma.

Weakness and confusion in patients with multiple myeloma may be exacerbated in the bedridden elderly and may be due to hypercalcemia. In addition to immobility, poor oral fluid intake can increase serum calcium levels. Weakness may be compounded by a normo-

cytic, normochronic anemia. Plasma cell proliferation in the bone marrow may result in thrombocytopenia and leukopenia, which in turn may lead to hemorrhagic and febrile episodes. Neuropathies complicating multiple myeloma raise the suspicion of amyloidosis, although they are also seen in cases in which the IgG protein binds to myelin.

The detection of multiple myeloma may be initiated by screening tests. A spot check of the urine with sulfosalicylic acid may reveal non-albumin proteinuria. A positive result should be followed with urine electrophoresis and a 24-hour quantitation of urine protein. Serum electrophoresis may reveal a monoclonal serum component in an otherwise asymptomatic patient. X-ray skeletal surveys must be done to detect lytic lesions. Nuclear bone scans are not appropriate in the detection of myeloma-related bone lesions because they frequently fail to detect the predominantly lytic lesions in the absence of osteoblastic reaction. Finally, a bone marrow study should be performed in the elderly when a constellation of signs and symptoms consistent with MM is present. Elderly people tolerate this procedure as well as younger patients, and there is no increased risk of complications due to age. Bone marrow plasma cells in excess of 30 percent or biopsy-demonstrable plasmacytoma is indicative of multiple myeloma.

Once the diagnosis of multiple myeloma has been established, it is useful to stage the disease, providing a gauge of its course and prognosis. Table 21-3 shows a staging scheme for multiple myeloma. In stage I tumor mass is low, and treatment may not be warranted until symptoms become manifest. Close followup is indicated, and evidence of disease progression becomes the basis for intervention. The natural course of multiple myeloma in the elderly is similar to that in younger disease groups. Clinical experience indicates that chemotherapy is at least as well tolerated by the elderly as by younger treatment groups.

Treatment involves combinations of from two to five drugs [99]. Melphalan and prednisone have become the standard regimen, generally given as monthly courses, and when calculated on a per weight or size basis they do not require further initial adjustment for age. Mel-

TABLE 21-3. *Staging scheme for multiple myeloma*

STAGE	CRITERIA
I	Hemoglobin > 10 gm/dl
	Calcium < 12 mg/dl
	Normal x-ray skeletal survey or solitary bone plasmacytoma
	Low M-protein value
	IgG < 5 gm/dl
	IgA < 3 gm/dl
	Urine light chain < 4 gm/24 hr
II	Criteria not contained in stages I or III
III	One or more of the following:
	Hemoglobin < 8.5 gm/dl
	Calcium > 12 mg/dl
	Extensive lytic bone lesions
	High levels of M-protein
	IgG > 7 gm/dl
	IgA > 5 gm/dl
	Urine light chains > 12 gm/24 hr

SOURCE: Data from B. G. M. Durie and S. E. Salmon. A clinical staging system for multiple myeloma. *Cancer* 36:842, 1975.

phalan 0.25 mg/kg per day for four days per month and prednisone 80 mg per day for seven days comprise the usual starting doses, titrated to maintain a slightly suppressed white blood cell count. Other drugs such as cyclophosphamide, carmustine (BCNU), vincristine, adriamycin, and vinblastine are utilized in combinations but do not appear to offer any significant advantage to the elderly patient.

WALDENSTRÖM'S MACROGLOBULINEMIA
Another B-cell disorder in the elderly akin to multiple myeloma is Waldenström's macroglobulinemia [100,101]. Macroglobulinemia occurs when there is an inappropriate elevation of serum IgM. A monoclonal IgM can be seen in a variety of disorders ranging from a MGUS to a diffuse lymphoma. Roughly 70 percent of the cases result from neoplasms, with the remaining cases occurring as a MGUS or cold agglutinin syndrome. In Waldenström's macroglobulinemia, the prototypical disorder of monoclonal IgM, the mean age at presentation is 66 years old. The disease is usually manifested by hepatosplenomegaly, lymphadenopathy, and dilated retinal veins. Epistaxis is common, as is polyneuritis. Blurred vision and Raynaud's phenomenon are also common complaints.

The findings and workup of macroglobulinemia are similar to those of multiple myeloma

with some exceptions. Osteolytic lesions occur infrequently in patients with macroglobulinemia; thus, skeletal x-rays are not as rewarding in the detection of the disease. Hyperviscosity syndrome occurs more frequently in macroglobulinemia than in myeloma.

Treatment generally involves alkylating agents, with chlorambucil and cyclophosphamide used most frequently. Standard initial doses for these agents are 0.1 to 0.2 mg/kg per day and 1.5 to 2.0 mg/kg per day for chlorambucil and cyclophosphamide, respectively. The white blood cell count should be monitored to maintain slight neutropenia as an indicator of active drug effect. In the older patient with urinary retention cyclophosphamide should be used with caution because of the occasional occurrences of hemorrhagic cystitis. As noted below, when hyperviscosity is a major component of the clinical picture, plasmapheresis may be required. In such cases, however, long-term control still depends on effective chemotherapy.

HYPERVISCOSITY SYNDROME
Because hyperviscosity is a potential complication of all the paraproteinemias associated with B-cell disorders, it is important to recognize the clinical manifestations of this syndrome [102]. Bleeding problems such as epistaxis and retinal hemorrhage may be present. Fundoscopic examination is critical because dilated, sausage-shaped blood vessels and papilledema can be observed. Vertigo, dizziness, and progressive loss of consciousness may occur. Furthermore, signs of hypervolemia may be prominent, and cardiac failure may ensue. Determination of plasma viscosity can be a useful guide to the clinician to judge the effectiveness of therapy and for longitudinal followup. Plasmapheresis is indicated when hyperviscosity syndrome occurs.

CHRONIC LYMPHOCYTIC LEUKEMIA
Chronic lymphocytic leukemia (CLL), a disorder usually of B-cell lineage, is a prominent neoplastic disorder in the elderly [103]. It is one of the most common leukemias and occurs at a mean age of 60 years. Like multiple myeloma, this predominantly B-cell disorder has a slowly progressive character.

Patients may be asymptomatic, and CLL is often discovered after a routine blood count that demonstrates lymphocytosis. Splenomegaly and lymphadenopathy may be found. Symptoms associated with CLL include fatigue, weight loss, and night sweats. As the disease progresses, symptoms related to neutropenia or anemia may emerge. CLL portends an immunodeficient state, and sinusitus, pneumonia, and herpes zoster infections are common.

Laboratory abnormalities in CLL include a lymphocytosis generally greater than 15,000 cells/mm^3 and anemia. Thrombocytopenia may also occur. Monoclonal antibodies such as Leu-1 as well as surface immunoglobulin may serve as markers for the B-cell leukemia. Hypogammaglobulinemia can usually be found, and in some instances a monoclonal gammopathy may arise.

Survival in CLL depends on the stage of the disease (Table 21-4). Early stages are thought to be associated with a 12- to 15-year survival, whereas, later stages have a one- to three-year survival. Blastic transformation of CLL can occur and has a very poor prognosis.

Current evidence does not support early intervention in the beginning stages of CLL. Indications for treatment might include progressive lymphadenopathy, hepatosplenomegaly, anemia, thrombocytopenia, neutropenia, and recurrent infections. Treatment predominantly involves the use of the alkylating agent chlorambucil, given as a daily dose of 0.08 to 0.2 mg/kg, or every four weeks at 0.4 to 0.8 mg/kg. The addition of prednisone may increase responses and is especially useful if autoimmune cytopenias are present. Supportive therapy in CLL includes antibiotics for infections and blood products for anemia and thrombocytopenia.

HAIRY CELL LEUKEMIA

Hairy cell leukemia (HCL) can be confused with CLL and is another form of a chronic neoplasm that appears to have a B-lymphocyte derivation. Hairy cell leukemia occurs mostly in men over the age of 50 years. In contrast to CLL, this disease is usually associated with a low leukocyte count rather than an elevated one. The immunoglobulins in HCL are not usually affected as they are in the other B-cell disorders, but infections play a prominent role in this disease. Hepatosplenomegaly with pancytopenia should raise the possibility of HCL. Peripheral blood smears may show finger-like projections from the surface membrane of these cells, but generally a bone marrow biopsy is required to confirm the diagnosis.

Patients with adequate blood counts and no splenomegaly generally require no therapy. Severe anemia, neutropenia, and thrombocytopenia warrant splenectomy in HCL. The peripheral blood counts in most of the patients respond favorably after this procedure. For the patient without splenectomy or who fails to respond to splenectomy, alpha-interferon has become the choice for systemic treatment [104]. It generally is given subcutaneously several times a week, and initial doses are 2 to 3 × 10^6 units. The severe flu-like symptoms that occur as a side effect may be particularly bothersome to elderly patients. Chlorambucil is a much less effective alternative. Successful treatment of HCL with alpha-interferon has special significance in the elderly because it represents application of an immunomodulatory substance in a setting that is thought to be immunodeficient [104]. The implications of therapy with immune-generated substances such as interferon are exciting and hold the promise that immunomodulation may be successfully applied to other immune disorders in the elderly.

LYMPHOMA

As a final consideration of B-cell disorders in the elderly it should be pointed out that these lymphocytes can be associated with malignan-

TABLE 21-4. *Staging and survival in chronic lymphocytic leukemia*

STAGE	DEFINITION	SURVIVAL
0	Lymphocytosis ~ 15,000/mm^3	~ 150 months
I	Lymphocytosis, lymphadenopathy	~ 101 months
II	Lymphocytosis, hepatomegaly, splenomegaly, or both, with or without lymphadenopathy	~ 71 months
III	Lymphocytosis and anemia, with or without stage II criteria	~ 19 months
IV	Lymphocytosis and thrombocytopenia (< 100,000 per μl), with or without above criteria	~ 19 months

SOURCE: Adapted from R. H. Stahl and R. Silber. Chronic lymphocytic leukemia. *Clin. Geriatr. Med.* 1(4):861, 1985.

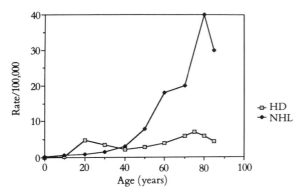

FIGURE 21-4. *Incidence of Hodgkin's disease (HD) and non-Hodgkin's lymphomas (NHL) per 100,000 population. (Adapted from J. H. Antin and D. S. Rosenthal. Acute leukemias, myelodysplasia, and lymphomas. Clin. Geriatr. Med. 1(4):795, 1985.)*

cies of lymph nodes. Categorization of lymphomas as strictly B- or T-cell lineage is not as straightforward as it seems. Consequently, review of lymphomas in the elderly is better approached by dividing these malignancies into Hodgkin's and non–Hodgkin's categories. Despite a paucity of studies on lymphomas in the elderly, some important facts about prognosis and treatment of elderly afflicted with lymphoma have come forth [105].

Non-Hodgkin's lymphomas (NHL) increase in incidence with increasing age [106]. Figure 21-4 graphically displays the importance of NHL as an age-associated problem. NHL are a diverse group of disorders with varied histologic and immunologic types and, unlike Hodgkin's disease, appear to be multicentric. Thus, they present with widespread disease early in their course. NHL may arise primarily in the gut and central nervous system as well as in the lymph nodes. Type B symptoms (fever, weight loss, night sweats, and pruritus) can be seen in non-Hodgkin's lymphoma but are less frequent than in Hodgkin's disease. It is not known whether the clinical manifestations of lymphoma in the elderly differ from those in a younger patient population.

In staging NHL, bone marrow aspirate and biopsy are performed as well as abdominal computed tomography (CT), but exploratory laparotomy is generally not required. Most patients manifest advanced disease. Prognosis is determined both by stage of disease and histol-

ogy. Bulky abdominal disease and a low hemoglobin level are particularly poor prognostic factors. Nodular pattern and well-differentiated lymphocyte histology are associated with a good prognosis. In this situation, elderly patients with few symptoms may be followed without treatment until problems develop. When required, treatment may be local with radiation therapy for symptomatic control, or it may be systemic, generally using alkylating agents such as chlorambucil or cyclophosphamide alone or in combination with vincristine and prednisone. These disorders are rarely cured but may be well controlled for long periods. The aggressive, or poor prognosis NHL, including the diffuse lymphocytic and histiocytic lymphomas, require aggressive therapy. Some NHL present locally and can be treated with radiation therapy. When systemic treatment is required, multiagent chemotherapy, including many of the drugs noted below for Hodgkin's disease, is utilized. Although both remissions and even cures can be obtained in the elderly, the overall rates are lower than in the younger adult, and toxicity with the aggressive regimens may be significant. Radiation therapy is limited in the elderly only by their ability to regenerate bone marrow elements and mucosa. Radiation doses above 3,000 rads increase the risk of complications in the elderly, and this point needs to be assessed by the radiation therapist [107].

Although not clearly either of B- or T-cell origin, Hodgkin's lymphoma has a bimodal incidence, and the second peak occurrence arises later in life [108]. For the elderly patient, the general principles of radiotherapy for localized disease and combination chemotherapy involving alkylating agents such as nitrogen mustard, cyclophosphamide, or chlorambucil and other agents including adriamycin, vincristine, prednisone, vinblastine, bleomycin, and procarbazine remain appropriate. Age seems to reduce the response rate and duration of remission after chemotherapy. Modified chemotherapy regimens and more advanced disease in the elderly may contribute somewhat to the impression that older patients with Hodgkin's lymphoma have a poor prognosis. One study suggested a prognosis in the elderly comparable to that in younger patients when there was an early stage Hodgkin's lymphoma [108]. Thus, while response and survival appear lower for elderly patients with Hodgkin's disease, treatment with a cure in mind should be considered for the older patients, especially with early stage disease and good functional status.

T-Cell Disorders

Since T-cells undergo important alterations with age, it is curious that they do not contribute more significantly to proliferative disorders in the elderly. Nevertheless, there are T-cell problems that may become an issue in geriatric practice. For instance, T-helper cell depression due to transfusion-induced acquired immune deficiency syndrome (AIDS) may play a larger role in the elderly population as more cases are being reported. A few cases of AIDS have been identified in men over 70 years old in New York [109], and even though the issue of elderly AIDS seems trivial, the question of whether elderly who were exposed to infected blood products mount the same antibody response to human immunodeficiency virus (HIV) as younger patients is not known. Lower immune responsiveness in the elderly could possibly lead to an underestimate of HIV-infected individuals. From a practical perspective, it would be prudent to test elderly patients for HIV antibody if they received blood products prior to HIV screening by local blood banks. The widespread practice of interstate blood shipments prevents assurance of a lower risk of transfusion-induced AIDS in areas where the prevalence of HIV is low.

Although HIV infections represent a selective suppression of T-cells, there are instances when overproliferation of T-cells poses clinical problems in the elderly. A small percentage of chronic lymphocytic leukemias are derived from T-cells, as are a small proportion of lymphomas.

Cutaneous T-cell lymphomas can also occur in the aged, although mycosis fungoides and Sézary syndrome generally occur during middle age. The finding of retrovirus genomes in T-cell leukemias and in cutaneous T-cell lymphomas has given recent support to the hypothesis that viral transformation is at the root of some lymphocytic neoplasms. Clearly, the interaction between external stressors such as the retrovirus and the aging immune system is an area that needs further exploration.

Although thymoma is infrequent and is not a T-cell disorder per se, its intimate association with T-cell development has special importance in the aged. The association of thymoma with many disease processes common to the elderly population deserves a parenthetical comment. Thymoma can be associated with thyrotoxicosis, myasthenia gravis, pemphigus vulgaris, hemolytic anemia, and neutrophil agranulocytosis. Thus, enlargement of the anterior mediastinum as detected by chest x-ray, especially in association with the aforementioned disorders, warrants CT or other imaging modalities.

Nutritional Impact on the Aging Immune System

The role of dietary habits in old age and the influence of nutrition on immune function have been recognized as important but are incompletely understood. The immune dysfunction that occurs in kwashiorkor syndrome has been cited as similar to the phenomenon that is thought to occur in protein-calorie malnutrition in the elderly. Perhaps an equally important consideration is the status of immune function in elderly patients who are under the stress of surgery and marginal nutritional intake. One study showed an age-related decrease in the leukocyte ascorbic acid level, and other studies have linked this finding to an increased risk of death in the elderly [10]. Alteration of protein stores, vitamin levels, and essential mineral content in the elderly can contribute further to the immunodeficiency of aging. Loss of cutaneous hypersensitivity, reduced lymphocyte responsiveness, and diminished quantities of white blood cells have been observed in elderly patients manifesting nutritional deficiency. Increased nutritional and vitamin intake improved all the immunologic parameters studied. Zinc supplementation in the elderly has been advocated on the basis of studies that show improvement of antibody production after immunization and increased responsiveness to intradermal skin testing in those given zinc.

Aside from overt malnutrition, the largest problem in addressing nutritional aspects of immune function in the elderly is not knowing the minimum levels of vitamins, minerals, and protein that would ensure maximal immune responsiveness. Furthermore, it is not clear whether aggressive nutritional advice and support will ameliorate some aspects of the immunodeficiency of aging [11]. Until better information is available, it is not possible to outline a cogent nutritional approach toward maintenance of immune function in old age.

Clinical Laboratory Evaluation of Immune Status

Laboratory investigation of immune status in old age can be accomplished in several ways [112]. A routine white blood cell count (WBC) and differential can provide the initial indication of immune status. The WBC ought to rise in response to infection in the elderly, and blunted elevations or even a decrease in the WBC may portend a poor prognosis. Lack of elevation of the WBC in response to infection may reflect overwhelming sepsis, poor nutritional status, chronic debilitation, or drug attenuation. Drug-induced neutropenia can occur insidiously in the elderly population, and although discontinuation of the offending agent will usually result in recovery of the white cell count, there is a 33 percent chance of death. Neuroleptics, especially the phenothiazines, are the class of drugs most likely to cause neutropenia.

Lymphopenia occurs frequently in sick elderly. Poor nutritional status has decided negative influence on lymphocyte counts. A clinical study showed that lymphopenia was a predictable result of acute bacterial infections in the elderly [13]. Furthermore, the prognosis of the acute bacterial infection decreased in proportion to the severity of lymphopenia. In fact, a mortality of 72 percent was observed in elderly patients with lymphocyte counts of less than 500/mm^3.

Lymphocytosis usually suggests chronic lymphocytic leukemia in the elderly, but this is not always the case. A "leukemoid lymphocytosis" can be associated with resolving tuberculosis as well as with solid tumors. To distinguish chronic lymphocytic leukemia from these other conditions, monoclonal antibody markers can be employed. Chronic leukemia will manifest a homogeneous cell population by cell marker study, whereas leukemoid lymphocytosis will result in a heterogeneous population.

Quantitative measurement of circulating monocytes in clinical geriatric practice has lim-

TABLE 21-5. *Conditions associated with monocytosis*

Tuberculosis	Listeriosis	Endocarditis
Syphylis	Inflammatory	Rheumatoid
Hemolytic	gut disease	arthritis
anemia	Immune	Post-
Agranulocytosis	thrombocytopenia	splenectomy
recovery	Hematologic and	
	solid malignancies	

SOURCE: Adapted from A. C. Allison. Macrophages and Neutrophils. In P. J. Lachmann, and D. K. Peters (eds.), *Clinical Aspects of Immunology.* Oxford: Blackwell, 1982. P. 125.

ited application. It is known that monocytopenia can occur after steroid administration, but perhaps an important consideration is the differential diagnosis of monocytosis. Table 21-5 outlines several conditions that are associated with elevated monocyte counts.

Elevations of other peripheral blood immunocytes such as eosinophils and basophils should prompt further investigation of infectious or neoplastic etiologies. Eosinophilia associated with atopy in the geriatric population is not as typical a finding as it is in the pediatric and young adult population. In fact, an alternative approach to assessing immediate hypersensitivity in the elderly population is skin testing. By this means it was found that the number of elderly patients with atopic histories who reacted to skin allergens was threefold less than in young adults [14]. Furthermore, skin reactivity to penicillin in patients allergic to this antibiotic appears to decrease with increasing age [115]. Loss of immediate hypersensitivity responses in the elderly does not mean that penicillin can be administered to elderly patients with a previous history of urticarial eruptions to this drug. Indeed, in life-threatening conditions in which penicillin or cephalosporin derivatives are required it is best to perform skin tests and desensitize elderly patients to penicillin. It is also important to note that drug desensitization does not confer lifelong protection from anaphylaxis. Thus, repeat courses of penicillin therapy require repetition of the desensitization process.

Skin testing in the elderly population is usually performed to evaluate delayed hypersensitivity reactions, especially in relation to the assessment of tuberculosis. Anergy, or the unreactivity to commonly recalled skin antigens, increases with increasing age. Thus, a negative response to intradermal administration of purified protein derivative does not necessarily preclude tuberculosis in the elderly (see Chap. 22). Delayed hypersensitivity reactions to agents such as *Candida* and *Trichophyton* decrease with age. Consequently, it is prudent to assess T-cell-mediated immunity in the elderly by intradermally testing for a battery of recall antigens in addition to the tuberculosis antigen. Some of these antigens include mumps, *Trichophyton, Candida,* and streptokinase-streptodornase. Skin test reactions ideally should be inspected within 24 hours to make certain that an accelerated reaction that may lead to skin sloughing has not occurred. This early inspection is particularly important when physicians choose to rechallenge a patient with purified protein derivative after a recent application.

Monoclonal antibodies can be helpful markers of immunoproliferative disorders in the elderly. Enumeration of clonal cell populations from blood and lymph nodes by cytoflotometry is a valuable tool, and the nomenclature for cell types detected by this technique will be referred to increasingly by a CD designation (clusters of differentiation). Measurement of T-helper (CD4) and T-suppressor (CD8) ratios in the aged, other than as an indicator of disease, does not appear to have much utility in this patient population.

Although not a measurement of immune function per se, the erythrocyte sedimentation rate may provide a nonspecific clue to disease in the aged. Elevation of a Westergren erythrocyte sedimentation rate (WESR) above 20 mm per hour cannot by itself be explained as an artifact of old age. Thus, depending on other clinical findings, a directed investigation of an elevated sedimentation rate in the elderly may increase the suspicion that a monoclonal gammopathy or other inflammatory condition may exist [116]. In conditions in which there is a persistently elevated WESR, there are some data to suggest that increased levels of C-reactive protein may be a nonspecific marker of an inflammatory condition superimposed on a chronic condition [117].

Quantitative and qualitative determinations of serum immunoglobulins in the elderly have special importance because of the increased incidence of paraproteinemias in old age. It is important to recognize that monoclonal gammopathies, both benign and malignant, can exist with normal levels of serum immunoglobulins. Another critical point is that light chain disease can occur without any evidence in the serum of this condition. Thus, urine immunoelectrophoresis is an ancillary test that is often necessary in the workup of paraproteinemias in the elderly.

Other serum components associated with the immune system can be measured and followed in immunoproliferative and inflammatory diseases. Beta$_2$-microglobulin (β_2M), a histocompatibility antigen sloughed from membranes of lymphocytes and plasma cells, has been associated with multiple myeloma and lymphoma [118]. Measurement of β_2M can be a helpful corollary to prognosis and therapy in the aforementioned disorders. Likewise, determination of serum complement levels can provide a guide to inflammatory disease activity in the elderly. Previously, the CH_{50}, or hemolytic assay, was used to detect alteration of complement levels, but current immunochemical determinations of C_3 and C_4 are preferred. Table 21-6 outlines diseases in the elderly that may be associated with elevated or reduced levels of serum complement.

Laboratory tests for autoantibodies are discussed in Chapter 31. In vitro assessment of immunocyte function in the elderly population currently does not have clear clinical applications, but future strategies geared toward im-

TABLE 21-6. *Complement levels in diseases encountered in the elderly*

HYPOCOMPLEMENTEMIA		
Systemic lupus erythematosus	Glomerulonephritis	Immune complex disease
Endocarditis	Myasthenia gravis	
Cryoglobulinemia	Lymphoma	Hepatitis/ cirrhosis
HYPERCOMPLEMENTEMIA		
Jaundice	Thyroiditis	Rheumatic fever
Rheumatoid arthritis	Diabetes	
Ulcerative colitis	Acute myocardial infarction	Gout

SOURCE: Adapted from D. P. Stites and R. P. Channing-Rodgers. Complement. In D. P. Stites, et al. (eds.), *Basic and Clinical Immunology.* Norwalk: Appleton & Lange, 1987.

TABLE 21-7. *Laboratory tests useful in the evaluation of the immune system*

TEST	NORMAL VALUES IN AGED	SIGNIFICANCE OF ABNORMAL TEST RESULTS
Westergren sedimentation rate	< 20 mm/hr	Elevated in monoclonal gammopathies, multiple myeloma, paraproteinemias, amyloidosis, and neoplastic and inflammatory conditions. Suppressed in red blood cell deformities (anisocytosis, spherocytosis) liver disease, and congestive heart failure.
C-reactive protein	0–23 mg/liter	Useful test for assessing acute inflammatory states, especially when Westergren sedimentation rate may be chronically elevated or falsely suppressed. May be elevated in active systemic lupus erythematosus when superimposed infection exists. Decreased levels in ulcerative colitis.
Antinuclear antibodies (ANA)	< 1:20	Important in drug-induced lupus, especially if signs and symptoms of vasculitis are present. ANA pattern in drug-induced lupus erythematosus is homogeneous (antibody reactive to DNA-histone complexes). Other diseases with positive ANA include cirrhosis, ulcerative colitis, CLL, AML, Waldenström's macroglobulinemia, hemolytic anemia. Up to 4% of healthy patients 65 years old and older may have elevated ANA.
Rheumatoid factor (RF)	< 1:40 latex fixation	Latex fixation RF titers of 1:40 or greater are considered elevated. Up to 24% of apparently healthy elderly over 60 years old have elevated titers. Some diseases associated with elevated titers include rheumatoid arthritis (~ 80%), systemic lupus erythematosus (15%), Sjögren's syndrome (96%), subacute bacterial endocarditis (48%), tuberculosis (11%), bronchitis (62%), cancer (22%), multiple myeloma (18%), and leukemia/lymphoma (19%) [49]. Also associated with cryoglobulinemia and transiently associated with immunization.
Immunoglobulins		
IgG	5–16 gm/liter	Decreased levels in protein-losing enteropathies, hematopoietic neoplasms, drugs.
IgA	0.5–4.25 gm/liter	Increased polyclonal levels in autoimmune diseases, malignancies, chronic liver disease.
IgM	0.5–1.8 gm/liter	Increased monoclonal levels in monoclonal gammopathy of unknown significance, multiple myeloma, chronic lymphocytic leukemia, lymphoma, Waldenström's macroglobulinemia.
IgD	~ 30 mg/liter	
IgE	0.3 mg/liter	
Parietal cell antibody		Elevated in pernicious anemia, iron-deficiency anemia, thyroid disease, atrophic gastritis, diabetes mellitus, and in 5–10% of normal elderly.
Antithyroid antibodies (Anti-thyroglobulin, anti-microsomal)		Elevated in thyroiditis, goiter, myxedema, thyroid carcinoma, and occasionally in normal elderly.
B_2 microglobulin		Elevated in lymphoproliferative disorders.

munologic reconstitution in the elderly could possibly add clinical utility to these tests.

Immune Reconstitution

In identifying many of the immune problems of old age, consideration has been given to interventional strategies. One possibility would be to reconstitute the senescent immune system, and another possibility would be to modulate selectively or upgrade certain activities of the immune system in response to problems with cancer, infection, or autoimmune disease. The complexity of the immune system is a sober reminder that a simple elixir is unlikely to remedy the immunodeficiency of aging [119]. Furthermore, the immune system probably readjusts itself to age-related changes in itself and other organ systems. Thus, any intervention will necessarily have to address the naturally occurring up-regulation and down-regulation of immune processes in old age. Given these caveats, what information can we glean from research that may provide insight into the possibility of improving the senescent immune system?

The first clear-cut example of interventional strategies in the aging immune system comes from immunization studies. Although immunization is covered in greater detail in Chapter 22, it is evident that immunization with pneumococcal and influenza vaccines can upgrade the immunoresponsiveness to these pathogens in the elderly. Unfortunately, immunization in the elderly does not ensure a more general improvement in humoral responsiveness to other infections. Future development of monoclonal antibodies to specific pathogens may hold the promise of passive immunization of the elderly against overwhelming infections, especially those of iatrogenic etiologies.

Positively influencing the aging immune system and its ability to mount a cellular response is the crux of any interventional strategy for the aged. The recent studies of improving antitumor capability by infusing autologous immunocytes previously incubated with interleukin-2 has opened new possibilities in the immunologic approach to cancer treatment. Although elderly patients have not been part of the lymphokine-activated killer cell protocol for the treatment of neoplasms refractory to chemotherapy, the application of immunomodulation in the aged patient, particularly with regard to tumor immunology, appears tenable.

In addition to possible supplementation with lymphokines, the aged may benefit from therapy that addresses thymic hormone depletion [120]. A recent study in humans has shown that the subcutaneous administration of thymopentin, the synthetic analogue of thymosin, improved responsiveness in antibody formation against the keyhole limpet hemocyanin antigen [121]. Another study has shown that TP-5, a five-amino acid analogue of thymic hormone, increased the amount of DNA synthesis in response to T- and B-lymphocyte mitogens. Furthermore, 1L-2 production was enhanced in lymphocytes from TP-5-treated subjects [122]. Delayed cutaneous hypersensitivity to common recall antigens was thought to improve in the TP-5-treated patients, but allowances were not made for a possible booster effect on antigenic rechallenge. The clinical ramifications of TP-5

therapy in the aged have not yet been studied, so improvement of in vitro tests may not translate into improved immune function in the elderly [123]. Whether other aspects of T-cell-mediated immunity are improved by thymopentin remains to be seen [124].

The impaired responsiveness of T-lymphocytes from the aged is partially reversible. In vitro addition of a phorbol ester and calcium ionophore seems to rejuvenate the lymphocyte's ability to incorporate radioactively labeled DNA much like its younger counterpart [125], suggesting that the DNA synthetic capacity is intact in aged cells but that the signaling systems for activating DNA replication are deficient. Although such information holds promise for improving DNA synthesis in aged cells, it will be important to determine whether this ability improves the immune response.

Immunomodulation of autoimmune diseases may also be possible. The finding in murine models that antibodies specific for class II histocompatibility antigens suppress the production of autoantibodies holds promise for controlling autoimmune disease in the elderly [126].

In conclusion, it appears that as more aspects of immunodeficiency and immune dysregulation of aging are identified, the ability to influence this system positively clinically becomes more feasible.

References

1. Felser, J. M., and Raff, M. J. Infectious diseases and aging. *J. Am. Geriatr. Soc.* 31:802, 1983.
2. Makinodan, T., et al. Immunologic basis for susceptibility to infection in the aged. *Gerontology* 30:279, 1984.
3. Kay, M. M. B. Aging of cell membrane molecules leads to appearance of an aging antigen and removal of senescent cells. *Gerontology* 31:215, 1985.
4. Kay, M. M. B. Age effects on colony-forming human peripheral blood T and B cells. *Gerontology* 31:278, 1985.
5. Duvall, E., and Wyllie, A. H. Death and the cell. *Immunol. Today* 7:115, 1986.
6. Good, R. A., and Yunis, E. Association of autoimmunity, immunodeficiency, and aging in man, rabbits,and mice. *Fed. Proc.* 33:2040, 1974.
7. Walford, R. L. *The Immunologic Theory of Aging.* Copenhagen: Munksgaard, 1969.

8. Horan, M. A., and Fox, R. A. Ageing and the immune response—a unifying hypothesis? *Mech. Ageing Dev.* 26:165, 1984.

9. Mathews, J. D., et al. Association of autoantibodies with smoking, cardiovascular morbidity, and death in the Busselton population. *Lancet* 2:754, 1973.

10. Roberts-Thomson, I. C., et al. Aging, immune response and mortality. *Lancet* 2:368, 1974.

11. Nagel, J. E., Yanagihara, R. H., and Adler, W. H. Cells of the Immune Response. In V. J. Cristofalo (ed.), *CRC Press Handbook of Cell Biology of Aging*. Boca Raton: CRC Press, 1985. Pp. 341–363.

12. Oppenheim, J. J., et al. There is more than one interleukin. *Immunol. Today* 7:45, 1986.

13. Adler, W. H., and Nagel, J. E. Clinical Immunology. In R. Andres, E. L. Bierman, and W. Hazzard (eds.), *Principles of Geriatric Medicine*. Philadelphia: Saunders, 986. Pp. 413–423.

14. Unanue, E. R., and Allen, P. M. The basis for the immunoregulatory role of macrophages and other accessory cells. *Science* 236:551, 1987.

15. Barrett, D. J., et al. Immunoregulation in aged humans. *Clin. Immunol. Immunopathol.* 17:203, 1980.

16. Bast, R. C. Tumor Immunology. In A. Devita (ed.), *Principles of Cancer Biology*. Philadelphia: Saunders, 1985.

17. Weksler, M. E. Biological Basis and Clinical Significance of Immune Senescence. In I. Rossman (ed.), *Clinical Geriatrics*. Philadelphia: Lippincott, 1986. Pp. 57–67.

18. Cinader, B. Immune Senescence: Individual Variation and Multicentricity. In A. deWeck (ed.), *Lymphoid Cell Functions in Aging*. Rijaswijk: Eurage, 1984. Pp. 3–16.

19. Steinmann, G. Changes in the human thymus during aging. *Curr. Top. Pathol.* 75:43, 1986.

20. Zauber, N. P., and Zauber, A. G. Hematologic data of healthy very old people. *J.A.M.A.* 257:2181, 1987.

21. DeViere, J., et al. Immune senescence: Effect of age and sex and health on human blood mononuclear subpopulations. *Arch. Gerontol. Geriatr.* 4:285, 1985.

22. Diaz-Jouanen, E., Strickland, R. G., and Williams, R. C. Studies of human lymphocytes in the newborn and the aged. *Am. J. Med.* 58:620, 1975.

23. Sparrow, D., Silbert, J. E., and Rowe, J. W. The influence of age on peripheral lymphocyte count in men: A cross-sectional and longitudinal study. *J. Gerontol.* 35:163, 1980.

24. Bender, B. S., et al. Absolute peripheral lymphocyte count and subsequent mortality of elderly men. *J. Am. Geriatr. Soc.* 34:649, 1986.

25. Nagel, J. E., Chrest, F. J., and Adler, W. H. Enumeration of T lymphocyte subsets by monoclonal antibodies in young and aged humans. *J. Immunol.* 127:2086, 1981.

26. Ohta, Y., et al. Normal values of peripheral lymphocyte populations and T cell subsets at a fixed time of day. *Clin. Exp. Immunol.* 64:146, 1986.

27. Tollefsbol, T. O., Cohen, H. J. Expression of intracellular biochemical defects of lymphocytes in aging. *Exp. Gerontol.* 21:129, 1986.

28. Brohee, D., et al. Specific effect of age on lectin-induced mitogenesis of lymphocytes from diseased patients. *Gerontology* 32:74, 1986.

29. Tollefsbol, T. O., and Cohen, H. J. Carbohydrate metabolism in transforming lymphocytes from the aged. *J. Cell. Physiol.* 123:417, 1985.

30. Tam, C. F., and Walford, R. L. Alterations in cyclic nucleotides and cyclase activities in T lymphocytes of aging humans and Down's syndrome subjects. *J. Immunol.* 125:1665, 1980.

31. Gutowski, J. K., et al. Impaired nuclear responsiveness to cytoplasmic signals in lymphocytes from elderly humans with depressed proliferative responses. *J. Clin. Invest.* 78:40, 1986.

32. Traill, K. N., et al. Age-related changes in lymphocyte subset proportions, surface differentiation, antigen density and plasma membrane fluidity. *Mech. Ageing Dev.* 33:39, 1985.

33. Rivnay, B., et al. Correlations between membrane viscosity, serum cholesterol, lymphocyte activation and aging in man. *Mech. Ageing Dev.* 12:119, 1980.

34. Jurivich, D. A., Rosen, G. M., and Cohen, H. J. Membrane organization of mononuclear blood cells from healthy young and old adults. *American Geriatric Society/American Federation of Aging Research Annual Meeting*, Abstract no. 19, 1987. P. 37.

35. Rao, K. M. K. Age-related differential effects of zinc on concanavalin A–induced capping of human lymphocytes. *Exp. Gerontol.* 17:205, 1982.

36. Chiricolo, M., et al. Alterations of the capping phenomenon on lymphocytes from aged and Down's syndrome subjects. *Gerontology* 30:145, 1984.

37. Noronha, A. B., et al. Changes in concanavalin A capping of human lymphocytes with age. *Mech. Ageing Dev.* 12:331, 1980.

38. Rosenberg, J. S., Gilman, S. C., and Feldman, J. D. Activation of rat B lymphocytes. II. Functional and structural changes in "aged" rat B lymphocytes. *J. Immunol.* 128:656, 1982.

39. Staiano-Coico, L., and Daryznkiewicz, Z. Increased sensitivity of lymphocytes from people over 65 to cell cycle arrest and chromosomal damage. *Science* 219:1335, 1983.

40. Johnson, R. C., and Wang, A. C. DNA repair, antibody diversity, and aging. *Gerontology* 31: 203, 1985.
41. Sokol, R. J., Hewitt, S., and Stamps, B. K. Autoimmune hemolysis. *Br. Med. J.* 282:2023, 1981.
42. Powell, R., and Fernandez, L. A. Proliferative responses of peripheral blood lymphocytes to polyclonal activation: A comparison of young and elderly individuals. *Mech. Ageing Dev.* 13: 241, 1980.
43. Gillis, S., et al. Immunological studies of aging: Decreased production of and response to T cell growth factor by lymphocytes from aged humans. *J. Clin. Invest.* 67:937, 1981.
44. Grossman, J., et al. The effect of aging and acute illness on delayed hypersensitivity. *J. Allergy Clin. Immunol.* 55:268, 1975.
45. Gianni, D., and Sloan, R. S. A tuberculin survey of 1285 adults with special reference to the elderly. *Lancet* 1:525, 1957.
46. Hausman, P. B., and Weksler, M. E. Changes in the Immune Response with Age. In C. E. Finch, and E. L. Schneider (eds.), *Handbook of the Biology of Aging* (2nd ed.). New York: Van Nostrand Reinhold, 1985. Pp. 414–432.
47. Menon, M., Jaroslow, B. N., and Koesterer, R. The decline of cell-mediated immunity in aging mice. *J. Gerontol.* 29:499, 1974.
48. Hollingsworth, J. W., and Gailotte, R. B lymphocyte maturation in cultures from blood of elderly men. *Mech. Ageing Dev.* 15:9, 1981.
49. Francus, T., et al. Effects of tobacco glycoprotein on the immune system. III. Effect of aging on the mitogenic response of human peripheral blood lymphocytes to TGP. *Cell Immunol.* 105:1, 1987.
50. Hefton, J. M., et al. Immunologic studies of aging. *J. Immunol.* 125:1007, 1980.
51. Bartfield, H. Distribution of rheumatoid factor activity in non-rheumatoid states. *Ann. NY Acad. Sci.* 168:30, 1969.
52. Ershler, W. B., et al. Interleukin-2 and aging. *Immunopharmacology* 10:11, 1985.
53. Wu, W. T., et al. The effect of aging on the expression of interleukin-2 messenger ribonucleic acid. *Cell Immunol.* 100:224, 1986.
54. Cheung, H. T., Two, J. R. S., Richardson, A. Mechanism of the age-related decline in lymphocyte proliferation: Role of IL-2 production and protein synthesis. *Exp. Gerontol.* 18:451, 1983.
55. Thoman, M. L. Role of interleukin-2 in the age-related impairment of immune function. *J. Am. Geriatr. Soc.* 33:781, 1985.
56. Weifeng, C., et al. The capacity of lymphokine production by peripheral blood lymphocytes from aged humans. *Immunol. Invest.* 15:575, 1986.
57. Bach, J. F. Immunosenescence. *Triangle* 25:25, 1986.
58. Lewis, M., et al. Age, thymic involution, and circulating thymic hormone. *J. Clin. Endocrinol. Metab.* 47:145, 1978.
59. Zatz, M. M., and Goldstein, A. L. Thymosins, lymphokines and the immunology of aging. *Gerontology* 31:263, 1985.
60. Ennist, D. L., et al. Functional analysis of the immunosenescence of the human B cell system. *J. Immunol.* 136:99, 1986.
61. Bender, B. S. B Lymphocyte function in aging. *Rev. Biol. Res. Aging* 2:143, 1985.
62. Mascart-Lemone, F., et al. Characterization of immunoregulatory T lymphocytes during ageing by monoclonal antibodies. *Clin. Exp. Immunol.* 48:148, 1982.
63. Wrabetz, L. G., et al. Age-related changes *in vitro* immunoglobulin secretion. *Cell Immunol.* 74:389, 1982.
64. Rosenberg, J. S., Gilman, S. S., and Feldman, J. D. Effects of aging on cell cooperation and lymphocyte responsiveness to cytokines. *J. Immunol.* 130:1754, 1982.
65. Zharhary, D., Klinman, N. R. Antigen responsiveness of mature and generative B-cell populations of aged mice. *J. Exp. Med.* 157:1300, 1983.
66. Buckley, C. S., III, Buckley, E. G., and Dorsey, F. C. Longitudinal changes in serum immunoglobulin levels in older humans. *Fed. Proc.* 33: 2036, 1974.
67. French, M. A. H., and Harrison, G. Serum IgG subclass concentrations in healthy adults. *J. Exp. Immunol.* 56:473, 1984.
68. Hallgren, H. M., et al. Lymphocyte phytohemagglutinin responsiveness, immunoglobulins, and autoantibodies in aging humans. *J. Immunol.* 111:101, 1973.
69. Fong, S., et al. Origin and age-associated changes in the expression of a physiologic autoantibody. *Gerontology* 31:236, 1985.
70. Ershler, W. B., Moore, A. L., and Socinski, M. A. Specific antibody synthesis in vitro. III. Correlation of in vitro and in nitro antibody response to influenza immunization in young and old subjects. *J. Clin. Lab. Immunol.* 16:63, 1986.
71. Makinodan, T., and Hirayama, R. Age-related changes in immunologic and humoral activities. *IARC Sci. Publ.* 58, 1980.
72. Gardner, I. D., Lim, S. T. K., and Lawton, J. W. M. Monocyte function in ageing humans. *Mech. Ageing Dev.* 16:233, 1981.
73. Braude, A. C., et al. Proportional analysis of respiratory cells obtained by bronchoalveolar lavage. *Can. Med. Assoc. J.* 126:1401, 1982.
74. Laviolette, M. Lymphocyte fluctuation in bron-

choalveolar lavage fluid in normal volunteers. *Thorax* 40:651, 1985.

75. Adler, W. H. Aging immune system. Presentation at the American Geriatric Society/American Federation of Aging Research Annual Meeting, Chicago, 1986.
76. Gilchrest, B. A. *Skin and the Aging Process.* Boca Raton: CRC Press, 1984.
77. Sauder, D. N. Effect of age on epidermal immune function. *Dermatol. Clin.* 4:447, 1986.
78. Schmucker, D. L., and Daniels, C. K. Aging, gastrointestinal infections and mucosal immunity. *J. Am. Geriatr. Soc.* 34:377, 1986.
79. World Health Organization. World Health Statistic Annual. I. *Vital Statistics and Cause of Death.* Geneva: World Health Organization, 1975.
80. Ries, L. G., Pollard, E. S., and Young, J. L. Cancer patient survival: Surveillance, epidemiology, and ERD results program. *J. Natl. Cancer Inst.* 70:693, 1983.
81. Crawford, J., and Cohen, H. J. Aging and neoplasia. *Ann. Rev. Gerontol. Geriatr.* 4:3, 1984.
82. Crawford, J., and Cohen, H. J. Relationship of cancer and aging. *Geriatr. Clin.* 3:419, 1987.
83. Prehn, R. T., and Prehn, L. M. The autoimmune nature of cancer. *Cancer Res.* 927, 1987.
84. Urban, J. L., and Schreiber, H. Rescue of the tumor-specific immune response of aged mice in vitro. *J. Immunol.* 133:527, 1984.
85. Bruley-Rosset, M., et al. Prevention of spontaneous tumors of aged mice by immunopharmacologic manipulation: Study of immune antitumor mechanisms. *J. Natl. Cancer Inst.* 66(6): 1113, 1981.
86. Ershler, W. B. The change in aggressiveness of neoplasms with age. *Geriatrics* 42:99, 1987.
87. Baranovsky, A., and Myers, M. H. Cancer incidence and survival in patients 65 years of age and older. *CA* 36:26, 1986.
88. Yancik, R., Ries, L. G., and Yates, J. W. Ovarian cancer in the elderly: An analysis of surveillance epidemiology. End results program data. *Am. J. Obstet. Gynecol.* 154:639, 1986.
89. Ershler, W. B. Why tumors grow more slowly in old people. *J. Natl. Cancer Inst.* 77:837, 1986.
90. Zanetti, M. New concepts on autoimmunity. *Immunol. Invest.* 15:287, 1986.
91. Bona, C. A. *Regulatory Idiotopes.* New York: Wiley, 1987.
92. Cammarata, R. J., Rodnan, G. P., and Fennell, R. H. Serum anti-globulin and antinuclear factors in the aged. *J.A.M.A.* 199:455, 1967.
93. Perry, H. M., Jr., et al. Relationship of acetyl transferase activity to antinuclear antibodies and toxic symptoms in hypertensive patients treated with hydralazine. *J. Lab. Clin. Med.* 76:114, 1970.
94. Jamshid, J. Immune hemolytic anemia in the aged. *Clin. Geriatr. Med.* 1:827, 1985.
95. Sohnle, P. G., Collins-Lech, C., and Huhta, K. E. Age-related effects on the number of human lymphocytes in culture initially responding to antigenic stimulus. *Clin. Exp. Immunol.* 47:138, 1982.
96. Westbrook, C. A., and Golomb, H. M. The Treatment of B-Cell Malignancy. In R. A. Thompson (ed.), *Recent Advances in Clinical Immunology.* Vol. 4. New York: Churchill Livingstone, 1987.
97. Kyle, R. A., Robinson, R. A., and Katzmann, J. A. Clinical aspects of biclonal gammopathies. *Am. J. Med.* 71:999, 1981.
98. Crawford, J., Eye, M. K., and Cohen, H. J. Evaluations of monoclonal gammopathies in the "well" elderly. *Am. J. Med.* 82:39, 1987.
99. Cohen, H. J. Multiple myeloma in the elderly. *Clin. Geriatr. Med.* 1:827, 1985.
100. Fudenberg, H. H., and Virella, G. Multiple myeloma and Waldenström macroglobulinemia: Unusual presentations. *Sem. Hematol.* 17:63, 1980.
101. Krajny, M., and Pruzanski, W. Waldenström's macroglobulinemia: A review of 45 cases. *Can. Med. Assoc. J.* 114:899, 1976.
102. Cohen, H. J., and Crawford, J. Disorders of Hyperviscosity. In S. E. Ritzman (ed.), *Protein Abnormalities.* Vol. 2. *Pathology of Immunoglobulins; Diagnostic and Clinical Aspects.* New York: Alan Liss, 1982. Pp. 237–259.
103. Stahl, R. L., and Silber, R. Chronic lymphocytic leukemia. *Clin. Geriatr. Med.* 1:857, 1985.
104. Golomb, H. M. The treatment of hairy cell leukemia. *Blood* 69:979, 1987.
105. Antin, J. H., and Rosenthal, D. S. Acute leukemias, myelodysplasia and lymphomas. *Clin. Geriatr. Med.* 1:795, 1985.
106. Greene, M. H. Multi-disciplinary approach to non-Hodgkin's lymphoma. *Ann. Intern. Med.* 94:218, 1981.
107. Fletcher, M. P. Immune function in the elderly. *Front Radiation Ther. Oncol.* 20:38, 1986.
108. Austin-Seymour, M. M., et al. Hodgkin's disease in patients over sixty years old. *Ann. Intern. Med.* 100:13, 1984.
109. Moss, R. J., and Miles, S. H. AIDS and the geriatrician. *J. Am. Geriatr. Soc.* 35:460, 1987.
110. James, S. J., and Makinodan, T. Nutritional Intervention During Immunologic Aging, Past and Present. In H. J. Armbrecht, J. M. Predergast, and R. M. Coe (eds.), *Nutritional Interven-*

tion in the *Aging Process*. New York: Springer-Verlag, 1984.

111. Hamm, M. W., Winick, M., and Schachter, D. Macrophage phagocytosis and membrane fluidity in mice: The effect of age and dietary protein. *Mech. Ageing Dev.* 32:11, 1985.

112. Brown, D. L. Interpretation of Tests of Immune Function. In P. J. Lachmann and D. K. Peters (eds.), *Clinical Aspects of Immunology*. Oxford: Blackwell, 1982.

113. Proust, J., et al. Lymphopenia induced by acute bacterial infections in the elderly. *Gerontology* 31:178, 1985.

114. Barbee, R. A., et al. Immediate skin-test reactivity in a general population sample. *Ann. Intern. Med.* 84:129, 1976.

115. Sullivan, T. J., et al. Skin testing to detect penicillin allergy. *J. Allergy Clin. Immunol.* 68:171, 1981.

116. Crawford, J., Eye-Boland, M. K., and Cohen, H. J. Clinical utility of erythrocyte sedimentation rate and plasma protein analysis in the elderly. *Am. J. Med.* 82:239, 1987.

117. Sliwinski, A. J., Weber, L. D., and Nashel, D. J. C-Reactive protein versus erythrocyte sedimentation rate. *Arch. Pathol. Lab. Med.* 107:387, 1983.

118. Alexanian, R., Barlogie, B., and Fritsche, H. Beta$_2$ microglobulin in multiple myeloma. *Am. J. Hematol.* 20:345, 1985.

119. Fauci, A. S., et al. Immunomodulators in clinical medicine. *Ann. Intern. Med.* 106:421, 1987.

120. Frasca, D., Adorini, L., and Doria G. Enhancement of helper and suppressor T cell activities by thymosin alpha 1 injection in old mice. *Immunopharmacology* 10:41, 1985.

121. Duchateau, J., et al. Modulation of immune response in aged humans through different administration modes of thymopentin. *Surv. Immunol. Res.* 4 (Suppl.):94, 1985.

122. Duchateau, J., et al. In vitro influence of thymopentin on proliferative responses and phytohemagglutinin-induced interleukin 2 production in normal human lymphocyte cultures. *Surv. Immunol. Res.* 4 (Suppl.):116, 1985.

123. Franchimont, P., and Bolla, K. Rationale for thymopentin as therapeutic agent in rheumatoid arthritis. *Surv. Immunol. Res.* 4 (Suppl.): 70, 1985.

124. Meroni, P. L., et al. In vivo immunopotentiating activity of thymopentin in aging humans: Increase of IL-2 production. *Clin. Immunol. Immunopathol.* 42:151, 1987.

125. Miller, R. A. Immunodeficiency of aging: Restorative effects of phorbol ester combined with calcium ionophore. *J. Immunol.* 137:805, 1986.

126. Klinman, D. M., et al. Suppression of Autoantibody Production with Anti-Class II Antibodies. In J. Brochier, J. Clot, and J. Sany (eds.), *Immune Intervention*. London: Academic, 1986.

22

Infections in the Elderly

RICHARD A. GARIBALDI
ELLEN G. NEUHAUS
BRENDA A. NURSE

RELATIVELY FEW DATA EXIST to support the widely held clinical impression that all elderly individuals are at increased risk for infection simply because they are old. Although physiologic changes occur over time in all organ systems, senescence of the immune system per se is not a major risk factor for infection. The elderly are not predisposed to infections with any single type of pathogenic organism. However, increased rates of infection occur in elderly patients with focal underlying diseases and chronic debilitation. The more severe the debility, the greater the risk of infection. The severely disabled elderly are at particularly high risk because they are unable to care for their personal hygiene and are often malnourished, immobile, incontinent, and institutionalized. Infections in these patients are associated with increased morbidity and mortality.

Infections usually present with typical signs, symptoms, and laboratory abnormalities. However, in the elderly the clinician must be alert to atypical presentations with nonspecific signs and symptoms. Evidence of focal infection is often absent or is obscured by underlying chronic conditions. In initiating antimicrobial therapy, the clinician must be aware not only of the array of pathogens that might be responsible for the infection but also of age-related physiologic changes in organ function that may affect antibiotic dosing. Strategies are available to prevent certain infections in the elderly. These include programs to help them maintain active life-styles, avoid risk factors for infection, and receive appropriate immunizations.

This chapter outlines the epidemiology and risk factors associated with infections in the elderly. It reviews the pathophysiology of infections at specific sites and points out the abnormalities associated with aging and chronic diseases that make the elderly susceptible to these infections. Finally, it stresses some of the unique features of infections in this population that challenge the clinician's diagnostic and therapeutic acumen.

Epidemiology
Population changes in the United States over the past fifty years and projections for the future have prompted a new interest in diseases of the elderly [1] (see Chap. 2).

INCIDENCE OF INFECTION
Relatively little cross-sectional or longitudinal data exist that document an increased incidence of infection in healthy, ambulatory elderly individuals. Comparisons of age-specific rates from different studies suggest that elderly patients may have higher rates of urinary tract infection as well as certain types of pneumonia and nosocomial infections. However, these studies

TABLE 22-1. *Rates of occurrences of selected acute infections by age group**

ACUTE INFECTION	AGE GROUPS (YEARS)			
	<5	5–24	25–64	>65
Common cold	76.5	36.4	23.3	14.3
Influenza	41.6	39.0	30.4	11.0

*Rate per 100
SOURCE: National Health Interview Survey, 1981.

do not take into account the impact of underlying chronic diseases that predispose the elderly to these infections. Thus, old age per se may not be responsible for the apparent increased rates of these infections. In fact, persons 65 years of age or older have lower rates than other age groups for certain infections such as the common cold and influenza (Table 22-1) [2].

Once infected, the elderly appear to be at increased risk for the more severe complications of infection. In the 1981 National Health Survey, the rate of hospitalization for acute pneumonia was 11.5 per 1,000 for patients 65 years of age or older compared with 2.0 per 1,000 for younger adults [3]. In 1983, elderly patients with pneumonia were hospitalized an average of 10.8 days and had a mortality of 12.8 per 100 hospital discharges compared with an average hospitalization of 7.5 days and a mortality of 1.5 per 100 discharges in younger patients [4]. Pneumonia/influenza is the fifth leading cause of death in persons over 65 years of age, with a rate of 148 deaths per 100,000 population.

Hospitalized elderly patients are at high risk for all types of nosocomial infections. In hospitalized patients between 70 and 90 years of age, rates of urinary tract infection, pneumonia, bacteremia, and wound infections are increased two- to fivefold compared with those in younger patients [5]. Descriptive epidemiologic studies confirm the importance of old age as a significant independent risk factor for hospital-acquired infections at each of these sites [6–8]. In fact, pneumonia accounts for 60 percent of the deaths attributed to nosocomial infection in seriously ill, elderly, hospitalized patients [9]. However, it is difficult in these studies to isolate the relative contribution of old age from the contributions of acute illness, chronic underlying diseases, impaired organ function, and ex-

posure to invasive diagnostic or therapeutic procedures that frequently complicate the hospital stays of older patients. For instance, elderly men and women are more likely than younger patients to require indwelling urinary catheters and are therefore at increased risk for urinary tract infections. They are more likely to have primary biliary tract disease, which predisposes them to ascending cholangitis. They are more likely to be bedridden or incontinent and are therefore at risk for decubitus ulcers and secondary skin infections.

RISK FACTORS

The susceptibility of the elderly to infection is influenced by several factors that are interrelated and perhaps work synergistically. The most important factor that predisposes to infection is the presence of chronic diseases that damage organ functions, impair clearance mechanisms, disrupt skin or mucous membrane barriers, and compromise cellular responses to infections. The degree of functional impairment or disability associated with underlying diseases has a direct impact on the risk of infection; the risk is highest in patients who are bedridden, malnourished, incontinent, catheterized, and institutionalized.

Physiologic Changes of Aging
Increasing age is accompanied by inevitable physiologic changes in organ function. Even relatively healthy elderly patients without identifiable chronic diseases undergo subtle changes due to the aging process [10] (see Chap. 1). For example, the aging lung loses elastic recoil because of changes in compliance and chest wall stiffness (see Chap. 20). These changes impair the effectiveness of the cough reflex and increase susceptibility to pulmonary infection. Age-related decreases in gastric acidity may predispose to infection with certain enteric pathogens. Aging skin has a decreased capacity for wound healing, greater likelihood for cracking or drying, and increased susceptibility to injury by ultraviolet light. Elderly patients with impaired memory and other subtle neurologic deficits are prone to accidents, errors in judgment, or misuse of medications that may indirectly increase their risk for infection. Subclinical physiologic impairments in renal and

liver function do not have a direct effect on the susceptibility to infection but may complicate therapy with antimicrobial agents.

Studies of the immune system and inflammatory responses in the elderly have revealed only subtle abnormalities that do not appear to play a major role in the pathogenesis of infection (see Chap. 21) [11,12]. The types of infections observed in the elderly do not suggest a particular type or severe degree of immunodeficiency. Reports of abnormal immune responses in elderly patients are difficult to interpret because of the possible confounding effects of nutritional deficits and other underlying disease conditions [13]. No important impairments have been reported in the function or numbers of polymorphonuclear leukocytes. T-lymphocyte numbers are also normal. However, T-lymphocytes collected from elderly patients have been shown to have a reduced ability to proliferate in vitro in response to challenges with specific antigens. This impairment is reflected in vivo by a decreased responsiveness to immunizing agents, including influenza and pneumococcal vaccines [14,15]. A diminution of cell-mediated immunity has also been noted in elderly patients. Functional impairments of cell-mediated immunity may be responsible for recrudescent herpes zoster infection or reactivated tuberculosis and may be related to increased activity of T-suppressor lymphocytes or a decreased production of interleukin-2, a lymphokine required for macrophage activation and natural T-killer cell activity [16]. However, skin test anergy and depressed cell-mediated immunity in this population may also be caused by malnutrition or other disease states rather than by old age per se. In fact, one study of non-hospitalized, elderly patients without chronic underlying diseases failed to show any depression in skin test reactivity compared with younger patients [17].

Diseases That Predispose to Infection

Many elderly persons are afflicted by chronic conditions that may predispose to infections. Diseases such as diabetes mellitus, chronic lung disease, cerebrovascular accidents, and cancer are known to impair host defenses and predispose to focal infections. More than 80 percent of adult patients with pneumonia have underlying emphysema, bronchitis, alcoholism, diabetes, or arteriosclerotic heart disease [18]. Drugs such as alcohol or tobacco and medications such as antidepressants or antihistamines may further impair cellular and mucociliary pulmonary defenses. Other drugs and neurologic diseases that depress mental acuity may predispose to aspiration pneumonia. Neurologically impaired patients are at increased risk for other infections by virtue of their immobilization, decreased sensory and motor function, incontinence, and poor personal hygiene.

Neoplastic diseases also predispose patients to infection. It is estimated that more than 50 percent of all cancers occur in patients over the age of 65. Cancer patients are at increased risk for pneumonia and other infections because of bronchial obstruction, generalized weakness, and malnutrition. Some malignancies have a direct effect on the bone marrow through invasion or involvement of specific cell types with a leukemic process. Conditions such as chronic lymphocytic leukemia and multiple myeloma are associated with diminished antibody production and a predictable risk of bacterial infection. Chemotherapeutic agents, prescribed as therapy for these malignancies, frequently damage skin and mucous membrane barriers, depress white blood cell numbers, impair granulocyte function, and compromise cell-mediated immunity. Other diseases such as diabetes mellitus or rheumatoid arthritis may further impair the functional capacity of white blood cells to react to bacterial pathogens. Thus, the presence of chronic diseases that impair the function of specific organ systems, including host cellular defenses, is a major risk factor for infection in the elderly.

Severity of Underlying Disease

The actual risk of infection in patients with chronic disease conditions is influenced by their overall level of disability. Severely ill patients are likely to have nutritional deficits that impair aspects of immunologic function, particularly cell-mediated immunity. Severely debilitated patients may be institutionalized, bedridden, incontinent of urine and feces, and unable to feed themselves or care for their personal needs. They are often treated with in-dwelling urethral catheters and nasogastric feeding tubes. Bed-ridden, incontinent patients are likely to have decubitus ulcers. Aspiration of oropharyngeal contents or food occurs frequently. Cough reflex and pain sensation are often impaired with increasing levels of neurologic dysfunction.

Because of their level of debility, elderly patients who need skilled nursing or medical care are often admitted to hospitals or nursing homes. In these settings they are frequently exposed to invasive therapies, antibiotics, and other infected patients. These exposures predispose them to colonization with potentially pathogenic microorganisms that subsequently may be responsible for infection. Increased rates of nosocomial infections at all sites are consistently reported for the elderly. High rates of infection are also reported for elderly residents of skilled nursing facilities. The prevalence of infection in these homes has ranged from 3 to 16 percent [19,20]. Skin, respiratory system, and urinary tract are the most common sites of infections in these patients. Like acute care hospitals, many skilled care nursing homes have problems with antibiotic-resistant bacteria and occurrences of epidemic infections.

Clinical Presentations of Infections in the Elderly

In most patients, both elderly and young, infections characteristically produce fever, tachycardia, and malaise as well as focal symptoms and signs of inflammation. However, in the elderly, clinical signs and symptoms are sometimes nonspecific, atypical, or absent (see Chap. 3). Temperatures may be normal, the tachycardic response may be blunted; anorexia and weakness may be ascribed to senility or chronic disease. The clinician must be aware of the possibility of infection whenever confronted with an elderly patient who presents with increased confusion, loss of appetite, new lethargy, unexplained tachycardia, or change in respiratory rate. Even the classic signs of focal infection may be missing in the elderly: the neck may be supple in patients with meningitis; pain and tenderness may be absent in patients with intra-abdominal infection; the temperature may be normal in patients with bacteremia [21]; leukocytosis may not be present in patients with

sepsis. In addition, many older patients are unable to communicate accurate histories of symptoms because of cognitive or affective disorders. These features of infections in the elderly are often responsible for delays in diagnosis and/or inappropriate therapeutic interventions.

In addition to their atypical presentations, infections in the elderly are often obscured by underlying chronic conditions. For instance, signs and symptoms of pneumonia may be difficult to interpret in elderly patients with chronic bronchitis or other pulmonary diseases in which cough and sputum production are invariably present. Clinical clues of urinary tract infection are frequently absent in patients with in-dwelling urinary catheters. The diagnosis of infected decubitus ulcers is often overlooked in bedridden elderly patients with abnormal mental status and diminished perception of pain. Septic arthritis may be difficult to distinguish from the primary disease in patients with severe rheumatoid arthritis or prosthetic joints. Elderly patients with neurologic disorders are predisposed to infection because of their immobility or cognitive dysfunction; in these patients, the diagnosis of infection may be obscured by blunted physiologic responses or an inability to perceive symptoms and communicate them effectively.

Infections at Specific Sites

Elderly patients are susceptible to infections at any site. However, some infections are particularly important in the elderly because of their frequency, morbidity, unique clinical features, or difficult differential diagnosis. Pneumonias, gastrointestinal infections, infections of the urinary tract, skin infections, meningitis, vascular infections, and fevers of unknown origin are some of the more common infectious disease problems of the elderly.

PNEUMONIA
Pathophysiology
Age-related changes in pulmonary defenses predispose elderly patients to lower respiratory tract infection [22] (see Chap. 20). Elastic tissue around the alveoli and alveolar ducts is decreased, and the anteroposterior chest diameter is increased. These factors, along with age-

related weakening of respiratory muscles, produce a less vigorous cough and a decreased ability to clear secretions. Changes have also been demonstrated in mucociliary function in the elderly, including a decrease in tracheal mucous velocity. Although it is unknown whether these findings reflect an abnormality of ciliary function or a change in the viscoelastic properties of mucus, the resultant effect is a relative inability to clear aspirated material effectively.

The presence of certain underlying diseases commonly encountered in the elderly further increases their risk for pneumonia. Patients with chronic bronchitis and obstructive pulmonary disease have damaged clearance mechanisms and altered pulmonary inflammatory responses. Smoking can also adversely affect mucociliary and macrophage function in these patients. Patients with cancer are predisposed to infection because of bronchial obstruction, malnutrition, bone marrow invasion, and quantitative or qualitative defects in white blood cell function. Patients with neurologic disease, esophageal problems, and alcoholism are at risk for aspiration pneumonia. Numerous medications are prescribed for the elderly that further increase their susceptibility to infection. Sedatives, tranquilizers, steroids, immunosuppressive agents, and anesthetics all affect components of the pulmonary defense system. The use of broad-spectrum antibiotics in hospitalized or institutionalized elderly can select for gram-negative bacilli, which are likely to be antibiotic-resistant.

Treatments with mechanical ventilators, nasogastric tubes, and nebulizers may further increase the likelihood of lower respiratory tract infection in severely ill hospitalized patients [23].

Diagnosis
The majority of elderly patients with pneumonia present with fever, cough, sputum production, dyspnea, and leukocytosis. However, atypical presentations are common and may cause dangerous delays in diagnosis and treatment. Mental status changes, lethargy, worsening of underlying congestive heart failure, anorexia, tachypnea, or acute respiratory failure may be the sole manifestations of pneumonia. In addition, the physical examination may yield few clues to suggest the diagnosis. As few as

25 percent of patients with documented pneumonia have rales on auscultatory examination [24]. Many elderly patients have preexisting chronic respiratory disease, which makes any findings on auscultation difficult to interpret.

Radiologic confirmation is essential for the diagnosis of pneumonia in the elderly. The absence of an infiltrate, even in the dehydrated patient, should prompt the clinician to search for another source of infection. The appearance of the pulmonary infiltrate, however, should not be used as the sole basis on which to choose antibiotic therapy; the x-ray is an unreliable predictor of the etiologic agent of pneumonia. Identification of a specific etiologic agent is always desirable and should be aggressively pursued. Obtaining expectorated sputum for Gram's stain and culture is often difficult in the elderly, especially if the patient is weak, dehydrated, or uncooperative.

Interpretation of sputum cultures is fraught with problems. Contamination with oropharyngeal flora is common, making accurate identification of anaerobic infection difficult. Gram-negative organisms, if present, overgrow other potential pathogens, especially when the specimen has not been cultured immediately. Delay in laboratory processing can also result in the death of fastidious organisms, such as pneumococci. Gram's stain of the expectorated sputum can enhance the reliability of the culture results. In addition, it can provide immediate information about the etiologic agent, making initial antibiotic choices more appropriate. The value of the sputum Gram's stain is greatest when it is examined by an experienced observer and when the specimen contains 10 or less epithelial cells and 25 or more white blood cells per high power field [25]. Columnar ciliated epithelial cells or macrophages, if present, are other indicators of an adequate specimen. Isolation of a single predominating organism is highly suggestive of its pathogenicity. A lack of growth or recovery of normal flora suggests aspiration pneumonia or an atypical pneumonia caused by virus, *Mycoplasma, Chlamydia,* or *Legionella.*

When expectorated sputum cannot be obtained or when the results are inconclusive or unsatisfactory, more invasive methods such as transtracheal aspiration, fiberoptic bronchoscopy, or open lung biopsy must be considered. Risks of complications from these procedures must be weighed against the risk of treating the patient with empiric or incorrect antibiotic therapy. The likelihood of identifying the etiologic cause of pneumonia can be enhanced by culturing blood and pleural fluid if present. Blood cultures should be drawn even if the patient is afebrile. Serologic tests are helpful to confirm the diagnoses of viral, *Mycoplasma,* or *Legionella* pneumonia. Throat and rectal swabs should be cultured for viral isolation, and sputum or lung tissue should be examined by direct fluorescent antibody techniques to identify *Legionella pneumophila.*

Pneumonia Syndromes
The causes of pneumonia in the elderly vary with the type and severity of the patient's underlying disease and the setting in which the infection occurs [26] (Table 22-2).

COMMUNITY-ACQUIRED PNEUMONIA
Streptococcus pneumoniae is the most common cause of community-acquired bacterial pneumonia in the elderly. However, sputum cultures are negative in as many as 50 percent of patients with x-ray evidence of pneumonia and positive blood cultures [27]. The lack of sensitivity of sputum cultures is due to the fastidious nature of the organism, inadequate collection or processing of the specimen, and the ease with which the organism is overgrown by other bacteria. Bacteremic pneumococcal pneumonia is more common in the elderly; the mortality approaches 60 percent in patients over 60 years of age [28]. Elderly patients are also more likely to experience empyema and extrapulmonary

complications, such as meningitis and endocarditis [29]. Penicillin G remains the treatment of choice for pneumococcal infection. Alternative agents include erythromycin, clindamycin, first-generation cephalosporins, and vancomycin. Although penicillin-resistant pneumococci have been described, they are not recognized as a major problem in the elderly. It is recommended, however, that all pneumococcal isolates from blood and cerebrospinal fluid be tested for penicillin susceptibility.

Hemophilus influenzae is a common colonizer of the respiratory tract in elderly patients with chronic pulmonary disease. It is often difficult to distinguish colonization from infection in patients with acute pulmonary symptoms. In elderly adults, pulmonary infections are most frequently caused by unencapsulated (nontypeable) isolates rather than encapsulated (type B) forms. In one study, 12 of 14 adults with documented *H. influenzae* pneumonia had nontypeable strains [30]. Most strains of *H. influenzae* are ampicillin sensitive. However, in recent years there has been an increase in the number of isolates that produce beta-lactamase, approaching 20 percent in some areas of the United States. Therefore, for serious infections in areas in which beta-lactamase-positive strains are common, initial therapy should include an agent such as chloramphenicol, trimethoprim-sulfamethoxazole, cefuroxime, or a third-generation cephalosporin pending laboratory evaluation for ampicillin sensitivity.

Legionella pneumophila is another important cause of community-acquired pneumonia in the elderly. Standing water is the principal reservoir of *L. pneumophila,* particularly water in air conditioner cooling towers. Cases of legionellosis occur in both sporadic and epidemic fashions in the community. Risk factors for infection include old age, smoking, alcohol intake, male sex, proximity to a construction site, and immunosuppression. The clinical spectrum of disease ranges from an upper respiratory infection characterized by fever, headache, and myalgia (Pontiac fever) to an atypical pneumonia to life-threatening infection. The more severe infections present with shaking chills, high fever, productive cough with mucoid or blood-tinged sputum, nausea, diarrhea, abdominal pain, and neurologic changes. The di-

TABLE 22-2. *Bacterial pathogens causing pneumonia in the elderly in descending order of frequency*

COMMUNITY-ACQUIRED INFECTION	HOSPITAL-ACQUIRED INFECTION
Streptococcus pneumoniae	Klebsiella pneumoniae
Enteric gram-negative bacilli	Other enteric gram-negative bacilli
Legionella pneumophila	Legionella pneumophila
Hemophilus influenzae	Streptococcus pneumoniae
Aspiration, including anaerobes	Staphylococcus aureus
Staphylococcus aureus	Aspiration, including anaerobes
	Hemophilus influenzae

agnosis of *L. pneumophila* pneumonia is made by comparing acute and convalescent serologic titers or by identifying the organism in sputum or lung tissue by direct fluorescent antibody staining. Erythromycin is the drug of choice for treatment.

Viral pneumonia with influenza A or B is an important cause of morbidity and mortality that are potentially preventable. Community-acquired outbreaks of influenza occur during each winter and spring season. Elderly persons, particularly institutionalized elderly patients with underlying cardiopulmonary disease, are at increased risk for pulmonary complications. The symptoms of influenza virus infection may resemble those of other respiratory viruses but are commonly characterized by a severe tracheo-bronchitis or atypical pneumonia syndrome. Patients with lower respiratory tract involvement are at risk for secondary infection with bacteria such as *S. pneumoniae, S. aureus,* or *H. influenzae.* Antiviral therapy with amantadine has been shown to be effective in modifying the disease course of influenza A infection if it is given within the first 24 to 48 hours of appearance of symptoms. Amantadine has also been shown to be useful as a prophylactic agent when given to susceptible uninfected elderly patients in an institutional setting during an outbreak of influenza A [31].

INSTITUTIONALLY ACQUIRED PNEUMONIA

Elderly patients frequently are institutionalized in nursing homes or hospitals. These patients are at increased risk for infection because of acute or chronic disease processes that may impair host defenses. Other contributory risk factors include the presence of altered neurologic function, tracheal intubation, exposures to antibiotics, and placement in intensive care units. Institutionalized patients who are most debilitated have a greater likelihood of colonization with gram-negative bacteria [32]. Thus, when they aspirate oropharyngeal contents, they frequently develop gram-negative rod pneumonias. Bacterial agents that are most commonly implicated in institutionally acquired pneumonias include the Enterobacteriaceae such as *Klebsiella pneumoniae, Escherichia coli,* and *Proteus* species. *Staphylococcus aureus* is another common isolate in these patients; in some hospitals and nursing homes, methicillin-resistant *S. aureus* infections are endemic. Patients who are intubated or receiving inhalation therapy are at increased risk of pneumonia with water organisms such as *Pseudomonas aeruginosa, Serratia marcescens,* or *Legionella pneumophila.* These infections are particularly difficult to treat because they are often resistant to first- or second-generation cephalosporins and penicillin.

The diagnosis of nosocomial pneumonia can be quite difficult in the elderly. Many patients already have underlying acute or chronic pulmonary disease and are producing purulent sputum. The diagnosis rests with such findings as the presence of a new fever, increased purulence of tracheal secretions, new auscultatory findings, or a new infiltrate on chest x-ray. However, the most reliable indicator of infection is the appearance of a new predominant organism on sputum Gram's stain [33]. The confirmation of pneumonia is particularly difficult in nursing home patients where x-rays, sputum Gram's stains, and cultures are usually not available. Gram's stain and culture of lower respiratory secretions are necessary to establish the cause of the pneumonia and guide the choice of antibiotics. Initial empiric therapy is given with a broad-spectrum agent to cover the array of gram-negative organisms and *S. aureus.* Aminoglycosides are not used as single agents in treating pneumonia because of their poor penetration into bronchial secretions. Usually aminoglycoside antibiotics are used in combination with a broad-spectrum penicillin, an antistaphylococcal antibiotic, or a third-generation cephalosporin. Concern about nephrotoxicity and ototoxicity in the elderly has prompted some clinicians to substitute other agents with broad gram-negative coverage for the aminoglycosides. The results of cultures and antimicrobial susceptibility testing should be used to guide the final selection of antibiotics.

ASPIRATION PNEUMONIA

Aspiration pneumonia can occur in elderly patients in either a community or institutional setting. Factors that predispose to aspiration are similar in both settings and include altered level of consciousness, depressed cough reflex, exposures to drugs or medications, periodontal disease, and disorders of swallowing. However, the etiologic agents responsible for aspiration pneumonias in a community setting are different from those causing infection in institutional settings [34]. Community-acquired aspirations are generally caused by a polymicrobial flora including gram-positive cocci and anaerobic bacteria such as *Bacteroides* species, fusobacteria, peptostreptococci, anaerobic streptococci, and occasionally *Actinomycetales*. In the hospital setting, aspiration with gram-negative organisms and staphylococci is more common.

The clinical presentation of patients with community-acquired aspiration pneumonia is often similar to that of other bacterial pneumonias. However, some patients experience a more indolent course with weeks or months of weight loss, low-grade fever, anorexia, and cough productive of putrid sputum. Any segment of the lung can be involved; however, the more common sites of infection are the superior segment of the right lower lobe and the posterior segments bilaterally. In the elderly, invasive methods of obtaining appropriate lower respiratory specimens for anaerobic culture are frequently contraindicated or not considered necessary. Parenteral penicillin or clindamycin are usually prescribed as empiric therapy. In addition to appropriate antibiotics, supportive therapy is recommended to aid breathing and to prevent recurrent aspiration and should include supplemental oxygen, chest physical therapy, proper positioning of the patient, avoidance of depressive medications, careful feeding, elimination of nasogastric tubes, and correction of predisposing underlying diseases that are amenable to treatment.

TUBERCULOSIS

Elderly patients, particularly those who are debilitated, continue to be at risk for pulmonary tuberculosis. Reactivation of upper lobe infection is the major presentation of disease in this population. However, as many as 80 percent of individuals older than 60 years of age now have negative tuberculin skin tests and are susceptible to primary tuberculosis. These patients may develop acute lower lobe pneumonia after exposure to an infectious case [35]. In the el-derly, tuberculosis needs to be considered in any patient with biapical pulmonary disease or an acute lower lobe pneumonia that does not respond to conventional antibacterial therapy. The diagnosis also needs to be considered in patients with symptoms of possible extra-pulmonary infection such as pyuria, vertebral osteomyelitis, meningitis, or fever of unknown origin. Most patients with active tuberculosis have positive skin test reactions. However, a negative skin test in a debilitated elderly patient should not exclude the diagnosis. In these patients, the diagnosis of tuberculosis must be made by a strong clinical suspicion, acid-fast stains, or appropriate cultures. Skin test reactivity may return after antituberculous therapy has been initiated and nutritional deficits have been corrected.

Active tuberculosis is treated with two or three drugs, depending on the severity of the infection and the debility of the patient. Isoniazid and rifampin plus or minus ethambutol or pyrazinamide are frequently prescribed combinations. Therapy for pulmonary infection is generally continued for at least nine months or six months after the sputum is negative for acid-fast organisms. Isoniazid-resistant tuberculosis is being diagnosed more frequently, particularly in patients from third world countries in which antituberculous drugs are available without prescription. In these patients, multi-drug regimens with as many as five agents are often prescribed. However, the final choice of specific drugs is usually determined on the basis of susceptibility testing and the patient's clinical response to therapy.

GASTROINTESTINAL INFECTIONS
Biliary Tract Infection
Biliary tract infection is one of the more common sources of intraabdominal sepsis in the elderly [36]. The pathophysiology of this infection in the elderly differs little from that in younger age groups. In more than 90 percent of cases, gallstones are responsible for obstructing the cystic duct, resulting in inflammation from trapped bile acids and subsequent infection. If left uncorrected, progressive cystic duct obstruction can compromise arterial, venous, and lymphatic flow, leading to further mucosal irri-

tation, inflammation, and tissue necrosis. This can result in perforation of the gallbladder wall with secondary peritonitis or intraabdominal abscesses. The elderly appear to be particularly prone to complications of cholecystitis such as empyema of the gallbladder and/or ascending suppurative cholangitis [37].

The classic clinical presentation of acute cholecystitis in both elderly and younger patients includes epigastric pain that migrates to the right upper quadrant accompanied by fever, nausea, and vomiting. However, in the elderly, classic signs, symptoms, and laboratory abnormalities may be absent in as many as 35 percent of patients [38]. Thus, the clinician must be alert to the possibility of gallbladder disease in patients without focal complaints. The diagnostic workup for biliary infection should include a complete blood count, liver function tests, and blood cultures. Abdominal x-rays detect gallstones in only 10 percent of cases; ultrasound examination of the right upper quadrant reveals stones in more than 90 percent of cases and is a more accurate method of identifying abscess formation. In patients with significant hyperbilirubinemia, neither cholecystograms (oral or intravenous) nor HIDA scans provide good visualization of the biliary tree. Computerized tomography of the abdomen is less sensitive than either ultrasound or cholecystography and does not assess gallbladder function [36].

Bile cultures taken at the time of surgery from patients with acute cholecystitis usually reveal aerobic enteric bacteria; the most common isolates are *E. coli, Klebsiella* species, *Enterobacter* species, and enterococci. Anaerobic organisms, either alone or in combination with enteric aerobes, are recovered from 15 to 30 percent of infected gallbladders [39]. Antibiotic therapy of patients with acute biliary sepsis should include drugs that cover the array of possible organisms that might be responsible for infection until the etiologic pathogen is identified. Treatment also includes the appropriate use of analgesics, intravenous fluids, and restricted oral intake. After medical stabilization, surgical intervention should be performed as soon as possible. Cholecystectomy is the procedure of choice for acute cholecystitis;

cholecystostomy and other drainage procedures should be reserved for those patients who may not tolerate a longer procedure [40].

Diverticulitis
Approximately 40 percent of patients 70 years of age and older have evidence of diverticular disease in autopsy studies [36]. The prevalence of diverticulosis increases with increasing age. Most diverticula are of the pulsion type with pockets of colonic mucosa bulging through the muscularis layers of the bowel wall and extending into the pericolic fat. Diverticulitis develops when fecal material obstructs the diverticular lumen, resulting in irritation, erosion, and leakage, often with perforation into the pericolic fat [41].

Most patients with diverticulitis complain of lower quadrant pain accompanied by fever, chills, and constipation; diarrhea is an infrequent presenting complaint. The physical examination usually reveals a palpable, tender, left lower quadrant mass with rectal tenderness or diminished bowel sounds. However, elderly patients are prone to atypical presentations such as absent or nonlocalized pain, nausea, or vomiting. The typical signs of peritonitis may be absent even when intestinal perforation has occurred. The organisms responsible for infection reflect the aerobic and anaerobic flora of the large bowel. In cases of intestinal perforation, early sepsis is likely to be caused by aerobic gram-negative bacilli. Individuals who survive the initial septic phase frequently develop intraabdominal abscesses with anaerobic organisms, particularly *Bacteroides fragilis* [42].

Many patients with mild diverticulitis can be managed medically with bowel rest; patients with more severe clinical disease who do not require surgery should be treated with intravenous antibiotics as well. Since a polymicrobial flora is often responsible for the infection, broad-spectrum antibiotics or antibiotic combinations are recommended for treatment. Patients who do not respond to conservative medical management, including those with signs of perforation or abscess formation, must be treated surgically. Mortality for these patients is related to delays in diagnosis, the extent of peritoneal soilage, and the presence of underlying conditions that may compromise the patient's ability to survive the intraabdominal infection.

Appendicitis

Appendicitis is an uncommon but clinically important site of intraabdominal infection in the elderly [43,44]. The elderly account for between 4 and 7 percent of all cases [39]. Normal aging changes include narrowing and obliteration of the appendix lumen, mucosal thinning, and arterial sclerosis. The latter can result in vascular thrombosis, gangrene, and perforation. The mortality of acute appendicitis in the elderly is as high as 16 times that of younger patients. The high mortality is due to delays in diagnosis and the presence of underlying medical problems. The symptoms of acute appendicitis in the elderly usually include abdominal pain, anorexia, and nausea with vomiting. Abdominal guarding and rebound tenderness in the right lower quadrant is present in only 50 to 75 percent [36]. Focal findings on abdominal x-ray or barium enema may sometimes be seen, but these modalities are neither sensitive nor specific indicators of the diagnosis. The treatment of patients with acute appendicitis includes surgery, supportive care, and appropriate intravenous antibiotics.

Hepatic Abscess

Although once considered a disease of young adults, as many as 30 percent of cases of hepatic abscess now occur in patients over 60 years of age [45–47]. In these patients infection is frequently secondary to prior biliary tract surgery, previous episodes of cholecystitis, or malignancies involving the pancreas of biliary tree. Other malignancies, abdominal infection, trauma, or previous bacteremic disease may also play a role in some patients. The clinical presentation of hepatic abscess in the elderly can be subtle or misleading. Most patients manifest fever, malaise, anorexia, and weight loss. However, in some patients the diagnosis is obscured by nonspecific symptoms, absent or atypical pain, and mental status changes. Some patients continue to have good appetites despite substantial intrahepatic infection. Laboratory abnormalities include a high white blood cell count, abnormal liver function studies, particularly the level of serum alkaline phosphatase, and an elevated right hemidiaphragm on chest x-ray. The diagnosis is usually confirmed by abdominal ultrasound, computerized tomography, isotopic liver scan, or gallium scan.

The treatment of intrahepatic abscess often requires a drainage procedure, which can be done percutaneously by a catheter if the abscess size and location permit or by open surgical drainage. Often both aerobic and anaerobic organisms are identified in aspirated specimens. The anaerobic organisms that are most commonly isolated include *Bacteroides* species, streptococci, and fusobacteria. The initial empiric antibiotic therapy must be broad-spectrum until a definitive etiologic agent is identified. Occasionally, antibiotics alone have been successful in treating patients who have multiple small abscesses or who cannot tolerate surgery [46,47].

Diarrheal Infection

As with other organ systems, certain changes occur in the aging gastrointestinal tract that may predispose to infection [48]. Atrophy of gastric acid-secreting cells and the presence of other diseases that delay intestinal motility can make the elderly susceptible to intestinal pathogens. Susceptibility may be further heightened by the administration of antacid medications, antibiotics, or drugs that delay intestinal transit. Despite these changes, there are no compelling epidemiologic studies that document an increased incidence of diarrheal diseases in the elderly compared to younger populations. In fact, elderly patients may be more likely to have acquired immunity to some enteroviral pathogens. However, the elderly, particularly those who are more debilitated, are at risk for severe dehydration or septic complications that may be life-threatening.

Gastrointestinal infections can be grouped into three broad clinical syndromes: acute food poisoning, noninvasive diarrhea, and invasive diarrhea. Episodes of food poisoning may occur as sporadic cases or clusters. The agents responsible for these episodes include *Staphylococcus aureus, Clostridium perfringens, C. botulinum, Vibrio parahaemolyticus,* and *Bacillus cereus.* The clinical manifestations of nausea, vomiting, and diarrhea associated with these pathogens are mediated by enterotoxins. The incubation periods of these diseases range from one to six hours for *S. aureus* to 48 to 72 hours for *C. perfringens*. Infections with longer incubation periods are characterized by lower gastrointestinal rather than upper gastrointestinal symptoms [49].

The noninvasive diarrheas are caused by a variety of agents including viruses, bacteria, and parasites. Of the viral agents, rotaviruses, Norwalk agent, and enteroviruses are the most commonly implicated pathogens. Occasionally, these agents are responsible for clustered outbreaks in nursing homes. Elderly patients are not at increased risk for infection with noninvasive bacterial pathogens such as enterotoxigenic *E. coli* or *Vibrio* species, or parasites such as *Giardia lamblia* or *Cryptosporidia*. The clinical syndromes associated with these infections include frequent loose stools or watery diarrhea without fever, abdominal pain, or systemic symptoms.

Salmonella, Shigella, and *Campylobacter* species cause invasive diarrheas that pose the most serious problems for the fragile elderly. The disease spectrum with these infections includes gastroenteritis, invasive colitis, bacteremia, sepsis, and death. Most often, patients present with bloody diarrhea, fever, and abdominal pain. Treatment of patients infected with any of these pathogens includes supportive therapy with fluid resuscitation, maintenance of electrolyte balance, and avoidance of antidiarrheal agents, which can increase the likelihood of tissue invasion and prolong the duration of symptomatic infection [50]. Usually, infections with these agents are self-limited, even in the elderly. For most cases, antibiotic therapy is not indicated and may prolong the carrier state, particularly with *Salmonella* infections. However, antibiotics are recommended for severely ill patients whose disease is complicated by profuse diarrhea, dehydration, systemic toxicity, bacteremia, or evidence of metastatic infection. The decision to initiate therapy is made on the basis of the clinical severity of infection, the epidemiologic setting, and the presence of other underlying diseases. Trimethoprim-sulfamethoxazole or aquinolone antibiotic is frequently prescribed for *Salmonella* and *Shigella* infections; erythromycin is the drug of choice for *Campylobacter*. It should be noted that recipients of antibiotics are themselves at risk for antibiotic-associated pseudomembranous colitis. This entity is caused by a gastrointestinal overgrowth with *Clostridium difficile* and is treated by stopping the offending agent and administering oral metronidazole or vancomycin.

URINARY TRACT INFECTION

Pathophysiology

The rates of asymptomatic bacteriuria and urinary tract infection increase with increasing age. The prevalence of bacteriuria ranges from 2 percent in young girls to 5 to 15 percent in sexually active women to more than 25 percent in healthy, elderly women. In men less than 50 years of age, infection is rare; the rate is 5 to 15 percent in elderly men. Rates of bacteriuria are as high as 25 to 50 percent for noncatheterized patients with chronic debilitating illnesses in institutional settings [51,52].

Several factors contribute to the higher rates of bacteriuria and urinary tract infection in the elderly [53]. With advancing age, the prostate gland may become chronically inflamed from microcalculi; prostatic secretions in these men have impaired bactericidal properties. In elderly women, a loss of pelvic support may result in urinary stasis. Postmenopausal estrogen deficiency causes changes in bladder and urethral mucosa and local antibody production that increase susceptibility to infection. Chronic vaginitis with bacterial overgrowth or fecal incontinence with perineal soilage are potential sources of urinary pathogens. Any condition that obstructs urinary flow can also predispose to infection. In the elderly, these processes include strictures, stones, tumors, prostatic hypertrophy, and sloughed papillae due to diabetes mellitus or drugs. Obstructed urinary tracts frequently require instrumentation or surgical procedures, further increasing the risk for infection [54].

Asymptomatic Bacteriuria

Bacteriuria is defined as the presence of bacteria in the urine, usually in concentrations of 10^5 or greater colony forming units (cfu) per milliliter of urine. Asymptomatic bacteriuria is more common in women than in men. The clinical significance of asymptomatic bacteriuria remains unclear. One study has reported that elderly, bacteriuric patients in a home for the aged had decreased survival compared with nonbacteriuric controls [55]. However, other studies have suggested that bacteriuria is only a marker for severe underlying disease rather than an independent risk factor for shortened survival [56]. Thus, the controversy regarding the significance of bacteriuria persists.

Data regarding the efficacy of treating asymptomatic bacteriuria with antibiotics are also controversial. Antibiotics have been unsuccessful in prolonging survival or preventing recurrent bacteriuria or symptomatic infection in noncatheterized men compared with untreated controls studied over a two-year period [57]. On the other hand, a study in elderly women has suggested a possible beneficial effect of therapy, but the follow-up period was only six months [58]. In addition, it must be remembered that repeated exposures to antibiotics may select for infections with resistant organisms.

Symptomatic Urinary Infection

Urinary tract infection is defined as bacteriuria with signs and symptoms of infection involving the kidneys, ureters, bladder, prostate, or urethra. Signs and symptoms of lower urinary tract infection in the elderly are similar to those in younger patients. However, urinary frequency and nocturia can be difficult to interpret in older persons. These symptoms can occur in the absence of infection and may be due to diabetes mellitus, medications, or neurogenic bladder dysfunction. On the other hand, some of the classic symptoms of infection, such as dysuria, may not be readily identified in patients with impaired neurologic function, indwelling catheters, or urinary incontinence. The localization of the site of infection to the upper or lower urinary tract by symptoms alone is unreliable. Infections at either site can sometimes present with chills, flank pain, and low back tenderness.

Laboratory findings suggestive of urinary tract infection at any site include pyuria with more than 10 white blood cells per high power field and bacteriuria with 10^5 or more cfu/ml urine. Occasionally, symptomatic infection can occur with urine colony counts as low as 10^3 or 10^4 cfu/ml [59]. The presence of white blood cell casts in urine sediment is diagnostic of renal involvement or pyelonephritis. Tests for antibody-coated bacteria are not widely available or well standardized. Invasive techniques are rarely indicated to identify the exact site of infection in the elderly. However, women with relapsing infection over a short period of time, patients with urosepsis, and men with infection who have not undergone prior instrumentation should be evaluated for underlying structural problems in the bladder, ureters, or kidneys. Ultrasonography can be an invaluable tool to rule out structural abnormalities, hydronephrosis, and intrarenal or perinephric abscesses that might require surgical correction. Intravenous pyelography (IVP) can detect calculi, anatomic anomalies, prostatic enlargement, and neurologic dysfunction. However, all elderly patients, especially those with poor renal function, must be hydrated vigorously prior to pyelography to avoid dye-associated nephropathy. Because of the sharp increase in adverse reactions and complications, IVP should be very carefully considered before use in the elderly.

In women, E. coli is responsible for more than 75 percent of symptomatic infections. In men, the range of potential urinary pathogens is much greater and includes the Enterobacteriaceae, enterococci, and Pseudomonas aeruginosa. In patients with polymicrobial urine cultures, the etiologic agent responsible for infection may sometimes be identified by positive blood cultures. Treatment of symptomatic infection should be directed against the most likely pathogen until final identification and sensitivities are known. The selection of appropriate empiric treatment is more difficult in patients who have had recurrent episodes of urinary tract infection and have received multiple prior courses of antibiotics that may predispose them to infection with resistant organisms.

Acute prostatitis usually presents with chills and fever, urgency, dysuria, and low back pain. On rectal examination the prostate is often swollen, extremely tender, and warm. Episodes of acute prostatitis are generally caused by gram-negative Enterobacteriaceae and are diagnosed by culture of midstream urine specimens. In chronic prostatitis urinary tract symptoms and signs may be minimal except for persistent perineal pain and dysuria. The diagnosis of chronic prostatic infection is generally made by culturing prostatic secretions obtained by massage, ejaculate fluid, or urine that is collected immediately after prostatic massage. The most likely causes of this infection are *E. coli* and other gram-negative bacilli, *P. aeruginosa,* and enterococci. Virtually all antibiotics penetrate into the acutely inflamed prostate; therefore, the choice of therapy for these infections is usually not difficult. On the other hand, relatively few antibiotics are able to penetrate into the noninflamed prostate, greatly restricting the choice of therapeutic agents. Trimethoprim-sulfamethoxazole is recommended for infections with susceptible organisms.

Catheter-Associated Urinary Tract Infections

More than 85 percent of episodes of hospital-acquired urinary tract infections are associated with urethral instrumentation or in-dwelling catheterization. In catheterized patients, the rate of new episodes of bacteriuria is 5 to 10 percent per day [8]. Catheter-associated infections are a major source of secondary gram-negative bacteremia and septic shock. Antibiotic-resistant Enterobacteriaceae, enterococci, *P. aeruginosa,* and *Serratia marcescens* are frequently responsible for these infections. Nursing home residents with chronic in-dwelling urethral catheters are also at risk for urinary tract infection and sepsis. Virtually all of these patients are colonized with multiple potential urinary pathogens [60]. In these patients the most commonly isolated organisms include *Proteus* species, *Providencia stuartii, E. coli, P. aeruginosa,* and enterococci. Generally, catheterized patients with asymptomatic bacteriuria should not be treated with antibiotics; these agents have only a transient effect on eradicating bacteriuria and predispose the patient to future infections with more resistant pathogens. Treatment should be restricted to patients with symptomatic infection. The choice of an appropriate antibiotic requires the identification of the responsible pathogen by culture and subsequent antimicrobial sensitivity testing.

SKIN INFECTIONS

Pathophysiology

The elderly are predisposed to skin infections because of physiologic changes in skin structure that occur with time [61]. The skin of old patients is strikingly different from that of younger patients. The epidermis is thinner, dryer, and more fragile and has fewer blood vessels. Poor wound healing in the elderly is a result of decreased vascularity and impaired collagen synthesis with slow epidermal turnover. Sensory nerve function is also diminished in the elderly, elevating their threshold for pain. These physiologic changes increase the susceptibility of the elderly to primary skin diseases, skin breakdown, diminished barrier function, and infection.

In addition to the physiologic changes affecting skin surfaces in the elderly, underlying diseases, malnutrition, medications (e.g, corticosteroids), and chronic exposure to noxious agents (e.g., ultraviolet light) are also important risk factors for skin infections. Certain conditions such as psoriasis, skin cancers, peripheral vascular diseases, and dependent edema have a direct effect on integumental barriers. Many primary underlying diseases affecting the elderly contribute to their increased risk for decubitus ulcers that may become secondarily infected. These include conditions that are associated with abnormal mental function, immobility, incontinence, and poor personal hygiene.

Specific Skin Infections

BACTERIAL INFECTIONS

The skin of the elderly is susceptible to a variety of bacterial infections. Elderly patients who undergo surgery have an increased incidence of postoperative wound infection; the likelihood of developing infection is related to the specific surgical procedure. The risk is as high as 25 to 30 percent in patients undergoing bowel resections [6]. In elderly patients with peripheral vascular disease secondary to arteriosclerosis or diabetes mellitus, small foot ulcers may become infected with both aerobic and anaerobic bacteria and develop into sites of focal necrosis that may progress to gangrene or bacteremia. Immobile, incontinent elderly are also at high risk for decubitus ulcers. These open, poorly vascularized skin lesions are common sites of infection with anaerobic and aerobic fecal flora. Infected decubitus ulcers can be quite extensive, undermining normal skin and spreading within fascial planes. They are difficult to treat because of the types of organisms involved and the overall debility of the patient. Surgical management with incision, drainage, and débridement is usually necessary. However, wound healing is poor in these patients, and the underlying disease processes are usually uncorrectable. Thus, the morbidity and mortality of decubitus ulcer infections are extremely high.

VIRAL INFECTIONS

Infections of the skin involving nonbacterial agents are relatively uncommon with the exception of herpes zoster virus infection. Contrary to earlier teachings, most of the elderly patients who are infected with this virus are otherwise healthy. The exact mechanisms by which varicella-zoster virus infections remain latent and the reasons for reactivation are not totally known. Reactivation may be precipitated by a variety of stimuli including stress, trauma, immunosuppressive therapy, and malignancy, particularly lymphoma or leukemia. Reactivation of herpes zoster may occur in up to 13 percent of patients with Hodgkin's disease [62]. However, zoster rarely antedates the diagnosis of malignancy.

The peak incidence of zoster infection occurs between 50 and 70 years of age. The clinical diagnosis is not difficult when dermatomal pain is followed by a band-like grouping of erythematous papules that progress to vesicles within 12 to 24 hours. These vesicles usually encrust within 10 to 12 days. The most perplexing complication of herpes zoster infection is postherpetic neuralgia, which affects between 25 and 40 percent of patients over 60 years of age. The incidence of postherpetic neuralgia is not affected by antiviral therapy with acyclovir. However, the risk of this complication may be decreased by the early initiation of high-dose corticosteroids [63].

BACTERIAL MENINGITIS

Although not a common infection, bacterial meningitis is frequently associated with a high degree of morbidity and mortality in the elderly.

Pathophysiology

As in younger patients, meningitis in the elderly can result from hematogenous spread from distant sites, direct inoculation from postsurgical or posttraumatic infection, or contiguous spread from sinusitis, otitis media, or mastoiditis. *Streptococcus pneumoniae* is the most common identifiable agent causing meningitis in the elderly. However, unlike the younger population, in which *Neisseria meningitidis* and *Hemophilus influenzae* are responsible for most of the other cases, bacterial meningitis in the elderly is also caused by unusual pathogens, such as gram-negative bacilli, *Listeria monocytogenes,* and *S. aureus;* these organisms are responsible for approximately 8 percent, 7 percent, and 6 percent of cases, respectively [64]. Tertiary care hospitals and Veterans Administration hospitals report even greater numbers of infections with unusual organisms.

Clinical Picture

Mental status changes, headache, fever, and nausea with vomiting are the most common presenting symptoms of patients with acute bacterial meningitis. Nuchal rigidity and other signs of meningeal irritation are frequently found on physical examination. However, these signs and symptoms may be totally absent in some elderly patients. Occasionally, a subtle change in neurologic function may be the only clue to suggest the presence of meningitis. In addition, other chronic diseases with signs or symptoms that obscure the diagnosis, such as cervical arthritis or preexistent neurologic disease, may be present. In these cases, the clinician must be alert to the possibility of meningitis and perform a lumbar puncture to examine the cerebrospinal fluid (CSF) for evidence of meningitis. Abnormalities in CSF are similar to those seen in younger patients. Gram's stain and culture are especially important in view of the high likelihood of unusual pathogens. Chest x-ray and cultures of blood, urine, and sputum should also be done to identify the possible source of infection.

Treatment

Rapid initiation of therapy is essential for maximum survival. The choice of antibiotic depends on its spectrum of activity against the most likely pathogens, its ability to penetrate into the CSF, and its toxicity. Gram's stain of CSF should be used to guide the selection of a specific antibiotic. Pneumococcal, meningococcal, and *Listeria* infection are best treated with high-dose penicillin. Semisynthetic penicillins, such as oxacillin, are the treatment of choice for *S. aureus* meningitis; when there is a high likelihood of methicillin-resistant staphylococci, vancomycin is recommended. The treatment of gram-negative bacillary meningitis has undergone considerable change since the introduction of the third-generation cephalosporins [65]. These agents have virtually replaced aminoglycosides alone or in combination with a broad-spectrum penicillin as first-line therapy unless a resistant pathogen is recovered. Chloramphenicol and trimethoprim-sulfamethoxazole are other agents that may be used in selected cases. The final choice of therapy should be directed by the results of cultures and sensitivity testing. There are no data to suggest that treatment with corticosteroids has any effect on morbidity or mortality.

Despite adequate antibiotic therapy, morbidity and mortality from bacterial meningitis in the elderly remain high. Severe neurologic sequelae, including deafness, hemiparesis, cranial nerve paresis, and dementia are common, particularly with pneumococcal meningitis. In older patients mortality rates of 44 percent have been reported, compared to 12.5 percent in younger patients [66]. Mortality rates as high as 70 to 80 percent have been reported with pneumococcal and *Listeria* meningitis.

INFECTIVE ENDOCARDITIS
Pathophysiology
An increasing proportion of patients with infective endocarditis are older than 60 years of age [67]. Not only does this age group comprise a greater percentage of the population but they also have an increased likelihood of underlying atheromatous or calcific valvular heart disease. Patients with degenerative valvular abnormalities, bicuspid aortic valve, longstanding rheumatic disease, and prosthetic heart valves are at increased risk for infection. These defects may serve as foci for platelet aggregates to which bacteria may adhere with subsequent formation of vegetations. Of note is the fact that no underlying cardiac abnormality can be found in up to 40 percent of elderly patients with infected valves [39].

As with other age groups, the source of primary infection is not identified in up to 50 per-

cent of cases of endocarditis in the elderly. However, elderly patients are at risk for bacteremias because of their increased exposures to invasive procedures. The organisms responsible for endocarditis in the elderly are similar to those observed in younger patients [68]. Streptococci account for more than 50 percent of diagnosed cases; preceding dental procedures are reported in up to 20 percent of patients infected with these organisms. Staphylococcal species, both *S. aureus* and *S. epidermidis,* account for 20 to 30 percent of cases; patients with prosthetic valves or intravenous catheters are at particularly high risk. As many as 10 to 30 percent of cases of infective endocarditis in the elderly are culture negative, a rate similar to that found in younger populations. The identification of *S. bovis* as an etiologic agent for endocarditis should alert the clinician to the possibility of colon carcinoma.

Clinical Picture
The clinical presentation of endocarditis in the elderly is similar to that in the young. Fever is found in most patients. Heart murmurs are heard in 60 to 100 percent of patients but may be unchanged from previous examinations or felt to be hemodynamically insignificant. Many elderly patients present with symptoms of a noncardiac nature, such as myalgia, anorexia, weight loss, or uremia [39]. Neurologic presentations are particularly common in the elderly and may range from minor aberrations of neurologic function to abnormalities in mental status, focal deficits, or coma.

The diagnosis is most apparent when blood cultures are repeatedly positive for a single organism, and the patient has either a murmur indicative of underlying cardiac pathology or peripheral manifestations of embolic disease. However, the lack of a murmur or negative blood cultures should not exclude the diagnosis if other suggestive findings are present. An elevated sedimentation rate is present in almost all patients. Other laboratory abnormalities include anemia, leukocytosis, microscopic hematuria, and proteinuria. Patients with longstanding disease may have a positive rheumatoid factor. An echocardiogram is a useful adjunct with a suggestive history, physical findings, and supportive laboratory data; in the absence of this information, the echocardiogram alone rarely makes the diagnosis.

Treatment

Treatment consists of intravenous bactericidal antibiotics directed against the organism isolated from the blood. Usually therapy is withheld until a definite pathogen is identified. If there are signs of clinical decompensation, such as congestive heart failure, rapid evaluation and empiric antibiotic therapy are warranted. Empiric coverage will usually include either penicillin G or ampicillin for streptococcal coverage or a penicillinase-resistant penicillin (oxacillin or nafcillin) to cover methicillin-sensitive staphylococci. If enterococcus is a possibility, aminoglycosides should be added for synergy. Vancomycin is the antibiotic of choice in patients who are penicillin allergic or in whom methicillin-resistant staphylococci are suspected, as with nosocomial line-related infection. The first-generation cephalosporins can provide broad-spectrum coverage, although they are not effective against enterococci or methicillin-resistant staphylococci. Depending on sensitivities, third-generation cephalosporins may be used to treat gram-negative endocarditis, eliminating the need for aminoglycoside therapy.

Factors that influence prognosis in patients with endocarditis include old age, the organism, the duration of illness, the extent of valvular injury or myocardial involvement, the presence of renal failure or congestive heart failure, and the occurrence of major emboli [68]. Indications for surgical intervention include progressive heart failure, infection that fails to respond to medical therapy, fungal infection, and repetitive embolic phenomena on appropriate therapy.

FEVER OF UNKNOWN ORIGIN

Fever of unknown origin (FUO) is identified as an illness of at least three weeks' duration with a temperature of 100°F or more and no established diagnosis after one week of investigation in the hospital. In recent years, neoplastic diseases have supplanted infections as the major underlying cause of this syndrome [69]. Among the neoplastic diseases, lymphoma is most commonly associated with FUO. This malignancy is often limited to retroperitoneal lymph nodes or the spleen. Fever, malaise, and weight loss may be the only manifestation of the underlying disease process; abdominal symptoms may be absent. Other carcinomas that cause FUO in the elderly are hypernephromas, hepatomas, and tumors that are metastatic to the liver. There may be no focal symptoms to draw attention to the site of the primary malignancy.

Intraabdominal abscesses, hepatobiliary infections, tuberculosis, and infective endocarditis are the infectious diseases that are most often cited as causes of FUO in the elderly [70]. A nonspecific clinical picture of fever, anorexia, wieght loss, malaise, and mental status changes may be the only manifestations of infection, making the diagnosis extremely difficult. Intraabdominal infection may be secondary to silent perforations of intestinal diverticula, inflamed appendices, or diseased gallbladders; there may be no history of prior surgery or inflammatory bowel disease. In patients with active tuberculosis, skin tests may be negative, miliary disease may not be detectable on chest x-ray, and sputum or other body fluids may be negative for acid-fast organisms on microscopic examination. With endocarditis, the classic signs are not always present. Murmurs may be absent or seemingly benign; focal skin lesions, eye findings, and splenomegaly are uncommon. This should not dissuade the clinician from obtaining blood cultures that may lead to the proper diagnosis.

Collagen vascular diseases account for relatively fewer cases of FUO in the elderly compared with younger patients. Diseases such as systemic lupus erythematosus and juvenile rheumatoid arthritis are rarely seen in the elderly. Instead, giant cell arteritis is the most common rheumatologic cause of FUO in these patients [71]. Fever may be the most prominent sign; headache, myalgia, and weakness may be subtle or absent. An elevated erythrocyte sedimentation rate is an important clue to this diagnosis.

Among the other conditions that can cause FUO in the elderly, the two most frequent are drug fevers and pulmonary embolic disease. Many medications that are prescribed for elderly patients have been implicated, including antihistamines, barbiturates, salicylates, ibuprofen, cimetidine, and dilantin. In addition, certain antihypertensives such as hydralazine and alpha-methyldopa, antibiotics, including penicillins and sulfa drugs, and antiarrhythmics such as procainamide and quinidine, can also cause fever. Factitious fever, acute thyroiditis, inflammatory bowel disease, sarcoidosis, and familial Mediterranean fever are unusual causes of FUO in this age group.

The diagnostic workup of FUO in elderly patients is similar to that in younger patients. A careful history and physical examination are essential. Routine screening tests are performed to rule out the more common causes of fever and to identify areas for more intense evaluation. A variety of noninvasive scanning techniques such as gallium or technetium scans, ultrasonography, computerized tomography, and nuclear magnetic resonance imaging are available to identify occult sites of inflammation, tumor, or abscess. More invasive tests such as digital subtraction angiography, arteriography, and tissue biopsies should be reserved for patients with focal signs in whom a specific etiologic cause is being sought. Therapeutic trials with antibiotics or corticosteroids should be avoided unless there is very strong evidence of a specific diagnosis and procedures to confirm the diagnosis are contraindicated.

Treatment

Prior to initiating antibiotic therapy, the clinician must be sure that appropriate specimens have been collected to establish a specific etiologic diagnosis. Empiric antibiotics are frequently indicated in life-threatening infections before the results of cultures are available. Once a pathogen is identified, every effort should be made to use the antimicrobial agent with the narrowest spectrum of activity and the least toxicity.

The clinician must take into account numerous variables when selecting an appropriate antibiotic regimen. For instance, the site of infection is an important determinant of antibiotic choice; some antibiotics penetrate poorly into the brain, cerebrospinal fluid, respiratory secretions, or prostatic tissue. Infections involving heart valves and bone are routinely treated with bactericidal agents. The setting in which the infection occurs may also affect the initial choice of antibiotics in that nosocomial

infections are more likely than community-acquired infections to be caused by resistant pathogens. The use of agents with broad-spectrum activity may either induce the development of resistance or select for antibiotic-resistant strains.

Pharmacokinetic considerations also play an important role in antibiotic selection. The presence of congestive heart failure, peripheral vascular disease, edema, diabetes, or hypotension may impair the absorption of antibiotics administered intramuscularly. Drug dosage or dosing interval should be modified for agents in patients with known renal dysfunction. A normal blood urea nitrogen (BUN) and creatinine are not reliable indicators of renal function; creatinine clearance decreases predictably with age. Aminoglycoside dosage should be calculated as outlined in Figure 22-1, and serum levels should be carefully monitored [72,73]. Penicillin and cephalosporins do not require dosing changes until the creatinine clearance is below 20 ml per minute. The presence of other chronic diseases may also predispose the elderly to antibiotic complications. Many of the penicillins (carbenicillin, ticarcillin, and oxacillin) contain as much as 5 mEq of sodium per gram and, when given in high doses, may exacerbate congestive heart failure. These drugs, as well as amphotericin B, are also associated with hypokalemic alkalosis, which may precipitate digitalis toxicity. Drugs such as trimethoprim-sulfamethoxazole, erythromycin, ampicillin, tetracycline, and the cephalosporins increase the anticoagulant effect of warfarin, whereas rifampin decreases its effect. Therapy with long-acting sulfa drugs may predispose patients receiving tolbutamide or chlorpropamide to hypoglycemia. The administration of erythromycin may induce theophylline toxicity.

The majority of untoward side effects from antibiotics occur regardless of age. However, certain direct toxicities are seen with greater frequency in the elderly. The risk of INH hepatotoxicity is rare in persons less than 20 years of age but occurs in 2 to 3 percent of patients over 50 years of age [74]. Agents such as isoniazid, minocycline, and amantadine may cause confusion or sedation in the elderly; amantadine-associated central nervous system toxicity is seen more frequently in patients with impaired

1. Select loading dose in mg/kg [LEAN WEIGHT] to provide peak serum level desired. Approximate peak levels from commonly used loading doses are indicated below:

LOADING DOSE	EXPECTED PEAK SERUM LEVEL BASED UPON ONE-HALF HOUR IV INFUSION
2.0 mg/kg	6 - 8 μg/ml
1.75 mg/kg*	5 - 7 μg/ml
1.5 mg/kg	4 - 6 μg/ml
1.25 mg/kg	3 - 5 μg/ml
1.0 mg/kg	2 - 4 μg/ml

*(Recommended for most moderate to severe systemic infections.)

2. Select maintenance dose (as percentage of chosen loading dose) to continue peak serum levels indicated above according to patient's creatinine clearance and desired dosing interval.

PERCENTAGE OF LOADING DOSE REQUIRED FOR DOSAGE INTERVAL SELECTED:

Cr. Clear.	8 hrs.	12 hrs.	24 hrs.
90	90%	-	-
80	88	-	-
70	84	-	-
60	79	91%	-
50	74	87	-
40	66	80	92%
30	57	72	88
25	51	66	83
20	45	59	75
15	37	50	64
10	29	40	55
7	24	33	48
5	20	28	35
2	14	20	25
0	9	13	25

A

(Shaded areas indicate suggested dosage intervals)

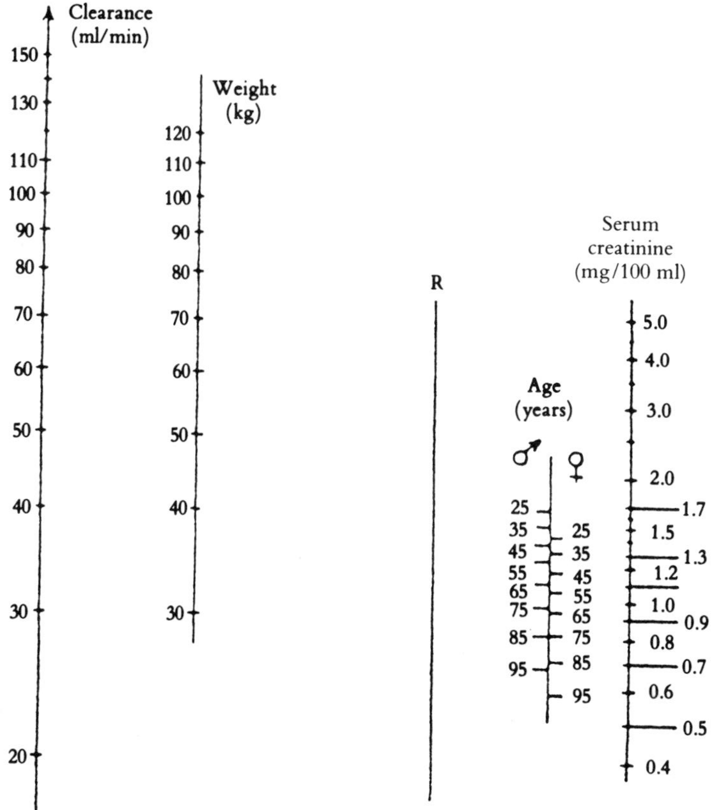

FIGURE 22-1. A. Gentamicin dosing chart. B. Nomogram for rapid evaluation of endogenous creatinine clearance. With a ruler, join weight to age. Keep ruler at crossing point of line marked R. Then move the right side of the ruler to the appropriate serum creatinine value and read the patient's clearance from the left side of the nomogram. (From J. Hull and P. G. Jones. Gentamicin serum concentrations: Pharmacokinetic predictions. Ann. Intern. Med. 85:183, 1976.)

B

renal function. Because of preexistent age-related decreases in renal function, the elderly are also at greater risk of aminoglycoside-associated nephrotoxicity, especially with the concurrent use of diuretics. Toxic levels of aminoglycosides may cause irreversible auditory or vestibular ototoxicity. Elderly patients are also at greater risk than younger patients for antibiotic-associated diarrhea [75].

Other considerations that may be important in the choice of antibiotics include patient compliance and drug cost. Most elderly patients take a variety of medications daily. The addition of a new agent may create confusion in dosing schedules, especially in patients with some degree of impaired memory. The cost of therapy must be taken into account as well, especially for elderly patients with fixed incomes or limited resources.

Prevention

A better understanding of the factors that predispose to infection in the elderly suggest a number of logical strategies that may be helpful in reducing the risks of infection. The elderly should receive help to enable them to maintain active life-styles, promote personal hygiene, and improve nutrition. Unnecessary medications that may dull mental function, alter normal flora, or impair mucosal barriers should not be used. Hospitalization and institutionalization should be avoided. But when they become necessary, appropriate precautions should be taken to minimize the risk of infection. Medications should be administered judiciously; invasive therapies, such as the insertion of urinary catheters, should be avoided, and physical activity should be maintained.

Immunization is another means of disease prevention in the elderly. Despite current recommendations for the use of influenza, pneumococcal, and tetanus/diphtheria vaccines in this population, these agents are underutilized in the United States. The protection achieved with influenza and pneumococcal vaccines in the ambulatory, healthy elderly is similar to that in younger populations.

However, the efficacy of vaccines in preventing infection in older, debilitated patients with multiple underlying diseases such as those found in nursing homes and Veterans Administration hospitals, is reduced [76,77]. The antibody response to vaccine in these patients is less than that observed in younger patients. Nonetheless, there is evidence that the influenza vaccine provides at least partial protection from the acquisition of infection and greatly reduces morbidity and mortality in those in whom symptoms develop [78]. The likelihood of at least some degree of protection imparted by these vaccines coupled with their safety and excellent patient tolerance support the continued administration in the elderly of yearly influenza vaccine, single dose pneumococcal vaccine, and boosters every five to ten years with tetanus/diphtheria vaccine (when the primary series has been given).

Influenza A infection can also be prevented by prophylactic administration of an antiviral agent, amantadine hydrochloride. For patients who have not received vaccine, amantadine in a dose of 100 mg per day can provide protection from clinical illness in more than 50 percent of cases [31]. However, its lack of protection against type B influenza disease, its relatively high cost, and its associated gastrointestinal and central nervous system toxicity limit its routine use as a prophylactic agent in the elderly. It may be used in conjunction with vaccine during occurrences of epidemic influenza A as interim protection until vaccine-associated antibodies develop. There is evidence to suggest a therapeutic effect of amantadine if it is given within the first 24 to 48 hours of symptoms. Amantadine may further reduce morbidity from infection in patients who have previously received vaccine. Studies of rimantadine, a close analogue of amantadine, have suggested decreased toxicity in the elderly compared with amantadine [79].

Tuberculosis is another preventable disease of increasing importance in the elderly. Prevention of tuberculosis, especially within the institutional setting, is best accomplished by identification of the susceptible population, appropriate isolation of patients with suspected or documented disease, and occasionally chemoprophylaxis. Although a positive tuberculin skin test is indicative of prior exposure to the disease, a negative test is often difficult to interpret. With increasing age, tuberculosis sensitivity may wane and may be detectable only by a second skin test done one week to one month after the original test ("booster phenomenon"). These patients do not require preventive therapy. On the other hand, patients with negative skin tests who subsequently convert to positive after exposure to tuberculosis or patients with positive skin tests receiving immunosuppressive therapy are at increased risk for development of acute disease. These patients should receive isoniazid as single agent preventive therapy despite the increased incidence of hypersensitivity hepatitis, which is as high as 2.5 percent in people older than 55 years of age [74]. Patients at high risk for hepatitis should be followed regularly throughout their period of treatment for clinical or laboratory evidence of liver disease.

Summary

The segment of our population that is elderly continues to grow at a rapid pace. In these patients, infection is associated with important morbidity and mortality. The relative importance of individual factors that contribute to infection, however, is difficult to delineate. Nonetheless, the presence of chronic underlying diseases appears to be a major risk factor predisposing to infection at specific sites. It is crucial that clinicians who care for the elderly are aware of both typical and atypical presentations of infection in these patients in order to diagnose problems and initiate appropriate interventions as soon as possible. In prescribing antibiotics for the elderly, the physician must take into consideration the impact of age-associated physiologic changes, other disease states, drug interactions, and compliance as well as the susceptibility of the agent responsible for the infection. The clinician also must be aware of the importance of preventive strategies in this population, including the optimal management of chronic diseases, maintenance of nutritional status, and avoidance of unnecessary medications and invasive procedures. Proper use of available immunizations may also reduce morbidity for some infections in the elderly.

References

1. Hodgson, T. A., and Lopstein, A. N. Health care expenditures for major diseases. Health and prevention profile, United States (U.S. Department of Health and Human Services, Public Health Service). Hyattsville, MD: National Center for Health Statistics, 1983. P. 79.
2. Current estimates from the National Health Interview Survey. United States 1982. Data from the National Health Survey, Series 10, No. 150 (Department of Health and Human Services Publication No. PHS 85-1578). Hyattsville, MD.
3. United States Department of Health and Human Services, National Center for Health Statistics. Utilization of short-stay hospitals. United States 1981, annual summary. Data from the National Health Survey, Series 13, No. 72 (DHHSS Publication No. PHS-83-1733). Washington, D.C.: U.S. Government Printing Office, 1983.
4. United States Department of Health and Human Services, National Center for Health Statistics. Utilization of short-stay hospitals. United States 1983, annual summary. Data from the National Health Survey, Series 13, No. 83 (DHHSS Publication No. PHS-85-1744). Washington, D.C.: U.S. Government Printing Office, 1985.
5. Haley, R. W., et al. Nosocomial infections in U.S. hospitals, 1975–1976: Estimated frequency by selected characteristics of patients. *Am. J. Med.* 70:947, 1981.
6. Cruse, P. Infection surveillance: Identifying the problems and the high-risk patient. *South. Med. J.* 70:4, 1977.
7. Garibaldi, R. A., et al. Risk factors for postoperative pneumonia. *Am. J. Med.* 70:677, 1981.
8. Garibaldi, R. A., et al. Factors predisposing to bacteriuria during indwelling urethral catheterization. *N. Engl. J. Med.* 291:215, 1974.
9. Gross, P. A., et al. Deaths from nosocomial infections. *Am. J. Med.* 68:219, 1980.
10. Goodman, R. Decline in Organ Function with Aging. In R. Rossman (ed.), *Clinical Geriatrics* (2nd ed.). Philadelphia: Lippincott, 1979. Pp. 23–59.
11. Gardner, I. D. The effect of aging on susceptibility to infection. *Rev. Infect. Dis.* 2:801, 1980.
12. Phair, J. P., et al. Host defenses in the aged: Evaluation of components of the inflammatory and immune responses. *J. Infect. Dis.* 138:67, 1978.
13. Chandra, R. K., et al. Nutrition and immunocompetence of the elderly: Effect of short-term nutritional supplementation on cell-mediated immunity and lymphocyte subsets. *Nutr. Res.* 2:223, 1982.
14. Ammann, A. J., Schiffman, G., and Austrian, R. The antibody responses to pneumococcal capsular polysaccharides in aged individuals. *Proc. Soc. Exp. Biol. Med.* 164:312, 1980.

15. Phair, J. P., et al. Failure to respond to influenza vaccine in the aged: Correlation with B-cell number and function. *J. Lab. Clin. Med.* 92:822, 1978.

16. Gilles, S., et al. Immunologic studies of aging: Decreased production of and response to T-cell growth factor by lymphocytes from aged humans. *J. Clin. Invest.* 67:937, 1981.

17. Kniker, W. T., et al. Multitest MCI for the standardized measurement of delayed cutaneous hypersensitivity and cell-mediated immunity. *Ann. Allergy* 52:75, 1984.

18. Sullivan, R. J., et al. Adult pneumonia in a general hospital. *Arch. Intern. Med.* 129:935, 1972.

19. Cohen, E. D., et al. Nosocomial infections in skilled nursing facilities: A preliminary survey. *Publ. Health Rep.* 94:162, 1979.

20. Garibaldi, R. A., Brodine, S., and Matsumiya, S. Infections among patients in nursing homes: Policies, prevalence and problems. *N. Engl. J. Med.* 305:731, 1981.

21. Denham, M. J., and Goodwin, G. S. The value of blood cultures in geriatric practice. *Age Ageing* 6:85, 1987.

22. Krumpe, P. E., et al. The aging respiratory system. *Clin. Geriatr. Med.* 1:143, 1985.

23. Reinarz, J. A., et al. The potential role of inhalation therapy equipment in nosocomial pulmonary infection. *J. Clin. Invest.* 44:831, 1965.

24. Osmer, J. C., and Cole, B. K. The stethoscope and roentgenogram in acute pneumonia. *South. Med. J.* 59:75, 1966.

25. Murray, P. R., and Washington, J. A. III. Microscopic and bacteriologic analysis of expectorated sputum. *Mayo Clin. Proc.* 50:339, 1975.

26. Niederman, M. S., and Fein, A. M. Pneumonia in the elderly. *Geriatr. Clin. North Am.* 2:241, 1986.

27. Barrett-Connor, E. The nonvalue of sputum culture in the diagnosis of pneumococcal pneumonia. *Am. Rev. Respir. Dis.* 103:845, 1971.

28. Austrian, R., and Gold, J. Pneumococcal bacteremia with special reference to bacteremic pneumococcal pneumonia. *Ann. Intern. Med.* 60:759, 1964.

29. Esposito, A. L., and Pennington, J. E. The pathogenesis of bacterial pneumonia. In R. A. Gleckman, and N. M. Gantz (eds.), *Infections in the Elderly.* Boston: Little, Brown, 1983. Pp. 53–62.

30. Verghese, A., and Berk, S. L. Bacterial pneumonia in the elderly. *Medicine* 62:271, 1983.

31. Advisory Committee on Immunization Practices. Prevention and control of influenza. *M.M.W.R.* 34:261, 1985.

32. Valenti, W. M., Trudell, R. G., and Bentley, D. W. Factors predisposing to oropharyngeal colonization with gram-negative bacilli in the aged. *N. Engl. J. Med.* 298:1108, 1978.

33. Tillotson, J. R., and Finland, M. Bacterial colonization and clinical superinfection of the respiratory tract complicating antibiotic treatment of pneumonia. *J. Infect. Dis.* 119:597, 1969.

34. Lorber, B., and Swenson, R. M. Bacteriology of aspiration pneumonia: A prospective study of community- and hospital-acquired cases. *Ann. Intern. Med.* 81:329, 1974.

35. Reichman, L. B., and O'Day, R. Tuberculous infection in a large urban population. *Am. Rev. Respir. Dis.* 117:705, 1978.

36. Glew, R. H. Abdominal Infections. In R. A. Gleckman, and N. M. Gantz (eds.), *Infections in the Elderly.* Boston: Little, Brown, 1983. Pp. 177–206.

37. Glenn, F., and Hays, D. M. The age factor in the mortality rate of patients undergoing surgery of the biliary tract. *Surg. Gynecol. Obstet.* 100:11, 1955.

38. Smith, J. K., and Wiener, S. P. Life-threatening infections in the elderly. Abdominal and pelvic infections. *Drug Ther.* 6:23, 1980.

39. Yoskikawa, T. T. Aging and infectious diseases. In M.S.J. Pathy (ed.), *Principles and Practice of Geriatric Medicine.* New York: Wiley, 1985. Pp. 221–238.

40. Marian, D. J., Thompson, J., and Wilson, S. E. Acute cholecystitis in the elderly. A surgical emergency. *Arch. Surg.* 113:1149, 1981.

41. Parks, T. G. Natural history of diverticular disease of the colon. *Clin. Gastroenterol.* 4:53, 1975.

42. Lorber, B., and Swenson, R. M. The bacteriology of intra-abdominal infections. *Surg. Clin. North Am.* 55:1349, 1975.

43. Owens, B. J., and Hamit, H. F. Appendicitis in the elderly. *Ann. Surg.* 187:392, 1978.

44. Peltohallio, P., and Jauhiainen, K. Acute appendicitis in the aged patient. Study of 300 cases after ages of 60. *Arch. Surg.* 100:140, 1970.

45. Butler, T. J., and McCarthy, C. F. Pyogenic liver abscess. *Gut* 10:389, 1969.

46. Lazarchick, J., de Souza Silva, N. A., and Nichols, D. R. Pyogenic liver abscess. *Mayo Clin. Proc.* 48:349, 1973.

47. Rubin, R. H., Swartz, M. N., and Malt, R. Hepatic abscess changes in clinical, bacteriologic and therapeutic aspects. *Am. J. Med.* 57:601, 1974.

48. Blacklow, N. R. Infectious Diarrhea. In R. A. Gleckman, and N. M. Gantz (eds.), *Infections in the Elderly.* Boston: Little, Brown, 1983. Pp. 159–175.

49. Hughes, J. M. Food Poisoning, In G. L. Mandell,

et al. (eds.), *Principles and Practices of Infectious Diseases*. New York: Wiley, 1985. Pp. 680–691.

50. Raudin, J. I., and Guerrant, R. L. Infectious diarrhea in the elderly. *Geriatrics* 38:95, 1983.

51. Kunin, C. M. An overview of urinary tract infections. In C. M. Kunin (ed.), *Detection, Prevention and Management of Urinary Tract Infections*. (2nd ed.). Philadelphia: Lea & Febiger, 1974. Pp. 1–52.

52. Kaye, D. urinary tract infections in the elderly. *Bull. N.Y. Acad. Med.* 56:209, 1980.

53. Cox, J. R., and Shalahy, W. A. Renal Diseases. In M.J.J. Pathy (ed.), *Principles and Practices of Geriatric Medicine*. New York: Wiley, 1985. Pp. 1121–1139.

54. Freedman, L. R. Urinary tract infection in the elderly. *N. Engl. J. Med.* 309:1451, 1983.

55. Dontas, A. S., et al. Bacteriuria and survival in old age. *N. Engl. J. Med.* 304:939, 1981.

56. Nordenstam, G. R., et al. Bacteriuria and mortality in an elderly population. *N. Engl. J. Med.* 314:1152, 1986.

57. Nicolle, L. E., et al. Bacteriuria in elderly institutionalized men. *N. Engl. J. Med.* 309:1420, 1983.

58. Boscia, J. A., et al. Therapy vs. no therapy for bacteriuria in elderly ambulatory non-hospitalized women. *J.A.M.A.* 257:1067, 1987.

59. Stamm, W. E., et al. Diagnosis of coliform infection in acutely dysuric women. *N. Engl. J. Med.* 307:463, 1982.

60. Warren, J. W., et al. A prospective microbiologic study of bacteriuria in patients with chronic indwelling urethral catheters. *J. Infect. Dis.* 146:719, 1982.

61. Gilchrest, B. A. Age-related changes in the skin. *J. Am. Geriatr. Soc.* 30:139, 1982.

62. Fulginiti, V. A. Herpes Zoster. In D. J. Demis, et al. (eds.), *Clinical Dermatology*. Vol. 3. Hagerstown, MD: Harper & Row, 1976. Pp. 1–8.

63. Keczkes, K., and Basheer, A. M. Do corticosteroids prevent post-herpetic neuralgia? *Br. J. Dermatol.* 102:551, 1980.

64. Schlech, W. F. III, et al. Bacterial meningitis in the United States, 1978 through 1981. The National Bacterial Meningitis Surveillance Study. *J.A.M.A.* 253:1749, 1985.

65. Cherubin, C. E., et al. Treatment of gram-negative bacillary meningitis: Role of the new cephalosporins antibiotics. *Rev. Infect. Dis.* 4:S453, 1982.

66. Gorse, G. J., et al. Bacterial meningitis in the elderly. *Arch. Intern. Med.* 144:1603, 1984.

67. Robbins, N., DeMaria, A., and Miller, M. Infective endocarditis in the elderly. *South. Med. J.* 73(10):1335, 1980.

68. Gantz, N. M. Infective Endocarditis. In R. A. Gleckman and N. M. Gantz (eds.), *Infections in the Elderly*. Boston: Little, Brown, 1983. Pp. 217–234.

69. Larson, E. B., Featherstone, H. J., and Petersdorf, R. G. Fever of undetermined origin: Diagnosis and follow-up of 105 cases, 1970–1980. *Medicine* 61:269, 1982.

70. Kauffman, C. A., and Jones, P. G. Diagnosing fever of unknown origin in older patients. *Geriatrics* 39:46, 1984.

71. Esposito, A. L., and Gleckman, R. A. Fever of unknown origin in the elderly. *J. Am. Geriatr.* 26:498, 1978.

72. Hull, J., and Sarubbi, F. A. Gentamicin serum concentrations: Pharmaco-kinetic predictions. *Ann. Intern. Med.* 85:183, 1976.

73. Siersbaek-Nielsen, K. Rapid evaluation of creatinine clearance. *Lancet* 1:1133, 1971.

74. Yoshikawa, T. T., and Fujita, N. K. Antituberculous drugs. *Med. Clin. North Am.* 66:209, 1982.

75. Gurwith, M. J., Rabin, H. R., Love, K., and the Cooperative Antibiotic Diarrhea Study Group. Diarrhea associated with clindamycin and ampicillin therapy. Preliminary results of a cooperative study. *J. Infect. Dis.* 135:S104, 1977.

76. Centers for Disease Control. Outbreaks of influenza among nursing home residents—Connecticut, United States. *M.M.W.R.* 34:478, 1985.

77. Simberkoff, M. S., et al. Efficacy of pneumococcal vaccine in high-risk patients: Results of a Veterans Administration Cooperative Study. *N. Engl. J. Med.* 315:1318, 1986.

78. Barker, W. H., and Mullooly, J. P. Influenza vaccination of elderly persons: Reduction in pneumonia and influenza hospitalizations and death. *J.A.M.A.* 244:2547, 1980.

79. Dolin, R., et al. Rimantidine prophylaxis of influenza in the elderly (Abstract 691). Proceedings 23rd Interscience Conference on Antimicrobial Agents and Chemotherapy. Washington, D.C.: American Society for Microbiology, 1983.

23

Cancer in the Elderly

MICHAEL S. RABIN
LOWELL E. SCHNIPPER

IT IS DIFFICULT to overstate the impact of malignancy on the elderly. No diagnosis conjures up the fear of debility, discomfort, dependence, or mortality as does cancer. Although great strides have been taken in understanding and treating cancer in recent decades, most of the progress has been in the area of cancer biology or in the treatment of those cancers that primarily afflict young patients.

Clinical gerontology and oncology have much in common. Cancer is an extraordinarily heterogeneous group of diseases whose treatment in the elderly patient demands attention to individual tumor biology, variable clinical pharmacology, nutrition, concurrent medical illnesses, and psychosocial support.

The goal of this chapter is to highlight some of the basic science and clinical issues relevant to the elderly cancer patient. Recent studies on aging, immunology, and cancer etiology are reviewed. Oncologic considerations uniquely relevant to the geriatric patient are examined, and these points are illustrated by using as examples cancer of the breast and prostate gland. Cancer screening, prevention, and early detection practices in older patients are presented. The reader is also referred to Chapter 21, which includes a detailed discussion of immunosenescence and related malignancies, including multiple myeloma and lymphomas.

Epidemiology of Cancer in the Elderly

More than 50 percent of cancers occur in persons who are 65 years or older, and approximately 60 percent of cancer deaths occur in this age group [1,2]. The five leading cancer sites for elderly white males are prostate, lung, colon, rectum, and bladder. Eighty percent of all prostate cancers present in this age group, as do 55 percent of lung cancers and 68 percent of colon cancers in males. Among females 65 and older, the major cancer sites (in descending order) are breast, colon, lung, uterus, and rectum. About 50 percent of lung, breast, and uterine cancers occur in this group, as do 70 to 75 percent of colorectal cancers in women [1].

Cancer incidence rises dramatically as people age. The chance of developing cancer between the ages 65 and 85 is 23 percent for men and 17 percent for women, compared with probabilities of 1 percent and 1.5 percent for men and women between 20 and 40 years old [3].

Aging, Immunology, and Cancer

Why does the incidence of malignancy rise so steeply with age? One possibility is that the biology of aging and cancer are intimately related, and some property of the aging cell and/or aging host defenses make neoplastic transformation more likely. An alternative explanation is predicated on the concept that the process of oncogenesis is multistep. A cell must sustain multiple carcinogenic insults, followed by a complex process of tumor promotion in order to be stably transformed. The implied time dependence of this process predicts that cancers will form late in life with an increasing incidence [4,5]. The alternatives are not mutually exclusive.

Several lines of evidence support the multistep model for increased cancer in aging individuals. Animal models of carcinogenesis [6] are consistent with carcinogenesis involving a minimum of two steps. The first, initiation, consists of introduction of irreversible changes in DNA by chemical or physical carcinogens (e.g., ultraviolet light, x-rays), and the second step, promotion, involves altered control of proliferation. Peto, et al. [4] painted benzpyrene on mice of various ages, and they found that tumors arose as a power of the duration of exposure independent of mouse age at first exposure. Doll [7], reviewing data on male smokers, showed that lung cancer incidence was a function of time elapsed smoking and was not dependent on the age at which smoking began. Similarly, the rate of mesothelioma in asbestos workers reflects the dose and duration of exposure but not the age of the worker [8].

What, then, is the evidence that age per se might increase susceptibility to carcinogenesis? Burnet [9] proposed that breakdown in "immune surveillance" with age allows for the proliferation of tumors. Aging humans have impaired or altered immune function in several respects, including decreased antigen–specific humoral responses [10], decreased production of and response to T-cell growth factors [11], and impaired delayed hypersensitivity (see Chap. 21 for detailed discussion). Drugs or diseases that cause immunosuppression are associated with an increase in malignancies, particularly lymphoreticular neoplasms [12]. Despite these observations, the data fall far short of implicating an aging immune system in gerontologic tumor excess.

Cancer cell genomes contain mutations (structural alterations) in DNA, some of which can be detected as gross karyotypic changes while others are as subtle as single changes in a base pair [13,14]. In the past decade a class of genes called oncogenes has been implicated in transformation because in many cases they express functions that are important in cell proliferation [15]. Activation of their diverse gene products generally requires either point mutation or translocation to another part of the genome to place it under the control of a DNA sequence that promotes overexpression of the gene [15].

Using techniques of molecular biology to study somatic cells, it is possible to detect changes including deletion of highly repetitive DNA sequences and amplification of certain extrachromosomal DNA sequences with advancing cell age [16,17]. Lymphocytes from people over 65 exhibit increased frequency of chromosomal damage when exposed to tritiated thymidine [18]. Although the authors infer that these examples of genomic lability in aging cells might link aging and cancer, there is as yet no etiologic proof.

Clinical Considerations of Cancer in the Elderly

GENERAL ASPECTS

The challenges in diagnosing and treating cancer in older patients are familiar to the gerontologist because they are not unique to oncology. Cancers may present with different symptoms than in younger patients, and tumors in the elderly may be more or less aggressive. Older patients are more likely to have intercurrent illnesses or utilize medications that compromise the administration of cancer therapy or intensify the adverse effects of cancer. Age-related functional deterioration in a number of organ systems may drastically alter pharmacokinetics and tolerance to chemotherapy, radiotherapy, or radical surgery. Elderly cancer patients may be further impaired or stressed by limited economic resources, lessened mobility, increased dependence on others, and distant or absent family supports.

This array of potential or actual problems has at times fostered a somewhat nihilistic, hands-off approach to cancer in the elderly. Yet it is increasingly clear that the elderly can tolerate surgery, radiotherapy, or chemotherapy, and that these modalities may cure some patients and substantially improve the outlook for others.

It is equally clear that individualized care is critical in older patients. Whereas one patient of 75 chronologic years might be physiologically much younger and can tolerate aggressive treatment as if he or she were 50 years old, another patient of 75 might have life-threatening heart disease that makes the same cancer clinically irrelevant from a therapeutic perspective.

DETECTION

Several factors may make the detection of cancer difficult in the elderly. Access to medical care may be inhibited by fear or by impaired mobility. In a patient with numerous medical problems who is taking multiple medications, the insidious onset of weight loss, malaise, or weakness may be more difficult to interpret than in a younger patient. Constipation is common in the elderly, but it may be the sole manifestation of colorectal carcinoma. Mild anemia may be the first sign of visceral malignancy.

Despite the diagnostic pitfalls, data from a large surveillance study suggest that cancers that present in old age are not generally more advanced than cancers presenting in middle age [19]. A notable exception is cervical cancer, which is often found to be more advanced in older patients [19]. A smaller study from New Mexico found significantly greater extent of disease at the time of diagnosis in older patients at several sites including breast, bladder, ovary, uterus, and cervix [20].

The geriatrician must compensate for problems in cancer diagnosis with heightened vigilance. Besides pursuing clues such as constipation or anemia, the physician should take advantage of regular cancer screening tests because early detection increases the likelihood of finding localized, curable disease. Current levels of detection are inadequate: One-third to one-half of new cancers are diagnosed at advanced stages for which the five-year survival is significantly decreased [19].

For asymptomatic persons over 65 years old, the American Cancer Society recommends a yearly digital rectal examination and stool test for occult blood and sigmoidoscopy every three to five years after two negative annual examinations. Women should have annual mammogra-phy, breast examination by a physician, and pelvic examination, and they should be educated in the technique of breast self-examination [21]. There is evidence from randomized, controlled trials that screening mammography reduces breast cancer mortality [22]. The carcinogenic risk of mammography has been reduced considerably by new techniques employing extremely low doses of x-rays, and this concern should no longer serve as an impediment [23]. Despite its presumptive value based on studies in younger populations, the beneficial impact of early detection on mortality in elderly patients has not yet been documented [24].

There is some controversy about the use of screening Pap smears in women over 65, in that they are not recommended by the American Cancer Society, whereas they are by the American Society of Obstetrics and Gynecology. The American Cancer Society's rationale was that in previously screened elderly women, the rate of positive tests was extremely low [25]. Given the fact that cervical cancer tends to be found at later stages in older women, it is sound practice to advocate the regular use of Pap smears in elderly patients, particularly women who have not been screened previously or who are at high risk for cervical cancer.

SURGERY

Surgery in the elderly is discussed in detail in Chapter 10. For a number of malignancies, among them skin, breast, stomach, endometrial, colorectal, and selected lung cancers, radical excision is the primary treatment of choice, offering at least a chance of a cure. In other circumstances surgery may offer palliation through debulking, relief of visceral obstruction, or interruption of pain afferents.

Surgical planning must be individualized and based on the patient's physiologic and clinical status, taking into account intercurrent illnesses and age-related decrements in cardiac, pulmonary, and renal function. Surgery may be performed safely on elderly patients given adequate preoperative preparation [26]. In one representative study, women over 70 years old undergoing mastectomy fared as well as their younger counterparts when actual five- and ten-year survivals were compared [27].

Certainly, chronologic age per se will not disqualify a patient from receiving optimal surgical management, but performance status and information about tumor biology must be considered. A bedridden 85-year-old with a low-lying rectal carcinoma might benefit from fulguration or radiotherapy rather than abdominoperineal resection with colostomy. Surgery on an otherwise healthy 80-year-old woman with a breast cancer need not include axillary lymph node dissection if there is no plan for adjuvant chemotherapy regardless of nodal status.

RADIOTHERAPY

A complete discussion of radiation oncology is obviously beyond the scope of this book. Radiotherapy is an enormously useful modality, particularly in some of the common geriatric cancers. It is currently applied as an adjunct to surgery in breast-sparing therapy of localized breast cancer, and in stages B2 and C rectal carcinoma [28]. Radiation may be used as primary (curative) or palliative treatment of tumors of the head and neck, lung, esophagus, bladder, prostate, central nervous system, female reproductive tract, and other sites.

Some side effects that may be particularly distressing to the older patient include xerostomia (following radiation to head and neck), nausea, and diarrhea resulting from radiation to the gastro-intestinal tract. Radiotherapy can diminish pulmonary function and impair bone marrow growth in treated fields, adding to preexisting disease- and age-related decrements. Radiation requires oxygen for maximal effect; therefore, preexisting deficits in the heart, lungs, blood, or blood vessels that lead to tissue hypoxia may theoretically reduce antitumor efficacy.

Skilled radiotherapists are often limited to major medical centers, and therapy is frequently administered in small daily doses over the course of weeks, therefore heightening difficulties in access to the hospital and impaired mobility experienced by many older patients.

CHEMOTHERAPY

Although most of the dramatic chemotherapeutic successes of the past quarter century affect tumors of childhood and young adulthood (e.g., acute lymphocytic leukemia, lymphomas, and testicular cancers), many of the tumors common in the elderly can be effectively palliated and occasionally cured, and long-term survival with a good quality of life is possible. Recognition of age-specific variables in pharmacokinetics, drug toxicity, and tumor responsiveness has helped establish some general guidelines for treatment.

Pharmacokinetics

The pathophysiologic changes with aging that affect drug action are discussed in detail in Chapter 9. Decrease in body water may change the volume of distribution of water-soluble agents such as methotrexate. Although hepatic reserve is great, the action of drugs metabolized in the liver such as 5-fluorouracil, doxorubicin, and etoposide may be affected. Robert and Hoerni [29] described age-dependent reduction in early clearance of doxorubicin (Adriamycin) in 37 patients, although there was considerable individual variation. Decrement in renal function with age is well recognized and may affect excretion of methotrexate, cis-platinum, and bleomycin.

Because multiple medications are often prescribed for the elderly for diverse problems, it is incumbent on care providers to recognize or anticipate drug interactions. As examples, agents such as diuretics that may impair renal perfusion may potentiate nephrotoxic drugs, or antiemetics may interact with previously prescribed sleep medications to produce additive sedation.

Toxicity

Apparent toxicity of chemotherapeutic agents is increased by diminished functional reserve in affected organs, particularly the heart, kidneys, and bone marrow. Accordingly, doxorubicin cardiomyopathy occurs more frequently in patients over 70 years old [30,31]. Other clinically important toxicities in the elderly include nephrotoxicity from cis-platinum and methotrexate and pulmonary toxicity from bleomycin. Peripheral neuropathy due to cis-platinum or vinca alkaloids may be particularly devastating in older patients. Cytosine arabinoside and 5-fluorouracil have the potential to be toxic to the central nervous system.

Many useful agents are myelosuppressive. Bone marrow cellularity is reduced in elderly patients, and at least one study demonstrates diminished hematopoiesis even in healthy elderly patients [32].

Begg and Carbone studied patterns of drug toxicity in patients over 70 years of age treated for various advanced solid tumors by the Eastern Cooperative Oncology Group (ECOG) [33]. Surprisingly, they found almost no difference in severe toxicity reactions in this older group compared to those in younger patients. The exception was slightly worse hematologic toxicity in several disease sites, which could be attributed to methotrexate and methyl-CCNU. Although participation in the ECOG trials implies a highly selected cohort, this study confirms that certain older patients tolerate intensive chemotherapy well.

Age and Response to Therapy
Because of intercurrent illnesses and compounding psychosocial factors, it is difficult to compare response to treatment in young and old patients with the "same" disease. In fact, there is relatively little information about the relative responses of most solid tumors in elderly patients. Breast cancer is one exception for which data favorably compare responses in old versus young patients, as is discussed in the next section.

The recent revolution applying bone marrow transplants to the treatment of acute myelocytic leukemia (AML) has been largely confined to those under 40. Nonetheless, there has been progress in the care of elderly leukemics. Elderly patients were shown to tolerate intensive chemotherapy, although rates of complete remission (CR) were lower than those of younger patients [34,35]. In 1981 UCLA reported identical rates of CR and median survival of 76 percent and 22 months, respectively, for patients above and below 60 treated intensively with daunorubicin, cytarabine, and thioguanine (DAT) [36]. In contrast, an ECOG study compared full-dose to attenuated-dose DAT in 40 patients older than 70. They noted comparable CR rates around 28 percent, but median survival was lower in the intensively treated group due to excess early deaths [37]. These reports are partly reconciled by an additional study of intensive therapy in AML in which patients 60 to 69 years old did as well as younger patients, but those over 70 fared poorly [38].

Elderly patients with advanced Hodgkin's disease have lower rates of response to combination chemotherapy and a lower duration of response than younger patients, although selected subgroups do well [39,40]. Armitage and Potter [41] demonstrated comparable response rates to chemotherapy in diffuse histiocytic lymphoma (DHL) in patients over versus those under age 70, but survival in the older group was diminished by an excessive number of treatment-related deaths. Dixon and colleagues [42] found a progressive decline in CR rates in DHL from 65 percent in those under 40 years to 37 percent in those 65 and older, although automatic dose reductions in the oldest group may have contributed to their inferior outcomes.

Interestingly, the relative survival rates for many cancer sites in patients 65 and older are only several percentage points below rates for those 45 to 64 years old [1]. In contrast, the relative survival of elderly patients is significantly reduced compared to that in younger patients with cancers of the bladder, thyroid, cervix, uterus, and ovary as well as with lymphoma and melanoma [1,43,44].

Breast Cancer
More than 50,000 American women over age 65 develop breast cancer each year. The example of breast cancer illustrates how tumor biology, therapeutic choices, and delivery of medical services may depend strongly on patient age.

The importance of cancer screening has been discussed previously. Women under 60 years of age who are formally taught self-examination find tumors that are smaller and less widespread compared to those found by women who examine themselves without instruction [45]. Women over 65 may be disinclined to examine their breasts because of fear, lack of physician encouragement, or difficulty interpreting the examination, but new lumps are more likely to be malignant than those in younger patients [23]. As stated earlier, breast self-examination must be coupled with physician examinations and mammography.

Considerable recent experience suggests comparable survival following either modified radical mastectomy or local excision, axillary sampling, and radiation therapy for many primary breast lesions. Most older women can physically tolerate either approach very well. Individualized decision making is necessary to weigh surgical risks, the importance of breast loss or preservation on self-image and sexuality, and the impact on life-style of either mastectomy or six weeks of radiotherapy.

The biology of breast cancer varies with patient age. Response of advanced cancers to hormonal therapy such as tamoxifen rises with advancing age. Postmenopausal women are more likely to have estrogen receptor-rich tumors, and the rate of receptor positivity continues to rise after the menopause. Examining tumors from women over age 75, von Rosen and colleagues [46] found that 70 percent had diploid karyotypes and 87 percent were estrogen receptor-positive, predicting slow tumor growth and likely response to antiestrogens. Despite these favorable tumor characteristics, women over age 75 fare no better than and in some reports much worse than younger women with breast cancer [47]. This observation emphasizes that outcome is a complex function of tumor biology and the host's ability to resist the tumor and tolerate antitumor therapy.

Although premenopausal women with positive axillary nodes benefit from adjuvant chemotherapy, most major studies have not demonstrated a significant survival benefit in postmenopausal women [48]. Bonadonna [49] subsequently noted that many elderly women in his trial had been given automatic dose reductions based on age alone, and that women over age 65 who receive full-dose combination chemotherapy derived survival benefit, suggesting a dose-response effect. Although Bonadonna found no increase in chemotoxicity with age, Gelman and Taylor [50] noted increasing hematologic toxicity in women with advanced breast cancers as age approached 65. They could eliminate this trend in hematologic toxicity in women over 65 by reducing doses according to creatinine clearance, but the trade-off was reduced response rate.

A 1985 National Cancer Institute Consensus Conference on adjuvant chemotherapy of breast cancer recommended tamoxifen for postmenopausal women with positive estrogen receptors and positive axillary nodes [51]. For women with negative estrogen receptors and positive nodes, no specific recommendation was made, but an informal 1987 physician survey suggests that many of these women receive adjuvant Cytoxan-methotrecate-5-fluorouracil (CMF). The treated group includes many of the "well elderly" without major concurrent illness.

Choice of CMF regimen may be very important. The "standard CMF" regimen involves daily oral cyclophosphamide for two weeks each month as well as two visits for intravenous methotrexate and 5-fluorouracil, and is a regimen with which the older patient may have compliance problems. The physician may elect to give "intravenous CMF," a simpler regimen in which all three drugs are administered intravenously every three weeks. There is evidence that the two CMF regimens are comparable in efficacy.

Hormonal therapy with tamoxifen may be particularly effective in the treatment of elderly women with metastatic breast cancer because of its effectiveness and relative lack of side effects. When tamoxifen fails after an initial response, other hormonal agents such as the progestational agent megestrol (Megace) may prove beneficial.

How does a woman's age influence the management of her breast cancer? Chu and colleagues [52] examined the effect of age on the care of women with breast cancer in 17 community hospitals. Elderly women were less likely to undergo biopsy prior to definitive treatment, see a medical oncologist, receive chemotherapy or radiotherapy, or be referred to a mastectomy support group. A UCLA group evaluated medical and surgical decision making in university and community hospitals, with attention to age and co-existing diseases [53]. Both patient age and co-morbidity status significantly and independently influenced treatment. In patients with minimal or no co-morbid disease, 96 percent of those aged 50 to 69 received what was deemed appropriate surgery, compared to 83 percent of patients over 70 years old. Treatment based on chronologic age alone may adversely affect outcome in otherwise healthy older women.

Prostate Cancer

Unlike breast cancer in women, which occurs throughout adulthood, cancer of the prostate in men is almost exclusively a disease of the elderly. Eighty percent of prostate adenocarcinoma presents after age 65, as previously noted. Interestingly, autopsy studies suggest that up to 70 percent of men over age 80 have prostate cancers, although most of these are clinically inapparent.

The digital rectal examination is the only reliable means of early detection. Subtle urinary symptoms may occur, but most cancers confined to the prostate (stages A and B) are asymptomatic. Locally advanced (stage C) or metastatic (stage D) tumors may present with impotence or relatively rapid onset of symptoms of urethral obstruction, or with evidence of bony or visceral spread. Unfortunately, 75 percent of patients present with clinical stage C or D, and half of stage C patients are found at surgery to have involved regional nodes (stage D1) [54]. Although measurement of serum acid phosphatase may be useful in diagnosing and staging individuals and in following their response to therapy, early excitement regarding its potential in screening for localized disease has not been borne out.

The prognosis for patients with prostate cancer depends on the extent of disease and the histologic grade, neither of which depends on age at diagnosis. Younger patients with prostate cancer are likely to succumb to it eventually, while older patients tend to die from problems other than prostate cancer [55].

Appropriate staging includes rectal examination, histologic examination of the prostate, acid phosphatase level, SMA-12, chest x-ray, and bone scan. Pelvic CT scan may be useful in delineating pelvic lymph node involvement. In cases of clinically localized disease with histologic features (e.g., poor differentiation), which suggests a significant likelihood of lymph node involvement, surgical exploration with lymphadenectomy may be undertaken because it may prevent a futile attempt at cure by local therapy.

Treatment must take into account both the behavior patterns of a particular tumor and the potential effects of therapy on the host. For example, a focal well-differentiated tumor detected only by transurethral resection (TURP) (stage A1) is very unlikely to disseminate or even recur; therefore, no further therapy is necessary. A poorly differentiated tumor found on TURP (clinical stage A2) involves the pelvic lymph nodes in 25 percent of patients, and even when demonstrated pathologically to be localized and treated appropriately, five- and ten-year survival rates are only 58 percent and 26 percent, respectively [56].

The two treatment options for localized disease are radical prostatectomy and radiation therapy, which offer comparable five- and ten-year survival rates of about 75 percent and 60 percent, respectively, for stage B, although surgical results are slightly better at 15 years [56]. The major adverse effects of retropubic prostatectomy are incontinence in 10 percent of subjects, bladder neck contracture, and impotence, which almost invariably occurs. A "nerve-sparing" prostatectomy has been introduced at Johns Hopkins University School of Medicine with encouraging decrease in the rate of erectile impotence [57]. Radiation therapy occasionally causes impotence as well as the possibility of proctitis, cystitis, bladder neck contracture, or urethral stricture.

Treatment of advanced prostate cancer is palliative, but it may be highly effective. For urinary obstruction either radiotherapy or TURP may be beneficial. The most effective treatment modality for disseminated prostate cancer is hormonal manipulation. Early treatment does not offer survival advantage; thus, systemic therapy may be reserved for symptoms such as pain. Androgen deprivation causes subjective improvement in 80 percent of patients and objective tumor regression in 50 percent [56].

The standard for androgen deprivation has been bilateral orchiectomy; it is a psychologically difficult approach for a man of any age to accept, but the benefit is rapid and is often sustained. Estrogen therapy with diethylstilbestrol (DES) proved comparable to orchiectomy in the large Veterans Administration study, but at a dose of 5 mg daily there was an unacceptable amount of cardiovascular mortality, particularly in older patients with underlying heart disease [58]. DES is usually given at 3 mg by mouth daily, which also achieves castrate levels of testosterone. Another agent that blocks androgen release and palliates prostate cancer as effectively as orchiectomy is leuprolide, an analogue of gonadotropin-releasing hormone [59]. Leuprolide has fewer side effects than DES, particularly cardiovascular effects. The major disadvantage of leuprolide is that it requires daily subcutaneous injection, but a monthly injectible form is being evaluated, which may make it tolerable for elderly patients.

When hormonal manipulations fail, some patients benefit from chemotherapy. Active agents include cyclophosphamide, 5-fluorouracil, Adriamycin, and cis-platinum. There are no age-dependent trends in response, although host factors such as renal or cardiac impairment affect tolerance to therapy.

Risk Reduction

Although treatment of advanced cancers may benefit patients, it is an increasing awareness of methods of prevention and early detection that is most likely to reduce the burden of cancer on individuals and on society in the coming decades. These methods are particularly relevant to the elderly because many 65-year-olds can reasonably expect to live 20 years or more. A patient's lifelong habits may be difficult to break, but it is the physician's responsibility to teach and encourage behavior that reduces cancer risk.

Cigarettes account for perhaps 30 percent of all cancer deaths, and the risk of lung cancer is diminished rapidly following cessation of smoking; hence, it is worth quitting at any age. The elderly must be wary of excessive sunlight. Unprotected sun exposure causes skin cancer, and people who are retired are perhaps more likely to sit in the midday sun or move to the sunbelt.

Diet may play a role in cancer prevention. Individuals should limit fat intake and lose weight because high fat diets or obesity may increase the incidence of cancers of the breast, colon, or prostate. A diet high in fiber may reduce the risk of colon cancer, as may a diet containing vegetables such as broccoli and Brussels sprouts. Alcohol consumption should be limited because ethanol may act as a carcinogen with tobacco in head and neck and visceral cancers. There is some information, albeit controversial, that suggests that foods rich in vitamins A and C may lower the risk for cancer of the larynx, esophagus, or lung.

A reasonable routine for cancer screening in

TABLE 23-1. *Recommendations for cancer screening in the elderly*

	PROCEDURE	FREQUENCY
All persons	History and physical examination, including rectal and skin examination	Once per year
	Stool for occult blood	Once per year
	Sigmoidoscopy	Once per year for three to five years after two negative annual examinations
Women	Breast self-examination	Once per month
	Physician breast examination	Once per year
	Mammogram	Once per year
	Pelvic examination	Once per year
	Pap smear	Once per year (see text)

SOURCE: Modified from American Cancer Society. Guidelines for the cancer-related checkup: Recommendations and rationale. *CA* 30:4, 1980.

the elderly is outlined in Table 23-1. Screening and early detection have been discussed earlier in this chapter, but their importance cannot be stressed enough.

References

1. Baranovsky, A., and Myers, M. H. Cancer incidence and survival in patients 65 years of age and older. *CA* 36:26, 1986.
2. Horm, J. W., et al. (eds.). SEER Program: Cancer incidence and mortality in the United States 1973–81. NIH Publication No. 85-1837. Bethesda, MD: National Cancer Institute, 1984.
3. Seidman, H., Silverberg, E., and Bodden, A. Probabilities of eventually developing and dying of cancer (risk among persons previously undiagnosed with the cancer). *CA* 28:33, 1978.
4. Peto, R., et al. Cancer and ageing in mice and men. *Br. J. Cancer* 32:411, 1975.
5. Cairns, J. Aging and the natural history of cancer. In R. Yancik, et al. (eds.), *Perspectives on Prevention and Treatment of Cancer in the Elderly*. New York: Raven, 1983. Pp. 19–23.
6. Berenblum, I., and Shubik, P. The role of croton oil applications, associated with a single painting of carcinogen, in tumour induction of the mouse's skin. *Br. J. Cancer* 1:379, 1947.
7. Doll, R. An epidemiological perspective on the biology of cancer. *Cancer Res.* 38:3573, 1978.

8. Peto, J., Seidman, H., and Selikoff, I. J. Mesothelioma mortality in asbestos workers: Implications for models of carcinogenesis and risk assessment. *Br. J. Cancer* 45:124, 1982.

9. Burnet, F. M. Immunological surveillance. Oxford: Pergamon, 1970.

10. Pahwa, S. G., Pahwa, R. N., and Good, R. A. Decreased in vitro humoral immune responses in aged humans. *J. Clin. Invest.* 67:1094, 1981.

11. Gillis, S., et al. Immunological studies of aging. *J. Clin. Invest.* 67:937, 1981.

12. Hoover, R. Effects of drugs: Immunosuppression. Cold Spring Harbor Conference on Cell Proliferation 4:369, 1977.

13. Rowley, J. D. Biological implications of consistent chromosome rearrangements in leukemia and lymphoma. *Cancer Res.* 44:3159, 1984.

14. Yunis, J. J. The chromosomal basis of human neoplasia. *Science* 221:227, 1983.

15. Bishop, J. M. The molecular genetics of cancer. *Science* 235:305, 1987.

16. Shmookler Reis, R. J., et al. Extrachromosomal circular copies of an 'inter-Alu' unstable sequence in human DNA are amplified during in vitro and in vivo ageing. *Nature* 301:394, 1983.

17. Lipschitz, D. A., et al. Cancer in the elderly: Basic science and clinical aspects. *Ann. Intern. Med.* 102:218, 1985.

18. Staiano-Coico, L., et al. Increased sensitivity of lymphocytes from people over 65 to cell cycle arrest and chromosomal damage. *Science* 219:1335, 1983.

19. Warnecke, R. B., Havlicek, P. L., and Manfredi, C. Awareness and use of screening by older-aged persons. In R. Yancik, et al. (eds.), *Perspectives on Prevention and Treatment of Cancer in the Elderly*. New York: Raven, 1983. Pp. 275–287.

20. Goodwin, J. S., et al. Stage of diagnosis of cancer varies with the age of the patient. *J. Am. Geriatr. Soc.* 34:20, 1986.

21. American Cancer Society. Guidelines for the cancer-related checkup: Recommendations and rationale. *CA* 30:4, 1980.

22. Shapiro, S. Evidence on screening for breast cancer from a randomized trial. *Cancer* 39:2772, 1977.

23. Synder, R. E. Detection of breast cancer in the elderly woman. In R. Yancik, et al. (eds.), *Perspectives on Prevention and Treatment of Cancer in the Elderly*. New York: Raven, 1983. Pp. 73–81.

24. Winawer, S. J., et al. Screening experience with fecal occult blood testing as a function of age. In R. Yancik, et al. (eds.), *Perspectives on Prevention and Treatment of Cancer in the Elderly*. New York: Raven, 1983. Pp. 265–274.

25. Fidler, H. K., et al. The cytology program in British Columbia. II. The operation of the cytology laboratory. *Can. Med. Assoc. J.* 86:823, 1962.

26. Greenburg, A. G., et al. Surgery in the aged. *Arch. Surg.* 116:788, 1981.

27. Herbsman, H., et al. Survival following breast cancer surgery in the elderly. *Cancer* 47:2358, 1981.

28. Gastrointestinal Tumor Study Group. Prolongation of the disease-free interval in surgically treated rectal carcinoma. *N. Engl. J. Med.* 312:1465, 1985.

29. Robert, J., and Hoerni, B. Age dependence of the early-phase pharmacokinetics of doxorubicin. *Cancer Res.* 43:4467, 1983.

30. Praga, C., et al. Adriamycin cardiotoxicity: A survey of 1273 patients. *Cancer Treat. Rep.* 63(5):827, 1979.

31. Von Hoff, D. D., Rozencweig, M., and Piccart, M. The cardiotoxicity of anticancer agents. *Sem. Oncol.* 9:23, 1982.

32. Lipschitz, D. A., et al. Effect of age on hematopoiesis in man. *Blood* 63:502, 1984.

33. Begg, C. B., and Carbone, P. P. Clinical trials and drug toxicity in the elderly. *Cancer* 52:1986, 1983.

34. Bloomfield, C. D., and Theologides, A. Acute granulocytic leukemia in elderly patients. *J.A.M.A.* 226:1190, 1973.

35. Gehan, E. A., et al. Prognostic factors in acute leukemia. *Sem. Oncol.* 3:271, 1976.

36. Foon, K. A., et al. Intensive chemotherapy is the treatment of choice for elderly patients with acute myelogenous leukemia. *Blood* 58:467, 1981.

37. Kahn, S. B., et al. Full dose versus attenuated dose daunorubicin, cytosine arabinoside, and 6-thioguanine in the treatment of acute nonlymphocytic leukemia in the elderly. *J. Clin. Oncol.* 2:865, 1984.

38. Rai, K. R., et al. Treatment of acute myelocytic leukemia: A study of cancer and leukemia group B. *Blood* 58:1203, 1981.

39. Peterson, B. A., et al. Effect of age on therapeutic response and survival in advanced Hodgkin's disease. *Cancer Treat. Rep.* 66:889, 1982.

40. Austin-Seymour, M. M., et al. Hodgkin's disease in patients over sixty years old. *Ann. Intern. Med.* 100:13, 1984.

41. Armitage, J. O., and Potter, J. F. Aggressive chemotherapy for diffuse histiocytic lymphoma in the elderly: Increased complications with advancing age. *J. Am. Geriatr. Soc.* 32:269, 1984.

42. Dixon, D. O., et al. Effect of age on therapeutic

outcome in advanced diffuse histiocytic lymphoma: The Southwest Oncology Group experience. *J. Clin. Oncol.* 4:295, 1986.

43. Peterson, B. A., and Kennedy, B. J. Aging and cancer management Part I: Clinical observations. *CA* 29:322, 1979.

44. Cohen, H. J., et al. Malignant melanoma in the elderly. *J. Clin. Oncol.* 5:100, 1987.

45. Mant, D., et al. Breast self examination and breast cancer stage at diagnosis. *Br. J. Cancer* 55:207, 1987.

46. Von Rosen, A., Gardelin, A., and Auer, G. Assessment of malignancy potential in mammary carcinoma in elderly patients. *Am. J. Clin. Oncol.* 10:61, 1987.

47. Adami, H. O., et al. The relation between survival and age at diagnosis in breast cancer. *N. Engl. J. Med.* 315:559, 1986.

48. Bonadonna, G., and Valagussa, P. Current status of adjuvant chemotherapy for breast cancer. *Sem. Oncol.* 14:8, 1987.

49. Bonadonna, G., and Valagussa, P. Dose-response effect of adjuvant chemotherapy in breast cancer. *N. Engl. J. Med.* 304:10, 1981.

50. Gelman, R. S., and Taylor, S. G., IV. Cyclophosphamide, methotrexate, and 5-fluorouracil chemotherapy in women more than 65 years old with advanced breast cancer: The elimination of age trends in toxicity by using doses based on creatinine clearance. *J. Clin. Oncol.* 2:1404, 1984.

51. Consensus Conference. Adjuvant chemotherapy for breast cancer. *J.A.M.A.* 254:3461, 1985.

52. Chu, J., et al. The effect of age on the care of women with breast cancer in community hospitals. *J. Gerontol.* 42:185, 1987.

53. Greenfield, S., et al. Patterns of care related to age of breast cancer patients. *J.A.M.A.* 257:2766, 1987.

54. Murphy, G. P., Joiner, J. R., and Saroff, J. Prostatic cancer: Evolution of treatment at a comprehensive center (1970–1974). *Urology* 8:357, 1976.

55. Correair, J. N., Curna, J. L., and Murphy, J. J. Prognosis in patients with carcinoma of the prostate. *Cancer* 25:911, 1970.

56. Garnick, M. B. Urologic cancer. In D. Federman, et al. (eds.), *Scientific American Medicine.* New York: Scientific American, 1985.

57. Walsh, P. C., and Mostwin, J. L. Radical prostatectomy and cystoprostatectomy with preservation of potency. Results using a new nerve-sparing technique. *Br. J. Urol* 56:694, 1984.

58. Blackard, C. E. The VACURG studies of carcinoma of the prostate: A review. *Cancer Chemother. Rep.* 59:225, 1975.

59. Leuprolide Study Group. Leuprolide versus diethylstilbestrol for metastatic prostate cancer. *N. Engl. J. Med.* 311:1281, 1984.

24

Neurologic Diseases

THOMAS M. WALSHE

TIME AFFECTS THE NERVOUS SYSTEM in two major ways. First, there is the involution of the nervous system that results from aging itself. The involutional changes of aging seldom provoke complaints but rather cause neurologic signs that confuse the physician, causing him or her to make an erroneous diagnosis. Second, neurologic diseases that accumulate over the years may leave only neurologic findings without symptoms. The two types of neurologic sign, one from aging alone, the other from quiescent disease, must be interpreted in the context of the patient's complaints. Involutional signs of aging are usually benign, but traces of previous illness may warn of preventable problems. Moreover, the neurologic signs from either source complicate the analysis of current neurologic complaints.

The nervous system components, peripheral nerve, spinal cord, and brain, change with age and suffer as the target of the disorders of long life.

Peripheral Nervous System

Nowhere in the nervous system is the separation of aging changes and changes of cumulative disease more difficult than in the peripheral nerve [1]. In old age the number of anterior horn neurons is reduced by 5 to 8 percent per decade. Fibers in the spinal roots also decline by almost one-third by age 90. Fiber number and the variety of fiber sizes also decline with age. The loss in heavily myelinated fibers is greater than in thinly myelinated fibers. The distance between the nodes of Ranvier is shorter in older individuals, and there is other evidence of demyelination and remyelination. The changes found in the nerves are similar to changes caused by recurrent trauma or vascular insufficiency. There is no way to know, therefore, whether the changes are a part of the aging process or are caused by other events. The intramuscular terminals and receptors of the peripheral nervous system also change with time. Nerve conduction drops in both sensory and motor nerves of elderly subjects. The loss of nerve conduction is as much as 0.16 meter per second per year of age greater than 40. The late responses (H reflex and F response) are also delayed in patients older than 50. The number of motor units is decreased in the elderly, indicating that fewer fibers are present. The anatomic and physiologic alterations of aging cause a decrease in vibration sensation on physical examination, especially in the feet.

The healthy elderly patient should have at most a minimal symmetric decline in vibratory sensation in the feet and reduced ankle reflexes. Any other findings should alert the physician to a process other than age alone.

POLYNEUROPATHY

Elderly patients suffer the same causes of chronic polyneuropathy [2] as younger patients. The syndrome of polyneuropathy consists of complaints of "numbness," "coldness," or subjective lack of sensation in the distal extremities. Some patients may complain of pain. In most polyneuropathies the feet are affected first, and the loss of sensation occurs in the stocking-glove distribution. The findings differ depending on the type of neuropathy, but examination usually shows loss of vibration, thermal, and pain sensations. The ankle reflexes are lost, and as the neuropathy becomes worse, the more proximal deep tendon reflexes disappear. Muscle wasting and weakness occur but usually after the sensory loss. Some primarily motor neuropathies such as Landry-Guillain-Barré disease can present with minimal sensory dysfunction.

Diabetes is by far the most frequent cause of polyneuropathy in old patients. The diabetes may be minimal and is easily treated with diet alone. Diabetes causes a sensory polyneuropathy that may be followed later by motor findings. Pain is a frequent complaint in diabetic polyneuropathy. Complications sometimes overshadow the neuropathy itself: Trophic ulcers of the feet and other painless sores may cause life-threatening infection, and Charcot joints may occur in some patients. Treatment of diabetic neuropathy consists of controlling the blood sugar, preventing complications with patient education and mechanical devices, and treating the pain. Pain treatment is usually the most challenging clinical problem and often fails. Use of narcotics is contraindicated since the patient will get at best temporary relief and will soon require massive doses of nontherapeutic narcotics. Carbamazepine (200–1,000 mg qid) is often tried and is successful in some patients.

Uremia, plasma cell dyscrasia, and other chronic disorders occur in elderly patients more often than in youth. Each has medical findings that usually overshadow the polyneuropathy.

Patients with malignancy may develop a polyneuropathy that evolves within six to ten months [3]. There are usually both sensory and motor findings, but a pure sensory neuropathy can be due to underlying malignancy. There may be cerebellar ataxia or other neurologic signs along with the neuropathy, and the neurologic syndrome may be detected before the neoplasm is diagnosable. Almost half the cases are caused by lung carcinoma.

Diseases causing *mononeuropathy syndromes* affect single large nerves. Diabetes again leads the list in elderly patients. The pathology of diabetic mononeuropathy is considered to be microinfarction of the nerve rather than axonal damage as in polyneuropathy. Weakness and loss of sensation appear with pain, but in some cases pain occurs alone. The control of the diabetes does not affect the course of mononeuropathy as it does in polyneuropathy. In most cases the pain improves in several weeks, and there is seldom a residual neurologic deficit. The femoral and sciatic nerves are most often affected, but mononeuropathy may affect almost any large nerve, including the cranial nerves. Diabetic mononeuropathy of the third cranial nerve is a cause of ophthalmoplegia that must be separated from compression of the third cranial nerve by a tumor or a posterior communicating artery aneurysm. The distinction can only be made by careful analysis of the whole set of clinical data. When the diagnosis is in doubt, the patient should be hospitalized and undergo angiography to identify the aneurysm. It is not always true that diabetic third nerve palsy spares the pupil, whereas the aneurysm causes dilation of the pupil. The sixth cranial nerve is also a target for diabetic mononeuropathy.

Diabetic amyotrophy is a syndrome of painful asymmetric multiple mononeuropathy that occurs in patients with mild diabetes. Muscle weakness and wasting occurs in the hips and thigh. There is less damage in the arms. The syndrome often improves in several months. Because the syndrome may recur over time, the patient is left with bilateral motor and sensory dysfunction. The syndrome may also occur gradually without pain as a prominent feature.

Another mononeuropathy that plagues the geriatric patient is peripheral nerve compression. With thinning of subcutaneous tissue and changes in the bony foramina, the nerves become exposed to compression and entrapment. The three syndromes most often found are (1) compression of the median nerve, (2) ulnar compression at the elbow, and (3) compression of the peroneal nerve at the head of the fibula.

Median nerve compression (carpal tunnel syndrome) causes tingling in the fingers with aching pains in the hand and wrist. The pain occurs at night and with repetitive movements of the wrist. There is reduced sensation in the middle and index fingers. The thenar muscles are wasted in advanced cases. The therapy is surgical separation of the volar ligament, which releases the entrapment.

Ulnar entrapment causes sensory signs and symptoms in the fourth and fifth fingers. The fourth finger is normal on the radial side but abnormal on the ulnar part. There may be weakness or wasting in the interossei. Surgical transposition of the nerve will resolve the complaints in most cases. Peroneal nerve compression causes aching and tingling in the upper-outer part of the involved leg. The problem can be caused by sitting with crossed legs or in chairs with hard edges that compress the legs at the fibular head. There may be weakness of foot dorsiflexion. The ankle jerk is preserved.

Spinal Cord

The spinal cord is the part of the central nervous system that contains nuclei for local reflex functions and the ascending and descending tracts that connect the brain to the body. Advanced age causes identifiable morphologic change in the spinal cord, but there is little in the way of clinical change in spinal cord function among healthy elderly [4]. It is therefore a reasonable rule to assume that a pathologic process, not aging, is at fault whenever a spinal cord sign or symptom is encountered.

The major changes seen with aging alone consist of neuronal loss, excess gliosis, and thinning of some myelinated tracts. The contribution of these changes to the thinning of muscle, benign fasciculation, and loss of vibratory sensation, well known in the elderly, is not easily clarified. The spinal cord houses many structures that are "passing through," and the seat of the lesion may be in the neurons either above in the brain nuclei or in the dorsal ganglia outside the cord.

Trauma is the major threat to the spinal cord at any age. In elderly patients, spinal cord trauma carries a high risk of mortality because of the fragility of the aged person and the frequency of concomitant illness. The syndromes of accidental trauma are the same at any age.

The elderly are more liable to trauma of the cord because of age-related abnormalities of the spinal canal. Osteoarthritis and other bone deformities that occur with age set the stage for the syndromes of cervical and lumbar compressions that occur in elderly patients.

CERVICAL SPONDYLOSIS

Patients with congenitally narrow spinal canals are more susceptible to cord and spinal root compression syndromes, but in old persons spinal canal deformity and narrowing may be the only causative factor [5, 6].

If the neuroforamina are narrow and irregular, the root that passes through either is compressed or its blood supply is disturbed, leading to development of a radiculopathy. The patient complains of pain and numbness that may radiate from the shoulder to the hand along the dermatome of the root involved. Muscle wasting, loss of segmental reflexes, and sensory loss are found in many cases. The findings are usually asymmetric and may be provoked by rotation or extension of the neck. The root syndrome is slow to develop, but because of the pain it may come to attention before there are objective signs of root dysfunction.

The syndrome of cord compression [7] follows the narrowing of the spinal canal itself either with degenerated disc material, ridge formations in the canal, or other bony deformities that narrow the canal enough to compress the cord [8, 9]. The patient may not have pain or may have neck, shoulder, or upper back pain. The deep tendon reflexes are hyperactive. There may be Babinski signs and sometimes a sensory disturbance to pin prick or vibration below the segment affected. The signs are often bilateral but may begin on one side. Cord compression develops insidiously, so there may be virtually no symptoms, but in these cases the neurologist may find slight hyperreflexia and Babinski signs on routine examination. Patients who have asymptomatic cervical stenosis are susceptible to sudden tetraplegia even with minimal trauma. Patients may develop the full-blown picture of spinal compression acutely and usually require immediate neurosurgical decompression. More often, the syndrome progresses to pain and weakness, causing the patient to complain.

Some patients experience a combined syndrome in which cord compression and root dysfunction create a mixed picture. These patients need to be separated from those who have progressive degeneration of the motor neurons. The cervical spondylosis patient usually has pain and sensory findings, signs absent in motor neuron disease. Radiographs of the cervical spine are useful in measuring the width of the spinal canal [10]. When the canal measures more than 13 mm from the posterior aspect of the vertebral body to the anterior aspect of the spine, compression is unlikely. The diagnosis of cervical spondylosis is made by using spinal cord imaging techniques. The myelogram is useful when the level is uncertain, but computerized tomography (CT) scan and especially magnetic resonance imaging (MRI) are fast becoming the best ways to image the cervical canal.

LUMBAR STENOSIS

Changes of bone also occur in the lumbar canal [10, 11, 12]. The structures at risk are the roots of the cauda equina, since the spinal cord itself ends at L-1. Lumbar stenosis causes multiple root complaints, and pain is almost always a prominent feature. The pain is crampy, bilateral, and asymmetric. Urinary incontinence, asymmetric loss of reflexes in the knees and ankles, muscle wasting, and loss of sensation in the affected dermatomes are the usual findings. The course is chronic and progressive. The diagnosis requires myelography or imaging with CT scan or MRI. In some cases the syndrome is so far advanced that surgery is not effective, but in early cases wide laminectomy is helpful.

In elderly patients the physician needs to separate the pain of lumbar stenosis from that of peripheral vascular disease [13, 14, 15]. The vascular cases may have bruits, and the pain is provoked with walking. In lumbar stenosis the pain is made worse on standing and when the back is extended.

OTHER SPINAL CORD SYNDROMES

There are other causes of spinal cord compression that occur in elderly persons. Tumors, cysts, or aneurysms in the area of the foramen magnum may mimic the syndrome of cervical spondylosis. Rheumatoid arthritis predisposes patients to acute spinal cord compression [16]. Foramen magnum tumors cause compression at the junction of the spinal cord and the medulla. They present bulbar signs and downbeating nystagmus, which does not occur in cervical spondylosis. The most common primary spinal tumor in older persons is meningioma, but even these are very infrequent in practice. More often, metastatic tumor causes compression of the spinal cord or the cauda equina. Imaging techniques will separate tumors from cervical or lumbar stenosis.

The syndrome of subacute combined systems disease caused by pernicious anemia is an uncommon disorder. It is a symmetric syndrome beginning with loss of vibratory sensation and paresthesia in the upper and lower extremities, followed in a few months by spasticity, hyperreflexia, and Babinski signs. The ankle reflexes may be absent. The disorder can be separated from cervical and lumbar spondylosis because of the distribution of the signs, megaloblastic marrow, gastric achlorhydria, and low serum vitamin B_{12} level. Pernicious anemia may affect the optic nerves and brain as well as the spinal cord. The pathology shows abnormalities of the myelin sheaths of the posterior columns and the tracts of the corticospinal paths. There is also myelin destruction in other areas. The axons are also affected. In fully developed cases gliosis and tissue destruction are present.

Disorders of the Brain

Neuronal depletion occurs as a consequence of normal aging in the brain. The loss of neurons is not uniform, and its clinical correlation remains evanescent. In normal aging, cell loss occurs in the substantia nigra, neocortex, limbic system, and other areas without obvious clinical signs; much of the loss of brain substance noted in elderly patients is a reduction in extracellular fluid of glial tissue. More important to the clinician are the pathologic neuronal degenerations that depopulate specific areas and cause the progressive neurologic disorders associated with late life.

PARKINSON'S DISEASE

Among the system degenerations, Parkinson's disease (PD) is second only to Alzheimer's disease in prevalence. The cause of PD is unknown. The neuropathologic features are specific and always include loss of cells in the substantia nigra. The locus ceruleus and other midbrain and diencephalic nuclei also show evidence of cell death. Small circular inclusions called Lewey bodies in the cytoplasm of the degenerating cells are found in idiopathic PD.

Although PD occurs in youth, the usual age of onset is 60 to 65 years. Normal elderly patients are known to have loss of substantia nigra neurons but not as much as parkinson patients. The relation of PD to normal aging remains unsettled.

The principal clinical finding in PD is bradykinesia or slowness of movement [17, 18]. There is no muscle weakness but rather a viscosity of motion that superficially may be mistaken for weakness. The slowness is often bilateral but may begin on one side so that a physician might suspect a hemiparesis. The history of onset and course will help because PD is a slowly progressive disease that usually takes years to become manifest. Moreover, PD frequently causes an increase in motor tone so that a limb, when moved passively, has an evenly rigid resistance. In many patients PD produces a distinctive tremor. The tremor and bradykinesia provide the basis for the venerable moniker paralysis agitans. The tremor of PD is a coarse, rhythmic movement, usually more obvious distally than proximally but present in both distributions. The tremor increases when the patient is in repose and attenuates with voluntary movement of the limb.

The tremor in repose of PD is separable from other tremors that are often found in elderly subjects [19, 20, 21]. Nonparkinsonian tremors are action tremors, that is, they increase with voluntary movement. Benign essential tremor is often familial and is faster than the tremor of PD [22, 23, 24]. Essential tremor interferes with eating and other actions much more than the tremor of PD. Patients with PD may have an essential tremor along with the tremor of PD [25]. The patient with PD almost always has bradykinesia as the major disabling sign, a feature not seen in essential tremor.

The bradykinesia interferes with gait and posture, producing the characteristic clinical picture of the parkinsonian patient [26]. The patient has a starched expression, is slow to respond and to execute motor actions, rises slowly, moves en bloc, is stooped forward, has little arm swing or associated movements when walking, and executes turns slowly with several steps. Other features, such as increasing forward speed when walking (propulsion), creates gait disturbances in some patients. All aspects of motor activity are affected, and the handwriting may change to a miniature version of the original (micrographia). Parkinson patients do not complain of falling early in the course of disease, but as the disease progresses postural stability is diminished. The voice is soft, and later the patient speaks in a whisper (hypophonia). The tremor and rigidity are grafted on the signs of bradykinesia to complete the nearly unmistakable clinical syndrome.

Other Causes of Extrapyramidal Signs

There are disorders other than degeneration of the substantia nigra that cause a syndrome similar to PD, but telltale differences help distinguish them [27]. Treatment with major neuroleptic tranquilizers (e.g., haloperidol, chlorpromazine) routinely induces the features of PD. Most patients have the fixed expression and generalized slowness of movement characteristic of PD. Tremor is also a feature in many patients. The syndrome is dose related and usually disappears when the drugs are stopped. Elderly patients are more likely to develop signs with low doses of neuroleptic drugs. Other drugs that are sometimes implicated in causing parkinsonism are the antihistamines.

Progressive supranuclear palsy is a degenerative disorder characterized by some of the signs of PD but with distinct features that allow it to be identified [30]. The course is usually shorter than that in PD. The patient complains of falling early in the course. Tremor is less common than in PD but occurs in both. Supranuclear palsy causes spastic paralysis of the tongue, pharynx, and other bulbar muscles. Dysarthria (not merely dysphonia) and dysphagia are common findings early in the disorder. There are other signs of spastic weakness such as Babinski signs and hyperactive reflexes.

The most telling feature is the onset of supranuclear ocular palsies. Patients have difficulty in moving the eyes vertically and later horizontally. Patients with PD also have limitations in upward gaze but to a much lesser degree than those with progressive supranuclear palsy. PD patients do not develop horizontal gaze palsies, although they have abnormalities in eye movement.

Other syndromes that also have features of PD are less common. Shy-Drager syndrome adds to the parkinson syndrome autonomic dysfunction, cerebellar ataxia, and other findings not seen in PD. Olivopontocerebellar atrophy adds ataxia and other signs to distinguish it from PD.

Alzheimer's disease (AD), especially in its late stages, often produces bradykinesia identical to that seen in PD. Tremor is almost never present in patients with AD alone, even with obvious bradykinesia. Moreover, in most but not all cases of AD the dementia occurs much before the onset of the movement disorder. Of course, patients with AD treated with neuroleptics develop the standard drug-induced parkinsonism described above.

Patients with PD have dementia that usually, but not always, begins well after the movement disorder. The dementia differs from that seen in AD mainly in that language is spared in PD but is almost universally affected in AD. The dementia of PD is somewhat less severe than that of AD [31, 32, 33].

AD is associated with the pathologic features of PD in about 20 to 30 percent of cases that come to autopsy late in the course. All patients with PD who are demented, however, do not have concomitant AD at postmortem examination. Patients with both diseases have the clinical features of both diseases.

Treatment

The rationale of treatment of PD arises from the information learned about the neurochemistry of the basal ganglia. The dopaminergic cells of the substantia nigra send axons to the striatum, where they synapse with cholinergic interneurons. The complete relay involves a number of cells and areas of the basal ganglia. The assumption is that dopaminergic input modulates the cholinergic neurons, which in turn alter basal ganglia function. The dopaminergic cells inhibit the cholinergic systems, so that lack of dopamine increases the cholinergic influence, which causes the signs of PD. Thus treatment has focused on (1) increasing dopamine effects, or (2) reducing cholinergic effects [34, 35, 36].

The mainstay of therapy is administration of L-dopa, which is transformed to the active dopamine in the brain. L-dopa passes the blood-brain barrier reluctantly, so large doses are needed to achieve adequate brain levels. L-dopa is combined with a dopadecarboxylase inhibitor, carbidopa, that prevents dopamine from forming. Since the inhibitor does not pass the blood-brain barrier, therapeutic levels of dopamine are reached in the brain with fewer systemic side effects. L-dopa is sold as combinations with 25 mg of carbidopa and 100 mg of L-dopa (25/100), 10/100, and 25/250. In elderly patients who have PD and are substantially bothered by the bradykinesia, the combination drug (Sinemet and others) should be started at 25/100 once or twice daily and gradually increased until the symptoms are improved. The maximum daily dose is determined by side effects but is usually 2 gm or less of L-dopa. Systemic side effects are nausea, hypotension, cardiac arrythmia, and diarrhea. The neurologic complication most bothersome in the elderly is the precipitation of acute psychosis. Some patients develop choreiform movements that may be tolerated if they do not interfere with function. The dose should be reduced with the onset of serious side effects and the patient maintained on the lower dose. The vagaries of L-dopa treatment are beyond this summary, but a key principle is to administer the drug before the patient needs to perform activities of daily living; a bedtime dose is helpful also. Nocturnal bradykinesia is most unpleasant, may lead to bedsores, and may cause incontinence because the patient cannot get out of bed easily. Small, frequent doses of L-dopa are usually best tolerated [37]. The treatment program depends entirely on the patient's response.

Bromocriptine, a dopamine agonist, is occasionally useful to add to L-dopa/carbidopa when there are periods during which the patient loses the effect of the L-dopa [38, 39]. Bromocriptine, used in doses of 20 to 70 mg daily, is particularly liable to cause psychosis in elderly patients.

The anticholinergic drugs (trihexyphenidyl, benztropine mesylate, and others) may relieve symptoms when used alone in PD. They are also useful if L-dopa/carbidopa fails to relieve symptoms adequately. The side effects are dry mouth, constipation, urinary retention, lethargy, and psychosis or a confusional state. The mental changes are most bothersome in the elderly and limit the use of anticholinergics. Amantadine (100 mg once or twice daily depending on renal function) has been used for years and is of help in some patients. Its mechanism of action is not totally clear, but it seems to inspire release of dopamine.

Other methods of treatment are almost as important as drug therapy, especially in patients who respond only partly to the medicines. Physical therapy helps to teach patients the best way to move and maintain gait. Walkers and other devices can be suggested by the therapists. Alterations of the home are also important to minimize physical obstacles that interfere with activities of daily living.

Complications of PD are related to the bradykinesia. Constipation and dehydration are frequent companions in PD because some patients are not able to maintain adequate hydration. A pitcher of water nearby helps the patient to maintain his needs. Slowness in eating may prevent adequate nutrition unless nursing staff or family allow the patient adequate time to eat. Aspiration of food is also a threat, especially in severely affected patients. Pressure sores can be prevented by ensuring that the patient changes position every few hours. Most patients with PD die of infections, usually during the late stages of the disease when they are immobile, bedridden, and in a near vegetative state.

HEAD TRAUMA AND SUBDURAL HEMATOMA

Acute head trauma is treated similarly in elderly and young patients. Cerebral contusion, lacerations, and skull fractures require neurosurgical care. The prognosis for recovery of function is worse in older patients. Acute subdural hematoma (SDH) is a sequel of head trauma that is seen mostly in young patients. The syndrome is not difficult to recognize because it follows the injury in a matter of hours.

Elderly patients have acute SDH but also suffer from a more elusive syndrome caused by subacute or chronic SDH [40, 41]. Because the brains of elderly patients are smaller, they have larger subarachnoid spaces. The veins that bridge the dura and subarachnoid membranes are stretched more than in youth. Almost any degree of trauma, therefore, may tear a vein, causing a subdural clot to form. Because of the extra subarachnoid space, the hematoma may not compress the brain to cause an immediate dramatic change. Over a period of days, however, the patient may have an indolent decline in neurologic function. The trauma may be so minor that it is not remembered, or it may be so remote that it appears unrelated to the current symptom.

The major complaint or problem associated with chronic SDH is decline in mental function. The historical features help to separate this entity from the many other causes of mental decline in elderly patients. The onset of the mental abnormality can usually be marked within a week or so. Some patients have focal headache. The course is usually short; complaints appear within a few months at most. With Alzheimer's disease and strokes a longer period usually elapses before the patient comes to medical attention. Chronic SDH almost always causes focal neurologic signs—brisk reflexes, a Babinski sign, or even a hemiparesis. Such signs are not found in Alzheimer's disease and should lead the physician to suspect another disease. Patients with chronic SDH have more dramatic fluctuations in mental status than most patients with stroke. Moreover, the patient with chronic subdural hematoma tends to be lethargic rather than alert, as one would expect in AD or vascular dementia.

Patients with AD and other brain atrophies are at high risk for SDH. One of the causes of sudden decline of neurologic function in a patient with AD is a subdural hematoma. The patient may become worse over several days and cause the family or physician to question the possibility of excess sedation. The patient usually develops some motor findings such as reflex asymmetry, a Babinski sign, or hemiparesis, but onset of obtundation may be the only sign. Bilateral SDH causes bilateral findings on neurologic examination and changes in mental status. The symmetry of the findings can be misleading and may suggest a degenerative disorder rather than a structural lesion. The SDH may expand to cause coma and death.

The diagnosis of chronic SDH in elderly patients is made by CT scan or MRI. With current technology it is unlikely that a SDH would be overlooked on either scan. The treatment is surgical evacuation of the clot if the patient can tolerate the procedure [42].

Elderly patients with hydrocephalus whose ventricles are decompressed with a shunt may develop a postoperative SDH. The change in mental status may be missed because the original deficit of hydrocephalus is replaced by that of the subdural, so there may be little clinical change.

HEADACHE

Headache in elderly patients causes more concern about serious underlying disease than headache in young patients [43]. Headache is a more frequent complaint in young than in old patients. In youth it is usually caused by benign disorders. When elderly patients complain of headache it must be evaluated systematically to identify the cause. Vascular headache, cervical radiculopathy, giant cell arteritis, and brain tumor are the most frequent causes.

Vascular Headache

Benign vascular headaches (migraine) usually cease to cause symptoms after the mid-fifties, but in some patients a flurry of headaches occur late in life. Patients with migraine may have headaches that are milder than those they had in youth, but they may have neurologic accompaniments not previously experienced. The diagnosis in these cases hinges on distinguishing the complicated migraine from transient ischemia of other causes. The separation depends on a reliable history of previous headaches, a deficit that develops sequentially, a visual scotoma or other visual phenomenon characteristic of migraine, and sometimes the demonstration of normal arterial anatomy. It is no simple matter to identify the elderly person having a benign migraine from one experiencing a prelude to a serious stroke. When a headache is accompanied by neurologic findings in patients of any age, the physician is required to search for a structural lesion. Headaches that have no neurologic findings are not always benign but do not require an immediate evaluation. Treatment of recurrent benign headaches in elderly patients is similar to that in young patients. Analgesics are the mainstay and must be used in lower doses in elderly patients. It is very unusual for a benign vascular headache to appear in patients over age 70.

Headache is almost never associated with ischemic stroke without other clear signs of stroke. Headache alone is almost unheard of as a transient ischemic symptom indicating carotid or basilar artery stenosis. Dissection of the carotid artery sometimes causes headache along with transient neurologic signs. A new carotid bruit may appear. Patients that have headache followed by a *transient* neurologic deficit need a thorough evaluation but may well have a migraine syndrome. Headache, either chronic or acute, does not herald the onset of an ischemic stroke. Ischemic stroke may cause a mild or moderate headache that accompanies the other signs of ischemia. The headache in stroke is caused by the abnormality in the vessel rather than the ischemia of the brain.

Some vascular syndromes almost always present with headache. Patients with subarachnoid hemorrhage invariably have an acute, severe headache [44,45]. They may lose consciousness after the onset of headache and awaken without neurologic signs. The headache of subarachnoid hemorrhage is usually more severe than a migraine but not in every case. Patients with intracranial bleeding may have a subhyloid retinal hemorrhage, which does not occur in migraine. Sudden severe headache in an elderly patient should suggest ruptured aneurysm as the first diagnosis. MRI, CT scan, or lumbar puncture will confirm the diagnosis [46]. Intracerebral hematomas also cause headache but almost never without other signs that make it clear that a cerebral lesion is at fault.

Cervical Radiculopathy

Elderly patients suffer from cervical radiculopathy, which may cause chronic occipital head pain and neck pain. The pain is usually made worse with movement of the neck and improves with rest. The shoulder may be painful also. The headache is usually less severe in the front than in the back of the head and neck. Most patients with head pain from cervical spondylosis show degenerative arthritis on spine films. The nature and location of the pain are, however, more important than the radiographic findings in making the diagnosis.

A cervical collar, neck traction, bed rest, and analgesics help most patients with head pain from cervical spine disease. Only when there is severe unrelenting pain or clear neurologic signs of cord or root compression causing fixed deficits should a laminectomy be considered.

Other Causes of Headache

Giant cell arteritis is a cause of headache that occurs almost exclusively in elderly patients [47]. The syndrome may occur with headache alone, but there are usually systemic complaints as well (see Chap. 31).

Brain tumor, either primary or metastatic, causes recurrent headache beginning in late life. There are often seizures, other neurologic signs, and a history of progressive worsening over weeks or months. CT scan and MRI make the diagnosis.

The evaluation of an elderly patient with recurrent headaches should include a CT or MRI head scan and an erythrocyte sedimentation rate. Other tests depend on the data collected in the history and neurologic examination. An acute headache requires evaluation for subarachnoid hemorrhage.

DIZZINESS

Dizziness is a term that patients use to describe a variety of discomforts [48, 49]. Sometimes it is used to connote a false sensation of motion or vertigo. The patient may perceive the environment to swirl or feel the sensation of falling. Dizziness does not always mean vertigo. Patients describe an unpleasant faintness or a sensation of imbalance without the illusion of motion as dizziness. Blurred vision, diplopia, orthostatic hypotension, among other things, also may be reported as dizziness by elderly patients. The analysis of a dizzy patient first re-

quires that the physician determine exactly what the patient means by the word *dizzy*. A careful history is the only way to determine the type of dizziness that is causing the complaint. Faintness, disequilibrium, lightheadedness, and vertigo, all reported as dizziness, require separate diagnostic approaches.

Vertigo

Stroke and transient ischemia in the vertebrobasilar circulation cause acute vertigo accompanied by other neurologic complaints. A careful history and examination uncover signs of diplopia, facial weakness, facial numbness, hemiparesis, quadriparesis, or other signs of brain stem dysfunction.

Acute cerebellar infarction or hemorrhage causes vertigo accompanied by limb ataxia or ataxia of gait [50]. There is almost always an abrupt onset, and the patient cannot walk. Vomiting is a frequent sign; headache is uncommon.

The first step in evaluation of acute vertigo is to look for focal neurologic signs. When signs other than vertigo are lacking, the localization usually lies outside the central nervous system, but not always. In patients with basilar ischemia and cerebellar lesions, additional signs usually appear in several hours, if not at onset, so careful follow-up examinations may lead to the diagnosis.

Acute vertigo without other neurologic signs is usually caused by disorders of the labyrinth [51, 52, 53]. Such disorders are not life-threatening but are disabling, especially in the elderly. Tinnitus is a frequent symptom of labyrinthine disease because the cochlea can also be affected. Another sign of labyrinthine (or eighth nerve) defects is nystagmus, in which the fast phase beats away from the lesion and the slow phase beats toward the lesion. The nystagmus does *not* change direction with direction of gaze. There may be a past history of similar vertiginous attacks. Patients with acute labyrinthine vertigo complain of spinning (away from the lesion), inability to walk, nausea, and vomiting. They are able to walk if forced, although they may find it unpleasant; patients with cerebellar ataxia of gait find it almost impossible to walk or even stand up. Elderly patients with acute vertigo require hospitalization for diagnostic evaluation and to ensure that they do not become dehydrated from the vomiting.

Elderly patients with chronic or recurrent dizziness complain of inability to balance, instability of gait, spatial confusion, and light-headedness. It is less common for such patients to complain of the environment moving about them. Patients with chronic labyrinthine disorders may not have a sense of motion but rather a sense of imbalance.

Other Dizzy Symptoms

Elderly patients with "dizziness" often are found to have a concatenation of problems that contribute to their failure to maintain comfortable spatial orientation. Problems of vision, hearing, and proprioception as well as the central processing of these modalities contribute to a multisensory syndrome that causes dizziness. The multiplicity of the problems interferes with the usual feedback mechanisms that allow the nervous system to remain aware of the body's position in space. When questioned, the dizzy patient will also complain of symptoms of neuropathy, visual loss, and the other independent deficits.

The treatment of elderly patients with multisensory dizziness is based on improvement of each separate deficit. Proper glasses and a hearing aid will help in some cases. A cane increases proprioceptive input and may improve the sense of stability. Medication is usually not very helpful and may even make the symptoms worse if it causes sedation. In patients with benign vertigo, small doses of meclizine or promethazine sometimes help.

SEIZURE DISORDERS

Diagnosis

The onset of seizures in the elderly, unlike that in youth, almost always means there is a pathologic lesion in the brain. Brain tumor occurs in 10 to 12 percent of late-onset seizure patients. When elderly patients complain of paroxysmal neurologic disturbances, a seizure disorder ranks high as the possible cause.

Brain damage from stroke is by far the most frequent cause of seizures in older persons [54, 55]. It is unusual for stroke to present with a seizure, but patients who have had stroke in the past develop seizures as a complication of the cerebral lesion left by the infarction.

A single seizure may indicate a serious occult problem such as acute subdural hematoma, ruptured aneurysm, brain tumor, or abscess. There are usually other neurologic features that help to identify the underlying cause [56, 57]. Laboratory tests such as MRI and CT scans are indispensible in diagnosis of tumor and other structural lesions.

Elderly patients sometimes have seizures that do not cause convulsions or other motor signs. Such patients may complain of paroxysmal sensory disturbances, loss of consciousness, vertigo, or other nonmotor problems. In such patients an electroencephalogram may show paroxysmal abnormalities that help to identify the symptoms as seizures.

An elderly patient with a new seizure needs a careful medical and neurologic evaluation to search for systemic disease. Patients with past brain lesions such as stroke may develop a seizure only when they become ill with a non-neurologic disease. A careful medical examination may turn up a urinary infection or other occult cause for the emergence of an otherwise quiescent seizure disorder.

Treatment

Chronic recurrent seizures in the elderly are treated using the same principles as are used in younger patients. A single drug is used until the seizures cease or signs of early toxicity occur [58, 59, 60]. Toxicity in elderly patients appears at lower doses than in young patients. Moreover, elderly patients become sedated from phenytoin much more easily than younger patients. Elderly patients with prior stroke or degenerative disorders are particularly liable to the sedative side effects of anticonvulsants. Phenytoin excess also causes ataxia, which may be overlooked in an elderly patient who begins to fall or becomes less secure in gait. The ataxia may occur even without excessive serum phenytoin levels.

When a single drug is inadequate to control seizures at tolerated levels, additional drugs are added. The drugs most often used are phenytoin, phenobarbital, and carbamazepine. The initial drug depends mostly on a guess at the patient's tolerance and the doctor's preferences. Seizures in most elderly patients are controlled with one drug.

Compliance may become a problem, especially if the patient experiences side effects. Rather than reduce the drug, the patient stops taking it. When a patient experiences toxic symptoms from an anticonvulsant, the drug need not be stopped entirely. It is best to skip a day's dose and reduce the daily dose. The toxic symptoms will abate slowly, and the patient will continue to be protected against seizure. If the anticonvulsant is stopped completely, there is a chance that the patient will have seizures and may develop status epilepticus.

Patients treated with anticonvulsants for a chronic seizure disorder should be followed at least yearly to ensure that the medicine is tolerated and that there are no new neurologic signs. While the dose of drug is being altered, the patient must be seen more frequently. Serum anticonvulsant levels are useful when there is a question of compliance. When the patient has a seizure, it is helpful to know the serum level that failed to prevent the seizures. Unless the seizure was provoked by a coincident systemic cause, the level measured just after a seizure is too low. Either another drug must be added or the single drug must be increased.

In patients who have seizures infrequently, the physician can use serum anticonvulsant levels to ascertain a reasonable dose of drug, but he cannot be sure it is the right dose unless a long seizure-free period ensues. It is of little use to measure the serum anticonvulsant level in a patient whose seizures are under control.

References

1. Dorfman, L. J., and Bosley, T. M. Age-related changes in peripheral central nerve conduction in man. *Neurology* 29:38, 1979.
2. Dyck, P. J., Thomas, P. K., and Lambert, E. H. (eds.). *Peripheral Neuropathy*. Philadelphia: Saunders, 1975.
3. Croft, P. B., Urich, H., and Wilkinson, M. Peripheral neuropathy of the sensorimotor type associated with malignant disease. *Brain* 90:31, 1967.
4. Morrison, R. L., Cobb, S., and Bauer, W. *The Effect of Advancing Age Upon the Human Spinal Cord*. Cambridge: Harvard University Press, 1959.
5. Brain, W. R., and Wilkenson, M. *Cervical Spondylosis and Other Diseases of the Cervical Spine*. Philadelphia: Saunders, 1967.
6. Ehni, G. Neurological disorders associated with skeletal changes. In W. S. Fields (ed.), *Neurological and Sensory Disorders in the Elderly*. Chicago: Year Book, 1975. Pp. 33–50.
7. Adams, C. B. T., and Logue, V. Studies in cervical spondylotic myelopathy. *Brain* 94:557, 1971.
8. Nurick, S. The pathogenesis of spinal cord disorder associated with cervical spondylosis. *Brain* 95:87, 1972.
9. Nurick, S. The natural history and the results of surgical treatment of the spinal cord disorder associated with cervical spondylosis. *Brain* 95:101, 1972.
10. Weinstein, P. R., Ehni, G., and Wilson, C. B. *Lumbar Spondylosis: Diagnosis, Management and Surgical Treatment*. Chicago: Year Book, 1977.
11. *Clin. Orthop. Rel. Res.* 115: 1976.
12. McIvor, G. W. D., and Kirkaldy-Willis, W. S. Pathological and myelographic changes in the major types of lumbar spinal stenosis. *Clin. Orthop. Rel. Res.* 115:72, 1976.
13. Blau, J. N., and Logue, V. The natural history of intermittent Claudication of the cauda equina. A long-term follow-up study. *Brain* 101:211, 1978.
14. Dyck, P., et al. Intermittent cauda equina compression syndrome. *Spine* 2:75, 1977.
15. Jellinger, K., et al. (eds.). *Handbook of Clinical Neurology*. Vol. 12. Amsterdam: North Holland, 1972. Pp. 504–547.
16. Nakano, K. K., et al. The cervical myelopathy associated with rheumatoid arthritis: Analysis of 32 patients with two postmortem cases. *Ann. Neurol.* 3:144, 1978.
17. Martin, W. E., et al. Parkinson's disease: Clinical analysis of 100 patients. *Neurology* 23: 783, 1973.
18. Hoehn, M. M., and Yahr, M. D. Parkinsonism: Onset, progression and mortality. *Neurology* 17:427, 1967.
19. Calzetti, S., et al. Effect of a single oral dose of propranolol on essential tremor: A double-blind controlled study. *Ann. Neurol.* 13:165, 1983.
20. Calzetti, S., et al. The response of essential tremor to propranolol: Evaluation of clinical variables governing its efficacy on prolonged administration. *J. Neurol. Neurosurg. Psychiatry* 46:393, 1983.
21. Chakrabarti, A., and Pearce, J. M. S. Essential tremor: Response to primidone. *J. Neurol. Neurosurg. Psychiatry* 44:650, 1981.

22. Critchley, E. Clinical manifestations of essential tremor. *J. Neurol. Neurosurg. Psychiatry* 35:365, 1972.
23. Fahn, S. Differential diagnosis of tremors. *Med. Clin. North Am.* 56:1363, 1972.
24. Shahani, B. T., and Young, R. R. Physiological and pharmacological aids in the differential diagnosis of tremor. *J. Neurol. Neurosurg. Psychiatry* 39:772, 1976.
25. Teravainen, H., and Calne, D. B. Action tremor in Parkinson's disease. *J. Neurol. Neurosurg. Psychiatry* 43:257, 1980.
26. Klawans, H. L., and Topel, J. L. Parkinsonism as a falling sickness. *J.A.M.A.* 230:1555, 1974.
27. Young, R. R. The differential diagnosis of Parkinson's disease. *Int. J. Neurol.* 12:210, 1977.
30. Steele, J. C. Progressive supranuclear palsy. *Brain* 95:693, 1972.
31. Hakim, A. M., and Mathieson, G. Dementia in parkinson disease: A neuropathologic study. *Neurology* 29:1209, 1979.
32. Ikeda, K., Hori, A., and Bode, G. Progressive dementia with "diffuse Lewy-type inclusions" in cerebral cortex. *Arch. Psychiat. Nervenkr.* 228:243, 1980.
33. Lieberman, A., et al. Dementia in Parkinson disease. *Ann. Neurol.* 6:355, 1978.
34. Bianchine, J. R. Drug therapy for parkinsonism. *N. Engl. J. Med.* 295:814, 1976.
35. Bosches, B. Sinemet and the treatment of parkinsonism. *Ann. Intern. Med.* 94:364, 1981.
36. Fann, W. E., and Whelan, J. C. Therapeutic principles in the management of movement disorders in elderly patients. *Interdiscipl. Top. Gerontol.* 15:194, 1979.
37. Fann, S. On-off phenomenon with levodopa therapy in parkinsonism. *Neurology* 24:431, 1974.
38. Lieberman, A., et al. Treatment of Parkinson's disease with bromocriptine. *N. Engl. J. Med.* 295:1400, 1976.
39. Teychenne, P. F., et al. Bromocriptine: Low-dose therapy in Parkinson's disease. *Neurology* 32:577, 1982.
40. Markwalder, T-M. Chronic subdural hematoma: A review. *J. Neurosurg.* 54:637, 1981.
41. Wintzen, A. R. The clinical course of subdural hematoma. *Brain* 103:855, 1980.
42. Bender, M. B., and Christoff, N. Nonsurgical treatment of subdural hematoma. *Arch. Neurol.* 31:73, 1974.
43. Raskin, N. Headaches associated with organic diseases of the nervous system. *Med. Clin. North Am.* 62:459, 1978.
44. Drake, C. G. Management of cerebral aneurysm. *Stroke* 12:273, 1981.
45. Walshe, T. M. (ed.). *Manual of Clinical Problems in Geriatric Medicine.* Boston: Little, Brown, 1985.
46. Weisberg, L. A. Computed tomography in aneurysmal subarachnoid hemorrhage. *Neurology* 29:802, 1979.
47. Huston, K. A., and Hunder, G. G. Giant cell (cranial) arteritis: A clinical review. *Am. Heart J.* 100:99, 1980.
48. Drachman, D. A., and Hart, C. W. An approach to the dizzy patient. *Neurology* 22:323, 1972.
49. Overstall, P. W., Hazell, J. W. P., and Johnson, A. L. Vertigo in the elderly. *Age Aging* 10:105, 1981.
50. Fisher, C. M. Vertigo in cerebrovascular disease. *Arch. Otolaryngol.* 85:529, 1967.
51. Smith, B. H. Vestibular disturbances in epilepsy. *Neurology* 10:465, 1960.
52. Stuart, W. H. Geriatric neurology for the otolaryngologist. *Otolaryngol. Clin. North Am.* 15:329, 1982.
53. Wolfson, R. J. (ed.). Symposium on vertigo. *Otolaryngol. Clin. North Am.* 6:1, 1973.
54. DeReuck, J., et al. Epilepsy in patients with cerebral infarcts. *J. Neurol.* 224:101, 1980.
55. Dodge, P. R., Richardson, E. P., and Victor, M. Recurrent convulsive seizures as a sequel to cerebral infarction: A clinical and pathological study. *Brain* 77:610, 1954.
56. Otomo, E. Convulsion in the aged. *Folia Psychiat. Neurol. Jpn.* 35:295, 1981.
57. Shigemoto, T. Epilepsy in middle or advanced age. *Folia Psychiat. Neurol. Jpn.* 35:287, 1981.
58. Penry, J. K., and Newmark, M. E. The use of antiepileptic drugs. *Ann. Intern. Med.* 90:207, 1979.
59. Wallis, W., Kutt, H., and McDowell, F. Intravenous diphenylhydantoin in treatment of acute repetitive seizures. *Neurology* 18:513, 1968.
60. Easton, J. D. Diphenylhydantoin and epilepsy management. *Ann. Intern. Med.* 77:421, 1972.

25

Stroke

THOMAS M. WALSHE

THE NEUROLOGIC ASPECTS OF CEREBROVASCULAR DISEASE depend on the underlying vessel pathologies and vary with the simple mechanical parameters of size of vessel affected, degree of ischemia, availability of collateral flow, and duration of ischemia. A reasonable approach to the diagnosis and treatment of stroke hinges on understanding the types of vascular lesion and the cerebrovascular anatomy. Certainly without some concept of the vascular anatomy there is little hope of correctly assessing patients with transient or progressive cerebrovascular syndromes.

Vascular Anatomy

The brain receives its blood flow from four major arteries: the right and left carotid arteries and the right and left vertebral arteries (Fig. 25-1).

The *common carotid artery* arises on the left from the aortic arch and on the right from the brachiocephalic artery. It continues in the neck to bifurcate into the *external carotid,* which flows to the face and into the *internal carotid* (IC), which passes to the brain through the carotid foramen at the base of the skull. At the base of the brain the IC bifurcates into the two vessels of the anterior cerebral circulation: the *middle cerebral artery* and the *anterior cerebral artery.*

The superior and inferior divisions of the *middle cerebral artery* supply blood to the lateral hemisphere, including the frontal and temporal lobes and most of the parietal lobe. Proximal branches of the middle cerebral artery arise just after it leaves the carotid and supply the deep structures anterior to the thalamus, including the putamen, globus pallidus, and internal capsule. The *anterior cerebral artery* supplies blood to the medial hemisphere and corpus callosum on each side. The *vertebral arteries* arise from the subclavian arteries, rise to the head via the vertebral canal, and enter the skull through the foramen magnum. Before the two vertebral arteries join to form the *basilar artery,* a vessel called the *posterior inferior cerebellar artery* (PICA) emerges to supply blood to the lateral medulla. The basilar artery supplies blood to the structures of the posterior fossa. Circumferential branches of the basilar artery supply the cerebellum and parts of the brain stem. Small branches of the basilar artery penetrate the upper medulla, pons, and midbrain, supplying them with blood. At the level of the midbrain the basilar artery bifurcates to form the right and left posterior cerebral artery.

The *posterior cerebral artery* supplies the posterior parietal lobe and the occipital lobe on each side. Proximal branches supply the deep structures of the diencephalon (thalamus).

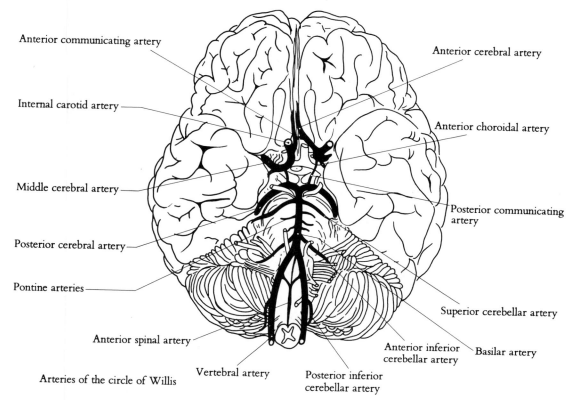

Anterior communicating artery

Internal carotid artery

Middle cerebral artery

Posterior cerebral artery

Pontine arteries

Anterior spinal artery

Arteries of the circle of Willis

Vertebral artery

Anterior cerebral artery

Anterior choroidal artery

Posterior communicating artery

Superior cerebellar artery

Anterior inferior cerebellar artery

Basilar artery

Posterior inferior cerebellar artery

FIGURE 25-1. *Vascular anatomy of the brain. (From S. J. DeArmond, et al.* Structure of the Human Brain: A Photographic Atlas. *New York: Oxford University Press, 1976.)*

At the base of the brain the anterior (carotid) and posterior (basilar) circulations are connected by the *posterior communicating arteries,* which connect the middle cerebral artery and the posterior cerebral artery on each side. The circulation on the right side is connected to that on the left through a short artery, the anterior communicating artery, between the right and left anterior cerebral arteries. The top of the basilar artery offers collateral flow in the posterior circulation. This system of connecting vessels, anterior communicating, posterior communicating, and top of the basilar, is called the arterial *circle of Willis.*

Under normal circumstances there is almost no flow across the communicating arteries. Blood from the right internal carotid flows to the right middle cerebral and anterior cerebral artery. Only when there is a decrease in pressure in one territory do the collateral channels (posterior or anterior communicating arteries) operate. For example, if flow is decreased in the right carotid so that the blood pressure is less than in the left, blood would flow across the anterior communicating artery from left to right, and across the right posterior communicating artery to fill the middle and anterior cerebral arteries from behind.

There are other potential anastomotic vessels that can provide flow when the cerebral vessels are occluded. The internal and external carotid have an anastomosis in the orbital vessels so that in some cases of internal carotid occlusion blood flows into the internal system via the orbital vessels. Meningeal and capillary anastomoses play a role in determining the size of an infarction but probably are not large enough to prevent a stroke unless the occluding process is unusually slow to develop.

Ideally, the circle of Willis and other collaterals should prevent strokes from occlusion of vessels below the circle. In fact, the circle of

Willis is not always complete because of anatomic variation or atherosclerotic occlusions. The vagaries of the cerebral circulation and its collaterals make the localization of stroke difficult and hamper the logical analysis of its prognosis and treatment.

Risk Factors

Collateral flow possibilities notwithstanding, cerebrovascular disease is the most frequent cause of neurologic dysfunction in elderly persons. For stroke of all types, advanced age is the most consistent risk factor [1, 2]. Hypertension is a major medical risk factor in causing both hemorrhagic and ischemic stroke, but other cardiac diseases and diabetes mellitus are also important. The incidence of all strokes has steadily declined during the last 20 years [3]. The reasons remain speculative, but almost all investigators agree that it is at least in part the result of widespread treatment of hypertension [4, 5]. Among patients older than 65, hypertension and cigarette smoking are associated with the highest mortality rates as well as the highest rates of stroke. Strokes in all groups have become less severe, and this factor has caused a 50 percent decline in stroke mortality in the last ten years. The incidence of embolic strokes has not been tracked separately, but one would assume a decline with recognition and treatment of the embolic sources.

Clinical Features

The hallmark of stroke is, as its name implies, a rapidly occurring neurologic deficit. There are several types of stroke, each having a distinct pathology and clinical profile [6]. Most strokes occur over minutes or hours, but in exceptional cases the syndrome may develop within a day or two. The clinician uses the history, neurologic findings, and laboratory tests to identify each type of stroke. Because each has a different treatment and prognosis, the diagnosis of the specific type is important to the care of the patient.

The vascular lesions that cause stroke can be divided into those that cause rupture of the vessel (hemorrhagic stroke) and those that cause occlusion of the vessel (ischemic stroke).

Within each main group there are several types of lesion.

Ischemic Stroke

THROMBOSIS

Thrombosis is the stationary coagulation of blood within the lumen of the artery. Thrombosis usually occurs in areas of atherosclerosis where the artery is abnormal [7]. An atherosclerotic vascular lesion may be stenotic, ulcerative, or both. Thrombosis that occludes the lumen of the artery occurs in arteries already narrow from atheromata. In ulcerative lesions the thrombosis may not occlude the lumen of the vessel but may be a source of cerebral embolism [8, 9]. Thrombosis of the cerebral vasculature usually involves the carotid, the vertebral, or the basilar artery. The distal cerebral vessels are usually spared from thrombotic cerebrovascular disease but are the prime targets for embolism. Hemorrhage into the atheromatous plaque has also been found to cause carotid artery occlusion.

The most frequent site of cerebral thrombosis is at the bifurcation of the common carotid artery [10]. The narrowing usually is not symptomatic until the lumen is at least 80 or 90 percent closed. When a stenotic carotid artery becomes occluded, the patient may not experience clinical change if there is adequate collateral circulation through the circle of Willis. The clinical syndrome and its severity depend on the availability of collateral circulation. If the obstruction develops slowly, there is a better chance that collateral circulation can compensate.

The variability of symptomatic carotid occlusion makes it difficult to describe a typical clinical picture, but certain features appear routinely [11, 12]. Large vessel thrombosis generally begins with a series of neurologic changes that wax and wane. Within a few hours the syndrome progresses in steps to the maximum deficit.

TRANSIENT ISCHEMIC ATTACKS

In some cases the neurologic deficit appears transiently and disappears completely, leaving the patient asymptomatic. Transient neurologic symptoms are highly suggestive of large vessel thrombosis and are called *transient ischemic at-*

tacks [13, 14]. It is, however, important to realize that all transient neurologic findings are not related to ischemia. Transient ischemic symptoms conform to deficits localized in the vascular territories. The transient ischemic attacks caused by large vessel thrombosis usually last less than an hour and often less than 20 minutes [10, 15]. Transient ischemia from stenosis or occlusion of the carotid artery usually causes a hemiparesis, hemisensory deficit, and hemianopsia. Ischemia of the dominant hemisphere causes aphasia and, in the nondominant hemisphere, apraxia. In many cases only parts of the syndrome occur transiently as a warning of an impending stroke. Transient numbness or weakness of the face and hand suggests an ischemic deficit in the distal territory of the middle cerebral artery, the so-called border zone between the middle and anterior cerebral arteries.

Thrombosis in the internal carotid or middle cerebral artery causes similar transient syndromes [16]. Cerebral angiography is the only sure method of separating the two possibilities [17]. Middle cerebral stenosis is much less frequent than carotid stenosis and has no effective surgical treatment [18].

Transient retinal ischemia that causes transient monocular blindness may occur with stenosis or obstruction of the internal carotid artery, obstruction or stenosis of the ophthalmic artery, or ischemia related to the central retinal artery. The blindness usually occurs briefly as a gradual fading of vision, sometimes with a shade-like effect. When a patient reports transient monocular blindness on one occasion and contralateral signs of hemispheric dysfunction on another occasion, there is a high probability of a carotid artery stenosis or obstruction. Transient monocular blindness that occurs without hemispheric findings or any other suggestion of brain dysfunction is usually related to abnormalities other than those in the carotid artery. Transient monocular blindness can also be caused by embolism to the branches of the retinal artery. Giant cell arteritis is another cause of visual symptoms in elderly patients.

Atherothrombosis occurs in the vertebral and basilar arteries, causing transient ischemic attacks with brain stem symptoms [7, 19]. Transient vertigo, diplopia, numbness of the face, and other cranial nerve signs are associated with basilar artery ischemia. There are usually bilateral motor and sensory deficits as well. Dizziness without other signs or symptoms is usually due to a labyrinthine disorder.

Thrombotic cerebrovascular disease occurs in the setting of risk factors for atherosclerosis. There may be arterial bruits either over the carotid arteries or over other large arteries. A bruit over the carotid artery, however, does not necessarily indicate immediate danger from a stroke.

Patients with transient ischemic attacks in the carotid artery territory are evaluated with cerebral angiography when surgical therapy is a consideration. Because elderly patients are at risk of dehydration following cerebral angiography, they should be well hydrated before the procedure and followed closely afterward. In fragile elderly patients who are not surgical candidates and in whom angiography itself is a risk, there are noninvasive tests that suffice if surgery or anticoagulation is not feasible. Doppler ultrasonography and real-time ultrasound of the carotid sometimes show the stenosis but may miss the lesion in a symptomatic patient. Digital intravenous subtraction angiography in experienced hands is somewhat safer than a conventional angiogram and shows the carotid artery sufficiently in many cases to direct therapy [20]. The technique is not as reliable in the distal cerebral vessels or in the posterior fossa. Intraarterial subtraction angiography is more accurate than intravenous studies. The risks of dehydration and renal failure from the contrast media are less than in conventional angiography because less contrast material is used. As digital subtraction angiography technique improves, there will be less need of conventional angiography.

TREATMENT

Treatment of thrombotic cerebrovascular disease depends on the details of the individual case. Old age alone is not a contraindication for treatment [21]. Several treatment options are available for atherothrombosis: surgical removal of the stenosis, anticoagulation, and antiplatelet treatment. For symptomatic carotid artery stenosis or for ulcerative plaques with symptoms of embolism, endarterectomy by experienced surgeons is our choice [22–25]. Elderly patients in relatively good health should not be excluded. Almost all patients with carotid atherothrombosis have significant heart disease and other medical problems that must temper the decision to operate. In patients who could not survive the surgery or who have multiple intracranial occlusions, anticoagulation provides a second choice for managing the carotid symptoms [26, 27]. Antiplatelet treatment has been shown to be effective in some men [28, 29] with transient neurologic deficits but would not be the choice of treatment for symptomatic carotid artery stenosis. In thrombosis of other vessels, for which endarterectomy is not possible, anticoagulation with warfarin sodium (Coumadin) is used widely. The risks of Coumadin therapy are greater in the elderly and must be weighed against the risk of stroke. Antiplatelet therapy is an alternative and may reduce the rate of stroke [30]. The controversy about treatment allows no easy generalizations, so each case must be considered in light of the medical, surgical, and neurologic details. Asymptomatic carotid stenosis (or bruit) requires careful follow-up; there is no need to treat the asymptomatic patient medically or surgically.

LACUNES

Lacunar stroke, named for its lake-like appearance in pathologic specimens, is a type of thrombotic stroke that occurs following occlusion of the small penetrating vessels that supply the basal ganglia, brain stem, and internal capsule [31, 32]. Although hypertension is the major risk factor for lacunar stroke, some patients without hypertension suffer from small vessel thrombosis. Transient ischemic attacks occur in about a quarter of lacunar cases and generally follow a slow, stepwise progression of a focal syndrome. Lacunes do not cause aphasia, apraxia, hemianopsia, or sudden alteration in mental status. Small lacunes, or those that occur in areas without clinical signs, do not cause immediate clinical syndromes until they accumulate, at which time the patient will develop a dementia and show signs of multiple infarctions.

There are many syndromes associated with lacunar stroke [33]. The clinical features depend on the site and size of the infarction. Pure motor hemiplegia is caused by a lacune in the internal capsule and is associated with a motor syndrome involving the face and the upper and lower extremities [34]. There are occasionally sensory complaints, but as a rule there are no sensory findings as would be expected with a cortical stroke. There is also a pure sensory stroke in which the patient presents with hemianesthesia of the face and body. The lesion has been found in the posterolateral nucleus of the thalamus. Other syndromes that are well known include ataxic hemiparesis, in which the patient has a mild weakness and an ipsilateral cerebellar ataxia. The dysarthria, clumsy hand, and facial weakness syndrome presents in patients who have a lacune in the basis pontis. The diagnosis of lacunar stroke is best made by using the clinical criteria, since the lesions may not show up on computed tomographic (CT) scan.

Prevention by controlling hypertension is the only valid treatment of a lacunar stroke. During the stroke there is little value in acute anticoagulation. Lacunar syndromes subside, leaving tolerable deficits in many instances.

EMBOLISM

The syndrome caused by cerebral embolism usually has a much more rapid onset than the syndrome caused by cerebral thrombosis. The infarction usually involves the cortex, and the lesion is often in the distal vascular territory of a single vessel. Occasionally a very large embolus will lodge in the carotid artery, causing a sudden onset of a complete carotid occlusion. More commonly, emboli pass distally into branches of the middle cerebral, anterior cerebral, or posterior cerebral arteries. The syndromes caused by emboli appear in minutes and are rarely preceded by transient signs. The rapid onset does not allow the collateral circulation to compensate as well as in thrombotic lesions. The most common site of cerebral embolus is the territory of the middle cerebral artery. Cerebral embolism usually leads to the sudden onset of a fixed hemiparesis, hemisensory loss, and hemianopsia. About 3 to 5 percent of patients have transient ischemic attacks or a stuttering course [35]. Embolism, however, may cause a stroke that lasts only several hours, so it is sometimes difficult to separate transient ischemic attacks caused by carotid or basilar artery thrombosis from cerebral emboli that cause deficits that last a very short time [10]. Cerebral angiograms may show the embolic occlusion in the distal vessel under scrutiny or may be normal. Unlike embolic occlusion, large vessel thrombotic lesions are easily seen on angiograms.

The heart is the source of cerebral embolism in cases of atrial fibrillation, valvular heart disease, myocardial infarction, cardiomyopathy, and other cardiac disorders [36]. Ulcerated atherosclerotic plaques in large arteries in which thrombus accumulates are also sources of cerebral embolism [9, 37]. In many patients with the syndrome of cerebral embolism there is no obvious source for the embolus.

Embolism to the proximal middle cerebral artery causes a hemiparesis, hemisensory deficit, and hemianopsia with aphasia or apraxia depending on which side the lesion occurs. If only the superior division of the middle cerebral artery is affected, there is no hemianopsia. When only the inferior division is affected, there is mild hemiparesis and hemianopsia; patients may have only a fluent aphasia when the lesion is in the left distal territory. Patients with anterior cerebral artery embolism have weakness and sensory changes in the lower extremity with less dysfunction in the upper extremity. Posterior cerebral artery embolism causes a hemianopsia without hemiparesis or other motor complaints.

Because embolism may recur [38], treatment should be aimed at preventing recurrence, not in correcting the existing lesion [39]. Treatment of embolic stroke requires identification of the source. If the source can be modified or removed to eliminate recurrent embolization, that is the only treatment needed. In many cases, a source is not obvious or cannot be removed (as in cardiomyopathy or after myocardial infarction [MI]), so chronic anticoagulation is needed. Anticoagulation with heparin followed by warfarin sodium should be continued until the risk of embolism has diminished. For instance, in patients with embolism following an MI, six months of treatment is enough to protect against embolism from the mural thrombus. In other cases, such as in patients with prosthetic valves, anticoagulation should be continued. Embolic infarctions sometimes change to hemorrhages with or without anticoagulants [40]. Moreover, small intracerebral hematomas may resemble the clinical picture of embolic strokes [41]. A CT scan will show the hematoma in every case and help to locate the embolic lesion. Some small cortical infarctions, however, may now show on the CT scan, especially in the first 24 to 48 hours.

Hemorrhagic Stroke
SUBARACHNOID HEMORRHAGE
The clinical syndrome of ruptured aneurysm is dramatic [42]. The sudden onset of severe headache is the constant feature of the syndrome. The patient may also lose consciousness at the onset or experience nausea, vomiting, diaphoresis, and general malaise. Often there are no neurologic signs other than drowsiness. The fundi show subhyaloid hemorrhages or papilledema in a few cases. Sudden coma or sudden death also occurs from ruptured berry aneurysm.

The vessels that rupture to cause subarachnoid hemorrhage are usually the medium-sized arteries that lie at the base of the brain in the subarachnoid space [43]. The rupture occurs because of an abnormality of the vessel, the so-called berry aneurysm, in which the muscular arterial layers become thin, causing the arterial wall to bulge. The only covering for the aneurysm is a thinned elastica and the intima of the artery. As a general rule, the larger the aneurysm, the more likely it is to rupture because the arterial defect thins as it enlarges. "Giant" aneurysms (over 25 mm) are more difficult to treat surgically, and although they rupture, they may present first as a mass lesion. Giant aneurysms also develop mural thrombus, which may be a source of cerebral embolism in distal territories. Small berry aneurysms can also cause focal signs (usually after rupture) when they are near a sensitive structure. The best known example is a berry aneurysm of the posterior communicating artery, which causes dysfunction of the third cranial nerve. There is usually headache in addition to ipsilateral ptosis, diplopia, and mydriasis.

Ninety percent of intracranial aneurysms are found in the anterior part of the circle of Willis. It is unusual to find an aneurysm distal to the main cerebral vessels. The other 10 percent occur in the posterior circulation. Ruptured an-

eurysms account for over 70 percent of subarachnoid hemorrhages. All aneurysms do not
rupture. In postmortem studies about 4 percent
of patients are found to have berry aneurysms.
Of these, about half are unruptured at the time
of death. The majority of patients with ruptured berry aneurysm are between 40 and 65
years old.

CT scan and magnetic resonance imaging
(MRI) usually show hematoma in the subarachnoid space but may miss some subarachnoid hemorrhages. The diagnosis can be made
by the finding of bloody spinal fluid. If there is
no blood in the cerebrospinal fluid, there is no
ruptured aneurysm.

The treatment of a ruptured aneurysm requires special surgical experience [44–47]. The
patient should be referred to a neurosurgical
center for care. Emergency care consists of putting the patient at rest, treating the headache
with analgesics, and watching for progression
of neurologic signs. Patients with subarachnoid
hemorrhage have high blood pressure due to
the increase in intracranial pressure. It is not
wise to reduce the blood pressure acutely even
though hypertension is a factor in causing the
aneurysm to rebleed. Maintaining the systolic
pressure at under 150 mm Hg is acceptable.
Prophylactic use of anticonvulsants is also wise
because there is a high risk of seizure.

Elderly patients who are in good health can
tolerate surgical treatment of an aneurysm [48].
Associated diseases are the largest postoperative
threat to the elderly, who do well through the
initial treatment.

INTRAPARENCHYMAL HEMORRHAGE

Intraparenchymal hemorrhage, caused in large
part by chronic hypertension, is more common
than subarachnoid hemorrhage in elderly patients [49]. The vessels that rupture are the deep
penetrating arterioles of 200 to 400 micra [50].
The most common site for hemorrhage is
the lenticulostriate arteries and their branches,
which lie in the area of the basal ganglia. The
vascular pathology is related to abnormalities of
the vessel wall caused by chronic hypertension.
There are cases, however, of intraparenchymal
hemorrhage without a history of chronic hypertension. Congophyllic angiopathy [51], a vascular change in which amyloid is deposited in

the arterial wall, increases with age and has been
identified as another substrate leading to intracerebral hemorrhage.

The clinical syndrome of intraparenchymal
hemorrhage [7] depends on the localization of
the hematoma [52, 53]. In general, most patients
with intracerebral hematoma have decreased
alertness. Vomiting is also a frequent sign, but
headache is not always present. Patients with
lesions in the putamen [54] or thalamus [55]
have a hemiparesis, and such lesions may resemble ischemic strokes except for the presence
of drowsiness and vomiting, which are not usually seen in ischemia. Hemorrhage in the brain
stem [56] causes bilateral signs related to that
area and causes coma.

Cerebellar hemorrhage [57, 58] requires
emergency treatment because the hematoma
rapidly compresses the brainstem, causing
coma and death. The cerebellar hemorrhage
presents as sudden ataxia of gait. Occipital
headache and vomiting frequently accompany
the other signs. Surgical removal of a cerebellar
hematoma is curative if done before the brainstem is compressed.

The diagnosis of intraparenchymal hemorrhage is made by CT scan or MRI [59]. Treatment, except for cerebellar hematoma, is aimed
at preventing aspiration, maintaining hydration, and treating underlying medical problems
[60]. High blood pressure should not be reduced precipitously during the acute stage. Patients with small supratentorial hematomas
often do well enough to return home. Those
who have large cerebral lesions die, and those
with hemorrhage in the brain stem are severely
impaired if they live.

Summary
The evaluation of a stroke begins with analysis
of the history and physical examination [61].
Once the clinician understands the syndrome,
he or she can make proper use of laboratory
tests that will support the diagnosis. If a large
vessel stenosis or occlusion is suspected, cerebral angiography is the only method of showing the vascular lesion. A suspected cerebral
embolism usually prompts the physician to
search for a cardiac source of the embolism or
to decide whether carotid angiography is neces-

sary to identify an artery-to-artery embolic source. A CT scan ensures that the syndrome that appears to be ischemic is not due to acute intraparenchymal hemorrhage. Patients who fit the clinical formula of a lacunar syndrome do not require angiography, although CT scan is useful to reduce the chance of missing a cortical stroke.

Once the diagnosis is established, the physician can use his or her experience and understanding of the individual case to choose the best treatment. It is not sufficient to ignore the possibility of making a specific diagnosis only because the patient is old. Indeed, when the stroke is mildest the stakes are highest, because a recurrence may mean death or a life of total dependency. The easiest decisions to be made involve elderly patients who have large strokes because there is little to do once the diagnosis is made. It is the minimally affected patient who needs the most aggressive evaluation and treatment planning.

References

1. Wolf, P. A. Risk factors for stroke. *Stroke* 16: 359, 1985.
2. American-Canadian Co-operative Study Group. Persantine Aspirin trial in cerebral ischemia— Part III: Risk factors for stroke. *Stroke* 17:12, 1986.
3. Garraway, W., et al. The declining incidence of stroke. *N. Engl. J. Med.* 300:449, 1979.
4. Kannel, W., et al. Components of blood pressure and risk of atherothrombotic brain infarction: The Framingham study. *Stroke* 7:327, 1976.
5. Shekelle, R., Ostfeld, A., and Klawans, H. Hypertension and risk of stroke in an elderly population. *Stroke* 5:71, 1974.
6. Siekert, R. G. (ed.). *Cerebrovascular Survey Report* (revised) (of the National Institute of Neurological and Communicative Disorders and Stroke) Bethesda, MD: National Institutes of Health, January 1980.
7. Fisher, C. M. Clinical syndromes in cerebral thrombosis, hypertensive hemorrhage, and ruptured aneurysm. *Clin. Neurosurg.* 22:117, 1975.
8. Bogousslavsky, J. and Regli, F. Delayed TIAs distal to bilateral occlusion of carotid arteries— Evidence for embolic and hemodynamic mechanisms. *Stroke* 14:58, 1983.
9. Pessin, M. S., et al. Mechanisms of acute carotid stroke. *Ann. Neurol.* 6:245, 1979.
10. Mohr. J. P., et al. The Harvard Cooperative Stroke Registry: A prospective registry. *Neurology* 28:754, 1978.
11. Castaigne, P., et al. Internal carotid artery occlusion. *Brain* 93:231, 1970.
12. Fisher, C. M. Occlusion of the internal carotid artery. *Arch. Neurol. Psychiat.* 65:346, 1951.
13. Jonas, S., and Hass, W. K. An approach to the maximum acceptable stroke complication rate after surgery for transient cerebral ischemia (TIA). *Stroke* 10:104, 1979.
14. Whisnant, J. P., et al. Carotid and vertebral-basilar transient ischemic attacks: Effect of anticoagulants, hypertension, and cardiac disorders on survival and stroke occurrence—A population study. *Neurology* 3:107, 1978.
15. Harrison, M. J. G., Marshall, J., and Thomas, D. J. Relevance of duration of transient ischemic attacks in carotid territory. *Br. Med. J.* 1:1578, 1978.
16. Jones, H. R., and Millikan, C. H. Temporal profile (clinical course) of acute carotid system cerebral infarction. *Stroke* 7:64, 1976.
17. Pessin, M. S., et al. Clinical and angiographic features of carotid transient ischemic attacks. *N. Engl. J. Med.* 296:358, 1977.
18. EC/IC Bypass Study Group. Failure of Extracranial-intracranial arterial bypass to reduce the risk of ischemic stroke: Results of an international randomized trial. *N. Engl. J. Med.* 313:1191, 1985.
19. Caplan, L. R. "Top of the basilar" syndrome. *Neurology* 30:72, 1980.
20. Furlan, A. J., et al. Digital subtraction angiography in the evaluation of cerebrovascular disease. *Neurolog. Clin.* 1:55, 1983.
21. Toole, J. F., et al. Transient ischemic attacks: A study of 225 patients. *Neurology* 28:746, 1978.
22. Mohr, J. P. Transient ischemic attacks and the prevention of strokes. *N. Engl. J. Med.* 299:93, 1978.
23. Sandok, B. A., et al. Guidelines for the management of transient ischemic attacks. *Mayo Clin. Proc.* 53:665, 1978.
24. Nunn, D. B. Carotid endarterectomy: Analysis of 234 operative cases. *Ann. Surg.* 182:733, 1975.
25. Siekert, R. G., Whisnant, J. P., and Millikan, C. H. Surgical and anticoagulant therapy of occlusive cerebral vascular disease. *Ann. Intern. Med.* 48:637, 1963.
26. Brust, J. C. Transient ischemic attacks: Natural history and anticoagulation. *Neurology* 27:701, 1977.
27. Fisher, C. M. Use of anticoagulants in cerebral thrombosis. *Neurology* (Minneap.) 8:311, 1958.
28. Canadian Co-operative Study Group. A ran-

domized trial of aspirin and sulfinpyrazone in threatened stroke. *N. Engl. J. Med.* 299:53, 1978.

29. Heikinheimo, R., and Jarvinen, K. Acetylsalicylic acid and arteriosclerotic-thromboembolic disease in the aged. *J. Am. Geriatr. Soc.* 19:403, 1971.

30. Grotta, J. C., et al. Does platelet antiaggregant therapy lessen the severity of stroke? *Neurology* 35:632, 1985.

31. Fisher, C. M. The arterial lesions underlying lacunes. *Acta Neuropathol.* (Berlin) 12:1, 1969.

32. Mohr, J. P. Lacunes. *Stroke* 13:3, 1982.

33. Fisher, C. M. Lacunar strokes and infarcts: A review. *Neurology* 32:871, 1982.

34. Rascol, A., et al. Pure motor hemiplegia: CT study of 30 cases. *Stroke* 13:11, 1982.

35. Fisher, C. M., and Pearlman, A. The non-sudden onset of cerebral embolism. *Neurology* 17:1025, 1967.

36. Hinton, R. C., et al. Influence of the etiology of atrial fibrillation on the incidence of systemic embolism. *Am. J. Cardiol.* 40:509, 1977.

37. Wood, E. H., and Correll, J. W. Atheromatous ulceration in major neck vessels as a cause of cerebral embolism. *Acta Radiol.* 9:520, 1969.

38. Koller, R. L. Recurrent embolic cerebral infarction and anticoagulation. *Neurology* 32:283, 1982.

39. Easton, J. D., and Sherman, D. G. Management of cerebral embolism of cardiac origin. *Stroke* 11:433, 1980.

40. Furlan, A. J., et al. Hemorrhage and anticoagulation after non septic embolic brain infarction. *Neurology* 32:280, 1982.

41. Cerebral Embolism Study Group. Immediate anticoagulation of embolic stroke: Brain hemorrhage and management options. *Stroke* 15:779, 1984.

42. Locksley, H. B. Report on the co-operative study of intracranial aneurysms and subarachnoid hemorrhage. Part II, Section V: Natural history of subarachnoid hemorrhage, intracranial aneurysms, and arteriovenous malformations, based on 6368 cases in the co-operative study. *J. Neurosurg.* 25:321, 1966.

43. Longstreth, W. T., et al. Risk factors for subarachnoid hemorrhage. *Stroke* 16:377, 1985.

44. Drake, C. G. Management of cerebral aneurysm. *Stroke* 12:273, 1981.

45. Hunt, W. E., and Hess, R. M. Surgical risk as related to time of intervention in the repair of intracranial aneurysms. *J. Neurosurg.* 28:14, 1968.

46. Sundt, T. M. and Whisnant, J. P. Subarachnoid hemorrhage from intracranial aneurysms: Surgical management and natural history of disease. *N. Engl. J. Med.* 299:116, 1978.

47. Whisnant, J. P., Phillips, L. H., and Sundt, T. M. Aneurysmal subarachnoid hemorrhage timing of surgery and mortality. *Mayo Clin. Proc.* 57:471, 1982.

48. Amacher, A. L., et al. (eds.). Aneurysm Surgery in the Seventh Decade. In *Present Limits of Neurosurgery*. Prague: Czechoslovak Medical Press, 1972. Pp. 263–266.

49. Furlan, A. J., Whisnant, J. P., and Elveback. L R. The decreasing incidence of primary intracerebral hemorrhage: A population study. *Ann. Neurol.* 5:367, 1979.

50. Herbstein, D. J., and Schaumberg, H. H. Hypertensive intracerebral hematoma: An investigation of the initial hemorrhage and rebleeding using Cr-51 labeled erythrocytes. *Arch. Neurol.* 30:412, 1974.

51. Tomonaga, M. Cerebral amyloid angiopathy in the elderly. *J. Am. Geriatr. Soc.* 29:151, 1981.

52. Ropper, A. H., and Davis, K. R. Lobar cerebral hemorrhages: Acute clinical syndromes in 26 cases. *Ann. Neurol.* 8:141, 1980.

53. Kase, C. S., et al. Lobar intracerebral hematomas: Clinical and CT analysis of 22 cases. *Neurology* 32:1146, 1982.

54. Hier, D. B., et al. Hypertensive putaminal hemorrhage. *Ann. Neurol.* 1:152, 1977.

55. Walshe, T. M., Davis, K. R., and Fisher, C. M. Thalamic hemorrhage. Computed tomographic-clinical correlation. *Neurology* 27:217, 1977.

56. Collomb, H., et al. Hemorragies primitives du tronc cerebral, étude, anatomique et clinique de 36 cas. *Rev. Neurolog.* 129:185, 1973.

57. Ott, K. H., et al. Cerebellar hemorrhage: Diagnosis and treatment. *Arch. Neurol.* 31:160, 1974.

58. Heros, R. C. Cerebellar hemorrhage and infarction. *Stroke* 13:106, 1982.

59. Muller, H. R., et al. The contribution of computerized axial tomography to the diagnosis of cerebellar and pontine hematomas. *Stroke* 6:467, 1975.

60. Crowell, R. M., et al. (eds.). Surgery for Brain Hemorrhage. In *Cerebrovascular Diseases, Twelfth Research (Princeton) Conference*. New York: Raven, 1981. Pp. 233–254.

61. Walshe, T. M. (ed.). *Manual of Clinical Problems in Geriatric Medicine*. Boston: Little, Brown, 1985.

26

Psychiatric Aspects of Aging

Benjamin Liptzin
Carl Salzman

As psychiatrists and other mental health professionals have gained exposure to geriatric patients, they have been compelled to discard their stereotypes of the elderly as senile, as unsuitable for psychotherapy, as treatment resistant, and as not interested in psychiatric care [1]. The high prevalence of psychiatric symptoms in this age group compels those working with the elderly to gain an understanding of the normal psychology of aging, psychopathology in the elderly, and the issues involved in managing the psychiatric problems of older patients.

Normal Psychology of Aging
COGNITIVE CHANGES

There is a substantial literature on the cognitive changes associated with normal aging [2]. This section highlights those findings that are of particular relevance for clinicians.

The concept of "intelligence" has been defined operationally using a variety of instruments. Early cross-sectional studies using the Wechsler Adult Intelligence Scale showed a peak of mental ability at age 24 with a decline after age 30 that continued into old age. In those studies, verbal performance was maintained, but performance on tests that required perceptual motor skills declined with increasing age. More recent longitudinal studies following the same elderly individuals over time have shown little or no change over a 14-year period [3]. This finding suggests that the difference in intelligence found in earlier cross-sectional studies may have been due to cohort differences in education, occupation, health status, and familiarity with tests. Although many intellectual functions show little or no decline in healthy individuals past the age of 60, there may be a decline in perceptual motor skills, particularly on timed tasks.

Studies of learning and memory, which generally have been conducted under artificial laboratory conditions, demonstrate decrements in performance with increasing age. Some of these decrements may be due to the speed of presentation or to motivational factors. In addition, older subjects may develop more anxiety in fast-paced test situations. Fear of failure may lead to fewer responses and withdrawal from the testing situation. Studies of factors that facilitate learning in the elderly suggest the value of slowing the rate of presentation or the expected speed of response, or helping the person develop strategies for learning. Improved understanding of learning mechanisms at advanced ages may lead to strategies that enhance the ability of older persons to adapt to new work or living conditions such as learning to drive a new car with high-tech controls or learning to use the thermostat in a new apartment.

Sophisticated studies of memory [4] indicate that older subjects have more difficulty than younger subjects with short-term memory tasks when asked to divide their attention or to reorganize the material presented. Mild forgetfulness, especially for names, is a normal experience for most people after the age of 35 and should not unduly alarm the patient or the clinician. Moderate or severe memory difficulties are not due to normal age-related changes, and a careful evaluation is indicated (see Chap. 4). This distinction between "physiologic" and "pathologic" memory loss is also important because persons with mild forgetfulness may function better if they are reassured that such mild changes do not mean they are suffering from Alzheimer's disease. As familiarity with this devastating disease increases, anxiety rises about any memory lapses, no matter how insignificant.

ADAPTATION AND COPING

Late life is a time of many changes. Any clinician dealing with an older person should assess that individual's ability to adapt to change and should assist the person to cope. Older persons, like younger people, have differing capacities for coping with life stresses and for coming to terms with their changing life situations. In his longitudinal studies of psychologic adaptation, Vaillant [5] has demonstrated consistency in the psychologic defense mechanisms used by individuals over time as well as some progression toward the use of more "mature" or "healthy" defense mechanisms.

A great deal of the psychodynamic literature on aging has focused on the losses experienced by older people, including loss of physical health, loved ones and friends, income, and social roles, and the ultimate loss that comes from contemplating one's own death. Neugarten [6] has shown that most people adapt well to life changes that are expected and occur "on time." These include menopause in women and extend through grandparenthood, retirement, widowhood, and the expectation of death. Elderly persons who do not adapt successfully to life transitions may benefit from professional help just as younger persons do.

Epidemiology of Mental Disorders in the Elderly

The Epidemiologic Catchment Area (ECA) project of the National Institute of Mental Health has provided a wealth of useful data on the prevalence of mental disorders in persons of all ages, including the group 65 years and older [7]. Persons dwelling in the community in Baltimore, New Haven, and St. Louis were interviewed in their homes using a structured diagnostic interview including the Mini Mental State Examination [8]. It has been assumed that depression was more common in the elderly because of their higher suicide rate (see below) and because of all the losses they experience. However, the ECA investigators found that for older men the rate of clinical depression was between 0.5 and 2.2 percent at the different sites, well below the 1.5 to 7.5 percent found in younger men. Similarly, for older women the rate was 3.1 to 5.0 percent compared to a range of 4.5 to 11.4 percent in younger women. As with younger age groups, the rate of depression was higher among older women than among older men. The only mental disorder that showed a higher rate among older (65+) than among younger (<65) persons was cognitive impairment. Older persons had about a 5 percent rate of severe cognitive impairment, and another 15 to 20 percent had mild cognitive impairment. The four most frequent psychiatric disorders for older men were severe cognitive impairment (4.6–6.3%), phobias (1.2–7.6%), alcohol abuse/dependence (3.0–3.7%), and dysthymia (mild but chronic depression, 0.5–1.8%). For older women, the four most frequent diagnoses were phobias (2.6–14.2%), severe cognitive impairment 3.6–4.8%), dysthymia (1.3–3.1%), and major depressive episode without grief (1.0–1.6%).

Suicide

National reporting of suicides has consistently shown that elderly white men have the highest rates of suicide, the rate increasing with each decade [9]. Figure 26-1 shows the rates by age for the United States population in 1980 and for white males. For women the highest rate occurs around age 50 with a gradual decline thereafter.

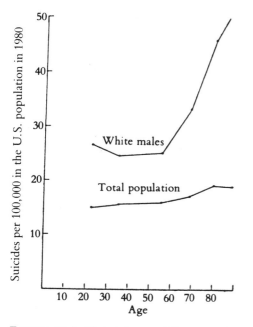

FIGURE 26-1. *United States suicide rates in 1980. (Reprinted with permission from the American Geriatrics Society, Suicide in late life, by D. G. Blazer, J. R. Bachar, and K. G. Manton.* Journal of the American Geriatrics Society, *34:519, 1986.)*

For blacks the peak rate occurs at age 30. Because the rate is so high for white males, however, the overall rate increases with age, and the elderly, who constitute 12 percent of the population, account for 25 percent of total suicides. A number of studies have attempted to elucidate the reasons for the high suicide rate among older white men. Depression, which might be a contributing factor, is less frequent among older men than among older women or younger persons, as noted above. Furthermore, the rate of suicide attempts is much higher in young persons than in the elderly, but there are fewer successful attempts and thus a lower suicide rate [10]. One major difference is that older white men tend to use more lethal methods (e.g., firearms, hanging, drowning) in suicide attempts and are therefore more likely to be successful. Any clinician who works with an older person should be alert to the possibility of suicide. Risk factors include living alone, failing health, alcohol abuse, and a history of previous suicide attempts.

Utilization of Health and Mental Health Services

For many years it was believed that the elderly had a higher prevalence of mental disorders than younger persons because of their higher rate of admission to and residence in state and county mental hospitals, which were the major sources of psychiatric care. By the mid-1960s, states began systematically to restrict admissions of older persons to state mental hospitals. By 1975, less than 1 percent of the population 65 years and over were admitted to inpatient services of state and county mental hospitals, private psychiatric hospitals, general psychiatric inpatient units, community mental health centers, and outpatient psychiatric services [11]. Persons 65 and over accounted for only 4.8 percent of admissions to this group of psychiatric services and for less than 2 percent of the patients seen in private psychiatrists' offices [12].

This change in utilization patterns had led to the assertion that the elderly are "underserved" by specialized mental health programs. However, many elderly persons with mental disorders receive some general health services for their mental condition. The ECA study found that, in contrast to all other age groups, older persons with psychiatric disorders were much less likely to consult a mental health specialist and were more likely to visit only a general medical provider for psychiatric problems [13]. Another important change has been the emergence of the nursing home as the major locus of institutional care for mentally impaired older persons [14]. Both of these changes emphasize the need for mental health outreach services. In addition, it is essential for general physicians and other health professionals to be able to recognize, diagnose, and treat mental disorders in their older patients.

Psychiatric Assessment of the Older Patient

Careful assessment is the first step in understanding the emotional, psychologic, behavioral, or cognitive difficulties presented by an older patient. Furthermore, ongoing assessment is essential for validating initial impressions or evaluating therapeutic interventions.

The psychiatric signs and symptoms presented by an older patient must be considered in relation to factors influencing their presentation or treatment, including medical illnesses and the medications used to treat them; neurologic disorders, especially those that produce cognitive deficits; sensory limitations, especially decreased vision or hearing; and the psychosocial support system available to the older person.

History-Taking

Some older persons seek psychiatric assistance on their own, but many are referred for psychiatric assessment by someone else—a family member, primary care physician, other health professional, neighbor, friend, police, or staff of the person's residence. The observations and concerns of those who stimulated the assessment need to be considered as well as those of the patient, especially in the case of patients who are poor historians because of impaired memory, denial of illness, or suspiciousness.

History-taking begins with a broad gathering of information about symptoms and the reasons why the patient is consulting the physician. Although a psychiatric assessment should be part of any comprehensive patient assessment, specific symptoms pointing to a problem that requires psychiatric evaluation include crying, suicidal thoughts, loss of appetite, weight loss, hypochondriasis, decreased energy, decreased interest or pleasure, memory difficulty, confusion, wandering, assaultiveness, agitation, irritability, excessive worrying, paranoid ideas, other delusions, hallucinations, or unexplained physical complaints. The following clinical examples illustrate the importance of probing for specific symptoms and not prematurely concluding that the presenting problem is one of "depression" or "dementia."

A woman was referred to inpatient treatment of "depression" so severe that she could not get out of bed. When seen, however, she was if anything inappropriately cheerful. A careful history uncovered the additional symptom of absent sense of smell. A computed tomographic (CT) scan confirmed the presence of a large olfactory meningioma. After removal of the tumor she recovered her ability to carry out complex tasks such as getting out of bed, making the bed, and preparing her own meals.

An elderly woman was referred for treatment of what seemed to be a moderately severe dementia characterized by complaints of poor memory and incontinence. A careful history indicated that the memory complaint was out of proportion to that documented on examination. For example, she was able to remember her doctor's name, including its unusual spelling. Kahn and associates [15] have suggested that memory complaint is more often a sign of depression than of dementia, and in this case, appropriate treatment for depression led to improvements in memory and control of incontinence.

The second step in history-taking is to explore the development over time of the presenting problem. Has it been a gradual process occurring over months or years, or did it appear abruptly? Sometimes the patient or family may date the onset of cognitive difficulties from a recent retirement or death of a spouse when in fact there were signs of slippage even earlier. The retirement may have been due to deteriorating job performance, or the deceased spouse may have been able to compensate for the patient's deficits. What other findings accompany the current problem? In trying to answer the question of why these particular symptoms have appeared and why now, it is essential to explore any recent changes in medication and in the patient's life situation. A relatively short history of confusion most likely represents an acute confusional state rather than a worsening of a dementing process as illustrated by the following case.

An elderly man who had been able to live alone became quite anxious and despondent after being swindled. His physician prescribed an antidepressant medication with strong anticholinergic properties, and within a few days he was completely disoriented and urinating on the floor. When the medication was discontinued, he returned to his baseline, well-oriented state and was able to deal with his problems.

The next step in history-taking is to explore the patient's past psychiatric and medical history. Has the person previously had problems similar to the current ones? If so, how were they diagnosed and treated? How successful was the treatment? A prior history of very similar problems suggests an affective disorder, since both depression and mania tend to be recurrent, whereas dementia tends to be slowly progressive. This clue is very important because the presence of cognitive symptoms in an elderly patient often leads to a diagnosis of dementia or, more recently, Alzheimer's disease and induces therapeutic nihilism. A case example illustrates this situation.

An 85-year-old female patient in a state mental hospital rarely spoke and was restrained in a chair all day because of contractures that had developed as a result of inactivity. The diagnosis on her record (and the one the staff accepted) was "chronic organic brain syndrome." Her chart, however, described numerous episodes of severe depression that had been treated successfully with electroconvulsive therapy until she reached the age of 80, when it was felt that she was too old for further treatments. After a trial of antidepressants, she became alert and was able to detail to her son the goings and comings of staff in the previous five years. Regrettably, her contractures were not as reversible as her "chronic brain syndrome."

A careful medical history, including a list of the patient's medications, is an essential part of the evaluation. Dementia or confusional states can be caused by a wide variety of medical conditions, as described in Chapter 27. In addition, symptoms of depression can be caused by a variety of medical disorders including anemia, hypothyroidism or hyperthyroidism, hypercalcemia, hyponatremia, diabetes with hyperglycemia, malignancies, dehydration, congestive heart failure, polymyalgia rheumatica, Parkinson's disease, brain tumors, subdural hematoma, or a cerebrovascular accident [16]. Drugs that can cause or mimic depression include antihypertensives such as reserpine, alphamethyldopa, or beta-blockers; steroids; histamine blockers such as cimetidine; digitalis; L-dopa; nonsteroidal antiinflammatory agents; neuroleptics; tranquilizers; alcohol; and hypnotic drugs.

A detailed family and social history is vital because a change in family relationships may either precipitate or signal a psychologic disturbance. Understanding the individual's cultural background and lifelong personality is essential to therapeutic planning. Furthermore, identification of changes in the individual's support system may explain why the problem is emerging or being referred now. Family history is also important in disorders that may have a hereditary component such as depression or Alzheimer's disease.

Mental Status Examination

Evaluation of mental status begins from the first contact, whether by telephone or in person with the identified patient or with the person referring the patient. The first observations of a patient involve appearance, including dress and grooming, followed quickly by observations of behavior including alertness, activity level, and reaction to the interviewer.

After the initial observations, it is important to evaluate the person's cognitive functioning, which begins with how the person relates the history of his or her problem. Is the story logical, coherent in proper temporal sequence, and in sufficient detail to make sense? Whether or not the person gives a coherent history, some formal assessment of cognitive functioning using a standardized instrument such as the 30-item Mini Mental State [8] is essential. This examination includes questions relating to orientation, registration of information, attention, calculation, recall, language, and visuoperceptual function (see Chaps. 4 and 27).

The next areas to consider are mood and affect, with the former the subjective state of the individual and the latter a state inferred by the listener. Any person who appears to be very depressed should be asked about thoughts of suicide. "Do you ever think you just can't go on anymore? Have you ever thought you would be better off dead? Have you ever tried to harm yourself?" The presence of serious suicidal intentions requires the clinician to take protective steps that may include hospitalization. One indicator of seriousness is whether the person has any future plans for trips, activities, or projects. Someone who is not planning anything for next week is more at risk than someone who is looking forward to a grandchild's wedding in six months.

Judgment, thinking, and perceptions are the last aspects to be covered in the mental status examination. A person's judgment may be affected either by cognitive deficits or by a psychotic illness. For example, a person may go out for a walk in winter without a coat because he can't remember what time of year it is or because he thinks he is the Messiah and needs no coat. Some patients may not bathe because they forget, are physically unable to get in and out of the tub, or, as one patient said, "I don't need to bathe. I am a self-cleaning model." Or a person may not eat because of a memory lapse, inability to cook, loss of appetite, or a belief that the food is poisoned. Delusions are false beliefs that are fixed and are not changed by arguments or facts. Paranoid delusions may be either persecutory or sexual in nature. Decreased vision and hearing may also lead to heightened vigilance and on occasion may be associated with frank paranoid delusions [17]. Perceptual disturbances include illusions, which are misperceptions of stimuli, or hallucinations, which are perceptions without external stimuli. The latter often occur with clouding of consciousness in confusional states [18] but can occur in an otherwise alert patient with a clear sensorium. It is important to assess whether the person understands the situation or not and whether any actions are dangerous to self or others.

Physical Assessment

To complete the data base for a psychiatric assessment, it is necessary to obtain the results of a complete physical examination including a neurologic examination and appropriate laboratory studies (for example, see the discussion in Chapter 27 on treatable dementias). In addition to the discovery of physical factors that may produce psychologic symptoms directly, a thorough physical assessment has three other purposes. First, it may identify treatable conditions, such as hearing loss, decreased vision, and decreased mobility, any of which may lead to social isolation and hence aggravate psychologic symptoms. Second, it may uncover areas of concern that the patient might otherwise not have expressed. Finally, knowledge of the patient's physical condition is an obvious precondition to treatment with any psychotropic medication.

Common Psychiatric Problems and Their Management

General issues in management will be highlighted in this section and will be followed by a more detailed discussion of psychopharmacologic and other somatic treatments of specific problems. The management of psychiatric problems in the elderly may involve multiple therapeutic approaches and involve professionals from different disciplines. Accurate diagnosis can help focus treatment or suggest possible therapeutic interventions. However, often patients have multiple problems and a precise diagnosis may be impossible. In such cases, a more useful therapeutic approach focuses on "treatable" problems and target symptoms. For example, a recent study of patients with dementia identified many treatable problems that could lead to improvements in the patient's functioning or well-being even though the primary memory deficit showed little change [19].

Appropriate changes in the physical or social environment of the individual may lead to improvements in functioning. It is possible to compensate for decreased hearing with a hearing aid, for unsteady gait with a cane or walker, for decreased vision with coded drawers or talking books, and so on. Often physicians focus on the "medical" aspects of the patient's problems when they could provide practical environmental or other suggestions or assistance [20]. Increased social contact in or outside the house and provision of supportive services such as Homemakers or Meals on Wheels are examples of practical changes that are very helpful to patients and their families.

The appearance of psychiatric problems in an older person can also lead to major stresses on close relatives or other caregivers [21]. Attention to the family's needs will not only improve their ability to cope but will also allow them to be more helpful to their relative.

The full range of individual and group psychotherapies can be useful to many older patients [22,23], although there are no specific controlled studies of psychotherapy in the elderly. In most cases it is appropriate to use the supportive techniques of listening, empathizing, and providing advice or reassurance in the context of a concerned professional relationship. This support may alleviate the patient's anxiety or enhance his or her self-esteem. Supportive psychotherapy can be carried out even with patients who have some cognitive deficit because such patients can often talk openly about the changes and losses they have experienced as well as take pride in their life accomplishments. In the past, psychodynamic psychotherapy was avoided in older patients, who were assumed to be too rigid to respond to it or because an extensive investment in personality change was thought to be not practical with so few years of life remaining. Recent publications, however, have provided anecdotal evidence that intensive therapy can be useful to some older persons [24,25].

TREATMENT OF PSYCHOSIS

A psychotic patient has lost touch with reality. The most prominent symptoms of psychosis are delusions and hallucinations. These symptoms may occur for the first time in late life, or they may have been present earlier in life and persist or recur in the older person. Psychotic symptoms may be associated with schizophrenia, paranoid disorders, major depression, mania, delirium, or dementia.

Schizophrenia is usually a chronic illness. Until recently, state mental hospitals had large numbers of elderly patients who had developed severe mental illness when young and were institutionalized then and never recovered. Many of these patients were actually manic or psychotically depressed and were misdiagnosed as schizophrenic when they were young. For that reason, any older "schizophrenic" should have a careful review of his or her history to rule out other psychotic illnesses that are more treatable than chronic schizophrenia.

The prevalence of paranoid symptoms in an elderly community population has been estimated to be 4 percent [26]. Paranoid thinking may be associated with depression, mania, or organic mental syndromes as well as schizophrenia. A small number of patients develops a late-onset paranoid disorder with no previous psychotic history, in contrast to schizophrenic patients whose illness must by definition arise before the age of 40. Sometimes called "late life paraphrenia," this disorder is generally not ac-

companied by the personality disintegration associated with schizophrenia, although the paranoid symptoms may be quite persistent. Sensory deficits may predispose a person to paranoid thinking although the evidence is still mixed [27]. Elderly paranoid patients frequently come to medical attention because of their unreasonable suspiciousness, threats, and accusations. Although suspiciousness may be a component of paranoid illness, some degree of suspiciousness may be adaptive for an older person to prevent victimization. Increased suspiciousness may also be a defensive response to changes in the individual that are unacceptable. For example, a patient may accuse others of stealing something to avoid acknowledging that he or she has misplaced it and cannot remember where it is.

Not every elderly psychotic patient requires treatment with an antipsychotic drug. Some psychotic patients are not disturbed by their abnormal thoughts or perceptions, are behaviorally appropriate, and do not disturb others. Psychotic elderly patients who are also medically ill, particularly patients with delirium, may become less psychotic or less behaviorally disturbed when their medical illness improves. Neuroleptic drugs are commonly used for older patients whose psychosis is severe enough to require pharmacologic treatment. Some older patients who require neuroleptic drugs during an acute exacerbation of their illness can be managed without medication when the acute episode is over.

Neuroleptic Drugs
CLINICAL PHARMACOLOGY

This chapter can provide only a brief overview of the psychopharmacology of the various drugs used to treat psychiatric illnesses. For more information, the reader should refer to the work by Salzman [28]. Several classes of neuroleptic drugs have been used to treat psychosis in the elderly including the phenothiazines (e.g., chlorpromazine, thioridazine, acetophenazine, perphenazine, trifluoperazine, and fluphenazine), the butyrophenones (e.g., haloperidol), the thioxanthenes (e.g., thiothixene), the dibenzoxazepines (e.g., loxapine), and the dihydroindolones (e.g., molindone). All these classes of drugs share certain pharmacologic characteristics. Age-related changes in absorption, protein binding, distribution, biotransformation, and clearance result in delayed onset of drug effect, elevated plasma levels, and prolonged drug effects. Increased sensitivity of central nervous system receptors to neuroleptic effects results in an increased risk of toxicity at lower doses than that seen in younger patients.

Neuroleptic drugs are all potent blockers of central dopamine transmission. Since animal models specifically designed to detect this effect have been used in the development of new neuroleptics, it is unclear whether this dopaminergic blockade is essential to their mechanism of action. Research in recent years has attempted to find more selective dopamine blockers or drugs with antipsychotic activity without any dopamine-blocking activity. The hope, still unrealized, is that a drug with antipsychotic activity can be developed that does not cause extrapyramidal side effects (see below).

All neuroleptic drugs are equally effective in controlling psychotic symptoms, and there is no selective therapeutic action of one drug compared with another. Some drugs are more convenient to use because they come in a wide range of dosage strengths, or in liquid or injectable form as well as in tablets or capsules. Long-acting injectable forms are available (e.g., fluphenazine and haloperidol) for patients who have difficulty taking medications daily. More important, neuroleptics differ in their ability to produce certain side effects. The selection of a neuroleptic for an elderly patient, therefore, depends more on a concern for their different toxicities than on their different clinical efficacy.

The therapeutic effect of neuroleptics is thought to correlate with the drugs' affinity for central nervous system (CNS) dopamine receptor sites. As the drug's receptor site affinity increases, milligram potency increases, and the dosage (number of milligrams necessary for clinical effect) decreases. Because of their affinity for dopamine receptors, higher potency neuroleptic drugs cause more extrapyramidal symptoms. However, they cause less sedation or orthostatic hypotension. The reverse pattern occurs with low-potency drugs. Table 26-1 compares the side effects of neuroleptic drugs, which are listed in order of increasing potency. The specific side effects of concern will be discussed individually.

Sedation. Sedation is a side effect that is sometimes used for therapeutic purposes. For the elderly patient who has trouble falling asleep because of psychotic fears at night, neuroleptic drugs with sedative side effects can induce sleep as well as reduce the psychotic fears. Sedating (low-potency) neuroleptics may also be used to quiet an agitated patient during the day. More commonly, however, daytime sedation is an unwanted side effect for an elderly patient. Daytime sedation may cause or aggravate nighttime insomnia and may also be associated with increasing disorientation, confusion, and agitation. This agitation is sometimes treated by an increased neuroleptic dose, which further ag-

TABLE 26-1. *Neuroleptic drugs*

GENERIC NAME	BRAND NAME	USUAL GERIATRIC DOSE RANGE (MG/DAY)	SEDATION	HYPOTENSION	EXTRAPYRAMIDAL SYMPTOMS	ANTICHOLINERGIC SYMPTOMS
Chlorpromazine	Thorazine	10–400	Marked	Marked	Mild	Marked
Thioridazine	Mellaril	10–400	Marked	Marked	Mild	Marked
Acetophenazine	Tindal	20–120	Mild	Mild	Mild	Moderate
Perphenazine	Trilafon	4–32	Mild	Mild	Moderate	Moderate
Loxapine	Loxitane	5–100	Mild	Mild	Moderate	Moderate
Molindone	Moban	10–100	Mild	Mild	Moderate	Moderate
Trifluoperazine	Stelazine	2–20	Mild	Mild	Marked	Mild
Thiothixene	Navane	2–20	Mild	Mild	Marked	Mild
Fluphenazine	Prolixin	0.5–15 (oral)	Mild	Mild	Marked	Mild
Haloperidol	Haldol	0.5–15 (oral)	Minimal	Minimal	Marked	Mild

gravates the agitation. Sedation and its consequences are more likely and more troublesome when sedating neuroleptics are combined with other sedating drugs (e.g., narcotics, analgesics, or hypnotics), as they often are in a general hospital.

Orthostatic Hypotension. Orthostatic hypotension is a consequence of blockade of the central vasoregulatory centers as well as of peripheral alpha-adrenergic blockade. Dizziness after standing up may be quite uncomfortable for an older person who is already somewhat unsteady. Sudden decreases in blood pressure after standing may also precipitate falls with secondary fractures, strokes, or even heart attacks. Orthostatic hypotensive episodes may be especially troublesome at night when the older person awakens to urinate. Older patients taking low-potency neuroleptics should be advised to change from a recumbent to a sitting position and then to rise slowly to a standing position. Any patient who is dizzy should be certain to have something to hold on to if they think they may fall. Supportive stockings are not very useful, and drugs that elevate blood pressure should be avoided.

Extrapyramidal Symptoms. Elderly patients treated with neuroleptic drugs are more likely than younger patients to experience extrapyramidal symptoms. Although the underlying neurochemical mechanism is unclear, it is likely that there is a greater reduction in dopamine than in acetylcholine in the extrapyramidal system in the brain. Patients who already have reduced dopaminergic transmission from Parkinson's disease may be especially sensitive to drug-induced dopamine reduction.

Neuroleptic-induced extrapyramidal symptoms include acute dystonia, akathisia, and parkinsonism. Acute dystonic reactions that result from rapid increases in neuroleptic dosage are uncommon in older patients. Akathisia is a motor restlessness that may be misinterpreted as agitation and may lead to an increase in the neuroleptic dosage rather than a decrease. Parkinsonism also commonly results from neuroleptic drugs prescribed to the elderly patient. Symptoms include rigidity, bradykinesia, tremor, shuffling gait, and drooling. In the older patient, bradykinesia can result in akinesia, a syndrome in which the patient appears anergic,

mute, and often immobile. Such patients are sometimes mistakenly thought to be depressed because they show little emotion or may acknowledge feeling sad. However, antidepressant treatment is not indicated; rather, a reduction in neuroleptic dose or a switch to a lower potency drug should be tried.

Tardive Dyskinesia. In contrast to the acute movement disorders described above, tardive dyskinesia appears after prolonged neuroleptic drug treatment. The risk of developing tardive dyskinesia increases with age [29] and with duration of neuroleptic treatment [30]. Symptoms include lip smacking, puckering movements, fly-catching tongue protrusions, rabbit-like snouting, or rhythmic, choreiform movements of the arms, hands, trunk, hips, or legs. These abnormal movements can be severe enough to be disabling or disfiguring and can lead to social isolation.

Currently there is no effective treatment for longstanding tardive dyskinesia. Some older patients respond to a dosage reduction or discontinuation of neuroleptic medication. Neuroleptic withdrawal, however, or an abrupt reduction in dosage may intensify the symptoms of tardive dyskinesia as well as those of psychosis. In the short run, restarting the neuroleptic or increasing the dose will suppress the abnormal movements, but in the long run, an increase in dosage makes the condition worse. The risk of developing tardive dyskinesia may be reduced by treating older patients with the minimum clinically effective dose of neuroleptics for as brief a time as possible. There is no evidence that any particular neuroleptic is more or less likely to cause tardive dyskinesia. At the first sign of these abnormal movements, a careful decision needs to be made as to whether the patient can be managed without neuroleptics to decrease the risk of severe, prolonged tardive dyskinesia.

CLINICAL PRESCRIPTION OF NEUROLEPTIC DRUGS
Clinicians who wish to prescribe a neuroleptic drug for an older patient are faced with a difficult choice. To avoid sedation and/or hypotension a high-potency drug can be used, but this selection increases the risk of extrapyramidal symptoms. To avoid extrapyramidal side ef-

fects, a low-potency drug can be used, but this will cause sedation and hypotension. It is usually preferable to reserve the use of low-potency neuroleptics for situations in which sedation is clinically necessary or when other higher potency drugs cannot be used. Table 26-1 suggests that middle-range neuroleptics, those that are neither extremely high nor low in potency, may be the best choice for the psychotic elderly patient. Perphenazine or acetophenazine, for example, are well tolerated and useful drugs for elderly patients.

Neuroleptics are equally effective in reducing psychotic symptoms in older patients. Thioridazine and haloperidol have been prescribed extensively for elderly psychiatric patients [31] and are the most commonly prescribed neuroleptic drugs for elderly medical patients in a general hospital [32]. The therapeutic effect of neuroleptics in controlling severe agitated behavior in the elderly, however, is modest, and some older patients become more confused, agitated, and psychotic when treated with these drugs [33].

Dose. The net result of the age-related alterations in neuroleptic pharmacokinetics as well as the increased receptor sensitivity that occurs with aging is that elderly patients often respond to very low doses of neuroleptics, whereas the usual therapeutic doses may be toxic. Starting doses should be low, particularly for the very frail, very old patient (e.g., 0.25 mg of haloperidol, 10 mg of thioridazine). Dosage increments should be equally small and should be made gradually and only as needed to reduce the target symptoms and only if the drug is well tolerated.

Treatment of Extrapyramidal Symptoms. Extrapyramidal symptoms are best treated by dose reduction or a change to a low-potency neuroleptic. Anticholinergic drugs (e.g., trihexyphenidyl or benztropine) are often used in younger patients to reduce the severity of extrapyramidal symptoms produced by high-potency neuroleptics by restoring a dopamine-acetylcholine balance centrally. In older patients, however, they may produce or add to already troublesome anticholinergic side effects and should be avoided if possible. (See the discussion of anticholinergic side effects in the next section.)

TREATMENT OF AFFECTIVE DISORDERS
Depression

As mentioned above, it was assumed until recently that depression was more common in the elderly than in younger adults. There were a number of reasons for this belief. First, the rate of successful suicides increases overall with age, as described above. Second, elderly persons experience many losses that are "depressing." Third, studies that ask about sadness or other dysphoric symptoms find a high prevalence of these symptoms (15%) among the elderly [34]. Despite these observations, ECA data cited earlier indicate that clinical depression is actually less common among the elderly than among younger adults. Depression in the elderly is, nevertheless, a common and serious problem that needs to be recognized and treated in older as in younger persons.

The differential diagnosis of depression is often more difficult in older than in younger patients. Many older patients have had recent losses that may lead to normal or pathologic grieving. A normal grief reaction may last up to 12 months and is characterized by many symptoms of dysthymia or mild depression, including depressed mood, loss of interest, loss of pleasure, loss of appetite, weight loss, and so on. However, if the symptoms do not resolve in 12 months, the patient may require treatment. Furthermore, patients whose symptoms are severe enough to meet the *Diagnostic and Statistical Manual of Mental Disorders* (third edition, revised) (DSM-III-R) [35] criteria for dysthymia or major depression in the first 12 months should be treated without waiting to see if the symptoms resolve over time. Drug reactions, systemic diseases, and central nervous system disorders as described in the section on history-taking must be considered in the differential diagnosis of the depressed older patient.

The diagnosis of a typical depression does not present much challenge. Few physicians would overlook the diagnosis of depression in a patient with complaints of sadness, crying, decreased energy, decreased appetite, weight loss, decreased libido, early morning awakening, and thoughts of suicide. However, many older depressed patients do not report feeling depressed or exhibit classic symptoms. Instead, they typically complain of not feeling physically well and may make repeated visits to their primary care physician with a variety of somatic complaints. Older depressed patients may also present with signs and symptoms that mimic or meet criteria for dementia, including apathy, decreased cognitive ability, memory complaint, loss of self-care skills, incontinence, confusion, and agitation. This presentation has been referred to as "pseudodementia" [36] or, more recently, as the "dementia syndrome of depression" [37]. Any demented patient with symptoms that could be due to depression should be given an empirical trial of an antidepressant to determine whether those symptoms improve.

Older depressed patients may also present with characteristic delusions. Somatic delusions, such as the delusion that one has cancer, a brain tumor, or rotting body viscera, are not unusual. These beliefs are much stronger and more immutable than occasional hypochondriacal preoccupations, which are fairly common as people get older and develop various illnesses. Delusions of poverty, such as the feeling that one has no money to eat or pay for other necessities of life, may occur. When confronted with documents showing a large bank balance,

the person will respond, "Banks make mistakes." Again, this belief is far beyond the normal concerns of the elderly about living on a reduced and often fixed income that is eroded by inflation. Delusions of guilt that one has committed some terrible sin and deserves to be punished also occur. To the outsider the transgression appears to be nonexistent or of little consequence, but the older person believes otherwise and is terrified. Such delusions may actually have a core of reality as the person reminisces about the successes and failures in his or her life.

Treatment of the older depressed patient includes the full range of psychotherapeutic, environmental, and behavioral approaches noted earlier. In addition, specific somatic therapy may be helpful.

ANTIDEPRESSANT DRUGS
Antidepressant drugs are the primary somatic treatment prescribed for depressed patients in all age groups, including the elderly. Table 26-2 lists the various drugs available, including the cyclic antidepressants, trazodone, monoamine oxidase inhibitors (MAOIs), and stimulants. *Clinical Pharmacology.* For cyclic antidepres-

TABLE 26-2. *Antidepressant drugs*

DRUG	USUAL GERIATRIC DOSE RANGE (MG/DAY)	INCIDENCE OF SIDE EFFECTS			ALTERED CARDIAC RATE AND RHYTHM
		SEDATION	HYPOTENSION	ANTI-CHOLINERGIC	
Cyclic antidepressants					
Imipramine	10–150	Mild	Moderate	Moderate-strong	Moderate
Desipramine	10–150	Mild	Mild-moderate	Mild	Mild
Doxepin	10–150	Moderate-strong	Moderate	Strong	Moderate
Amitriptyline	10–150	Strong	Moderate	Very strong	Strong
Nortriptyline	10–100	Mild	Mild	Moderate	Mild
Maprotiline	10–150	Moderate-strong	Moderate	Moderate	Mild
Amoxapine	25–200	Mild	Moderate	Moderate	Moderate
Triazolopyridine antidepressant					
Trazodone	25–300	Moderate-strong	Moderate	Mild	Mild-moderate
MAO inhibitors					
Phenelzine	15–60	Mild	Moderate	Mild	Mild
Tranylcypromine	10–30	Mild	Moderate	Mild	Mild
Stimulants					
Methylphenidate	5–40	None	None	None	Mild

sants, age-related changes in protein-binding, distribution, biotransformation, and clearance result in higher proportions of unbound drug, increased total accumulations with elevated drug plasma levels, and prolonged time for elimination of the drug. Altered pharmacokinetics are of particular importance for the tertiary tricyclics (e.g., imipramine and amitriptyline), which undergo N-demethylation to active desmethyl metabolites (desipramine and notriptyline). This process partially explains the finding that steady-state plasma levels of amitriptyline and imipramine are increased with age whereas levels of desipramine are not [38].

Age-related changes in the biotransformation of MAOIs are less well studied. The MAO inhibition produced by tranylcypromine is rapidly reversed when the drug is stopped, in contrast to phenelzine, whose effects may persist for a week or more [39]. In considering the pharmacology of these drugs in the elderly, it is noteworthy that of the two types of MAO that have been described, MAO-A levels remain constant, but MAO-B levels increase with age in both platelets and brain [40]. The increase in MAO-B provides a theoretical physiologic rationale for the use of MAOIs in elderly depressed patients.

In recent years, a number of new antidepressant drugs with different chemical structures (e.g., trazodone, nomifensin, bupropion) have been developed in the hope of improving effectiveness, accelerating response, which generally takes three to four weeks, or reducing side effects. These new drugs have also raised questions about the underlying neurochemical defect in depression and the basis for the effectiveness of antidepressants [41]. Although it was hoped that these drugs would be safer than older, well-established drugs, nomifensin was withdrawn from the market shortly after its release because of frequent reports of hemolytic anemia, and bupropion was not released because of case reports of seizures.

Choice of Antidepressant Drug. There are many antidepressants available to the clinician. All currently available drugs are about equally efficacious. Despite many attempts to develop predictors of response, there is no symptom pattern or biologic measure that predicts response to one drug rather than another. Like the neu-

roleptics, antidepressants differ from each other in side effect profiles. An antidepressant drug, therefore, is selected based on the side effect profile that will be least dangerous or intolerable to the older patient.

Cyclic antidepressants have been the most commonly prescribed antidepressants in the United States. However, MAOIs such as tranylcypromine or phenelzine are also effective antidepressants that have been available for many years and are more widely used in Europe. They have not been as popular in the United States because of concern for the rare hypertensive crisis that can occur if a patient ingests food or medication containing tyramine or other pressor amines while taking an MAOI. In an elderly patient with fragile, arteriosclerotic cerebral vessels, a hypertensive episode would be especially hazardous.

Among the most serious common side effects of antidepressant drugs are orthostatic hypotension, alterations in cardiac rhythm, and anticholinergic effects. As noted in the earlier discussion of neuroleptic drugs and in the detailed discussion in Chapter 15, orthostatic hypotension is a troublesome and potentially dangerous side effect in older patients. Elderly patients with preexisting bundle branch block or other arrhythmias who receive cyclic antidepressants are at increased risk of developing complete heart block or ventricular arrhythmias because of the quinidine-like effect of these drugs [42]. Trazodone, which was originally thought to be less "cardiotoxic" than tricyclics, has been reported to cause ventricular arrhythmias [43]. From a cardiac point of view, the secondary (demethylated) amines, desipramine and nortriptyline, appear to be the best tolerated tricyclic drugs. One group of investigators has suggested that nortriptyline may be less likely to cause hypotension [44]. MAOIs do not affect cardiac rhythm but do cause orthostatic hypotension and are not recommended in patients with serious cardiac disease, particularly because they may suppress anginal pain that would warn of cardiac ischemia. Some studies have suggested that a stimulant drug may also be safe and effective in the treatment of medically ill depressed patients, even following cardiac surgery [45,46].

Anticholinergic toxicity is also a potentially

serious consequence of use of antidepressants in the elderly. Peripheral anticholinergic side effects include dry mouth, constipation, urinary retention, blurred vision, and aggravation of narrow angle glaucoma. Dry mouth not only can be unpleasant but also can lead to ill-fitting dentures and decreased food intake. Constipation is a more troublesome anticholinergic side effect in older patients and can be distressing enough to cause noncompliance. Urinary retention, in addition to its acute presentation, may predispose older patients to bladder and kidney infections and is especially troublesome for men with enlarged prostates. Elderly patients may also develop a central anticholinergic delirium with disorientation, confusion, hallucinations, restlessness, and agitation. Antidepressants must be stopped for any patient who becomes delirious but may be restarted at a lower dose when the symptoms of anticholinergic toxicity subside. Trazodone is free of anticholinergic activity but does cause some dry mouth and constipation because of its alpha-adrenergic-blocking effect. MAOIs have mild anticholinergic effects and stimulant drugs have none.

Sedation is also a potentially unwanted side effect of antidepressant drug therapy. As noted in the discussion of neuroleptics, sedation can be quite troublesome in older patients. Sedating antidepressants (e.g., amitriptyline or doxepin) are sometimes used for depressed older patients who have difficulty sleeping at night. However, in addition to causing daytime sedation, these drugs are more likely to cause anticholinergic side effects. Trazodone is very sedating in some patients, which can limit its use. Phenelzine is somewhat sedating, but tranylcypromine is activating, as are stimulants. Activating drugs can cause insomnia if they are given in the afternoon or evening.

On the basis of differential side effect profiles, the cyclic antidepressants that are likely to be best tolerated in older patients are nortriptyline and desipramine; the former is a little more sedating and the latter a little more activating. The tertiary amine tricyclics, imipramine, amitriptyline, doxepin, and trimipramine, should not be the first choice antidepressant for elderly patients. Maprotiline, another secondary amine, has a favorable side effect profile but in younger patients has been associated with a higher risk

of seizures than other antidepressants [47]. As noted above, trazodone can be overly sedating and has also been associated in younger patients with painful priapism [48]. Amoxapine is not recommended because it is metabolized to the neuroleptic loxapine and therefore can cause extrapyramidal side effects or tardive dyskinesia. MAO inhibitor antidepressants are often very helpful and are generally well tolerated by the elderly. Any patient treated with an MAOI should be given a list of dietary restrictions and medications to avoid. The patient's primary care physician should also be informed of these restrictions. Stimulant drugs (e.g., methylphenidate) are often used in general hospitals to activate withdrawn, apathetic, depressed patients. Administration of stimulant drugs is sometimes used as a diagnostic test to determine whether depression is "treatable," but it does not predict whether a patient will respond to a different antidepressant. Although stimulants can lead to dramatic improvement in such patients after just a few doses, long-term effectiveness is uncertain, and the possibility of tolerance and dependence limit their usefulness. Electroconvulsive therapy (to be discussed later) is probably the safest, most effective, and fastest acting treatment for patients who are severely depressed.

Clinical Prescription of Antidepressants. Starting doses of an antidepressant should be low (e.g., 10–20 mg of nortriptyline or desipramine) in an elderly patient because of the risk of toxicity. Dosage increases should also be small (e.g., 10 mg) and gradual and should be prescribed only if the patient tolerates the medication and if the target symptoms for which the drug was prescribed still persist. Clinical benefits may not appear for ten days to three weeks. All older patients must have a pretreatment electrocardiogram (ECG), which should be repeated periodically during the course of treatment if there is any abnormality on the initial tracing. Blood pressure, taken with the patient seated and standing, should be obtained before treatment is started and repeated with dosage increases, particularly if the patient complains of lightheadedness on standing. A large blood pressure drop should be a cause for concern but does not require stopping the drug unless the patient is lightheaded or dizzy.

Anticholinergic side effects in older patients

may be quite bothersome, and their management can challenge the physician's ingenuity. Sugarless hard candies are sometimes helpful for dry mouth. A peripheral cholinergic agonist (e.g., bethanechol) is sometimes needed if patients have difficulty initiating urination. Use of a bulk laxative or a stool softener may relieve distressing constipation.

ELECTROCONVULSIVE THERAPY

Electroconvulsive therapy (ECT) has been found to be safe, effective, and well tolerated by geriatric patients [49]. Generally reserved for patients with severe depression who require hospitalization, it is more effective than an antidepressant alone in the treatment of delusional depression [50]. Present techniques of ECT administration have reduced or eliminated many of its undesirable features. Modifications of technique include the use of general anesthesia, muscle blockade with succinylcholine, and pretreatment with atropine to reduce the risk of arrhythmias. All patients require a careful medical evaluation prior to treatment. If the patient has serious cardiopulmonary disease, it is advisable to conduct the treatments in a medically supervised hospital setting. Memory complaints are common during and after a course of treatments but can be reduced somewhat by the use of unilateral electrode placements to the nondominant hemisphere [51]. Treatments are generally given three times a week on alternate days. If the patient becomes very confused, treatments may be given only once or twice a week. Most older patients show a response after three to six treatments and then receive an equal number of additional treatments. Patients with previous episodes of depression may be less likely to relapse if ECT is followed by maintenance treatment with an antidepressant drug or with lithium (see below under Treatment of Mania).

TREATMENT OF MANIA

Since mania is considerably less common than depression in the elderly, many physicians are unfamiliar with the typical picture of elated mood, hyperactivity, decreased sleep, and flight of ideas. In addition, elderly patients may present with atypical features, including confusion at the outset, more pronounced paranoid fea-

tures, more labile affect, irritability, and mixed depression and elation [52]. It is highly unusual for mania to present for the first time after age 65, and a previous history of depression is generally found. Some patients may present with a manic picture secondary to some other illness [53], or the syndrome may be precipitated by antidepressant treatment.

The treatment of an acute manic episode may involve the use of neuroleptics, of sedative drugs, or of lithium or carbamazepine, which may also have prophylactic mood-stabilizing effects. ECT may also be useful in unresponsive manic patients. Studies in younger manic patients have suggested that valproic acid, clonidine, clonazepam, and verapamil may be clinically effective, but no studies have been done of these drugs in the elderly.

Lithium

The use of lithium in the last 20 years has dramatically improved the outlook for patients with bipolar affective disorders [54]. Lithium is effective in acute mania and, in some depressed patients, can potentiate the effectiveness of an antidepressant drug. In addition, lithium reduces the frequency and severity of future episodes of mania or depression in bipolar patients and may also be effective prophylactically in some unipolar depressed patients.

Lithium is excreted entirely by the kidney and is indistinguishable from sodium ions in the proximal tubule. Since glomerular filtration rate decreases with age [55], the elimination half-life of lithium is prolonged in older patients. Sodium-depleting diuretics or low-salt diets result in further lithium retention. For these reasons, oral doses of lithium should be considerably lower in the elderly than in younger adults.

Prior to initiating lithium therapy, it is essential to obtain a careful medical history and perform a physical examination, paying special attention to the presence of cardiovascular or renal disease. Patients should be asked whether they are on a low-salt diet or take medication for hypertension. Laboratory studies include an ECG, urinalysis, serum electrolytes, blood urea nitrogen (BUN), serum T4, and thyroid-stimulating hormone (TSH). Creatinine clearance is more meaningful than a simple serum creatinine determination as a measure of renal function in patients with suspected kidney disease. It is essential that the patient's primary care and other treating physicians know that the patient is taking lithium.

Lithium should be used cautiously in older patients, particularly those with cardiovascular or renal disease. Patients with preexisting cognitive impairment should not be treated with lithium unless the medication is closely supervised and administered. The starting dose is 150 mg or less with increases as tolerated to achieve a blood level of 0.3 to 0.7 mEq/liter, in contrast to a target level of 0.8 to 1.2 mEq/liter in younger patients. For an acute manic episode, an occasional older patient will require and tolerate blood levels as high as 1.3 mEq/liter under close observation.

Older patients are more susceptible than younger patients to side effects from lithium. Common side effects are gastrointestinal distress, diarrhea, a fine resting tremor, and mild ataxia. In the older patient, however, neurotoxicity, manifested by confusion, disorientation, and memory impairment, is often the first sign of lithium toxicity. Severe tremor and ataxia are also more likely in older patients and may prevent the patient from reaching a therapeutic level of lithium. Nephrogenic diabetes insipidus with polydipsia, polyuria, and hypernatremia may develop. These symptoms may respond to dose reduction, but some patients may require the addition of a thiazide diuretic to treat this complication. Determination of blood levels of the drug is essential when lithium is first started. Blood levels can be taken infrequently in patients on maintenance treatment if they are reliable or are under supervision, since increased tremor or unsteadiness or confusion will usually identify patients who are becoming toxic. Some patients on lithium develop hypothyroidism, which in the elderly may be confused with depression or dementia. Follow-up thyroid studies should be done annually to check for this possibility.

Carbamazepine
In recent years, the anticonvulsant drug carbamazepine has been shown to be a safe and effective alternative for some bipolar patients who do not respond to or tolerate lithium therapy [56]. It has been suggested that patients who are "rapid cyclers" (i.e., who complete more than three full cycles in a 12-month period) may respond better to carbamazepine than to lithium. Carbamazepine has not been studied in elderly biopolar patients. In younger patients its therapeutic and prophylactic effects are enhanced when it is prescribed in conjunction with lithium.

As with lithium, a complete history and physical examination are essential prior to initiating therapy with carbamazepine. Pretreatment laboratory tests should include a complete blood count, platelet count, serum iron, liver function tests, and urinalysis.

The starting dose of carbamazepine is 100 mg or less, and the dose should be increased as tolerated to achieve a blood level of 4 to 8 μg/ml. Because carbamazepine induces hepatic enzymes, the dose will usually need to be increased again after the patient has achieved a therapeutic level.

The side effects of carbamazepine are similar to those of imipramine, with a few important additions. There is a higher incidence of bone marrow suppression, hepatotoxicity, or ataxia in patients treated with carbamazepine. For that reason, complete blood counts, platelet counts, and liver function tests should be obtained regularly. Elderly patients are also more susceptible than younger adults to neurotoxicity (confusion and disorientation).

TREATMENT OF ANXIETY DISORDERS
Anxiety, a common symptom in older patients, often arises from actual experiences. For example, an older patient may be anxious about her own health or that of her husband and children, about their financial situation, or about where they will live. Anxiety in these situations is usually manageable without specific treatment or with simple support, encouragement, and practical assistance. More serious, debilitating anxiety may require pharmacologic intervention. The differential diagnosis of anxiety in an older person includes physical illnesses, phobias, panic disorder, generalized anxiety disorder, depressive disorders, delirium, dementia, or schizophrenic disorders.

Any physical illness in an older person is likely to be accompanied by some anxiety. In addition, specific disorders can cause anxiety or symptoms that often accompany anxiety such as sweating, tachycardia, or tremor. These disorders include angina, mitral valve prolapse, pulmonary disease, hyperthyroidism, hypoglycemia, alcohol withdrawal, or pheochromocytoma. Careful medical evaluation to rule out these disorders is essential.

According to ECA data [7], phobias are the most common disorder in older as in younger people. Mild phobias do not usually require treatment, especially if the person is able to avoid the feared situation or object. More serious phobias, such as agoraphobia, can severely impair a person's functioning and make one a prisoner at home. Such patients may seek specialized treatment, which can include the use of behavioral techniques, psychotherapy, or medication. In addition to antianxiety medication (to be discussed later), some patients may respond to beta blockers, which reduce the peripheral symptoms of anxiety and allow them to face the feared stimulus.

Panic disorder was diagnosed in about 1 percent of older people in the ECA sample [7]. In this serious disorder the person is overcome by an overwhelming sense of dread in addition to the autonomic symptoms of anxiety. Panic disorder may lead to agoraphobia as the patient becomes afraid to leave home because of fear of a panic attack. The usual antianxiety drugs are not very effective in panic disorder. Rather, the drugs of choice appear to be antidepressants such as imipramine or phenelzine, or alprazolam, a benzodiazepine.

If the anxiety symptoms accompany a depressive disorder, an antidepressant is the treatment of choice rather than an antianxiety drug. If the anxiety symptoms are part of a schizophrenic disorder, a neuroleptic is usually the drug of choice. The treatment of patients with dementia or delirium is discussed in Chapter 27.

Benzodiazepines
For generalized or specific anxiety that is so distressing that the patient requests pharmacologic treatment, the benzodiazepines have virtually replaced all other treatments, and their use will be discussed at length. Recently, buspirone, a new antianxiety agent with a different mechanism of action, has become available. It appears to be effective in reducing anxiety without producing tolerance of sedation [57]. To date, no studies of its use in the elderly have been reported.

CLINICAL PHARMACOLOGY
The biotransformation of benzodiazepines changes with age. All benzodiazepines bind extensively to plasma albumin. Elderly persons, who are more likely than younger persons to have reduced plasma protein levels, may be at risk for increased levels of unbound drug at the usual therapeutic dose.

Table 26-3 lists the benzodiazepines in order of duration of action or half-life. Benzodiazepines with active metabolites (e.g., diazepam, chlordiazepoxide, or flurazepam) have greater

TABLE 26-3. *Antianxiety and hypnotic drugs*

GENERIC NAME	BRAND NAME	USUAL GERIATRIC DOSE RANGE (MG/DAY)	DURATION OF ACTION
Benzodiazepines			
Triazolam	Halcion	0.125–1	Very short
Oxazepam	Serax	10–60	Short
Temazepam	Restoril	15–60	Short
Lorazepam	Ativan	0.5–4	Short
Alprazolam	Xanax	0.5–4	Medium
Chlordiazepoxide	Librium	10–100	Long
Diazepam	Valium	2–30	Long
Clorazepate	Tranxene	3.75–15	Long
Flurazepam	Dalmane	15–60	Very long
Barbiturates		Not recommended	
Antihistamines			
Diphenhydramine	Benadryl	25–100	Moderate
Chloral hydrate	Noctec	250–1,000	Long

age-related decreases in hepatic metabolism than those without active metabolites (e.g., oxazepam, lorazepam, temazepam, or triazolam). These decreases prolong the elimination half-life and the time needed to reach steady-state blood levels. Hepatic metabolism may be further reduced by liver disease or by other medications that interfere with the biotransformation of these drugs.

The clinical consequences of decreased protein-binding and prolonged duration of action include unwanted and prolonged sedation, impaired motor coordination, confusion, disorientation, and apathy. The elderly may also be at greater risk than younger people for side effects due to increased receptor sensitivity [58]. These effects are made worse by interactions with other CNS depressants (e.g., alcohol, analgesics, or narcotics). Paradoxically, some older patients become more agitated when given benzodiazepines.

CHOICE OF BENZODIAZEPINE
All benzodiazepines are effective at reducing anxiety, although some are marketed primarily as hypnotics (e.g., temazepam, triazolam, and flurazepam). As noted earlier, alprazolam may have some unique advantages in treating panic disorder. Selection of a benzodiazepine in an older patient must consider the pharmacokinetic characteristics of each drug. Long-acting drugs (e.g., diazepam and chlordiazepoxide) may be used if a single bedtime dose is sufficient to provide an antianxiety effect in the daytime. These drugs may be less likely to cause withdrawal symptoms because of their prolonged elimination time. However, the shorter-acting drugs (e.g., oxazepam and lorazepam) are generally preferred for the treatment of anxiety in older patients because they allow more flexibility in dosage scheduling and are less likely to accumulate and cause unwanted side effects. Shorter-acting drugs may, however, lead to more severe withdrawal reactions (e.g., seizures) than the longer-acting drugs [59]. For any of the benzodiazepines, the usual starting dose for an older patient should be one-third to one-half that prescribed for younger patients. The dose should be increased slowly to achieve the desired antianxiety effect without causing undesirable side effects. Benzodiazepines are recommended only for short-term treatment of anxiety because of the possibility of tolerance, dependence, and withdrawal reactions. Some patients, however, do not need an increased dose even after several years on the drug and are very reluctant to discontinue it. Furthermore, patients who have been stabilized on a long-acting benzodiazepine may resist attempts to switch to a shorter-acting drug.

TREATMENT OF SLEEP DISORDERS
There are important changes in sleep patterns with age [60]. Older people sleep a bit less at night, but, more important, they experience more nocturnal waking periods that disrupt sleep and spend less time in both REM and deeper stages of sleep. A healthy older person typically lies awake for one-fifth of the night. Perhaps because of these frequent awakenings, by age 75 one-third to one-half of healthy people complain of insomnia. Some patients respond to reassurance that their experience of altered sleep is not abnormal or unhealthy. Other patients need instruction in good sleep hygiene, which includes going to sleep and arising at about the same time each day, avoiding daytime naps, getting some regular exercise during the day, avoiding caffeine or nicotine, and sleeping in comfortable, familiar surroundings with one's usual partner if possible. Alcohol should be avoided because it disrupts sleep during the night even though it may help induce sleep at first. Antihypertensive drugs may cause nightmares or otherwise disrupt sleep. Patients should avoid stressful activities just prior to bedtime.

A variety of physical symptoms can disrupt sleep, including itching, angina, arthritic or musculoskeletal pain, nocturnal dyspnea, or heartburn. Treatment of these physical symptoms may improve sleep. Many older patients also suffer from nocturia and subsequent difficulty returning to sleep, which can be aggravated by disease or by treatment with diuretics. Elderly patients may have central or obstructive sleep apnea. Severe obstructive sleep apnea is uncommon. However, obstructive sleep apnea not only disrupts sleep but is potentially dangerous if the apnea is prolonged and may require uvulopharyngoplasty after careful evaluation in a sleep laboratory. Sleep disturbances in the elderly are commonly due to depression and can be relieved with specific antidepressant treatment.

In a hospital setting, disturbed sleep is common due to unfamiliar surroundings, anxiety, pain, lack of exercise, and irregular hours with daytime naps. For older hospitalized patients who experience disturbed sleep, short-term prescription of hypnotics may be useful during the hospital stay. Long-term use of hypnotic medication, in contrast, should be avoided for several reasons. First, the goal is daytime alertness and energy. Many patients who take sleeping pills for long periods find they are more sluggish and dull the next day even though they sleep better at night. Second, tolerance and dependence can develop with prolonged use of all sleeping pills and can lead to uncomfortable and potentially dangerous withdrawal reactions. Furthermore, as tolerance develops, the drug is no longer effective in inducing sleep. Finally, hypnotics may disrupt normal sleep architecture by suppressing REM sleep, which may be unhealthy.

Choice of Hypnotic Medication

The benzodiazepines have become the drugs of choice for short-term treatment of insomnia because of their high margin of safety and their combination of antianxiety and sedative effects. In older patients the short-acting benzodiazepines are preferable to longer-acting drugs such as hypnotics. They are less likely to cause daytime sedation, confusion, or ataxia or to accumulate in the body. Clinical experience suggests, however, that triazolam is too short-acting and can quickly lead to dependence and severe withdrawal reactions.

Occasionally, sedating antidepressants are used to induce sleep in older patients. Unless the patient is depressed, however, this strategy is not recommended because of the associated anticholinergic and cardiovascular side effects. Similarly, sedating neuroleptics should generally not be used simply to induce sleep. As an alternative to benzodiazepines, chloral hydrate is sometimes used, although it may cause gastric irritation. An antihistamine (e.g., diphenhydramine) may be helpful for short-term use because of its sedative effect, but it can also cause confusion. Barbiturates are not recommended because they have a lower margin of safety than benzodiazepines, induce hepatic enzymes, lead to tolerance, and can cause paradoxical agitation.

TREATMENT OF COGNITIVE DISORDERS AND ASSOCIATED BEHAVIOR PROBLEMS

As indicated in Chapter 27, a variety of agents have been used to enhance memory in normal older people and in patients with dementia. Most late-life dementia is senile dementia of the Alzheimer's type. Until a specific successful treatment for Alzheimer's disease is developed, what help can the clinician offer these patients and their families? Patients with cognitive deficits should be carefully evaluated as discussed in Chapter 4. Even without significant improvement in memory function, treating associated medical conditions may enhance the patient's well-being [19]. Of particular interest is the identification of treatable depression in patients with cognitive deficits. Such patients may improve dramatically with antidepressant treatment. Some demented patients can also make use of psychotherapy to help them work through and accept the changes in their lives.

Demented patients are sometimes restless, agitated, or screaming. These behaviors are very difficult to manage at home or in a nursing home setting. Increased daytime activity such as walking may tire the person and improve the sense of well-being and nighttime sleep. However, often caregivers request medication to calm the patient. Neuroleptics are the most commonly prescribed drugs for behavioral control of agitated, demented patients, although their effectiveness is modest and they cause a variety of side effects [61]. Benzodiazepines may also be cautiously used if the goal is simply to calm the patient or induce sleep, although they may paradoxically aggravate agitation. Beta blockers (e.g., propranolol) can reduce the agitation of demented patients [62]. With doses of 20 to 160 mg per day and with careful monitoring of cardiovascular function, side effects are minimal.

Family caregivers need considerable support to deal with the burden of caring for a demented relative [63,64]. Support may include support groups, respite services, and treatment of the patient's troublesome behaviors such as incontinence, paranoia, or wakefulness at night. Support for caregivers not only makes them feel better but can also enhance the care of the demented patient.

References

1. Butler, R. A. Psychiatry and the elderly: An overview. *Am. J. Psychiatry* 132:983, 1975.
2. Birren, J. E., and Schaie, K. W. (eds.). *Handbook of the Psychology of Aging* (2nd ed.). New York: Van Nostrand Reinhold, 1985.
3. Schaie, K. W., and Labouvie-Vief, G. Generational versus ontogenetic components of change in adult cognitive behavior: A fourteen-year cross sequential study. *Develop. Psychol.* 10:305, 1974.
4. Poon, L. W. Differences in Human Memory with Aging: Nature, Causes and Clinical Implications. In J. E. Birren and K. W. Schaie (eds.), *Handbook of the Psychology of Aging* (2nd ed.). New York: Van Nostrand Reinhold, 1985. P. 427.
5. Vaillant, G. E. *Adaptation to Life*. Boston: Little, Brown, 1977.
6. Neugarten, B. L. Time, age, and the life cycle. *Am. J. Psychiatry* 136:887, 1979.
7. Myers, J. K., et al. Six month prevalence of psychiatric disorders in three communities. *Arch. Gen. Psychiatry* 41:959, 1984.
8. Folstein, M. F., Folstein, S., and McHugh, P. R. Mini-mental state: A practical method for grading the cognitive state of patients for the clinician. *J. Psychiatr. Res.* 12:189, 1975.
9. Blazer, D. G., Bachar, J. R., and Manton, K. G. Suicide in late life. *J. Am. Geriatr. Soc.* 34:519, 1986.
10. Weissman, M. M. The epidemiology of suicide attempts, 1960 to 1971. *Arch. Gen. Psychiat.* 30:737, 1974.
11. Alcohol, Drug Abuse and Mental Health Administration. *The Alcohol, Drug Abuse, and Mental Health National Data Book*. Publication No. 80-938. Rockville, MD: U.S. Department of Health and Human Services, Public Health Service, 1980.
12. Marmor, J., Scheidemandel, P. S., and Kanno, C. K. *Psychiatrists and Their Patients: A National Study of Private Office Practice*. Washington, D.C.: Joint Information Service of the American Psychiatric Association and the National Association for Mental Health, 1975.
13. Shapiro, S., et al. Utilization of health and mental health services. *Arch. Gen. Psychiatry* 41:971, 1984.
14. Borson, S., et al. Psychiatry and the nursing home. *Am. J. Psychiatry* 144:1412, 1987.
15. Kahn, R. L, et al. Memory complaint and impairment in the aged. *Arch. Gen. Psychiatry* 32:1569, 1975.
16. Klerman, G. L. Problems in the Definition and Diagnosis of Depression in the Elderly. In L. D. Breslau, and M. R. Haug (eds.), *Depression and Aging: Causes, Care and Consequences*. New York: Springer, 1983.
17. Cooper, A. F., et al. Hearing loss in paranoid and affective psychoses of the elderly. *Lancet* 2:851, 1974.
18. Lipowski, Z. J. Transient cognitive disorders (delirium, acute confusional states) in the elderly. *Am. J. Psychiatry* 140:1426, 1983.
19. Larson, E. B., et al. Dementia in elderly outpatients: A prospective study. *Ann. Intern. Med.* 100:417, 1984.
20. Stetten, D. Coping with blindness. *N. Engl. J. Med.* 305:458, 1981.
21. Liptzin, B., Grob, M. C., and Eisen, S. B. Family burden of demented and depressed elderly psychiatric in-patients. *Gerontologist* (in press).
22. Kahana, R. J. Strategies of dynamic psychotherapy with the wide range of older individuals. *J. Geriatr. Psychiatry* 12:71, 1979.
23. Yesavage, J. A., and Karasu, T. B. Psychotherapy with elderly patients. *Am. J. Psychother.* 36:41, 1982.
24. Myers, W. A. *Dynamic Therapy of the Older Patient*. New York: Jason Aronson, 1984.
25. Nemiroff, R. A., and Colarusso, C. A. *The Race Against Time: Psychotherapy and Psychoanalysis in the Second Half of Life*. New York: Plenum Press, 1985.
26. Christenson, R., and Blazer, D. Epidemiology of persecutory ideation in an elderly population in the community. *Am. J. Psychiatry* 141:1088, 1984.
27. Watt, J. A. G. Hearing and premorbid personality in paranoid states. *Am. J. Psychiatry* 142:1453, 1985.
28. Salzman, C. (ed.). *Clinical Geriatric Psychopharmacology*. New York: McGraw-Hill, 1984.
29. Smith, J. M., and Baldessarini, R. J. Changes in prevalence, severity, and recovery in tardive dyskinesia with age. *Arch. Gen. Psychiatry* 37:1368, 1980.
30. Toenniessen, L. M., Casey, D. E., and McFarland, B. H. Tardive dyskinesia in the aged: Duration of treatment relationships. *Arch. Gen. Psychiatry* 42:278, 1985.

31. Stotsky, B. A. Psychoactive Drugs for Geriatric Patients with Psychiatric Disorders. In S. Gershon and A. Raskin (eds.), *Aging*. Vol. 2: *Genesis and Treatment of Psychologic Disorders in the Elderly*. New York: Raven, 1975.

32. Salzman, C., and Van der Kolk, B. A. Psychotropic drug prescriptions to elderly patients in a general hospital. *J. Am. Geriatr. Soc.* 28:18, 1980.

33. Salzman, C. Treatment of the elderly agitated patient. *J. Clin. Psychiatry* 48 (5 Suppl.): 19, 1987.

34. Blazer, D., and Williams, C. D. Epidemiology of dysphoria and depression in an elderly population. *Am. J. Psychiatry* 137:439, 1980.

35. American Psychiatric Association. *Diagnostic and Statistical Manual of Mental Disorders* (3rd ed., revised). Washington, D.C.: American Psychiatric Association, 1987.

36. McAllister, T. W. Overview: Pseudodementia. *Am. J. Psychiatry* 140:528, 1983.

37. Folstein, M. F., and McHugh, P. R. Dementia Syndrome of Depression. In R. Katzman, R. D. Terry, and K. L. Bick (eds.), *Alzheimer's Disease*. New York: Raven, 1978.

38. Nies, A., et al. Relationship between age and tricyclic antidepressant plasma levels. *Am. J. Psychiatry* 134:790, 1977.

39. Jenike, M. A. The use of monoamine oxidase inhibitors in the treatment of elderly, depressed patients. *J. Am. Geritatr. Soc.* 32:571, 1984.

40. Robinson, D. S., et al. Monoamine metabolism in human brain. *Arch. Gen. Psychiatry* 34:89, 1977.

41. Charney, D. S., Menkes, D. B., and Heninger, G. R. Receptor sensitivity and the mechanism of action of antidepressant treatment. *Arch. Gen. Psychiatry* 38:1160, 1981.

42. Glassman, A. H., and Bigger, J. T., Jr. Cardiovascular effects of therapeutic doses of tricyclic antidepressants. *Arch. Gen. Psychiatry* 38:815, 1981.

43. Janowsky, D., et al. Ventricular arrhythmias possibly aggravated by trazodone. *Am. J. Psychiatry* 140:796, 1983.

44. Roose, S. P., et al. Comparison of imipramine- and nortriptyline-induced orthostatic hypotension: A meaningful difference. *J. Clin. Psychopharmacol* 1:316, 1981.

45. Katon, W., and Raskind, M. Treatment of depression in the medically ill elderly with methylphenidate. *Am. J. Psychiatry* 137:963, 1980.

46. Kaufmann, M. W., et al. The use of methylphenidate in depressed patients after cardiac surgery. *J. Clin Psychiatry* 45:82, 1984.

47. Dessain, E. C., et al. Maprotiline treatment in depression. *Arch. Gen. Psychiatry* 43:86, 1986.

48. Lansky, M. R., and Selzer, J. Priapism associated with trazodone therapy. *J. Clin. Psychiatry* 45:232, 1984.

49. Karlinsky, H., and Shulman, K. I. The clinical use of electroconvulsive therapy in old age. *J. Am. Geriatr. Soc.* 32:183, 1984.

50. Glassman, A. H., Kantor, S. J., and Shostak M. Depression, delusions, and drug response. *Am. J. Psychiatry* 132:716, 1975.

51. Horne, R. L., et al. Comparing bilateral to unilateral electroconvulsive therapy in a randomized study with EEG monitoring. *Arch. Gen. Psychiatry* 42:1087, 1985.

52. Shulman, K., and Post, F. Bipolar affective disorder in old age. *Br. J. Psych.* 132:26, 1980.

53. Krauthammer, C., and Klerman, G. L. Secondary mania. *Arch. Gen. Psychiatry* 35:1333, 1978.

54. Liptzin, B. Treatment of Mania. In C. Salzman (ed.), *Clinical Geriatric Psychopharmacology*. New York: McGraw-Hill, 1984.

55. Rowe, J. W., et al. The effect of age on creatinine clearance in men: A cross-sectional and longitudinal study. *J. Gerontol.* 31:155, 1976.

56. Ballenger, J. C., and Post, R. M. Effects of carbamazepine in manic-depressive illness: A new treatment. *Am. J. Psychiatry* 137:782, 1980.

57. Goldberg, H. L. Buspirone hydrochloride: A unique new anxiolytic agent. *Pharmacother.* 4:315, 1984.

58. Calderini, G., and Toffano, G. Phospholipid methylation H-diazepam, and H-GABA bonding in the cerebellum of aged rats. In E. Giacobini, et al. (eds.), *The Aging Brain: Cellular and Molecular Mechanisms of Aging in the Nervous System*. New York: Raven, 1982.

59. Howe, J. G. Lorazepam withdrawal seizures. *Br. Med. J.* 280:1163, 1980.

60. Miles, L., and Dement, W. Sleep and aging. *Sleep* 3:119, 1980.

61. Barnes, R., Veith, R., and Okimoto, J. Efficacy of antipsychotic medications in behaviorally disturbed dementia patients. *Am. J. Psychiatry* 139:1170, 1982.

62. Greendyke, R. M., Schuster, D. B., and Wooton, J. A. Propranolol in the treatment of assaultive patients with organic brain disease. *J. Clin. Psychopharmacol.* 4:282, 1984.

63. Mace, N. L., and Rabins, P. V. *The 36-Hour Day*. Baltimore: Johns Hopkins University Press, 1981.

64. Gwyther, L. P., and George, L. K. Caregivers for dementia patients: Complex determinants of well-being and burden. Introduction. *Gerontologist* 26:245, 1986.

27

Dementia and Delirium

Richard W. Besdine

HUMAN BRAIN FUNCTION is precious and unique, and deranged intellect is feared more than death by most people. Yet disruption of cognition is a common but misunderstood phenomenon in older persons. Dementia and delirium—both disturbances of all or most higher cortical functions—occur increasingly with advancing age. Both have numerous possible etiologies and require careful, prompt evaluation to yield optimal therapeutic outcomes. In addition to their morbidity, these disorders are among the most emotionally devastating to friends, families, and caregivers of the afflicted, and any benefit achieved from medical intervention is as gratifying and desirable as the most heroic technologic "save" in health care.

Delirium is among the most important disorders of the aged. The frequent occurrence of transient confusion in physically ill old persons hospitalized for acute care justifies calling delirium "the very stuff of geriatric medicine" [1]. Acute confusional states (delirium) are widely neglected and cause substantial morbidity and mortality in older patients. Often the first sign of illness, delirium occurs either as a prominent presenting feature of life-threatening disease or as a complication of another disorder.

Senile dementia is a prevalent, highly morbid, and costly chronic disability among the elderly [2-4]. In those aged 75 to 84, new cases of dementia occur as frequently as heart attacks

and more frequently than strokes [5]. *Senile dementia* is a term used to describe progressive decline in cognitive function resulting in impairment of memory, orientation, reasoning ability, judgment, and social adjustment [6]. The most common cause of senile dementia is Alzheimer's disease (AD). First described in 1835 by James Pritchard [7], senile dementia or "incoherence" was characterized by "forgetfulness of recent impressions, while the memory retains a firm hold of ideas laid up in the recesses from times long past." In a landmark publication, Alois Alzheimer [8] reported the neuropathologic findings in the brain of a woman who died at age 55 after four years of progressive dementia. The clinical picture of her deterioration was described with remarkably contemporary precision and relevance.

After mention of intellectual changes of normal aging, this chapter considers global cognitive disturbances of older persons (dementia and delirium), primarily from clinical and biologic perspectives, with brief observations on the social aspects of the disorders.

Definitions

Because both dementia and delirium are global cognitive disturbances and occur more commonly with advancing age, clinicians may confuse or fail to differentiate between them. In view of the major differences in etiology and therapeutic approach, separation is crucial, and thus the following elaborate definitions are offered.

Dementia, a Latin word literally meaning "without mind," is loss of intellectual capacity in a mature adult that is severe enough to interfere with social or occupational function. Diagnostic criteria [9] include (1) memory impairment; (2) at least one of the following: (a) impaired abstract thinking, (b) impaired judgment, (c) other higher cortical disturbances (agnosia, aphasia, apraxia, visual–spatial impairment), or (d) personality change; and (3) *un*impaired level of consciousness. When detected, dementia has usually been present for months to a year or longer. Although this definition is multidimensional and specific, it is crucial to remember that dementia, and delirium as well, are only syndromes, and each has a long and diverse array of potential etiologic diseases that is even further expanded in older persons.

Delirium, like dementia, is a global disturbance of cognitive function, meaning that all modalities of intellect are probably disturbed but not necessarily with equal severity. In addition, delirium is accompanied by alteration and often fluctuation in the level of attentiveness and usually consciousness. Diagnostic criteria for delirium [9] are summarized in Table 27-1. Table 27-2 compares and contrasts dementia and delirium. Although documentation of dementia cannot be established in the presence of clouded consciousness, since the cognitive losses could be attributable solely to delirium under these circumstances, dementia and delirium can certainly coexist. The common sequence is that a demented person acquires a superimposed illness, which then provokes delirium. Only in retrospect, when the delirium has lifted and an obvious dementia remains, can the concurrence of the two be ascertained with certainty, unless a precisely accurate history is available at presentation.

Although delirium and dementia are very different disturbances, with numerous different characteristics, humility and an open mind are essential in approaching evaluation of an older person with disturbed cognition. Several of the key differential points (onset, duration, progression) between delirium and dementia are

TABLE 27-1. *DSM-III-R diagnostic criteria for delirium*

A. Reduced ability to maintain attention to external stimuli and to appropriately shift attention to new external stimuli
B. Disorganized thinking as indicated by rambling, irrelevant, or incoherent speech
C. At least two of the following:
   (1) Reduced level of consciousness
   (2) Perceptual disturbances: misinterpretations, illusions or hallucinations
   (3) Disturbance of sleep-wake cycle with insomnia or daytime sleepiness
   (4) Increased or decreased psychomotor activity
   (5) Disorientation to time, place, or person
   (6) Memory impairment (e.g., new material or past material)
D. Clinical features that develop acutely (hours to days) and fluctuate over the course of a day
E. Either (1) or (2):
   (1) Evidence from the history, physical exam, or laboratory tests of an organic etiology
   (2) In absence of such evidence, an etiologic organic factor can be presumed if the disturbance cannot be accounted for by any nonorganic mental disorder

SOURCE: Reprinted with permission from the *Diagnostic and Statistical Manual of Mental Disorders, Third Edition, Revised.* Copyright 1987 American Psychiatric Association.

TABLE 27-2. *Delirium versus dementia*

DELIRIUM	DEMENTIA
1. Develops abruptly	1. Develops slowly
2. Nonprogressive	2. Progressive
3. Short duration	3. Present for many months or years
4. Fluctuating consciousness	4. Rarely altered consciousness
5. Precise time of onset	5. Uncertain date of onset

SOURCE: T. Wetle (ed.). *Handbook of Geriatric Care.* E. Hanover, N.J.: Sandoz, 1982.

based exclusively on history, and accurate historical information is usually insufficient at the time of detection and presentation of a cognitively impaired older person. Additionally, the hectic and dynamic features, ubiquitous in young patients with delirium, may be dampened or absent in an older person, who may show only cognitive loss and blunted consciousness. Dementia and delirium will be considered separately in this chapter.

Cognitive Changes of Normal Aging

The definition, measurement, and theoretical framework of intellectual change that occurs in healthy aging humans are fraught with controversy and are beyond the scope of this chapter. Reviews, monographs, and books of high quality on this subject are available, and they should be consulted [10-13]. Observations of modest decrement in short-term memory, speed of information retrieval, willingness to make a guess, reaction time, and fluid intelligence have been described with age, but many argue that even these observations are spurious due to cohort differences and contamination of performance by the sensory, motor, and endurance deficits so common among healthy aged subjects. One especially well-done cross-sectional study [14] demonstrated a decline in adult intelligence (on five tests) of one-third to one-half a standard deviation over a 14-year period, beginning at about age 60. More important, longitudinal follow-up of the same subjects showed that cognitive training techniques could improve test performances to predecline levels for nearly two-thirds of the subjects who had declined [15]. Additionally, more than half the subjects did not decline at all, and when trained, these stable individuals actually improved their intellectual performance late in life. These data strongly suggest that disuse is a major factor in age-related intellectual decline.

It is clear that only minor cognitive declines can be attributed to age, and in these circumstances, if disease is not playing a role, function can be improved or restored by increased participation in intellectually challenging tasks. Cognitive impairment that interferes with leading a normal life is never part of normal aging, and its appearance should provoke suspicion of disease and prompt medical evaluation.

Dementia

EPIDEMIOLOGY

Important studies of the epidemiology of dementing disease in older persons are currently in progress through the Established Populations for Epidemiologic Studies of the Elderly program, initiated by the National Institute on Aging and based at the East Boston Senior Health Project, the Iowa 65-Plus Rural Health Study, and the Yale Health and Aging Project [16]. These studies are the first prospective projects that follow community-dwelling populations of representative elders in the United States, and they are measuring a broad array of physical, functional, social, and cognitive variables over time. In the absence of data from these studies we must summarize currently available studies of dementia. Most studies report a 5 percent prevalence of severe dementia among community-dwelling persons over 65 years of age and an additional 10 percent with mild to moderate impairment [17]. Ranges of 0.6 to 12.0 percent for severe impairment, and 1.5 to 22.0 percent for mild dementia have been reported [17], but the outliers are from age-extreme populations.

Incidence data for dementia have been presented indicating rates of 0.3 percent per year in more than 4000 Swedes over 60 years of age [18], 1.5 percent of more than 600 persons over 65 in England [19], and 1.0 percent per year in Baltimore among volunteers over age 65 [20]. One highly regarded long-term longitudinal study [21,22] reported annual incidence rates of 0.7 percent and 0.5 percent for men and women, respectively, aged 70 to 79 years, and rates of 1.9 percent and 2.5 percent for men and women over the age of 80. It is obvious that incidence and prevalence rates for dementia will be greatly influenced by the age composition of the population being studied, and thus age-specific rates are of greatest interest. In summary, it is rather surprising how similar the reported incidence and prevalence rates are in view of the heterogeneity and pitfalls of the various studies, suggesting that the data may be more reliable than previously supposed.

Although many studies state that their rates for senile dementia approximate the rates for AD, these speculations are not supported by robust diagnostic criteria in most cases. One report from the Baltimore Longitudinal Study that uses reasonable clinical criteria calculates the age-specific incidence and prevalence rates of AD [23] based on ascertainment of 27 cases in 519 subjects (Table 27-3). Other estimates of prevalence of AD have suggested 3 to 5 percent of persons 65 to 74 and more than 30 percent of those over age 80 [3,20,24,25,26]. It is estimated that the risk for developing AD doubles every five years between ages 60 and 80 [27]. But preliminary results from the East Boston NIA study site suggest that more than 11 percent of those 65 and over have AD, a prevalence

TABLE 27-3. *Age-specific rates calculated for Alzheimer's disease (per 1,000 subjects)*

AGE	INCIDENCE	PREVALENCE
65	1.7	6.0
70	3.3	17.8
75	6.7	41.1
80	13.4	86.2
85	26.8	170.3
90	53.7	316.3
95+	107.7	536.1

SOURCE: R. B. Sayetta. Rates of senile dementia-Alzheimer's type in the Baltimore Longitudinal Study. *J. Chronic Dis.* 39:271, 1986.

double previous estimates [28], and people over age 85 are almost as likely as not to have AD. Based on estimates that two-thirds of all senile dementia is AD (recent studies suggest an even higher proportion), it seems likely that there are more than 2.5 million community-dwelling American victims of AD. Since the nursing home population of 1.4 million Americans is estimated to contain a minimum of another half million demented persons, and an autopsy study revealed AD in more than half of 100 consecutive examinations in one nursing home [5], the total of Americans in institutions and the community afflicted by AD may exceed 3 million persons.

Age has been clearly identified as a risk factor for AD for several decades by virtually every epidemiologic study published. In addition, a family history of AD or Down's syndrome [29-34], head injuries [33,35], and thyroid disorder [33] have all been suggested as well, but controversy has arisen around most of these factors (see below). Most studies also indicate that the disease has a predilection for women, even after adjustment for the greater longevity and higher institutionalization rates for women.

CLINICAL CHARACTERISTICS

The initial presentation of dementia in older persons commonly involves memory loss, both short- and long-term. Associated intellectual deficits in reasoning, judgment, abstraction, calculation, and orientation are usually less obvious at first, but, depending on the demands of the patient's life, these may eventually dominate the picture. The overall tempo tends to be extremely slow, and thus the confident appraisal

that something is definitely wrong is often protracted and painful in the family setting. Although it has been a clinical saw that rate of progression in dementing illness is inversely proportional to the age at onset [36], one persuasive report documents no difference in slope of intellectual decline by age, at least in a sample of demented persons with carefully clinically diagnosed AD [37]. In 165 patients recruited from a Memory Disorders Clinic and followed for five years, increasing age actually correlated weakly with rapidity of progression, and duration of dementia was shorter for the oldest group at diagnosis. Severity at the time of detection did not correlate with rate of decline.

The first signs of dementia may be difficult to distinguish from the very modest and subtle cognitive alterations of normal central nervous system (CNS) aging (see earlier section on cognitive changes of normal aging). Need for repetition to remember new information in daily life (addresses, phone numbers, names of new people) and hesitancy in answering direct questions can be the earliest changes. Progression to forgetting previously remembered information and occurrences in the previous day or two raise more concern. Neglecting initiated tasks, such as forgetting to comply with medical regimens, to close the door in winter, or to turn off the oven or running water can be hazardous. Primary dementia does not produce lethargy or other alteration of consciousness.

Defects in reasoning and abstraction first produce reluctance to enter new situations, and reports of emotional upset and frustration in unusual events involving complex adjustments, such as reunions and parties, are typical. Calculation, particularly mental arithmetic, is disturbed early and usually interferes with handling money. Personality changes are typical, but no one type is especially characteristic. Change from docility to aggressiveness or vice versa certainly may occur, but more common is a blunting of whatever had been the previous personality traits, although exaggeration of premorbid personality also occurs. Dampening of affect, shallowness of interaction, and withdrawal are frequent. Emotional state is closely related, and apathy is common. Depression or, less often, paranoia can complicate the early stages of dementia and may dominate the clinical picture. Overemphasis on pseudodementia (pure depression presenting as cognitive impairment) may lead to misidentifying the early depression of true dementia as pseudodementia, thus producing devastating subsequent disappointment (see below).

Poor judgment is usually part of the middle if not early stages of dementia. Bizarre or inappropriate social behavior, hypersexuality, unwise financial decisions, and slovenly dress with neglect of personal hygiene are reflections of loss of judgment in dementing illness. A variety of other higher cortical functions may be impaired, depending on the etiology of the dementia. Visual-spatial or constructional abilities are usually impaired, but aphasia, apraxia, and agnosia are variably present.

DETECTION

The major element in early and successful detection of dementia in older people—the alertness and sensitivity of friends and family to the signs of dementia—is beyond the physician's control. Once the patient or other referring person has struggled with perceived deficits and made the decision to report a problem, the remaining steps are relatively simple. The initial physician approach must be neutral, acknowledging both the concerns of the patient or others as well as the data that a majority of older persons never develop dementia and that there are modest normal age-related changes in cognition. The first step is a pragmatic, formal, objective assessment of cognitive function, using one of the several practical and sensitive instruments available to test mental status. The Mini-Mental State [38] and the Dementia Rating Scale [39] are both suitable for routine clinical use (see Chap. 4). Clinical impressions, "gestalt," and "seat-of-the-pants" perceptions have no place in determining whether or not dementia is responsible for the observations that brought the patient to the doctor. Because baseline intelligence, experience, and education play such a crucial role in differentiating intellectual function among human beings, objective information (work or recreational history, previous evaluations) concerning prior cognitive status is of inestimable value in early or borderline cases. As part of a thorough mental status examination, functional assessment of cognitive capac-

ity also helps to determine whether dementia-related deterioration is present.

One caveat deserves special emphasis. When the family brings an older person for evaluation and the initial physician screening does not detect difficulty, beware. For example, if the patient knows the President's name and can spell "world" backwards but no longer remembers any of the dozen stocks in his portfolio that he used to follow avidly each day in the *Wall Street Journal,* chances are that important cognitive losses have occurred. Families spend their entire lives with the older person, while an assessment, in the most conscientious hands, lasts minutes to an hour or so. If the family is firm in its resistance to reassurance and insists that their relative is impaired, a careful search for factors that have improved performance and prevented expression of the problem at the doctor's office is worthwhile. Contributory factors include missed doses of drugs previously interfering with cognition, fluctuating depression, intermittent sleep deprivation, or inadequately rigorous questions. In addition, support in the interview by a loving relative, a "good day," and many other phenomena can make an old person with early dementia transiently perform better. Respect for the family's perception is not only good manners but also usually leads to the correct clinical determination. In cases of uncertainty, referral for more elaborate neuropsychologic testing is essential. Once the presence of dementia has been ascertained with some confidence, the next and crucial step is a comprehensive clinical evaluation to determine which of the myriad causes of dementia is the specific culprit.

EVALUATION

Although often regarded as a diagnosis, cognitive impairment is a symptom or a syndrome. It has been called senile dementia, senility, hardening of the arteries, and many other names, but whatever intellectual impairment is called, it is not a disease or diagnosis. It is a symptom when the patient or family complains, or it is a syndrome when a number of characteristic features are described together. This syndrome, like any other, has its own differential diagnosis, including reversible and irreversible diseases. The potential causes must be sifted and evaluated to identify the one afflicting each impaired individual person. An incorrect historical assumption has persisted that dementia syndromes are irreversible and hopeless, and only delirious states are reversible and curable. But curable diseases can provoke a classic dementia syndrome that is reversible when the disease is treated [40,41]. The crucial point is that the dementia syndrome in older individuals is often a nonspecific response to many medical illnesses that occur in the absence of primary neuronal degeneration.

Thus, thorough evaluation of the cognitively impaired elderly patient is as essential as the workup of the patient with unexplained fever, chest pain, or any other important symptom complex. Although few patients would accept the diagnosis of "chest pain of early middle age" from their physician to explain substernal distress, most health consumers and many professionals may be satisfied with no investigation of mental decline in the elderly and may accept a label of "senility," "hardening of the arteries," or "old age." Different presenting syndromes suggest different specific diagnostic evaluations, but often a distinction between dementia and delirium or determination of whether both are present cannot be made at presentation, especially when the history is scanty or unavailable. In these instances, comprehensive diagnostic screening is necessary to uncover the underlying cause of the impairment [42,43].

As complete a history as possible, including identification of recent environmental events and losses relevant to mental health, should be taken of every cognitively impaired patient. A comprehensive physical examination, including rectal, genital, neurologic, and mental status examination, should also be performed. Several studies [44,45,46] have suggested that the history and physical examination alone, or with the addition of only the simplest screening blood and other laboratory tests, are sufficient to rule out the contribution of a reversible or curable condition to the patient's dementia. Currently, however, most experts agree with our and Katzman's [5] recommendations, as follows: a complete blood count; measurement of sedimentation rate; study of the stool for occult blood; thyroid tests; mea-

surements of electrolytes, creatinine, blood urea nitrogen, calcium, and phosphorus; urinalysis and culture; serum vitamin B_{12} and folate measurements; tests of liver function and blood sugar; syphilis serology; chest x-ray; and electrocardiogram (ECG) should all be performed routinely. If initial screening tests are uninformative, additional diagnostic studies specifically aimed at each of the many causes of cognitive impairment must be undertaken. Further tests should be done in stages, starting with the least invasive, as directed by any clinical or preceding laboratory data that suggest a possible etiology. Studies undertaken may include checking blood levels of toxins or therapeutic drugs, plain or contrast x-rays, lumbar puncture, tuberculin skin test, measurement of blood gases, blood culture, electroencephalogram (EEG), diagnostic ultrasound, and magnetic resonance imaging (MRI) brain scanning.

Psychiatric evaluation of the demented patient is another central and routine component of assessment. In addition to the possible detection of pseudodementia (see below, under Relationship to Depression), affective disorders often complicate primary dementia, and detection and treatment of the complication can be quite beneficial. Less commonly but still important enough to consider, various psychotic disorders such as paraphrenia can present elements that may resemble dementia.

A CT scan of the head should be performed in demented older persons for whom a definite diagnosis has not been established with the initial assessment. CT scanning can reliably detect subdural and epidural hematoma, tumor, intracerebral hemorrhage, brain abscess, subdural empyema, hydrocephalus, and nonhemorrhagic stroke. In addition to these focal lesions, the CT scan delivers information about ventricular size and width of cortical sulci. Unfortunately, these measurements have been used in attempts to identify brain shrinkage as the cause of clinical dementia. Although it is true that group differences of statistical significance do emerge in comparisons of brain volume, sulcal widening, and ventricular size between large numbers of demented and nondemented older persons, the presence of atrophy shows substantial overlap in the two groups, making the CT scan not useful in establishing a diagnosis of primary dementia [47,48].

The CT scan is useful in either establishing the diagnosis of one of the focal intracranial diseases previously enumerated or ruling them out and prompting other diagnostic studies. The CT scan cannot verify or exclude AD, a clinical and pathologic diagnosis. Timing of CT scanning in the evaluation of cognitively impaired patients will vary, depending on the clinical presentation and neurologic examination, but it should be done early unless the diagnosis is quickly obvious. Because of the patient's limited ability to cooperate, the pursuit of a medical diagnosis in the presence of mental impairment must often rely disproportionately on laboratory and radiologic tests to find a reversible cause of the impairment. If comprehensive laboratory and radiographic screening is not undertaken in elderly, cognitively impaired patients, medical disease presenting as mental impairment will remain undiagnosed, and the patient will be irretrievably lost.

CAUSES OF DEMENTIA

Many individual causes of cognitive impairment in the elderly are reversible, although a majority of cases are irreversible. Reversible causes are defined as diseases with specific treatments that, when applied, allow the return of previous intellectual function. Irreversible causes are brain diseases that have no known specific treatment. Current best estimates for previously unscreened older people with dementia are that 10 to 20 percent have reversible disease, and the remaining majority, 80 to 90 percent of cognitively impaired older persons, have an irreversible primary dementia [41,44,45,49,50,51]. *Irreversible* does not mean hopeless, however, and there is substantial literature documenting successful techniques for making patients with irreversible brain disease more comfortable and more manageable [6,52-57]. Reversible causes, in spite of their relative rarity, are a crucial focus. If reversible causes of cognitive impairment are untreated, they result either in death or in the eventual establishment of fixed dementia. Because most causes of delirium are reversible, a common misconception is that the causes of dementia are irreversible. Certainly there is abundant evidence to the contrary, and, perhaps more important, many patients with mild or modest cognitive loss experience chronic or episodic complicating but treatable illness that exacerbates their slowly progressive dementia. Awareness of and sensitivity to this phenomenon of "reversible superimposed on irreversible" can have major benefits for cognitively impaired older persons and reduce excess disability.

Reversible Dementia

It is crucial to identify reversible causes of dementia promptly. If untreated, these disorders often allow the patient to survive, but the dementia may become fixed and irreversible, even if the underlying disorder is eventually discovered and treated. Furthermore, if untreated, these diseases usually result in costly institutionalization and much shortening of lifespan. Accordingly, it is urgent to evaluate the patient with newly discovered dementia, in spite of the apparent adynamic nature of the disorder. Those syndromes due to reversible diseases are sometimes called secondary dementias, to emphasize that the primary disease process is outside the brain itself and is exerting a secondary detrimental effect on cognitive function. Conditions most likely to produce global organic mental disorders in the elderly, both dementia and delirium, are listed in Table 27-4 in decreasing order of frequency. Also noted is whether dementia or delirium or both can be expected.

Irreversible Dementia

Although there has been extensive emphasis on reversible dementia [40,49,58], there is no question that the large majority (80 to 90 percent) of older persons presenting with dementia will be found, after adequate evaluation, to have a primary, irreversible (at present) brain disease. A relatively small number of etiologic conditions, dominated by AD (Table 27-5), is responsible. AD, multiple infarcts, and Parkinson's disease together probably account for 95 percent or more of primary dementia in old age. The remaining handful of disorders are exceedingly uncommon, with the exception of alcoholic dementia, which has probably been underreported by patient selection bias in most studies.

TABLE 27-4. *Reversible causes of organic mental disorders in the elderly*

CAUSES	DEMENTIA	DELIRIUM	EITHER OR BOTH
Therapeutic drug intoxication			×
Depression	×		
Metabolic factors			
Azotemia/renal failure (dehydration, diuretics, obstruction, hypokalemia)			×
Hyponatremia (diuretics, excess ADH, salt wasting, intravenous fluids)			×
Hypernatremia (dehydration, intravenous saline)		×	
Volume depletion (diuretics, bleeding, inadequate fluids)			×
Acid–base disturbance		×	
Hypoglycemia (insulin, oral hypoglycemics, starvation)			×
Hyperglycemia (diabetic ketoacidosis or hyperosmolar coma)		×	
Hepatic failure			×
Hypothyroidism	×		
Hyperthyroidism (especially apathetic)	×		
Hypercalcemia			×
Cushing's syndrome	×		
Hypopituitarism	×		
Infection and/or fever			
Viral			
Respiratory or gastrointestinal		×	
Bacterial			
Pneumonia		×	
Pyelonephritis		×	
Cholecystitis		×	
Diverticulitis		×	
Tuberculosis (TB)			×
Endocarditis			×
Cardiovascular			
Acute myocardial infarction		×	
Congestive heart failure			×
Arrhythmia			×
Vascular occlusion		×	
Pulmonary embolus		×	
Brain disorders			
Vascular insufficiency			
Transient ischemia		×	
Stroke			×
Trauma			
Subdural hematoma			×
Concussion/contusion		×	
Intracerebral hemorrhage		×	
Epidural hematoma		×	
Infection			
Acute meningitis (pyogenic, viral)		×	
Chronic meningitis (TB, fungal)			×
Neurosyphilis	×		
Subdural empyema			×
Brain abscess			×
Tumors			
Metastatic to brain			×
Primary in brain			×
Pain			
Fecal impaction			×
Urinary retention		×	
Fracture		×	
Surgical abdomen		×	
Sensory deprivation states such as blindness or deafness	×		
Hospitalization			
Anesthesia or surgery			×
Environmental change and isolation			×

TABLE 27-4. *continued*

CAUSES	DEMENTIA	DELIRIUM	EITHER OR BOTH
Alcohol toxicities			
Lifelong alcoholism	×		
Alcoholism new in old age			×
Decreased tolerance with age, producing increasing intoxication			×
Acute hallucinosis		×	
Delirium tremens		×	
Anemia			×
Tumor: systemic effects of nonmetastatic malignancy			×
Chronic lung disease with hypoxia or hypercapnia			×
Deficiency states such as vitamin B_{12}, folic acid, or niacin	×		
Normal pressure hydrocephalus	×		
Accidental hypothermia		×	
Chemical intoxications			
Heavy metals such as arsenic, lead, or mercury			×
Consciousness-altering agents			×
Carbon monoxide			×

SOURCE: National Institute on Aging Task Force. Senility reconsidered: Treatment possibilities for mental impairment in the elderly. *J.A.M.A.* 244:259, 1980. Copyright 1908, American Medical Association.

TABLE 27-5. *Causes of irreversible dementia in older persons*

	PERCENT
Alzheimer's disease	70
Multiinfarct dementia	10
Mixed	10
Parkinson's disease	5
Creutzfeldt-Jakob disease	
Alcoholic dementia	
Progressive supranuclear palsy	
Progressive multifocal leukoencephalopathy	
Human immunodeficiency virus infection	
Kuru	5
Gerstmann-Straussler-Scheinker disease	
Pick's disease	
Multiple system degeneration	
Dementia pugilistica	

ALZHEIMER'S DISEASE

In 1906, at a meeting of the Southwest German Society of Alienists, Alois Alzheimer recounted the unique neuronal degenerative changes seen in the brain of a 55-year-old woman who suffered rapid and devastating cognitive decline that terminated in death after four years [8]. During the next 50 years, the characteristic pathology of AD was confirmed, including: (1) the neurofibrillary tangles (NFT) uniquely identified by Alzheimer, now known to be paired helical protein filaments (PHF), which are dif-

ferent from normal neurofilaments; (2) the characteristic neuritic or "senile" plaque, composed of an amyloid core surrounded by abnormal coalescent degenerating axons and dendrites (neurites); (3) cerebral vascular amyloid angiopathy; (4) cytoplasmic neuronal granulovacuolar bodies; (5) loss of dendritic spines; and (6) Hirano bodies (extraneuronal elongated eosinophilic structures). The characteristic lesions predominate in the neocortex, especially the hippocampus, and although plaques and tangles appear and increase modestly with normal brain aging, sharp quantitative distinctions are made easily between the normal brain and the brain with AD.

For the half-century following Alzheimer's original description, AD was defined as a rare, presenile (patients younger than 65 years of age) cause of dementia unrelated to the senile dementias of aging. However, a series of painstaking and meticulous clinicopathologic studies [59–62] has convinced most investigators that the most common form of senile dementia and AD share a specific identical pathology. Accordingly, the single name AD is given to both.

Diagnosis. Because there is still no definitive diagnostic test for AD other than the presence of characteristic neuropathology at postmortem or brain biopsy examination, substantial attention has focused on the accuracy of clinical determinations. Although substantial clinical uncertainty may appear to pervade the assessment process, there are reports of 90 percent specificity in making a determination of AD [63]. The agreement on and publication of criteria for the clinical diagnosis of AD is a major step toward better care of the individual patient as well as toward standards for more comparable research work [64]. In summary, criteria for a *probable* diagnosis of AD include (1) typical dementia, ascertained by objective mental status examination, (2) deficits in at least two cognitive functions, (3) progression without altered consciousness, and (4) exclusion of other diseases, by adequate evaluation, that could cause the dementia. *Possible* AD can be determined when criteria for probable AD are met except (1) there is variation in onset, presentation, or clinical course, or (2) a disease is detected that could cause the dementia but is felt not to be the cause of the observed cognitive losses. *Definite* AD may be determined only in the presence of clinical criteria for probable AD and characteristic brain histopathology. The reader is referred to the original source [64] for clinical use of these standards. Use of the criteria for probable disease can generally produce a 90 percent specificity of diagnosis, as validated by postmortem follow-up examination [5], but by these criteria, half the patients thought not to have AD subsequently show its neuropathology at autopsy. Unusual presentations of AD as documented by neuropathology include isolated memory loss, personality alterations, progressive aphasia, and visual agnosia [65] that have persisted in isolation or at least as the major clinical finding for years before appearance of the more typical clinical picture.

Because of the need for standardization and the difficulty in assembling sizable numbers of AD victims for study using clinical criteria, a vigorous hunt for peripheral markers of AD has been underway, but at least one major voice in the field regards the findings published as of 1986 as "nonspecific" [5] based on (1) subtlety of changes, with considerable overlap between subjects and controls, and (2) the general good health of many AD victims at the onset of illness. Since then, one report of specific brain-directed antivascular antibodies in sera from AD patients has raised hopes for a peripheral marker and in addition suggests a pathogenetic

mechanism [66]. Most promising thus far is a report of immunologic detection of a protein, designated A68, from AD brains and in spinal fluid of AD patients [67,68]. In addition, A68 appears to be associated with neurofibrillary tangles, although the antibody identifying A68 (Alz 50) also reacts with Tau and other brain proteins (Selkoe, personal communication).

Another arena in which more definite diagnostic certainty for AD has been sought is through imaging techniques. Although ordinary clinical CT scanning cannot separate individual AD victims from aged controls with normal cognition [47,48], refinements of the technique with newer scanners and the use of volumetric analysis allowed statistically significant identification of AD patient groups; however, the clinical utility of these techniques for individual cases remains uncertain. Positron emission tomography (PET) scanning measures the glucose metabolism of the brain in vivo, and reports of substantial diminution of metabolic activity in the temporal–parietal cortex of AD victims have produced optimism about its diagnostic utility [69]. Ischemia is not the culprit, since oxygen extraction ratios are not increased, and glucose metabolism from biopsy tissue is actually increased [70]. MRI scanning is the latest contender for noninvasive brain examination in the diagnosis of AD.

Clinical Features. The clinical features of AD are obviously those of dementia (see above discussion of clinical characteristics of dementia), with some additional specific factors. Besides the typical insidious, slowly progressive memory loss usually seen in elderly AD victims, other cortical deficits abound. Language disorders are often present, with prominent difficulty in naming and consequent circumlocution. Overall paucity of spontaneous speech and meaningless repetition of words or movement (stereotypy) are also frequent. Apraxia and agnosia may occur somewhat less often. Myoclonic jerks have been reported and even seizures, but these rarely occur early in the course and should raise suspicion of Creutzfeldt-Jakob disease.

Earliest signs may be very difficult to distinguish from the circumscribed small declines associated with normal aging (see above, Cognitive Changes of Normal Aging), but most victims of AD do not present at this early stage. Family or colleagues may first notice forgetfulness, loss of initiative and interest, irritability, and a decline in ability to perform previously managed tasks. Distractibility and decreased clarity and speed of thought follow. Deteriorating memory may dominate, although social and behavioral lapses may be most disturbing. Loss from memory of entire important events or even periods of time is characteristic, and by then language ability is usually quite impaired. Visual-spatial or constructional abilities are obviously impaired on formal testing, and these losses also influence visual motor coordination activities. Double incontinence, mutism, and akinesia characterize the last stages, and death usually results from infection brought on by immobility. A severity staging scale, which describes the common sequences in the trajectory of decline in AD victims, is useful for following individuals and for matching patients for comparison [71].

Mesulam [72] has suggested that there are definable recurring clinical subgroups within the demented elderly population and that the phenotype of dementia can be helpful in etiologic narrowing (differential diagnosis). Patients with predominating memory loss are most likely to have AD. The second group, characterized by major apraxias-agnosias-aphasias, appears to include AD, Pick's disease, and a mixture of other cortical degenerations. The third group, who show problems principally in motivation and behavior, Mesulam states, rarely show AD findings at postmortem, but a characteristic neuropathology has not been defined for them. It is very likely that, based on differences in pathologic neuroanatomy and transmitter neurochemistry, there are distinct phenotypes within the large group of demented older persons who show typical Alzheimer tangles and plaques. But definition and analysis of these populations must await better assessment instruments and a "gold standard" diagnostic test in living patients.

From onset of disease to death may span a decade or more in victims of AD, even when the disease begins in the seventh and eighth decades of life [71]. Although several early studies document a 50 percent or more reduction in remaining life expectancy following the diagnosis of AD [73,74], at least one more recent report reaches a different conclusion [23]. During 20 years of follow-up of 519 volunteers by the Baltimore Longitudinal Study, screening for new-onset AD was carried out. Life expectancies with and without disease were estimated, and survival analysis showed no premature mortality among AD victims. Death rates were strictly determined by chronologic age and were uninfluenced by AD acquisition, duration, or age at onset.

Relationship to Depression. Often in the early phases of AD, family and friends report that the quality of their relationship with the patient is deteriorating. The patient may show a decreased attention span, less concern about hygiene and appearance, a dislike for change, less involvement in daily activities, and even withdrawal. He or she may show a flattened affect. Since these symptoms are also attributable to depression, the differentiation between depression and dementia is crucial for the clinician (Table 27-6). One way to distinguish the two is by means of a careful history, which usually shows a more gradual and progressive deterioration with dementia and a more abrupt or cyclic course with depression. Patients with dementia do not usually have the dysphoric mood commonly seen in depression. Patients with a personal or family history of depression are more likely to become depressed in old age. Although the initial cognitive impairment is likely to be severe in the depressed patient, progressive decline is unusual. A useful differential clinical point is that the depressed patient, though complaining of severe memory loss, will perform better than expected on careful mental status examination. If the depression/dementia dilemma persists, treatment for depression may allow retrospective diagnostic certainty by evidence of improvement in the symptoms of the "dementia."

TABLE 27-6. *Depression presenting as pseudodementia*

1. Rapid onset of intellectual loss
2. Little or no progression of deficit
3. Family or prior history of depression
4. Objective testing shows better memory than patient's complaint
5. Recent provocative stress

SOURCE: T. Wetle (ed.). *Handbook of Geriatric Care.* E. Hanover, N.J.: Sandoz, 1982.

In addition, the neuropsychologist can usually help to differentiate dementia from depression. The person with mild early dementia may be aware of the impairment and may respond to the deficit by becoming anxious, angry, frustrated, agitated, and depressed. Since all such emotional reactions, if prolonged and intense, add to the dysfunction of the individual, they must be diagnosed and treated promptly.

There has been appropriate emphasis on the detection and treatment of pseudodementia, the presentation of depression in older people primarily or exclusively with cognitive loss [75]. It is interesting that Kiloh's original description of pseudodementia included patients with disorders other than depression [76], but current usage confines the term solely to elderly persons presenting with poor cognition who turn out to be depressed and usually respond to treatment. It is gratifying and dramatic to identify the intellectually blunted, dysfunctional old person who is restored to normal and productive life by treatment for depression. But recently it has become clear that elderly patients who appear to have pseudodementia are in fact frequently in the very early stages of AD [77, 78], and although they improve when treated with antidepressants, intellectual decline recurs, often within a year, and a diagnosis of AD is then made. Thus it appears that one early presentation of AD may be through its complicating depression, and although treatment is certainly indicated and beneficial, a proclamation of cure by detection of pseudodementia may be premature and intensely disappointing later on to both patient and family.

Pathology. Gross examination of the AD brain reveals a striking picture of diffuse atrophy, but it must be kept in mind that the normal aged brain is 8 to 15 percent lighter than in youth [79,80]. Nevertheless, in AD there is asymmetric atrophy of gyri serving the cortical association areas compared with the visual, motor, and somatosensory cortices [81].

Microscopic examination of the AD brain is the final arbiter of diagnosis. The unique observation reported by Alzheimer in 1906 and 1907 was of the argentophilic NFT, using the newly available Bielschowsky (1902) stain. These cytoplasmic inclusions dominate the neurons in which they appear and consist of filamentous proteins 8 to 13 nm in diameter with unique configurations, which are wound about one another with 80-nm periodicity to form paired helical filaments (PHF) [82]. Although resembling the normal cytoskeletal neurofilaments microscopically, the extraordinary abundance and spiral wrapping of PHF are unique. Although there are reports of immunologic similarities between PHF and normal neurofilaments [83], most investigators believe that PHF have unique chemical and immunologic characteristics [84]. Besides AD, tangles with morphologically identical PHF appear in dementia pugilistica, Down's syndrome, postencephalitic Parkinsonism, and the Guam-Parkinsonism dementia complex [85].

The fellow traveler of tangles in AD, described by Hirano a decade before Alzheimer's work, is the neuritic or "senile" plaque, composed of degenerating neurites (axons and dendrites) around a core of beta amyloid protein. Some of the presynaptic neurites show a marked decrease in spines, but others appear to pass unaffected through the plaque. A 28-amino acid fragment of beta amyloid from human plaques is immunologically identical to neuritic plaque and cerebrovascular amyloid obtained from aged primates and four other mammalian species [86]. In addition to its central presence in neuritic plaques, the same beta amyloid is extensively deposited in the walls of capillaries, arterioles, and small arteries in the cerebral cortex, and one study identified a capillary with amyloid at the basement membrane associated with every neuritic plaque examined from six AD brains [87]. Plaques and tangles are found in small numbers with increasing age in humans of normal intellect, primarily in the hippocampus, amygdala, and adjacent temporal cortex [79,88], but their wider strategic distribution in many association areas of the brain and much larger numbers make it clear that plaques and tangles in AD victims' brains represent far more than an exaggerated dose of normal aging [5]. Numbers of plaques and tangles correlate closely with the severity of dementia [62,89], and in the AD brain they cluster in the hippocampus, entorhinal cortex, and amygdala as well as the olfactory bulb [81,90].

Other characteristic pathologic changes in AD include granulovacuolar degeneration and peculiar cytoplasmic inclusion bodies found only in large pyramidal hippocampal neurons [91]. The final microscopic marker of AD is the Hirano body, an elongated eosinophilic structure usually found in filamentous aggregates that are more often associated with neurites than with the cell body; when they occur, they are usually found in the hippocampus.

Neuronal loss is certainly well documented with increasing age in normal human brains [92,93], but artifacts and pitfalls related to postmortem specimens abound [94]. The aggregate data point to an asymmetric loss of Golgi type II cells of layers II and IV (predominantly in the superior frontal, superior temporal, precentral, and striatal regions) with preservation of glial cells. Most studies report a modest 5 to 10 percent loss of neurons as a result of aging. For a complete discussion, the reader is urged to consult a review of the changes associated with aging [94]. Whatever the baseline, AD brains show substantial neuronal loss by comparison. The greatest losses are of large neurons with cross-sectional surface areas greater than 90 μm^2. Compared with matched controls, AD brains lose an additional half of these neurons [95], and cortical losses are greatest in the hippocampus, locus ceruleus, nucleus basalis, and entorhinal cortex [5]. Although AD brains show total cell losses of only an additional 10 percent compared with controls, it appears that the specific cell groups involved are those that connect the memory areas with numerous other key cognitive regions and produce chaos and disruption in higher cortical function when damaged [96].

Neurochemistry. Neurotransmitter measurements in AD correlate strikingly with earlier anatomic observations and indicate a reliable, specific regional deficit in cholinergic neurotransmission among AD victims that is not found in matched controls. Earliest observations of deficiencies in acetylcholine (ACh), choline acetyltransferase (CAT—an enzyme involved in ACh synthesis), and acetyl cholinesterase (the degrading enzyme for ACh) [97] were quickly followed by quantitative correlations between neuropathologic indicators of cholinergic losses and the severity of dementia [98]. Furthermore, these deficiencies have been noted in biopsy (not postmortem) specimens

from AD victims obtained within the first year of illness [70]. It appears that postsynaptic muscarinic receptors are normal in AD [99] and that cholinergic deficits arise from presynaptic cholinergic neuronal damage and eventual death, although one report of M_2 subtype loss in AD raises uncertainty [100]. The major anatomic lesion that correlates with AD cholinergic deficiency is loss of a majority of ACh-releasing neurons, whose cell bodies lie in the basal forebrain, the nucleus basalis of Meynert in the substantia innominata, just above the optic chiasm. It is here that three-fourths of the cholinergic innervation to the cerebral cortex originates, and it is the cholinergic axons of nucleus basalis neurons that appear to terminate in hippocampal neuritic plaques [101].

Many other neurotransmitters have been studied in AD brains, including dopamine, norepinephrine, serotonin, gamma–amino–butyric acid (GABA), and a variety of neuropeptides. It appears that there are no reliable reductions in any of these [5] except somatostatin, a neuropeptide found in the same large hippocampal and cortical neurons that are most affected in AD [102].

The cholinergic hypothesis of AD, modeled on the dopamine deficiency of Parkinson's disease, postulates that the deficit results from a reduction of ACh release in the prime memory association areas with preservation of postsynaptic receptors. Accordingly, if ACh repletion could be accomplished pharmacologically, just as dopamine supplementation has been accomplished within the basal ganglia by administration of L-dopa and carbidopa in Parkinson's disease, then AD might be similarly palliated [103]. Therapeutic efforts using cholinergic repletion strategies are summarized below (see under Management).

Genetics. Initial reports of rare individual family lines with high numbers of AD victims suggested that inheritance of a rare autosomal dominant AD gene might be a causative factor [104,105]. Studies of such families revealed that rates of AD approached 50 percent among first-degree relatives, and age at onset was generally younger than that in average victims. Analysis of more typical sporadic disease initially revealed a far lower rate of AD among relatives, and confidence that AD onset over age 70 carried little or no increased risk for family members was expressed [106]. Yet victims with autopsy-proven disease whose illness began before age 70 conferred on siblings a nearly 50 percent chance of affliction with AD by age 84 [31], suggesting that age-dependent expression of an autosomal dominant gene might underlie more common varieties of AD. A careful study of the families of 50 unrelated demented individuals with probable AD revealed a 46 percent cumulative incidence of AD by age 86 among first-degree relatives [34]. The risk was fourfold greater for AD in these families than in controls, suggesting the presence of a relatively common autosomal dominant gene whose expression is delayed into old age and completed by age 90.

The genetically intriguing observation of classic AD neuropathology in brains of Down's syndrome patients who reach mid-life [107] has led to the discovery of substantial epidemiologic associations between the two disorders [31,32]. Furthermore, the similar neuropathology carries with it the same neurochemical cholinergic deficiency [108] and the same amyloid deposition [109], but there is evidence that dementia does not uniformly accompany these neuroanatomic and chemical changes [110]. In view of the AD-Down's syndrome relationships, the report of mapping the genetic defect of AD to chromosome 21 (trisomy of Down's syndrome) is intriguing [111]. Using genetic linkage to DNA markers to study four different familial AD pedigrees, the location of the AD-associated gene has been mapped to a region of the long arm of chromosome 21, closer to the centromere than the region associated with Down's syndrome. In related work, the complementary DNA coding for the beta amyloid protein of AD and Down's syndrome was cloned and localized to chromosome 21 in the same region containing the AD gene [112,113]. Although it was transiently suggested that the beta amyloid gene might be duplicated in both AD and Down's syndrome cells and be the "Alzheimer gene," it has been proven not to be true [114].

Cause. Numerous causes for AD have been suggested during two decades of increasing attention paid to the disorder. These have included aluminum accumulation in neurons, autoimmune attack on the nervous system, and slow virus infection, as well as neurotransmitter deficiencies, genetic disorders, and the interaction of an environmental insult with a genetic predisposition. It is accurate to say that we do not yet know the cause of AD or even whether it is likely that there is a single cause or a series of causes. Yet accumulating research data do now allow construction of a plausible hypothesis that can be subjected to rigorous analysis.

It is reasonable, based on the latest data, to suggest that plaque amyloid, cerebrovascular basement membrane amyloid, and PHS protein may have similar primary structures or at least share areas that have similar amino acid sequences. One could imagine that the usual two copies of the gene coding for beta amyloid are derepressed and expressed late in life, leading to modest amyloid accumulation with a few plaques and tangles but with no important clinical consequences. In AD and Down's syndrome, excessive turning on of the gene produces far more amyloid and many more damaged neurons. One revitalized old theory [115] suggests that susceptible or afflicted neurons synthesize the abnormal protein or subunit, which aggregates to form PHS and, in some neurons, neurofibrillary tangles. The PHF migrates or is transported to neurites and is extruded, where, in the extracellular space, further aggregation occurs into the familiar beta amyloid configuration. This beta amyloid then either remains trapped by and does damage to the adjacent neurites or is taken up by contiguous blood vessels, adheres to the basement membrane, and becomes vascular amyloid.

One additional observation deserves mention. Discovery of prions, or infectious proteins, as the mediators of several CNS slow virus diseases in humans (kuru, Creutzfeldt-Jakob disease) and animals (scrapie) has led to speculation about their potential role in AD [116]. Several lines of evidence are suggestive: (1) prion preparations from scrapie-infected sheep brains and human cases of Creutzfeldt-Jakob disease meet electron microscopic and tinctorial characteristics of amyloid; (2) anti-neurofilament antibodies produced to kuru, Creutzfeldt-Jakob disease, and scrapie prions cross-react with neurofibrillary tangles of AD; and (3) monoclonal antibody to scrapie fibrils reacts with AD tangle protein. When considered in the light of Gajdusek's [117] hypothesis that CNS diseases of prions and plaques/tangles/PHF may share a common pathogenesis of disrupted axonal transport, it is plausible that prions could be that pathogen.

Management. Without preventive or curative therapy for AD, the current best advice for physicians is that most of their beneficial interventions for AD victims and their families will consist of managing complications, aiding the family with accurate information and sensible advice, and preventing harm. Numerous excellent publications can be consulted for detailed recommendations for management strategies [6,52–57].

1. Managing complications. Careful surveillance of the AD victim in the early and middle stages of disease may detect complicating medical or psychiatric illness promptly, and treatment may prevent discouraging secondary declines in cognitive and functional capacity. AD rarely causes abrupt or precipitous drops in intellect or self-care capacity, and when these do occur, rapid evaluation will probably discover a treatable problem. When behavioral disorders with agitation occur, transient low doses of a neuroleptic can be helpful over the hard spots (see below, Treatment of Delirium) [118].

2. Providing information. At the time of diagnosis, accurate information and a realistic prognosis about AD should be provided to at least one responsible family member and to the victim, if appropriate. Referral to the Alzheimer's Disease and Related Disorders Association (ADRDA) or other local resources for further support and counseling is wise as well. One text, *The Thirty-Six Hour Day,* is particularly helpful for families managing at home [119]. Making oneself available for problems or questions over the long term can be very reassuring and may reduce demands along the way. At some point for many victims, respite or permanent institutional care is necessary and proper, and helping a family recognize and accept that reality is most easily accomplished by the physician.

3. Preventing harm. Keeping the victim and family away from "snake oil" cures and marginal therapies is unfortunately still necessary, especially in light of the large and growing number of victims, the desperation produced by the disease, and the absence of specific curative medical treatment.

Specific Treatment. Although no breakthrough therapies are currently in routine clinical use for AD victims, several agents and groups of drugs can be mentioned under specific pharmacotherapy.

1. Cholinergic repletion. Soon after documentation of the uniform cholinergic deficit in AD, studies using some form of choline in an attempt to increase brain synthesis and availability of ACh were undertaken with high enthusiasm. Seventeen such studies were reviewed, and all but one acknowledged little benefit [103]; not surprisingly, precursor enrichment strategies have been abandoned.

Prevention of degradation of existing or natural ACh is a different path to the same objective. Intravenous or oral physostigmine, an inhibitor of acetyl cholinesterase (the enzyme that degrades ACh), has been reported to improve memory in some AD patients, but its toxicity and limited benefit are discouraging. In the most enthusiastically received report of cholinomimetic therapy oral tetrahydroaminoacridine (THA), a potent centrally acting acetyl cholinesterase inhibitor, was administered over many months to 12 clinically diagnosed AD victims; improvement in memory and self-care skills on certain scales devised by the authors was noted [120]. These results were sufficiently provocative to initiate a large prospective trial by the NIA. Another strategy is to give a muscarinic agonist of ACh, and one study reported subjective improvement of several AD patients following neurosurgical administration of intraventricular bethanechol [121], only to have the author later recommend that the procedure not be used.

2. Ergoloid mesylates. This group of dehydrogenated ergot alkaloids, marketed most often under the brand name Hydergine, is the only drug with FDA approval as "indicated" for treatment of senile dementia, including AD. One review summarized nearly two dozen controlled trials that documented statistical benefits, and in 18 of these, improvement was considered of practical importance [122]. On further analysis it was concluded that if a physician wants to try a drug, Hy-

dergine is the only one approved for treatment of AD; it is quite safe and is therefore worth trying [123]. Although its mechanism of action is unknown and its effects probably relate more to alertness than to cognition, a trial of it, especially in the early stages of disease when small gains may make life better for the victim and family, is reasonable. Although it was initially used in doses of 1 to 3 mg daily, the greatest benefits have been documented when doses of 4.5 to 9.0 mg per day were administered. Starting with 1 mg daily, the dose should be increased by 1 mg per day each week until a dose of 6 mg per day is reached. Benefit, if it occurs, generally can be recognized within a month or two after reaching the target dose and may last as long as a year or longer. At higher doses, the only important (but rare) side effect is postural hypotension, and only if symptoms of this occur should the dose be reduced.

3. Monoamine oxidase (MAO) inhibition. CNS monoamines decline with age and MAO levels increase with age, and because of some reports of exaggerated decline of monoamines with AD it is hypothesized that some symptoms of AD may improve with MAOI therapy. The selective increase of MAO-B in aging brains led to a clinical trial in AD victims of L-deprenyl, a selective inhibitor of MAO-B at low doses (10 mg per day) [124]. In a double-blind, placebo-controlled, serial study, statistically significant objective improvement occurred in anxiety/depression, tension, and excitement, with practical clinical benefit and better cognitive performance in half the patients. It should be remembered that MAO inhibition is a standard treatment for depression, and although subjects were free of major psychiatric illness, improvement in depressive symptoms could have contributed to the benefits seen.

MULTIINFARCT DEMENTIA

Multiinfarct dementia (MID) accounts for approximately 10 percent of cases of progressive dementia, although some studies count far fewer cases [41]. MID is more common in men and tends to begin at a younger age than AD. Emphasized by Hachinski [125], MID is the result of repeated strokes, and postmortem examination shows multiple areas of infarcted, softened brain. A threshold phenomenon has been demonstrated, showing that dementia correlates with more than 50 ml of infarcted brain tissue. Most patients have antecedent hypertension or diabetes, and numerous characteristics of MID differentiate it clinically from AD [126], including (1) rapid onset, (2) stepwise fluctuating mental decline, (3) associated atherosclerotic pathology elsewhere in the body, (4) focal or lateralizing signs or symptoms, (5) diabetes or hypertension, (6) male sex, (7) marked emotional lability, and (8) pseudobulbar palsy. Certain patients show clinical features of both, and the brains of such patients may show features of both AD and MID at postmortem examination. Treatment of MID is limited primarily to prevention by detecting and controlling antecedent diabetes and hypertension. The recent decline in stroke incidence should reduce the future prevalence of MID.

MIXED DISEASE

Although patients with a mixed clinical picture of MID and AD may be easy to imagine, they are difficult to identify antemortem unless strokes are superimposed on previously diagnosed dementia in situations of prolonged clinical follow-up. Thus, a diagnosis of mixed disease is usually included only in autopsy series, and the findings are usually a surprise to clinicians. Mixed disease accounts for about 10 percent of cases in such series.

PARKINSON'S DISEASE

Although at one time there was debate about whether Parkinson's disease (PD) and AD, as two common diseases in old age, simply coincided frequently, it is now generally acknowledged that up to one-third of advanced PD patients will become cognitively impaired. Insidious in onset, the dementia is alleged to begin with nocturnal disorientation and progress to vivid hallucinations; it is often exacerbated by L-dopa and thus limits treatment.

CREUTZFELDT-JAKOB DISEASE

Creutzfeldt-Jakob disease (CJD) is a rare cause of the dementia syndrome that generally occurs in middle aged patients, although there is considerable variation in presenting age. In addition to dementia, patients commonly manifest cerebellar ataxia, myoclonic jerks, and seizures. Progression to death is rapid, usually within six months or less, although there is a variant of the disease in which patients survive up to a year or two following diagnosis. The brain shows spongiform degeneration (CJD is characterized as one of the spongiform encephalopathies). Senile plaques are found in CJD, but the abnormal filaments and thickened neurites of AD are absent. CJD has come to prominence in spite of its rarity because it is the first North American dementia proved to be caused by a slow virus, one that has been transmitted from human material to higher apes and other experimental animals, and it has subsequently been shown to be caused by a prion (see above under discussion of causes of AD).

Reports of accidental contagion, combined with the hardiness of the agent, have provoked discussion of precautions needed in dealing with afflicted patients [127]. Recommendations include careful handling of and avoiding exposure to CNS tissue, cerebrospinal fluid, and blood of victims. Skin contact requires only washing, but inoculation should be scrupulously guarded against. Postmortem central nervous specimens should be regarded as highly infectious. Patient isolation is not recommended. Although transmitted by a prion that is related to the agents of kuru and scrapie, an autosomally dominant mechanism of heritability has been documented as well, possibly suggesting an underlying genetic predisposition to infection.

KURU

Kuru is a progressive and lethal CNS degenerative disease found among the Fore tribespeople of eastern New Guinea. Earliest signs are ataxia, tremor, involuntary movements, and severe strabismus, followed later by dementia. Death from infectious complications usually occurs within a year. The pathology is of profound neuronal loss, glial proliferation, loss of myelinated fibers, and plaques with central amyloid. A prion etiology has been confirmed. Transmission, primarily among women, occurs by means of cannibalism, especially of undercooked brain; with increasing westernization, both cannibalism and kuru are disappearing.

PROGRESSIVE SUPRANUCLEAR PALSY

Progressive supranuclear palsy usually presents with severe balance and gait disorders, secondary falls, truncal rigidity, and progressive ophthalmoplegia. Whether patients truly have Parkinson's disease as a substrate or only appear to is uncertain. Dementia is generally mild and of secondary prominence. Neuropathology includes neurofibrillary tangles, but the helical filaments are not paired. Neuronal losses in the vestibular and ocular nuclei and in the midbrain are widespread. Anti-parkinsonian drugs may be helpful only on rare occasions.

PICK'S DISEASE

Pick's disease, a very rare disorder, is clinically indistinguishable from AD, but the pathology is unique. Atrophy is severe and grossly obvious, though it is confined in a highly visible, sharply marginated fashion to the anterior parts of the frontal and temporal lobes. Neurofibrillary tangles of unpaired filaments occur as in progressive supranuclear palsy. Densely packed argentophilic Pick bodies are seen in the cytoplasm, and in spite of microscopic disparities between them and AD tangles, they react with the same monoclonal antibody [128].

GERSTMANN-STRAUSSLER-SCHEINKER DISEASE

Gerstmann-Straussler-Scheinker disease is a familial disorder of midlife that has a protracted course lasting from many months to a decade, beginning with spinocerebellar ataxia and producing dementia later. The neuropathology includes extensive amyloid and spongiform degeneration.

DEMENTIA PUGILISTICA

The punch-drunk syndrome is a dementia afflicting boxers, usually well after cessation of prize fighting. A latent period of ten years or more has been documented. Although it is assumed that repeated brain trauma provokes this irreversible dementia, the brain pathology is not dominated by evidence of injury but rather by the appearance at postmortem examination of typical AD neurofibrillary tangles. AD plaques, however, are not found with increased frequency.

COST OF DEMENTIA CARE

The cost of care for AD victims alone, who account for more than two-thirds of those with primary dementia, has been emphasized appropriately in discussions urging more funding for research and training focused on dementia. Figures for 1986 range from 25 billion dollars [5] to 40 billion dollars [129], but these do not approach the 77 billion dollar figure calculated by the NIA, which considers indirect as well as direct service costs [28]. All of these are small compared with Stone's projection of 750 billion dollars in the year 2030, based on 7 percent inflation and 22 percent population over age 65 [129]. Between now and the year 2000, the number of individuals over the age of 80, those most likely to become demented, will double [130], thus placing a tremendous strain on the current service delivery system. Demented patients are at high risk for nursing home admission, and once admitted, they rarely leave before death. Sixty percent of nursing home residents are estimated to have dementia [5,131], and while still living in the community before nursing home admission, victims are more likely to require in-home supervision and services, resulting in increased demand for community-based services and increased burdens on family caregivers [132].

The true cost of dementia cannot be limited to dollar calculations for institutional care. This condition has devastating financial and social-psychologic impact on the family and friends who care for the victim as well as on the victim personally [132,133]. One study of family caregivers indicated that 87 percent reported fatigue, anger, or depression; 56 percent reported family conflicts; 29 percent reported troubles in assuming new roles and responsibilities; and only 7 percent reported no problems in caring for the victim [132]. Other studies cite a litany of mental and physical health symptoms resulting from the demands of caregiving, including depression, anxiety, frustration, helplessness, sleeplessness, lowered morale, alcohol and drug abuse, physical abuse, cardiac problems, and ulcer disease [134,135,136]. Contrary to popular myth, family caregivers are not rushing to dump impaired elders into nursing homes; 80 percent of community care is provided informally by family and friends. Unfortunately, little in the way of support for the care provider is currently available in most communities [134], and family providers may care for the elder at home until personal and emotional resources have been exhausted.

Delirium

DETECTION

Delirium is frequently misdiagnosed, often because its clinical picture is mistaken for dementia. Although both dementia and delirium are global disturbances of cognition, the two conditions reveal different patterns in onset and natural history, as shown in Table 27-2 [6]. The detection of delirium, even with an adequate history, can be complicated by the frequent concurrence of dementia and delirium [137]. Estimates indicate that approximately one-third of demented hospitalized geriatric patients are likely to have delirium superimposed on their dementia [46]. Lipowski [138] suggests that symptoms of confusion may be modified in the demented patient because the concurrent dementia limits the patient's ability to elaborate symptoms such as complex hallucinations, dream-like mentation, and confabulations. The demented patient may simply sink quietly and apathetically into an unresponsive state. The *Diagnostic and Statistical Manual of Mental Disorders* (third edition, revised) (DSM-III-R) definition is long (see Table 27-1), but one can usually assume that a patient is suffering from an acute confusional state if he or she has functioned well intellectually and then abruptly develops a cognitive-attentional disorder that fluctuates in severity during the day and worsens at night [138].

EPIDEMIOLOGY

Although the importance of acute confusional states among the aged is increasingly acknowledged, consistent epidemiologic data are not available. Incidence estimates vary widely because of the lack of precise diagnostic criteria, inconsistent use of terms, varying methods of case finding, and the different settings in which patients are studied [139]. Moreover, during the

25 years in which acute confusion has been studied, the terminology used by the American Psychiatric Association to define the syndrome has changed. Despite these methodologic problems, it appears that the disorder is highly prevalent among the hospitalized elderly. For a complete review of the epidemiology of delirium, a comprehensive review is suggested [140].

COURSE AND OUTCOME

The natural history of acute confusion is not well documented. By definition, the onset of the disorder is rapid, occurring over a few days or even hours. Kral [141] has suggested that the onset varies, depending both on the severity of the stress and on the stress resistance of the patient. During the day, the mildly confused patient may conceal deficits. A patient often first experiences the full-blown disorder during the night, perhaps being frightened after waking from a dream. The patient may become confused about place and often attempts to get out of bed. As the patient becomes more confused, symptoms are experienced more consistently, and inattention and disorientation are the rule. Although the majority of cases of acute confusion clear within one to two weeks after the underlying problem is detected and treated, episodes can last as long as a month. Prognosis is good for survivors, because the transition from an acute syndrome to dementia appears uncommon [138]. However, since the delirium may signal the onset or exacerbation of life-threatening physical illness, failure to diagnose and adequately treat the underlying disease can result in death.

More recent studies have also attempted to delineate the natural history of the condition. In a British multicenter study, 25 percent of individuals with an acute confusional state had died within one month of admission, 35 percent had been discharged, and 40 percent remained in the hospital, compared to 12 percent, 47 percent, and 41 percent, respectively, for mentally normal patients [142].

CAUSES

The potential causes of confusion include most clinical disorders as well as some not within the traditional confines of medicine [143]. By definition, the disorder requires cerebral dysfunction due to systemic or CNS disease, to ex-

ogenous physical or chemical agents, or to withdrawal from certain substances of abuse. However, little is known about the mechanisms producing delirium. Etiologic conditions are listed in Table 27-4.

Intoxication with drugs, particularly those with anticholinergic properties, is perhaps the single most frequent cause of acute confusion. Age-related changes in the metabolism, distribution, and excretion of drugs, coupled with high drug consumption and polypharmacy, are clearly related to the high incidence of drug-related acute confusion (see Chap. 9). Some of the drugs most often implicated in producing acute confusional states among the aged are included in Table 27-7.

PATHOPHYSIOLOGY

Although the literature identifies numerous clinical precipitants, little is known about the

TABLE 27-7. *Drugs associated with delirium in the elderly*

I. Psychoactive
  A. Sedatives/hypnotics
    1. Long-acting benzodiazepines (flurazepam [Dalmane], diazepam [Valium], chlordiazepoxide [Librium])
    2. Short-acting benzodiazepines (less often a problem)
    3. Barbiturates
  B. Antidepressants
    1. Heterocyclics, especially sedating (amitriptyline [Elavil], doxepin [Sinequan], trazadone [Desyrel])
    2. Lithium
  C. Neuroleptics (less common)
II. Medical agents
  A. Cardiac
    1. Digitalis glycosides
    2. Diuretics
    3. Antiarrhythmics (most)
    4. Calcium channel blockers
    5. Antihypertensives
      a. Beta blockers
      b. Alpha methyldopa
  B. Gastrointestinal
    1. H_2 antagonists (cimetidine, ranitidine)
    2. Metaclopramide (Reglan)
  C. Analgesics, especially narcotics and derivatives
  D. Antiinflammatory
    1. Corticosteroids
    2. Nonsteroidal antiinflammatory agents
III. Over-the-counter drugs
  A. Cold remedies (antihistamines, pseudoephedrine)
  B. Sedatives (antihistamines)
  C. Stay-awakes (caffeine)
  D. Antinauseants
  E. Alcohol

precise mechanisms by which these disorders cause acute confusion in the older patient. In 1959 Engel and Romano [144] postulated that a general reduction of cerebral metabolism, evidenced by a concurrent clouding of consciousness and slowing of EEG activity, may represent the final common pathway for most cases of acute confusion. It is probable that the aged are predisposed to acute confusion because of a number of age-related changes in psychologic, physiologic, anatomic, and biochemical factors in the brain as well as a number of nonneural factors [145]. Age-related psychologic changes, such as a reduced ability to process new information presented rapidly, increase the older patient's susceptibility to acute confusion. Structural changes of the aging brain, in which populations of nerve cells have fallen to a level critical for maintaining function, may allow a mild disorder to reduce function below the threshold at which clinical signs and symptoms of confusion develop [145].

Another interesting recent hypothesis [146] suggests a possible role for interleukin-1 (endogenous pyrogen) in the delirium of febrile and possibly other acute illnesses. Interleukin-1 (Il-1) is produced by numerous cells in response to varied toxic, infectious, and inflammatory stimuli. Among the many actions of Il-1, beyond producing hypothalamically mediated fever, is its capacity to increase slow wave sleep in experimental animals. The EEG pattern in slow wave sleep is similar to that seen in delirium, and thus Il-1 may be one mediator of delirium.

MANAGEMENT

Successful management of the acutely confused patient depends first on the correct identification of the clinical picture of delirium and second on the correct diagnosis of its specific etiology. Once a delirium is detected, it is imperative to look for all possible causes, because more than one etiologic factor may be implicated. A mnemonic, SUNDOWNERS, is offered by the author to identify factors that put patients at high risk for delirium (Table 27-8).

The value of the SUNDOWNERS mnemonic is severalfold. First, it reminds us that acute confusion, sometimes referred to as "sundowning," often begins at night, when reduced

TABLE 27-8. *Mnemonic: Sundowners*

Sick
Urinary retention/fecal impaction
New environment
Demented
Old
Writhing in pain
Not adequately evaluated
Eyes and ears
Rx—therapeutic drug intoxication
Sleep deprived

lighting and activity, combined with nadirs of several circadian hormones, conspire to make the aged brain even more vulnerable to misinterpretation of reality. Second, the mnemonic is a useful reminder that there may be remediable risk factors that, if addressed early in the course of hospitalization, may prevent or ameliorate an impending delirium. Thus, the mnemonic becomes a checklist, suggesting that to prevent delirium, one should begin by (1) treating *sickness,* (2) ruling out or relieving *urinary retention* or *fecal impaction,* (3) being sensitive to the psychic needs of the *newly admitted* elder in a new environment, (4) promptly identifying the patient with preexisting *dementia* and reducing confusing stimulation, (5) realizing that the very *old* patient is at high risk, (6) being particularly attentive to analgesics for the patient *writhing in pain,* (7) recognizing that patients *not adequately worked* up can have discoverable conditions whose treatment may prevent delirium, (8) supplying adequate sensory inputs to those with impairments in *eye or ear* function, (9) being aware of the great potential of many *therapeutic drugs (Rx)* in producing or contributing to delirium, and (10) preventing *sleep deprivation.* A third value of the mnemonic is to alert the clinical team to those patients who have risk factors for delirium that, although identified, are not remediable and therefore mark those individuals as especially likely to become acutely confused. Whether delirium can be prevented is uncertain and merits further investigation.

Treatment of the underlying pathology is the first and foremost action in management of delirium. A principle of geriatric medicine is that the classic presentation of disease is commonly replaced by nonspecific symptoms, and this is especially true for delirium (see Chap. 3). Whenever an older person presents with confusion, the search for physical illness, either acute or chronic with acute exacerbation, should begin immediately. Many acutely confused patients with reversible disorders go untreated because they are not properly worked up. The misidentification of the clinical picture of delirium as chronic dementia aborts the search for and treatment of an underlying reversible physical illness. Misdiagnosis of causation, such as the attribution of confusion to a psychosis brought on by a recent change in life events or psychosocial stress, can be disastrous by provoking the wrong treatment.

Drug toxicity is one of the most common preventable causes of acute confusion. Careful examination of all drugs taken by the patient is critical, and those drugs that can produce delirium should be eliminated to the extent possible. When the drug is considered essential, a reduction in the dosage may be sufficient to eliminate adverse effects. A useful strategy in the delirious old patient is to stop all drugs and resume those for which a clinical indication emerges, and then only at lower doses. It must always be kept in mind that the underlying cause of the acute confusional episode may be multifactorial; for example, drug toxicity could be implicated along with concomitant urinary infection that results from urinary retention and incontinence from fecal impaction. Maintenance of fluid and electrolyte balance and sound nutrition are important to prevent dehydration, hyponatremia or hypernatremia, malnutrition, and vitamin deficiencies, all of which can potentially contribute to acute confusion.

While identifying and treating the underlying cause or causes of delirium, symptomatic and supportive measures must be given equal attention because it often requires hours to days for treatment of the underlying cause to relieve delirium. Measures should be instituted to avoid extremes of sensory input, including deficient or excessive stimulation, since either is likely to exacerbate delirium and both are potentially preventable [147]. Eyeglasses and hearing aids, often left at home or in the nursing home during the hectic transfer to the acute care hospital, should be retrieved and provided to the patient as quickly as possible. Loud, disruptive noise should be eliminated when possible, but manageable sensory stimulation can help. Hospital staff should assume a calm and consistent approach toward confused patients, providing frequent reorientation and reassurance. Family members and friends should be encouraged to visit.

The physical environment of the patient also merits special attention. Abrupt relocation, especially at night, to a new and unfamiliar environment should be avoided. The patient should be placed in a safe and ordered environment with familiar personal objects, such as toiletries, bedclothes, photographs, and family mementos. The patient should rest in a quiet, well-lighted private room during the day and a dimly lighted room at night. Minimizing demands on impaired function can be achieved through the use of orienting devices such as written signs that give the place, date, time, and other necessary information. Staff should attempt to make the immediate environment as constant as possible, avoiding room changes and providing labels for the bathroom, the patient's closet, and even the bed or other pertinent objects. Nursing routines and personnel should be adjusted to make them as consistent as possible. Safety precautions such as bed side rails and close observation are imperative during periods of confusion. In some cases, restraints may be unavoidable to protect the patient; when considered necessary, they should be accompanied by frequent explanations of their purpose and by close monitoring [148].

Drug therapy is an important aspect of the management of the acutely confused agitated patient, and several different classes of drugs are commonly employed. Benzodiazepines should be used only for minor degrees of agitation or anxiety because they themselves may cause excessive drowsiness or paradoxical agitation. Shorter acting agents, including lorazepam and oxazepam, are preferred when a benzodiazepine is tried.

The neuroleptics are usually preferred in delirious patients because they help organize thinking and diminish hallucinations and delusions. Individual agents can be selected for varying degrees of sedation as required by the patient's condition. These drugs have a prolonged clearance time in the aged, and elderly individuals show earlier and greater sensitivity to adverse effects, necessitating lower doses than those used in younger individuals. The aged are more susceptible to the side effects of neuroleptics, perhaps in part because of reduced CNS levels of acetylcholine and dopamine. The choice of drug depends on the side effects that are most necessary to minimize and the degree to which certain side effects are desirable. Some agents have higher anticholinergic potential and sedating effects and may cause orthostatic hypotension. Other drugs, with a lower anticholinergic potential, have serious extrapyramidal side effects, including akathisia, parkinsonism, and tardive dyskinesia.

For the elderly hospitalized patient with underlying dementia who becomes acutely confused, a sedating neuroleptic is generally desirable because of the high degree of agitation usually accompanying delirium; thioridazine (Mellaril) is a reasonable choice. Concern over an anticholinergic effect should not be excessive with use of thioridazine. Although thioridazine is the most anticholinergic of the currently used neuroleptics, its atropine equivalence is only 0.003 mg per mg; thus each 10-mg dose of thioridazine yields the effect of 0.03 mg atropine. For comparison, the least anticholinergic agent among the tricyclic antidepressant drugs, desipramine, is used with enthusiasm in elderly patients, in part because of its minimal anticholinergic side effects, yet its atropine equivalence is identical with that of thioridazine, 0.003 mg per mg. Accordingly, it seems reasonable to use thioridazine if its sedating side effects are indicated, especially in the agitated, delirious, already demented elderly patient. The initial dose should be 5 mg, and the behavioral and physiologic effect should be carefully observed. If the liquid concentrate is used, the dose may be doubled as early as 20 to 30 minutes after the first administration in urgent clinical situations. If the patient weighs more than 100 pounds, 10 mg usually may be given safely as the first dose. Most patients will respond to a dose of 10 to 30 mg during the delirious episode, but 50 mg or more may be required in some instances. These dose ranges are much lower than those commonly used in younger adult psychotic patients, but they are usually quite sufficient in frail and previously demented elderly who most often exhibit sundowning in the acute care hospital. Patients frequently require administration of the neuroleptic drug for several days following the first episode, and common sense titration is the rule. In the high-risk patient, it may be a useful strategy to give a small dose (5–10 mg) of thioridazine in the afternoon or early evening if mild agitation or confusion begins to appear in an attempt to prevent the development of a more florid syndrome.

For the patient who has had no previous cognitive impairment or in whose delirium agitation is not prominent, an agent without sedating effect may be preferred. Haloperidol (Haldol) is the least anticholinergic, least sedating of the neuroleptics, but it has the most intense and frequent extrapyramidal side effects. If thioridazine is too sedating and haloperidol not sufficiently sedating, acetophenazine (Tindal), an agent midway between the poles of the first two, may provide the desired effect. When oral administration is prevented by combativeness or lack of cooperation, thorazine in 5- to 10-mg increments, or haloperidol in 0.25- to 1.0-mg increments, can be given intramuscularly.

Several general principles are useful in administering neuroleptic drugs to elderly delirious patients:

1. The initial dose should be half of the smallest dose supplied by the manufacturer, followed by careful continuing assessment of the effect.
2. Expect that the effective dose, if administered for more than a few days consecutively, will probably lead to side effects, especially excess sedation, and will need to be reduced.
3. The beneficial effect on behavior is limited to the period during which delirium is present, and thus the neuroleptic should usually be stopped during hospitalization as delirium abates.

The beta blockers may be valuable in treating chronic confusional states. They are particularly useful in patients with outbursts of rage. The therapeutic range for propranolol may be as high as 80 to 200 mg per day, but the starting dose should be 10 mg three times a day.

Thus, a variety of management strategies are useful for the acutely confused patient, both during evaluation and after treatment of the underlying cause is begun. Supportive and symptomatic measures should be given as much attention as drug therapy. Only when all measures are employed in a coordinated and sensible way can success be anticipated in managing these most challenging and vulnerable elderly patients.

References

1. Brocklehurst, J. C., and Hanley, T. *Geriatric Medicine for Students.* Edinburgh: Churchill Livingstone, 1976.
2. Cowell, D. Senile dementia of the Alzheimer's type: A costly problem. *J. Am. Geriatr. Soc.* 31(1):61, 1983.
3. Gurland, B., and Cross, P. Epidemiology of psychopathology in old age. *Psychiatr. Clin. North Am.* 5:11, 1982.
4. Brody, J. An epidemiologist views senile dementia—facts and fragments. *Am. J. Epidemiol.* 115 (2):155, 1982.
5. Katzman, R. Alzheimer's disease. *N. Engl. J. Med.* 314:964, 1986.
6. Wetle, T. (ed.). *Handbook of Geriatric Care.* New Jersey: Sandoz Pharmaceuticals, 1982.
7. Prichard, J. C. *A Treatise on Insanity and Other Disorders Affecting the Mind.* London: Sherwood, Gilbert and Piper, 1835.
8. Alzheimer, A. Über eine eigenartige Erkrangkung der Hirnrinde. *All. Z. Psychiatr.* 64:146, 1907.
9. American Psychiatric Association. *Diagnostic and Statistical Manual of Mental Disorders* (3rd ed., revised). Washington, D.C.: American Psychiatric Association, 1987.
10. Wolman, B. B. *Handbook of Developmental Psychology.* Englewood Cliffs, NJ: Prentice-Hall, 1982.
11. Birren, J. E., Cunningham, W. R., and Yamamoto, K. Psychology of adult development and aging. *Ann. Rev. Psychol.* 34:543, 1983.
12. Birren, J. E., and Schaie, K. W. (eds.). *Handbook of the Psychology of Aging* (2nd ed.). New York: Van Nostrand Reinhold, 1985.
13. Poon, L. W. (ed.). *Aging in the 1980's: Psychological Issues.* Washington, D.C.: American Psychiatric Association, 1980.
14. Schaie, K. W., and Hertzog, C. Fourteen-year cohort sequential analyses of adult intellectual development. *Dev. Psychol.* 19:531, 1983.
15. Schaie, K. W., and Willis, S. L. Can decline in adult intellectual functioning be reversed? *Dev. Psychol.* 22:223, 1986.
16. Cornoni-Huntley, J., et al. *Established Populations for Epidemiologic Studies of the Elderly.* National Institute of Aging, U.S. Department of Health and Human Services, NIH Publication No. 86-2443, 1986.
17. Henderson, A. S. The epidemiology of Alzheimer's disease. *Br. Med. Bull.* 42:3, 1986.
18. Akesson, H. O. A population study of senile and arteriosclerotic psychoses. *Hum. Hered.* 19:546, 1969.
19. Bergman, K., et al. A Follow-up Study of Randomly Selected Community Residents to Assess the Effects of Chronic Brain Syndrome and Cerebrovascular Disease. In R. de la Fuente and M. N. Weisman (eds.), Psychiatry 2. Proceedings of the Fifth World Congress of Psychiatry, Mexico, 1971. Amsterdam: Excerpta Medica, 1973. P. 856.
20. Mortimer, J. A., Schuman, L. M., and French, L. R. Epidemiology of Dementing Illness. In J. A. Mortimer and L. M. Schuman (eds.), *The Epidemiology of Dementia.* New York: Oxford University Press, 1981.
21. Hagnell, O., et al. Does the incidence of age psychosis decrease? A prospective, longitudinal study of a complete population investigated during the 25-year period 1947–1972: The Lundby study. *Neuropsychobiology* 7:201, 1981.
22. Hagnell, O., et al. Current trends in the incidence of senile and multi-infarct dementia. *Arch. Psychiatry Neurol. Sci.* 233:423, 1983.
23. Sayetta, R. B. Rates of senile dementia-Alzheimer's type in the Baltimore longitudinal study. *J. Chronic Dis.* 39:271, 1986.
24. Gilmore, A. Community Surveys and Mental Health. In W. Anderson and T. Judge (eds.), *Geriatric Medicine.* New York: Academic Press, 1974.
25. Katzman, R. The prevalence and malignancy of Alzheimer disease: A major killer. *Arch. Neurol.* 33:217, 1976.
26. Gruenberg, E. M. Epidemiology of Senile Dementia. In B. S. Schoenberg (ed.), *Advances in Neurology.* New York: Raven, 1978.
27. United States Senate, Subcommittee on Aging of the Committee on Labor and Human Resources. *Oversight on Treatment of Alzheimer's Disease.* Washington, D.C.: U.S. Government Printing Office, 1983.
28. U.S. Department of Health and Human Services. Progress report on Alzheimer's Disease: III. National Institute on Aging, Public Health Service, NIH Publication No. 86-2873, 1986.
29. Larsson, T., Sjögren, T., and Jacobson, G. Senile dementia. A clinical, sociomedical and genetic study. *Acta Psychiatr. Scand.* Suppl. 167:1, 1963.
30. Sjögren, T., Sjögren, H., and Lindgren, A. G. H. Morbus Alzheimer and Morbus Pick. A genetic, clinical and patho-anatomical study. *Acta Psychiatr. Neurol. Scand.* 82 (Suppl.):1, 1952.

31. Heston, L. L., et al. Dementia of the Alzheimer type: Clinical genetics, natural history and associated conditions. *Arch. Gen. Psychiatry* 38:1085, 1981.

32. Heyman, A., et al. Alzheimer's disease: Genetic aspects and associated clinical disorders. *Ann. Neurol.* 14:507, 1983.

33. Heyman, A., et al. Alzheimer's disease. A study of epidemiological aspects. *Ann. Neurol.* 15:335, 1984.

34. Mohs, R. C., et al. Alzheimer's disease: Morbid risk among first-degree relatives approximates 50% by 90 years of age. *Arch. Gen. Psychiatry* 44:405, 1987.

35. Mortimer, J. A., et al. Head injury as a risk factor for Alzheimer's disease. *Neurology* 35:264, 1985.

36. Seltzer, B., and Sherwin, I. A comparison of clinical features in early- and late-onset primary degenerative dementia: One entity or two? *Arch. Neurol.* 40:143, 1983.

37. Huff, J. F., et al. Age at onset and rate of progression of Alzheimer's disease. *J. Am. Geriatr. Soc.* 35:27, 1987.

38. Folstein, M. F., Folstein, S. E., and McHugh, P. R. "Mini-mental state": A practical method for grading the cognitive state of patients for the clinician. *J. Psychiatr. Res.* 12:189, 1975.

39. Vitaliano, P. P., et al. The clinical utility of the dementia rating scale for assessing Alzheimer patients. *J. Chronic Dis.* 37:743, 1984.

40. National Institute on Aging Task Force. Senility reconsidered: Treatment possibilities for mental impairment in the elderly. *J.A.M.A.* 244:259, 1980.

41. Larson, E., et al. Diagnostic evaluation of 200 elderly outpatients with suspected dementia. *J. Gerontol.* 40:536, 1985.

42. Kampmeier, R. H. Diagnosis and treatment of physical disease in the mentally ill. *Ann. Intern. Med.* 86:637, 1977.

43. Robinson, R. A. Differential diagnosis and assessment in brain failure. *Age Ageing* (Suppl.) 6:42, 1977.

44. Larson, E. B., et al. Dementia in elderly outpatients: A prospective study. *Ann. Intern. Med.* 100:417, 1984.

45. Fox, J. H., Topel, J. L., and Huckman, M. S. Dementia in the elderly—a search for treatable illness. *J. Gerontol.* 34:557, 1975.

46. Organic impairment in the elderly. *J. R. Coll. Physicians Lond.* 15:141, 1981.

47. Ford, C. V., and Winter, J. Computerized axial tomograms and dementia in elderly patients. *J. Gerontol.* 36:164, 1981.

48. Gado, M., et al. Volumetric measurements of the cerebrospinal fluid spaces in demented subjects and controls. *Radiology* 144:535, 1982.

49. Beck, J. C., et al. Dementia in the elderly: The silent epidemic. *Ann. Intern. Med.* 97:231, 1982.

50. Freemon, F. R. Evaluation of patients with progressive intellectual deterioration. *Arch. Neurol.* 37:658, 1976.

51. Freemon, F. R., and Rudd, S. M. Clinical features that predict potentially reversible progressive intellectual deterioration. *J. Am. Geriatr. Soc.* 30:449, 1982.

52. Lawton, M. P. Psychosocial and Environmental Approaches to the Care of Senile Dementia Patients. In J. O. Cole and J. E. Barrett (eds.), *Psychopathology in the Aged*. New York: Raven, 1980.

53. Cassell, C. K., and Jameton, A. L. Dementia and the elderly: An analysis of medical responsibility. *Ann. Intern. Med.* 94:802, 1981.

54. Winograd, C., and Jarvik, L. Physician management of the demented patient. *J. Am. Geriatr. Soc.* 34:295, 1986.

55. Glosser, G., Wexler, D., and Balmelli, M. Physicians' and families' perspectives on the medical management of dementia. *J. Am. Geriatr. Soc.* 33:383, 1985.

56. McEvoy, C. L., and Patterson, R. L. Behavioral treatment of deficit skills in dementia patients. *Gerontologist* 26:475, 1986.

57. Rabins, P. V. Management of irreversible dementia. *Psychosomatics* 22:591, 1981.

58. Cummings, J., Benson, D. F., and LoVerme, S., Jr. Reversible dementia: Illustrative cases and review. *J.A.M.A.* 243:2434, 1980.

59. Roth, M. The natural history of mental disorder in old age. *J. Mental Sci.* 101:281, 1955.

60. Kidd, M. Paired helical filaments in electron microscopy of Alzheimer's disease. *Nature* 197:192, 1963.

61. Terry, R. D., Gonatas, N. K., and Weiss, M. Ultrastructural studies in Alzheimer's presenile dementia. *Am. J. Pathol.* 44:269, 1964.

62. Blessed, G., Tomlinson, B. E., and Roth, M. The association between quantitative measures of dementia and of senile change in the cerebral grey matter of elderly subjects. *Br. J. Psychiatry* 114:797, 1968.

63. Ron, M. A., et al. Diagnostic accuracy in presenile dementia. *Br. J. Psychiatry* 134:161, 1979.

64. McKhann, G., et al. Clinical diagnosis of Alzheimer's disease: Report of the NINCDS-ADRDA Work Group. *Neurology* 34:939, 1984.

65. Shuttleworth, E. C. Atypical presentations of dementia of the Alzheimer type. *J. Am. Geriatr. Soc.* 32:485, 1984.

66. Fillit, H. M., et al. Antivascular antibodies in the

sera of patients with senile dementia of the Alzheimer's type. *J. Gerontol.* 42:180, 1987.

67. Wolozin, B. L. A neuronal antigen in the brains of Alzheimer patients. *Science* 232:648, 1986.

68. Amato, I. Alzheimer's disease: Scientists report research advances. *Science News* 130:327, 1986.

69. Foster, N. L., et al. Cortical abnormalities in Alzheimer's disease. *Ann. Neurol.* 16:649, 1984.

70. Francis, P. T., et al. Neurochemical studies of early-onset Alzheimer's disease: Possible influence on treatment. *N. Engl. J. Med.* 313:7, 1985.

71. Reisberg, B., et al. Global deterioration scale (GDS) for age-associated cognitive decline and Alzheimer's disease. *Am. J. Psychiatry* 139:1136, 1982.

72. Mesulam, M. M. Dementia: Its definition, differential diagnosis and subtypes (editorial). *J.A.M.A.* 253:2559, 1985.

73. Peck, A., Wolloch, L., and Rodstein, M. Mortality of the aged with chronic brain syndrome. *J. Am. Geriatr. Soc.* 21:264, 1973.

74. Vitaliano, P. P., et al. Dementia and other competing risks for mortality in the institutionalized aged. *J. Am. Geriatr. Soc.* 29:513, 1981.

75. Arie, T. Pseudodementia (editorial). *Br. Med. J.* 286:1301, 1983.

76. Kiloh, L. G. Pseudo-dementia. *Acta Psychiatr. Neurolog.* 37:336, 1961.

77. Reding, M., Haycox, J., and Blass, J. Depression in patients referred to a dementia clinic: A three-year prospective study. *Arch. Neurol.* 42:894, 1985.

78. Reifler, B. V., et al. Dementia of the Alzheimer's type and depression. *J. Am. Geriatr. Soc.* 34:859, 1986.

79. Tomlinson, B. E., Blessed, G., and Roth, M. Observations on the brain in non-demented old people. *J. Neurol. Sci.* 7:331, 1968.

80. Dekaban, A. S., and Sadowsky, D. Changes in brain weights during the span of human life: Relation of brain weights to body heights and body weights. *Ann. Neurol.* 4:345, 1978.

81. Terry, R., and Katzman, R. Senile Dementia of the Alzheimer Type: Defining a Disease. In R. Katzman and R. Terry (eds.), *Neurology of Aging.* Philadelphia: F. A. Davis, 1983.

82. Terry, R. D. The fine structure of neurofibrillary tangles in Alzheimer's disease. *J. Neuropathol. Exp. Neurol.* 22:629, 1963.

83. Anderton, B. H., et al. Monoclonal antibodies show that neurofibrillary tangles and neurofilaments share antigenic determinants. *Nature* 298:84, 1982.

84. Ihara, Y., Abraham, C., and Selkoe, D. J. Antibodies to paired helical filaments in Alzheimer's disease do not recognize normal brain proteins. *Nature* 304:727, 1983.

85. Iqbal, K., et al. Neurofibrillary Pathology: An Update. In K. Nandy and I. Sherwin (eds.), *The Aging Brain and Senile Dementia.* New York: Plenum, 1977.

86. Selkoe, D., et al. Conservation of brain amyloid proteins in aged mammals and humans with Alzheimer's disease. *Science* 235:873, 1987.

87. Miyakawa, T., et al. The relationship between senile plaques and cerebral blood vessels in Alzheimer's disease and senile dementia. *Virchows Arch. [B]* 40:121, 1982.

88. Peress, N. S., Kane, W. C., and Aronson, S. M. Central nervous system findings in a tenth decade autopsy population. *Progr. Brain Res.* 40:473, 1973.

89. Katzman, R., et al. What is the Significance of the Neurotransmitter Abnormalities in Alzheimer's Disease? In J. B. Martin and J. Barchas (eds.), *Neuropeptides in Neurologic and Psychiatric Disease.* New York: Raven, 1986.

90. Brun, A. The structural development of Alzheimer's disease. *Dan. Med. Bull.* 32:(Suppl. 1) 25, 1985.

91. Ball, M. J., and Lo, P. Granulovacuolar degeneration in the ageing brain and in dementia. *J. Neuropathol. Exp. Neurol.* 36:474, 1977.

92. Anderson, J. M., et al. The effect of advanced old age on the neurone content of the cerebral cortex. Observations with an automatic image analyser point counting method. *J. Neurol. Sci.* 58:235, 1983.

93. Brody, H., and Vijayashankar, N. Anatomical Changes in the Nervous System. In C. E. Finch and L. Hayflick (eds.), *Handbook of the Biology of Aging.* New York: Van Nostrand, 1977.

94. Creasy, H., and Rapoport, S. I. The aging human brain. *Ann. Neurol.* 17:2, 1985.

95. Terry, R. D., et al. Some morphometric aspects of the brain in senile dementia of the Alzheimer type. *Ann. Neurol.* 10:184, 1981.

96. Hyman, B. T., et al. Alzheimer's disease: Cell-specific pathology isolates the hippocampal formation. *Science* 225:1168, 1984.

97. Davies, P., and Maloney, A. J. F. Selective loss of central cholinergic neurons in Alzheimer's disease. *Lancet* 2:1403, 1976.

98. Perry, E. K., et al. Correlation of cholinergic abnormalities with senile plaques and mental test scores in senile dementia. *Br. Med. J.* 2:1457, 1978.

99. Davies, P., and Verth, A. H. Regional distribution of muscarinic acetylcholine receptor in normal and Alzheimer's-type dementia brains. *Brain Res.* 138:385, 1977.

100. Mash, D. C., Flynn, D. D., and Potter, L. T. Loss of M2 muscarine receptors in the cerebral cortex in Alzheimer's disease and experimental cholinergic denervation. *Science* 228:1115, 1985.

101. Coyle, J. T., Price, D. L., and Delong, M. R. Alzheimer's disease: A disorder of cortical cholinergic innervation. *Science* 219:1184, 1983.

102. Davies, P., Katzman, R., and Terry, R. D. Reduced somatostatin-like immunoreactivity in cerebral cortex from cases of Alzheimer disease and Alzheimer senile dementia. *Nature* 288:279, 1980.

103. Bartus, R. T., et al. The cholinergic hypothesis in geriatric memory dysfunction. *Science* 217:408, 1982.

104. Nee, L., et al. A family with histologically confirmed Alzheimer's disease. *Arch. Neurol.* 40:203, 1983.

105. Goudsmit, J. A. A. P., et al. Familial Alzheimer's disease in two kindreds of the same geographic and ethnic origin: A clinical and genetic study. *J. Neurol. Sci.* 49:79, 1981.

106. Harris, R. Genetics of Alzheimer's disease. *Br. Med. J.* 284:1065, 1982.

107. Burger, P. C., and Vogel, F. S. The development of the pathologic changes in Alzheimer's disease and senile dementia in patients with Down's syndrome. *Am. J. Pathol.* 73:457, 1973.

108. Yates, C. M., et al. Alzheimer-like cholinergic deficiency in Down syndrome. *Lancet* 2:979, 1980.

109. Glenner, G. G., and Wong, C. W. Alzheimer's disease and Down's syndrome: Sharing of a unique cerebrovascular amyloid fibril protein. *Biochem. Biophys. Res. Commun.* 122:1131, 1984.

110. Karlinsky, H. Alzheimer's disease in Down's syndrome. *J. Am. Geriatr. Soc.* 34:728, 1986.

111. St. George-Hyslop, P. H., et al. The genetic defect causing familial Alzheimer's disease maps on chromosome 21. *Science* 235:885, 1987.

112. Goldgaber, D., et al. Characterization and chromosomal localization of a cDNA encoding brain amyloid of Alzheimer's disease. *Science* 235:877, 1987.

113. Tanzi, R. E., et al. Amyloid B protein gene: $_c$DNA, $_m$RNA distribution, and genetic linkage near the Alzheimer locus. *Science* 235:880, 1987.

114. St. George-Hyslop, P. H., et al. Absence of duplication of chromosome 21 genes in familial and sporadic Alzheimer's disease. *Science* 238:664, 1987.

115. Divry, P. Considerations sur le viellissement cerebral. *J. Belge. Neurol. Psychiatry* 47:65, 1947.

116. Prusiner, S. B. Some speculations about prions, amyloid, and Alzheimer's disease. *N. Engl. J. Med.* 310:661, 1984.

117. Gajdusek, D. C. Hypothesis: Interference with axonal transport of neurofilament as a common pathogenetic mechanism in certain diseases of the central nervous system. *N. Engl. J. Med.* 312:714, 1985.

118. Stotsky, B. Multicenter study comparing thioridazine with diazepam and placebo in elderly, non-psychotic patients with emotional and behavioral disorders. *Clin. Ther.* 6:546, 1984.

119. Mace, N. L., and Rabins, P. V. *The 36-Hour Day: A Family Guide to Caring for Persons with Alzheimer's Disease.* Baltimore: Johns Hopkins University Press, 1981.

120. Summers, W. K., et al. Oral tetrahydroaminoacridine in long-term treatment of senile dementia, Alzheimer type. *N. Engl. J. Med.* 315:1241, 1986.

121. Harbaugh, R. E., et al. Preliminary report: Intracranial cholinergic drug infusion in patients with Alzheimer's disease. *Neurosurgery* 15:514, 1984.

122. Yesavage, J. A., et al. Vasodilators in senile dementias: A review of the literature. *Arch. Gen. Psychiatry* 36:220, 1979.

123. Hollister, L. E., and Yesavage, J. Ergoloid mesylates for senile dementias: Unanswered questions. *Ann. Intern. Med.* 100:894, 1984.

124. Tariot, P. N., et al. L-Deprenyl in Alzheimer's disease. *Arch. Gen. Psychiatry* 44:427, 1987.

125. Hachinski, V., Lassen, M. A., and Marshall, J. Multi-infarct dementia. *Lancet* 2:207, 1974.

126. Hachinski, V., et al. Cerebral blood flow in dementia. *Arch. Neurol.* 32:632, 1975.

127. Gajdusek, D. C., et al. Precautions in medical care of, and in handling materials from, patients with transmissible virus dementia. *N. Engl. J. Med.* 297:1253, 1977.

128. Rasool, C. G., and Selkoe, D. J. Sharing of specific antigens by degenerating neurons in Pick's disease and Alzheimer's disease. *N. Engl. J. Med.* 312:700, 1985.

129. Stone, J. H. Editorial. *Business and Health.* Sept. 1986, p. 34.

130. Brody, E., Lawton, M., and Liebowitz, B. Senile dementia: Public policy and adequate institutional care. *Am. J. Public Health* 74(12):1381, 1984.

131. Kay, D., and Bergman, K. Epidemiology of Mental Disorders Among the Aged in the Community. In J. Birren and B. Sloane (eds.), *Handbook of Mental Health and Aging.* Englewood Cliffs, NJ: Prentice-Hall, 1980.

132. Rabins, P., Mace, N., and Lucas, M. The im-

pact of dementia on the family. *J.A.M.A.* 248:333, 1982.

133. Campbell, A., et al. Dementia in old age and the need for services. *Age Ageing* 12:11, 1983.

134. Brody, E. Parent care as a normative family stress. *Gerontologist* 25(1):19, 1985.

135. Cantor, M. Strain among caregivers: A study of experience in the United States. *Gerontologist* 23:597, 1983.

136. Deimling, G., and Bass, D. Symptoms of mental impairment among elderly adults and their effects on family caregivers. *J. Gerontol.* 41:778, 1986.

137. Wolfson, L. I., and Katzman, R. The Neurologic Consultation at Age 80. In R. Katzman and R. D. Terry (eds.), *The Neurology of Aging*. Philadelphia: F. A. Davis, 1983.

138. Lipowski, Z. J. Transient cognitive disorders (delirium, acute confusional states) in the elderly. *Am. J. Psychiatry* 140(11):1426, 1983.

139. Lipowski, Z. J. Acute Confusional States (Delirium) in the Elderly. In M. L. Albert (ed.), *Clinical Neurology of Aging*. Boston: Oxford University Press, 1984.

140. Levkoff, S. E., Besdine, R. W., and Wetle, T. Acute confusional states (delirium) in the hospitalized elderly. *Ann. Rev. Gerontol. Geriatr.* 6:1, 1986.

141. Kral, V. A. Confusional States: Description and Management. In J. G. Howells (ed.), *Perspectives in the Psychiatry of Old Age*. New York: Brunner/Mazel, 1975.

142. Hodkinson, H. M. Mental impairment in the elderly. *J. R. Coll. Physicians Lond.* 7:305, 1973.

143. Arie, T. Confusion in old age. *Age Ageing* (Suppl.) 7:72, 1978.

144. Engel, G. L., and Romano, J. Delirium, a syndrome of cerebral insufficiency. *J. Chronic Dis.* 9:260, 1959.

145. Blass, J. P., and Plum, F. Metabolic Encephalopathies. In R. Katzman and T. D. Terry (eds.), *The Neurology of Aging*. Philadelphia: F. A. Davis, 1983.

146. Krueger, J. M. Sleep-promoting effects of endogenous pyrogen (interleukin-1). *Am. J. Physiol.* 246(15):994, 1984.

147. Trockman, G. Caring for the confused or delirious patient. *Am. J. Nurs.* 78:1495, 1978.

148. Boss, B. J. Acute mood and behavior disturbances of neurological origin: Acute confusional states. *Neurosurg. Nurs.* 14(2):61, 1982.

28

Endocrine Systems

GRAYDON S. MENEILLY
SUSAN L. GREENSPAN
JOHN W. ROWE
KENNETH L. MINAKER

Thyroid Function and Disease

The prevalence of thyroid disease in the elderly population is approximately twice that of the younger population, with estimates of 3 to 4 percent for both hypothyroidism and hyperthyroidism [1,2]. In hospitalized elderly patients up to 9 percent may have overt thyroid disease [3]. Thyroid disease in the elderly differs from that in the young because the symptoms and presentations are nonspecific, atypical, often confused with nonthyroidal illness, and usually attributed to old age. These age-related differences are based on physiologic, pathologic, and pharmacologic factors. Because of homeostenosis (reduction in reserve capacity of each organ system), the physiologic presentation of thyroid disease often centers around the most compromised organ system. Elderly patients often have multiple concurrent diseases with signs that can *mimic* or *mask* thyroid disease. For example, tachycardia in a young patient is a sensitive indicator for hyperthyroidism. However, tachycardia in an older subject is more often related to underlying coronary artery disease and conduction disturbances. Coarse hair, dry skin, and constipation are common in euthyroid elderly, and when hyperthyroidism develops in this age group the fine hair, moist skin, and diarrhea that are characteristic in the younger hyperthyroid population are often not seen. Finally, elderly patients are much more likely to be taking pharmacologic agents that confuse the presentation of hyperthyroidism, such as beta blockers, sympathomimetics, and benzodiazepines.

In general, normal aging has no significant effect on thyroid function. The hypothalamus releases thyrotropin-releasing hormone (TRH), which stimulates the anterior pituitary gland to produce thyrotropin or thyroid-stimulating hormone (TSH). TSH release is pulsatile [4] and stimulates thyroidal synthesis and release of thyroxine (T_4) and triiodothyronine (T_3). Although T_4 is produced only in the thyroid gland, only about 20 percent of the more physiologically potent T_3 is of thyroid origin; 80 percent of T_3 originates from peripheral conversion of T_4 to T_3. The circulatory levels of T_4 and T_3 then feed back in a negative fashion at the level of the pituitary and hypothalamus to regulate thyroid hormone.

THYROID FUNCTION TESTS

With normal aging there is no significant change in serum levels of T_4, T_3RU (T_3 resin uptake), free T_4, or the free T_4 index (FT_4I) [5]. Although T_4 clearance is decreased, it is coupled with a decrease in synthesis of serum T_4, resulting in no major overall change in serum levels [6]. There is a minor age-related decrease in serum T_3; however, values remain within the range of normal limits [5]. Basal serum TSH,

402

the most sensitive test of thyroid status, is either unchanged or slightly increased (but still within normal limits) [5]. There is no consensus on the influence of age on TRH-stimulated TSH. Most recent evidence indicates that the test does not vary with age.

The 24-hour test of thyroid uptake of radioiodine is unchanged with age. Thyroid antibodies occur more commonly in the elderly population [7], but antibodies are not a good screening test for thyroid disease because up to one-third of patients with hypothyroidism do not have antibodies [8].

HYPERTHYROIDISM
Clinical Evaluation
Elderly hyperthyroid patients are more likely to present with symptoms focusing on the most frail organ system. In general, they present with cardiovascular symptoms (atrial fibrillation, congestive heart failure, angina, acute myocardial infarction), central nervous system symptoms (apathy, depression, confusion, lassitude), or gastrointestinal symptoms (constipation, failure to thrive, anorexia). Weight loss, anorexia, and weakness often initiate lengthy and unnecessary workups for occult malignancy. Older patients are much less likely to present with symptoms commonly found in younger adults such as sinus tachycardia (because of conduction system disease or beta blockers) and diarrhea (constipation is more common) [9,10].

The physical examination of an elderly hyperthyroid patient is very different from that of a young patient. Resting tachycardia is less common, and ophthalmopathy is rare because of the etiology of hyperthyroidism. Although Graves' disease, an autoimmune-induced hyperthyroidism, occurs in the elderly and may produce ophthalmopathy, toxic multinodular goiter and the toxic nodule are much more common in this age group and do not result in the impressive eye findings characteristic of younger adults. In contrast to the young, who almost uniformly have enlarged thyroid glands, two-thirds of elderly patients have thyroid glands that are normal or not palpable. Finally, tremor, which is a sensitive indicator of disease in the young, is common in older patients and usually is not related to thyroid disease.

TABLE 28-1. *The effects of medications and dyes on thyroid function tests*

DRUG	SERUM T_4	SERUM T_3	T_3RU	SERUM TSH
Propranolol	N or ↑	↓	N	N
Dilantin	↓	N or ↓	N or ↑	N or ↓
Estrogens	↑	↑	↓	N
Glucocorticoids	N or ↓	↓	N or ↑	↓
Dopamine	↓	↓	N	↓
Radiopaque dyes	N or ↑	↓	N	↑, N, ↓*

Key: N = no change.
*If subjects become hyperthyroid the serum TSH will be depressed.

Laboratory Evaluation
The diagnosis is confirmed by obtaining elevated values for the serum T_4, T_3RU, and total T_3 tests. The serum TSH should be undetectable. Although usually unnecessary, a flattened TRH test will also confirm the diagnosis. The etiology can then be clarified with a radioactive iodine uptake test. However, there are potential difficulties in making the diagnosis. T_3 toxicosis may be more difficult to diagnose because nonthyroidal illness will depress T_3 first. The diagnosis can be confusing in patients who have chemical hyperthyroxinemia due to nonthyroidal illness (see later section, Nonthyroidal Illness—High T_4 Syndrome). Elderly patients may be taking medications (e.g., propranolol) that can iatrogenically elevate T_4 (Table 28-1). However, the most common confounding event occurs after a radiocontrast study; T_4 may then be temporarily elevated due to iodine-induced hyperthyroidism.

Treatment
Radioiodine (^{131}I) therapy is the most efficient, uncomplicated, and inexpensive definitive treatment in this age group. Radiation-related concerns are not issues in this age group, and radiation thyroiditis can be avoided by a short pretreatment course with antithyroid agents such as propylthiouracil or methimazole. Following treatment with radioactive iodine, patients usually become euthyroid over a period of 6 to 12 weeks. They should then be followed carefully, checking the free T_4 index and serum TSH levels once or twice a year because hypothyroidism will ultimately develop in 80 per-

cent or more of patients who are treated adequately. Antithyroid agents do not provide definitive treatment and are potentially more toxic in this age group when used for long-term treatment. Beta blockers can be used adjunctively for symptoms of hyperthyroidism until a euthyroid state is achieved. Surgery has a much smaller role because of the increased risks in the elderly. Once hyperthyroidism has been treated, the metabolic clearance rate of other medications may then decrease and drug levels may increase, requiring dosage adjustments.

HYPOTHYROIDISM

Clinical Evaluation

The clinical presentation of hypothyroidism in older persons is confounded by the fact that many euthyroid elderly patients complain of nonspecific symptoms of fatigue, cold intolerance, weakness, constipation, dry skin, depression, and lethargy, all symptoms that would be key to the diagnosis of hypothyroidism in younger patients. Elderly hypothyroid patients are more likely than their younger counterparts to present with cardiovascular symptoms (congestive heart failure or angina occurs in 25 to 50 percent) or central nervous system symptoms (psychosis, mental confusion, depression, paresthesias, deafness, or coma). The physician must be particularly suspicious and think of the diagnosis whenever a patient's clinical status, behavior pattern, or cognitive abilities change. *Subclinical hypothyroidism,* defined in a clinically euthyroid patient with a normal T_4 and T_3RU and an elevated TSH, is also common in the elderly, with prevalence estimates ranging from 4 to 14 percent [3,11].

Physical examination is also often misleading because dry skin and coarse hair are common features in euthyroid elderly subjects. However, a puffy face, delayed deep tendon reflexes, and myoedema are helpful clinical findings that support the diagnosis. Results of the serum T_4, T_3RU, and the free T_4 index should all be depressed in primary hypothyroidism. The diagnosis is best confirmed by an elevated serum TSH level. The TSH level is the most sensitive and single best screening test for hypothyroidism. Measurement of serum T_3 is useless and unnecessary because it is the hormone most likely to decrease in nonthyroidal illness. The most common cause of primary hypothyroidism is Hashimoto's disease or autoimmune thyroiditis. Hypothyroidism following radioactive ablative therapy for hyperthyroidism is the second most common cause. Low serum T_4, T_3, and TSH levels suggest pituitary hypothyroidism, which is usually accompanied by other signs of pituitary failure. This uncommon entity can be confirmed by a flat TSH response to intravenous TRH.

Treatment

Thyroid hormone replacement requirements decrease with age [12,13]. Elderly patients should be started on low doses of thyroid hormone replacement (L-thyroxine 25–50 μg/day) and replaced gradually (L-thyroxine increased by 25 μg every three to four weeks). Particular caution must be used in patients with underlying cardiovascular disease. In these patients initial replacement should be 12.5 to 25 μg per day, and the ultimate replacement dose may depend on the cardiac disease rather than on normalization of TSH. Preparations of desiccated thyroid hormone should be avoided because of the variable hormone content, and preparations containing T_3 should not be given to elderly subjects because T_3 is rapidly absorbed and rapidly disappears from the bloodstream. Once the hypothyroidism is corrected, the metabolic clearance rate of other drugs may change and require adjustment. Proper management of subclinical hypothyroidism in the elderly has not been examined. In this group of patients, in whom the cardiovascular and central nervous systems are more sensitive to supplementary thyroxine, patients should initially be followed and observed closely for development of overt hypothyroidism.

THYROID NODULES AND CANCER

Multinodular goiters are more common in the elderly. If an enlarged gland does not compromise swallowing or breathing functions and thyroid function tests are normal, the goiter can be followed without treatment. However, if the goiter produces obstructive symptoms, which may occur particularly if there is substernal extension, then surgical removal may be necessary. L-thyroxine suppression rarely shrinks the gland but may prevent it from growing larger. However, caution must be exercised. Occasionally multinodular goiters develop areas of autonomous function. When L-thyroxine therapy is then added, the previously euthyroid elderly patient may become thyrotoxic. An isolated palpable nodule often represents a more prominent nodule in a multinodular goiter but deserves careful workup if it has recently changed in size. A newly discovered isolated nodule in an elderly patient deserves the same careful evaluation that would be given to such a finding in a younger person and should include a thyroid scan and fine needle aspiration or large needle biopsy.

Although thyroid carcinoma usually presents as an isolated palpable nodule that is "cold" (unable to take up iodine) on radioiodine uptake scan, 90 to 95 percent of cold nodules are benign. Papillary thyroid cancer accounts for more than one-half of all types of thyroid cancer. It more commonly occurs in young to middle-aged subjects and rarely causes death. However, papillary thyroid carcinoma carries a poor prognosis in the elderly. Follicular thyroid carcinoma comprises approximately 15 percent of thyroid cancers, generally occurs in middle-aged to older individuals, tends to be more invasive, and has a worse prognosis. Anaplastic carcinoma of the thyroid gland is almost exclusively found in middle-aged to elderly people. It presents as a rapidly growing mass, is locally invasive, often has metastatic lesions on presentation, and carries a very poor prognosis. Primary lymphoma of the thyroid gland may present in a similar manner as a rapidly expanding neck mass. However, it may respond more favorably to radiation and chemotherapy [14].

Nonthyroidal Illness

Nonthyroidal illness or the euthyroid-sick syndrome is even more common than thyroid disease in the elderly population and is often confused with true thyroid pathology. By definition, the patient is clinically euthyroid but has an alteration in thyroid function tests due to sickness or medications (see Table 28-1). The term *nonthyroidal illness* is broad and comprises a heterogeneous group of clinical situations but can be divided into three syndromes: the low T_3, low T_4, and high T_4 syndromes [15,17].

TABLE 28-2. *Thyroid function tests in nonthyroidal illness*

	Low T_3 SYNDROME	Low T_4 SYNDROME	High T_4 SYNDROME
Total T_3	↓	↓	↑ or N
Free T_3	↓ or N	↓	↓ or N
Total T_4	N	↓	↑
Free T_4 dialysis	N or ↑	N or ↑	N
Free T_4 index	N	N or ↓	N
T_3 RU	N or ↑	N or ↑	↓
Total rT_3	↑ or N	↑ or N	↑ or N
TSH	N	N	N
TRH stimulated TSH	N	N or ↓	N

Key: N = no change.

Low T_3 Syndrome

The low T_3 syndrome is the most common and is defined as a clinically euthyroid patient with a low serum T_3 level and normal serum T_4 and T_3RU concentrations (Table 28-2). The syndrome is acute, reversible, and occurs commonly after surgery, during fasting, in many acute febrile illnesses, in renal failure, congestive heart failure, or after an acute myocardial infarction. A low serum T_3 value is found in up to 40 percent of subjects during an acute illness and in up to two-thirds of patients in an intensive care unit [18]. This condition results from a decrease in 5′monodeiodinase, the enzyme responsible for peripheral conversion of T_4 to T_3, resulting in a lowering of serum T_3. Glucocorticoids, propranolol, amiodarone, propylthiouracil, and radiographic contrast agents are drugs that may also produce a low T_3 level (see Table 28-1).

Low T_4 Syndrome

The low T_4 syndrome describes a clinically euthyroid patient with low serum T_3 and T_4 concentrations (see Table 28-2). This syndrome is found in the sickest patients and has the worst prognosis [19]. The prevalence of a low serum T_4 value during an acute illness is approximately 20 percent and doubles if a patient is in an intensive care unit setting [18]. These very sick patients have a decrease in all the thyroid hormone-binding proteins, leading to a low serum T_4 and a normal or elevated T_3RU. There is also an inhibitor of T_4-binding that is released into the circulation by peripheral tissues [20]. In addition, dopamine, phenytoin (Dilantin), and glucocorticoids, medications often used in very sick patients, can depress TSH. The diagnosis can usually be confirmed by low serum T_4 and normal or elevated T_3RU, a normal free T_4 index ($T_4 \times T_3RU$), and normal TSH levels (see Table 28-2). A rT_3, although not necessary, may be elevated. TSH measurement is the best test to differentiate between euthyroid sick (normal TSH) versus primary hypothyroid sick (elevated TSH).

High T_4 Syndrome

The high T_4 syndrome or euthyroid hyperthyroxinemia (elevated serum T_4 value in the presence of low or normal T_3RU [see Table 28-2]) has multiple etiologies but is usually caused by an increase in thyroid-binding globulin. Such an increase can be seen in patients taking estrogen, tamoxifen, or methadone or in patients with hepatitis or familial disorders. Iodine-containing compounds (medications or contrast agents) can cause hyperthyroxinemia from iodine-induced hyperthyroidism, known as the Jodbasedow effect. This occurs occasionally in elderly subjects who have multinodular goiters with areas of autonomous function. When they are given an iodine load, the gland produces an excess of thyroid hormone. Acute psychiatric illness can also cause hyperthyroxinemia from an unknown cause.

The diagnosis of nonthyroidal illness in all instances can be confirmed by careful evaluation of the individual thyroid function tests. When the total T_4 and T_3RU are abnormal in the same direction, a true thyroid hormone production abnormality is present. If the total T_4 and T_3RU are abnormal in opposite directions (low T_4, high T_3RU), there is likely to be a thyroid-binding globulin abnormality (Table 28-3). A normal FT_4 index and normal TSH value suggest a state of nonthyroidal illness. Patients with nonthyroidal illness should not be treated with thyroid hormone [21]. Once their underlying illness is treated or the incriminating medication is stopped, the thyroid function tests will return to normal.

Carbohydrate Metabolism and Diabetes Mellitus

An age-related impairment in the capacity to maintain carbohydrate homeostasis after glucose challenge has been recognized for over 60 years. For the past two decades, many gerontologists have focused their attention on elucidation of the underlying mechanisms, and a general consensus is now emerging. Increasing age in individuals without evidence or family history of diabetes is associated with a progressive decline in carbohydrate tolerance. Many studies indicate a very slight (approximately 1 mg/dl/decade) increase after maturity in fasting blood glucose levels [22], which is accompanied by a rather striking increase in blood sugar after oral glucose challenge. In an extensive review of the English literature, Davidson found that the average postchallenge glucose increase in blood sugar with advancing age was 9.5 mg per dl per decade at one hour, and 5.3 mg per dl per decade at two hours. Using the National Diabetes Data Group criteria for impaired glucose tolerance (Table 28-4), approximately 9.2 percent of people over the age of 65 have impaired carbohydrate tolerance (Table

TABLE 28-4. *National Diabetes Data Group criteria for the classification and diagnosis of glucose intolerance and diabetes mellitus*

Normal
  Fasting plasma glucose level: < 115 mg/dl
  OGTT* ½–1½ hr glucose level: < 200 mg/dl
  OGTT 2 hr glucose level: < 140 mg/dl
Impaired glucose tolerance
  Fasting plasma glucose level: < 140 mg/dl
  OGTT ½–1½ hr glucose level: ≥ 200 mg/dl
  OGTT 2 hr glucose level: 140–200 mg/dl
Diabetes mellitus
  Classic symptoms and elevated plasma glucose
    Fasting plasma glucose level: ≥ 140 mg/dl on two occasions
    OGTT ½–2 hr glucose level: ≥ 200 mg/dl
    Meeting any one of the above criteria is sufficient for the diagnosis

*OGTT = 75-gm oral glucose tolerance test.
SOURCE: National Diabetes Data Group. Classification and diagnosis of diabetes and other categories of glucose intolerance. *Diabetes* 28:1039, 1987.

TABLE 28-3. *Thyroid function tests in thyroid disease states versus thyroid-binding globulin (TBG) abnormalities*

	↓ TOTAL T_4	↑ TOTAL T_4
↓ T_3 resin uptake	Hypothyroidism	TBG excess
↑ T_3 resin uptake	TBG deficiency	Hyperthyroidism

TABLE 28-5. *Prevalence of various classes of glucose intolerance, United States, 1976–1980**

	PERCENT OF POPULATION			
	AGE 20–44	AGE 45–54	AGE 55–64	AGE 65–74
Diagnosed diabetes	1.1	4.3	6.6	9.3
Undiagnosed diabetes	0.9	4.2	6.2	8.4
Impaired glucose tolerance	2.1	7.0	7.4	9.2
Totals	4.1	15.5	20.2	26.9

*National Diabetes Data Group criteria used to define each class; data includes all races and both sexes.
SOURCE: M. I. Harris, et al. Prevalence of diabetes and impaired glucose tolerance and plamsa glucose levels in U.S. population aged 20–74 years. *Diabetes* 36:523, 1987.

28-5). Distribution of blood glucose levels at one and two hours after glucose challenge in the elderly is unimodal, which suggests that the change does not reflect the increasing prevalence of a second population of diabetics who are skewing the data. The higher postprandial glucose levels seen with aging are reflected in an increased level of hemoglobin A1C [23].

Pathogenetic mechanisms postulated to explain these age-related changes in carbohydrate tolerance include changes in body composition, diet, activity, and insulin secretion and action [22]. Age-associated changes in body composition may also play an important role in determining age effects on carbohydrate metabolism. Elahi and his colleagues [24] studied normal volunteers aged 23 to 93 and found that fatness but not aging was associated with increases in basal insulin, glucagon, and fasting glucose. Decreases in lean body mass with age have also been shown to correlate with reduced glucose tolerance [22]. In addition, marked limitation of physical activity or ingestion of low-carbohydrate diets have been shown to impair glucose tolerance.

Most studies in well-nourished subjects on ad lib diets show that in response to oral or intravenous glucose challenges, the elderly have insulin levels equivalent to and in many cases slightly greater than the levels found in their younger counterparts [22]. Recently, Chen et al. [25] have shown that in subjects on low-carbohydrate diets insulin levels were reduced in the elderly compared to those in younger subjects, suggesting that glucose intolerance was due

both to impaired insulin secretion and peripheral insulin resistance. In young and old subjects on high-carbohydrate diets, insulin levels were equivalent and carbohydrate intolerance persisted, suggesting that glucose intolerance was due primarily to peripheral insulin resistance. The higher insulin levels reported after oral glucose tolerance tests by some authors may be due to impaired insulin clearance with age [26]. There is no effect of age on basal hepatic glucose production, and the regulation of hepatic glucose production by insulin is unchanged with age [27].

It appears that the major effect of age on carbohydrate metabolism is a decrease in the effectiveness of insulin to induce glucose uptake in peripheral tissues [28] (Fig. 28-1). When corrected for lean body mass, these differences persist. There is no change in insulin receptor number or affinity with age, and it appears that the insulin resistance is due to a postreceptor defect in the action of the hormone [29].

As discussed in Chapter 1, the carbohydrate intolerance of aging may be an example of *usual* aging and may carry substantial risk. A recent report from the Honolulu Heart Study evaluated the 12-year risk of stroke in 690 diabetics and 6,908 nondiabetics who were free of stroke on entry in the study. Diabetes was associated with a clearly increased risk of stroke [30]. Additionally, in nondiabetics the risk of stroke was moderately age related and was statistically significantly higher for those at the eightieth percentile of serum glucose than for those at the twentieth percentile. Studies focusing on postprandial hyperinsulinemia, a cardinal feature of the insulin resistance of aging, have shown that an increase in insulin levels is a significant independent contributor to the incidence of coronary artery disease [31,32]. In addition to these effects, increases in insulin level are associated both with increases in triglyceride level and with decreases in high-density lipoprotein cholesterol levels, both of which are known risk factors for heart disease.

Attempts have been made to determine which components of the age-related alterations in carbohydrate tolerance are related to aging per se and which might be related to factors such as diet, exercise, medications, and body composition. For example, in a study of Italian factory

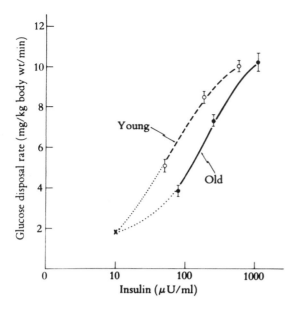

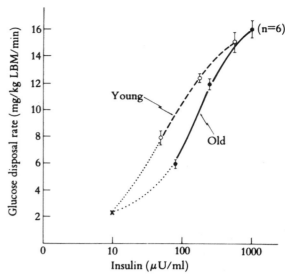

FIGURE 28-1. *Dose response curves for insulin-mediated glucose disposal in young (---) and old (———) subjects. In the panel on the left, glucose disposal is expressed as milligrams per kilogram of body weight. In the panel on the right, glucose disposal rates are normalized for lean body mass. (From J. W. Rowe, et al. Characterization of the insulin resistance of aging. J. Clin. Invest. 71:1581, 1983. By copyright permission of the American Society for Clinical Investigation.)*

workers aged 22 to 73, Zavaroni et al. [33] evaluated the relative contributions of obesity, physical activity, family history of diabetes, and use of diabetogenic drugs to age-related increases in glucose and insulin levels after an oral glucose tolerance test. The initial strong correlation between age and both postprandial glucose and insulin levels became so much weaker when the effects of exercise, diet, and drugs were taken into account that the correlation between glucose and age was limited to marginal statistical significance, and there was no longer an effect of age on insulin levels. Hollenbeck et al. [34] showed a direct significant relationship between physical fitness as reflected in maximum oxygen consumption and insulin-stimulated glucose metabolism in nonobese healthy older men. Seals and coworkers [35] found that the performance of older, physically trained men on an oral glucose tolerance test was identical to that of young athletes and significantly better than that of untrained older men.

These findings clearly suggest that much of the observed carbohydrate intolerance and insulin resistance of older people may be caused by factors other than biologic aging per se [36]. Dietary or exercise modifications may substantially blunt the emergence with age of carbohydrate intolerance and insulin resistance. The latter view is supported by earlier studies demonstrating improvements in glucose tolerance in young adults [37] and diabetics after exercise regimens [38], as well as recent studies suggesting that exercise programs and dietary manipulations can also improve the glucose tolerance and insulin resistance of older people [25,39,40].

Although the glucose intolerance of aging is common and is clearly associated with an increased risk of vascular disease, there is no evidence at present that treatment of glucose intolerance, as opposed to frank diabetes, will decrease the risk of these complications. Nonetheless, it would be prudent to recommend moderate exercise and weight loss to older individuals with greater degrees of glucose intolerance.

Diabetes Mellitus

The prevalence of symptomatic and asymptomatic diabetes mellitus increases substantially with age. The Health and Nutrition Examination Survey (HANES) shows that about 18 percent of people over the age of 65 are diabetic [41] (see Table 28-5). This figure increases to 25 percent in studies of individuals over age 85. Age-related changes in insulin action, exercise, diet, and body composition are the substrate on which diabetes develops. Several factors appear to predispose the elderly individual with age-related impairment in carbohydrate tolerance to the development of overt diabetes. These factors include a clear genetic predisposition, obesity, illness-induced changes in diet and activity, and drug therapy, which complicate the insulin resistance seen in normal elderly subjects. Patients with type II diabetes also have impaired insulin secretion, a reduction in insulin receptors, an elevation of basal hepatic glucose production, and resistance to the suppression of hepatic glucose production by insulin.

The presentation of diabetes is often insidious in the elderly and may be asymptomatic. Polyuria and polydipsia secondary to hyperglycemia may not develop until the disease is far advanced because the reduced glomerular filtration rate in the elderly reduces osmotic diuresis by reducing the salt and water losses normally associated with hyperglycemia. Additionally, the renal threshold for spilling glucose into the urine increases with age, and thus glycosuria often does not appear until the plasma glucose level reaches 300 mg per dl. Patients may complain of weakness, fatigue, weight loss, and nonspecific failure to thrive, or they may present with a minor skin or soft tissue infection—for example, *Candida vulvovaginitis*. Frequently, neurologic abnormalities, either cranial or peripheral neuropathy, are the initial presenting symptoms. Patients rarely develop ketoacidosis but may instead slip into a nonketotic hyperosmolar state and present with confusion, coma, or focal neurologic signs.

DIAGNOSIS

The best marker for the diagnosis of diabetes is a fasting blood sugar greater than 140 mg per dl on two separate occasions (see Table 28-4). Glycosuria is unreliable in view of the increase in renal threshold with age noted earlier. If the fasting blood sugar is between 120 mg per dl and 140 mg per dl and postprandial sugars are consistently high (for example, greater than 200 mg/dl), it is reasonable to proceed to a two-hour glucose tolerance test. A glucose tolerance test should be performed with the patient in the basal state after receiving an adequate carbohydrate intake of at least 200 gm per day for at least three days. The National Diabetes Data Group criteria for interpreting glucose tolerance tests are outlined in Table 28-4.

TREATMENT

Is treatment beneficial in this illness? Diabetics in the United States have a 29 times greater frequency of blindness, a 17 times more frequent incidence of renal failure, a five times more frequent amputation rate, and a two- to sixfold increased risk of coronary artery disease and stroke [42,43,44]. In addition, 40 to 50 percent of men who have diabetes for more than 10 years become impotent. It now appears that patients with type II diabetes are no less susceptible to target organ complications than patients with type I diabetes [45]. That diabetes may in some ways represent a state of accelerated aging is suggested by the findings of decreased proliferative capacity of cultured fibroblasts, increased thickening of capillary basement membranes, and increased collagen cross-linking, all of which occur in the normal aging process [46]. These changes may be due to nonenzymatic glycation of a wide variety of proteins.

Just because diabetes is associated with increased risks does not necessarily mean that therapy is helpful. However, several compelling reasons are offered for treating the elderly diabetic. Polyphagia and polyuria should be treated to control the symptoms. In animals, controlling diabetes results in a decreased risk of complications, particularly vascular complications. There are also some data in humans [47] suggesting that good control of blood sugar results in a decreased risk of complications, although a definitive answer to this question will be provided by the Diabetes Control Complications trial currently underway. Hyperglycemia adversely affects white cell function, which can predispose to infections in elderly persons who already have an age-related decline in immune system function. Accumulation of sorbitol with uncontrolled hyperglycemia can lead to the progression of cataracts and worsen age-related changes in nerve conduction. Most important, if an uncontrolled blood sugar level is combined with cognitive impairment, infection, or an inability to maintain proper food intake, the patient may develop nonketotic hyperosmolar coma, which has a mortality of 15 to 20 percent in this age group.

If a decision is made to treat the elderly diabetic, therapy may have to be less aggressive than in younger individuals because the complications of therapy, particularly hypoglycemia, may not be well tolerated by the aged. The goal should be to keep the fasting blood sugar level below 150 mg per dl and postprandial glucose less than 220 mg per dl with no evidence of glucosuria.

Several considerations must be borne in mind when specific therapy is initiated. Elderly diabetics frequently have reduced acuity of the special senses and poor dentition, which may affect dietary therapy. Arthritis or other chronic disease may limit their ability to comply with an exercise program. Chronic diseases, such as neoplasms, may make the blood sugar level harder to control. Social factors such as poverty, depression, dementia, or poor dietary knowledge may affect compliance with a therapeutic program. Finally, the elderly may be taking a number of drugs that may affect therapy. Steroids, hydrochlorothiazide, and beta blockers may all decrease glucose tolerance. In addition, nonsteroidal anti-inflammatory agents or warfarin sodium (Coumadin) may interact with the older oral agents, resulting in an increased incidence of adverse drug reactions.

Several options are available for therapy [42, 48,49], including diet, exercise, oral agents, and insulin. In general, if fasting blood sugar is less than 300 mg per dl initially, a diet and exercise regimen can be tried for a period of two to three months and then reassessed. If fasting blood sugar is greater than 300 mg per dl initially, diet and insulin should be started from the beginning.

The first and most important goal in the management of the elderly diabetic is to control other risk factors. The Framingham Study has shown that the development of vascular complications may be more related to associated risk factors, such as smoking and hypertension, than to the actual level of blood sugar [44]. Careful attention to other factors, such as foot care, is also critical.

The next step is diet. Although dietary modification may be difficult to institute in the elderly, a number of studies have shown that even modest weight loss, on the order of 10 to 15 pounds, may result in significant improvement in diabetic control [38]. The diet recommendation of the American Dietary Association is a diet high in complex carbohydrates and fiber and low in fat and simple sugars. Fat should generally be less than 30 percent of total caloric intake, with an increase in polyunsaturated fats and a decrease in saturated fats. Carbohydrates should make up about 50 to 60 percent of the total caloric intake. A professional dietician can be engaged in the dietary prescription for older people to facilitate education and compliance. Although diet may reduce fasting blood sugar in many individuals, it is successful as the sole method of therapy in only about 10 to 20 percent of patients. An exercise program has also been shown to improve glucose tolerance and reduce the need for oral agents and insulin [38]. It should be undertaken in a gradual, sequential manner tailored to the patient's physical capabilities and disabilities. In addition to improving insulin action, it will aid in weight reduction, improve the general sense of well-being, and help control blood pressure. Even modest degrees of exercise, such as walking at a moderate pace 15 to 20 minutes four to five times a week may improve glucose tolerance.

If two to three months of diet and exercise fail, then it is reasonable to begin therapy with a sulfonylurea agent. First-generation agents became available in the 1950s, and the second-generation agents glyburide and glipizide became available in the United States in 1984 [50]. Sulfonylurea agents decrease fasting hepatic glucose production, increase insulin secretion, increase insulin receptors, and increase the post-receptor action of insulin (Table 28-6). Because second-generation agents have few active metabolites and less protein binding than first-generation agents they are less likely to interact with other drugs such as warfarin sodium (Coumadin) and nonsteroidal antiinflammatory agents. They are unlikely to cause alcohol-induced flushing and inappropriate antidiuretic hormone secretion. Finally, they are more potent than first-generation agents. Of the new

TABLE 28-6. *Mechanisms of action of the sulfonylureas*

Increase endogenous insulin secretion in the presence of
  high glucose levels during both acute and chronic usage
Reduce hepatic glucose production when used chronically
May increase insulin receptors in chronic usage
May potentiate insulin action and increase insulin
  responsiveness

agents, glipizide has a shorter half-life than glyburide and has been shown to result in a lower incidence of hypoglycemia [51]. It should be considered the agent of first choice in elderly diabetics.

If blood sugar is well controlled, the patient should not be switched from the older agents unless one of these is chlorpropamide. Chlorpropamide has a high likelihood of causing severe hypoglycemia and hyponatremia, with most case reports of severe reactions occurring in elderly diabetics. If a first-generation agent fails, a second-generation agent can result in acceptable control in 10 to 20 percent of cases and negate the need for insulin. If diabetes has been present for less than five years and insulin requirements are less than 30 units per day, insulin can sometimes be replaced by one of the newer agents. Finally, in some type II diabetic patients taking insulin, oral agents have been shown to be helpful in improving control and reducing insulin requirements. These agents can be considered adjunctive therapy when the insulin requirements are greater than 60 units per day.

The second-generation agents are about 70 percent effective as primary therapy in achieving an acceptable degree of control of blood sugar. The starting dose of glipizide or glyburide is 2.5 mg before breakfast; the dose can be increased in 2.5-mg increments every five to seven days until control of blood sugar is achieved. Maximum dose is 20 mg per day; when dose requirements are over 10 mg per day the drug should be given in divided doses.

The University Group Diabetes Project (UGDP) [52] reported in 1970 that patients treated with tolbutamide had a higher death rate from myocardial infarction than patients treated with insulin or placebo. A number of studies since that time have not confirmed that the risk of vascular complications is increased with oral agents, and in fact, some studies have suggested that the use of oral agents may actually decrease cardiovascular risk. The general consensus today is that there is scant evidence to incriminate sulfonylureas as a cause of myocardial infarction.

If an acceptable degree of control is not achieved with oral agents or if initial fasting blood sugar is greater than 300 mg per dl, insulin therapy should be given. Ultrapure porcine or human insulin should be used to prevent the development of antibodies that may make control more difficult. The starting dose is 15 to 30 units of NPH insulin. In most older diabetic subjects, only one injection of a short- or intermediate-acting insulin is required unless the total dosage is greater than 50 units per day. Decreases in memory, vision, and motor coordination may decrease the patient's capacity to self-administer insulin. Therefore, patients should be managed with one daily insulin dose whenever possible. A family member or visiting nurse can draw up the syringes on a weekly basis if the patient is unable to draw them up.

Hypoglycemia may be particularly treacherous in the elderly because it may go unrecognized and unwitnessed in some patients. The elderly frequently have no peripheral symptoms such as sweating, hunger attacks, and palpitations, and symptoms may not be reported by patients with dementia. For this reason, stringent control of blood sugar should not be attempted in older diabetics.

Urine testing is not helpful in monitoring the elderly diabetic because of the increase in the renal threshold for glucose. All elderly diabetics taking insulin or their caretakers should be taught how to monitor blood glucose levels at home unless their blood sugar levels are very stable [42]. These measurements will give the physician a good means of assessing control and making sure that dangerous hypoglycemia is avoided. A hemoglobin A1C is a monitor of glucose tolerance during the last eight to ten weeks and should also be done periodically in elderly diabetic patients. A hemoglobin A1C value of less than 9 percent indicates an acceptable degree of blood sugar control in the elderly diabetic.

Nonketotic Hyperosmolar Coma

The hallmark of acute uncontrolled diabetes mellitus in the elderly is the syndrome of the hyperosmolar nonketotic coma, which is characterized by marked elevations in blood glucose concentration that are often greater than 1,000 mg per dl compared with the approximately 300 mg per dl that is usually seen in diabetic ketoacidosis. In this syndrome plasma osmolality is higher than 325 mOsm per kg, and marked extracellular fluid volume depletion may occur. Hyperosmolar coma can be termed a geriatric syndrome because it is almost exclusively present in individuals over age 65 [53]. A recent study of elderly subjects with this syndrome revealed that risk factors include female sex, newly diagnosed diabetes, and acute infection [54]. Management differs in several important ways from that of uncontrolled diabetes in the younger adult, who more commonly experiences diabetic ketoacidosis.

In this syndrome inadequate insulin levels result in a decreased utilization of glucose by peripheral tissues and an increase in hepatic glucose production. This condition in turn results in uncontrolled hyperglycemia. Sufficient insulin is present, however, to prevent the production of ketones by the liver, and ketoacidosis does not develop.

Because of the increase in renal threshold with age, an osmotic diuresis does not occur until the blood glucose level is markedly elevated. When the renal threshold is exceeded, an osmotic diuresis ensues that results in extracellular fluid volume depletion. However, large amounts of glucose cannot be excreted by the kidneys because of the age-related decrease in renal function, and the blood sugar continues to increase.

The syndrome usually presents in a patient with known type II diabetes, but in one-third of cases it is the initial presentation of diabetes. There may be a several-week history of weakness, polyuria, or polydipsia. Nursing home patients may gradually become confused, withdrawn, obtunded, and even comatose. Neurologic findings are often prominent, and the focality of these findings may prompt the diagnosis of stroke or other acute neurologic event. These patients generally have marked depletion of extracellular fluid volume with decreased tissue turgor, lack of sweating, orthostatic hypotension, and prerenal azotemia.

As noted earlier, although water loss is usually greater than sodium loss, it may not be reflected in serum sodium values, since hyperglycemia, by virtue of its osmotic effect on cells, will draw water from the intracellular space to the extracellular space, thus depressing the serum sodium concentration. Ketosis is usually absent, and acidosis, when present, is mild in degree and is associated with increased levels of plasma lactate.

Once the diagnosis is made, appropriate treatment includes administration of intravenous insulin in small amounts and prompt repletion of the extracellular fluid volume. Despite the hypertonic state, therapy should be instituted with rapid intravenous infusions of isotonic (0.9 percent) saline. Although some authors favor the use of hypotonic (0.45 percent) saline, this use will incur the risk of inducing too rapid shifts in the levels of plasma osmolality. Isotonic saline will have some effect in decreasing plasma osmolality, since, although the solution is isotonic, it will be significantly hypotonic compared with the patient's plasma. In general, these patients usually have an extracellular fluid volume deficit of 5 to 7 liters or greater. One-half of the deficit should be repleted within the first 24 hours of hospitalization. Too rapid correction of the volume deficit may precipitate pulmonary edema, especially in elderly individuals with preexisting cardiac disease. To avoid worsening the neurologic status due to too rapid correction of plasma osmolality, when blood glucose reaches 250 mg per dl, 5 percent dextrose in water should be added to the saline infusion and blood glucose maintained at approximately 250 mg per dl for 24 hours while volume repletion is completed. The initial dose of insulin should be a 10-unit intravenous bolus followed by a continuous intravenous infusion at between 3 and 5 units per hour. Potassium deficits in these patients are less than those in patients with diabetic ketoacidosis because of the age-related impairments in renal function. If the potassium concentration is normal and the patient is producing urine, 10 mEq of potassium should be added to the first liter of intravenous fluid and none thereafter. Most of these patients, particularly if they have cardiac disease, will require insertion of a central venous pressure catheter or Swan-Ganz catheter for precise monitoring of cardiac filling pressures.

As in the case of a younger patient with uncontrolled diabetes, a thorough evaluation including a history and physical examination is important to discern the precipitating event. Common precipitating events in old people include stroke, myocardial infarction, infections, and use of drugs such as thiazides or steroids.

Patients with hyperosmolar coma are generally stuporous or comatose on admission and may, particularly if they are very old or have pre-existing central nervous system disease, recover to their previous neurologic state very slowly despite prompt correction of volume deficits and hyperosmolality. In some cases, the patient's mental status may not clear for a week or more after correction of the metabolic abnormalities. In the absence of focal signs or evidence of worsening neurologic status, it is best to observe the patient rather than subject him or her to a series of neurologic studies to detect the basis of the abnormal mental status. Following an episode of hyperosmolar coma, many patients will require insulin therapy, although some can be managed with oral agents, diet, and exercise.

Parathyroid Gland

PHYSIOLOGY

Recognition of the importance of parathyroid hormone in the maintenance of calcium homeostasis and skeletal integrity has focused considerable interest on possible age-related alterations in parathyroid function. Studies of healthy men and women across the adult age range show increased circulating levels of parathyroid hormone with advancing age [55,56]. As parathyroid hormone is metabolized, fragments accumulate in the blood and are excreted by the kidney. Radioimmunoassays that detect intact hormone as well as these inactive fragments indicate an 80 percent increase in the circulating level of parathyroid hormone from age 30 to 80. When assays sensitive only for intact hormone are employed, the increase is limited to 30 percent (Fig. 28-2). This discrepancy probably relates to the decrease in renal function that ac-

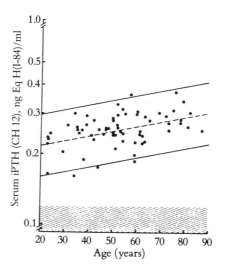

FIGURE 28-2. *Serum parathyroid hormone levels in normal women measured by an assay specific for the intact hormone. (From J. C. Gallagher, et al. The effect of age on serum immunoreactive parathyroid hormone in normal and osteoporotic women. J. Lab. Clin. Med. 95:373, 1980.)*

companies normal aging and the associated reduced excretion of the nonbiologically active fragments of parathyroid hormone. The modest increase in circulating levels of parathyroid hormone is not accompanied by a change in total serum calcium but rather by a slight reduction in ionized calcium. This increase in parathyroid hormone in the elderly results in increased levels of urinary cyclic AMP [57] and also explains the slight decrease in serum phosphate with age.

The slight decrease in ionized calcium with age contributes to the increase in parathyroid hormone level. The well-documented age-related decrease in intestinal calcium absorption [58] probably causes the decrease in ionized calcium. Decreases in circulating levels of 1,25-hydroxyvitamin D are responsible for the decreases in calcium absorption with age [59]. The increase in parathyroid hormone necessary to augment intestinal calcium absorption may need to be greater in the elderly because of the known age-related impairment in the ability of parathyroid hormone to stimulate the renal production of 1,25-hydroxyvitamin D. The decreased response of 1,25-hydroxyvitamin D to parathyroid hormone infusion correlates with both age and glomerular filtration rate, but it appears that the decrease in renal function is the most important determinant of this abnormality [60].

HYPERPARATHYROIDISM

Primary Hyperparathyroidism

Primary hyperparathyroidism, once thought to be a rare disease, is now known to occur commonly in the middle and late years [61]. The detection of the disease has increased dramatically in recent years with the use of automated blood screening. Recent studies show that the incidence of the disease is less than 10 per 100,000 in patients under the age of 40, but in females over the age of 60 the incidence is approximately 190 per 100,000 [62]. Fifty percent of all cases of hyperparathyroidism now occur in people over the age of 65, particularly women.

In the past, the most common presentations of hyperparathyroidism were renal failure or renal stones and metabolic bone disease. Currently, most cases are asymptomatic and are detected on routine screening of blood calcium levels [63]. In symptomatic patients there are important differences in the presentation of hyperparathyroidism between young and old adults. Symptoms are often vague and insidious in the elderly, and the clinical presentation is frequently dominated by alterations in mental status. Modest elevations in serum calcium to levels of between 11 and 12 mg per dl may result in substantial alterations of mental function in the elderly, particularly in the presence of preexisting mild central nervous system disease. Patients may complain of fatigue, depression, weakness, personality change, and memory failure [64–69]. Anorexia and constipation are also common early complaints. It is important to note that patients who were considered asymptomatic in older reports would now be considered symptomatic on the basis of the above neuromuscular symptoms. Most studies suggest that renal problems such as renal stones or renal failure, gastrointestinal problems such as peptic ulcer disease or pancreatitis, and skeletal problems such as osteoporosis, fractures, and bone pain are present in less than 50 percent of elderly people at presentation. Hypertension is frequent in primary hyperparathyroidism, and the incidence in elderly patients may be twice that of age-matched controls without the disease.

The diagnosis of primary hyperparathyroidism rests on a number of factors. The serum calcium level can fluctuate between high normal and slightly abnormal and may need to be repeated on several occasions. Elderly people frequently suffer from hypoproteinemia, and the serum calcium measurement should be corrected using the following formula:

$$\text{Serum Ca (corrected)} \atop (\text{mg/dl}) = \frac{\text{Serum Ca (mg/dl)}}{0.55 + \dfrac{\text{T prot (g/dl)}}{16}}$$

In addition to hypercalcemia, patients generally have hypophosphatemia and a high normal or increased serum chloride. Alkaline phosphatase will also be increased in many patients, but it is a common finding in elderly people even without hyperparathyroidism and is thus nonspecific. Reliable determinations are now available for urinary cyclic AMP, but it may also be elevated in hypercalcemia of malignancy. Parathyroid hormone levels are elevated but may be hard to evaluate in view of the normal age-related increase in the level of the hormone. However, values over 50 percent above normal using hormone-specific assays are considered diagnostic. The best test to confirm the diagnosis is a measurement of parathyroid hormone level performed with a good assay.

A high index of suspicion for other causes of hypercalcemia should be present when evaluating an older person with hypercalcemia. In particular, multiple myeloma or other malignancies, thyroid disease, vitamin D intoxication, and the use of various drugs such as thiazide diuretics should be considered.

In general, patients with primary hyperparathyroidism who have an elevated serum calcium level greater than 1 mg per dl above the upper limit of normal for the laboratory, or who have symptoms or signs regardless of the degree of hypercalcemia, should undergo parathyroid surgery [70]. In addition to the classic symptoms related to renal failure and renal stones, bone disease, and gastrointestinal symptoms, the mental symptoms described earlier should be considered indicative of symptomatic hypercalcemia in the aged and should suggest a surgical referral.

Parathyroid surgery is well tolerated by the elderly, and the clinical results are often gratifying. Tibblin et al. [69] recently reported on a series of 140 cases over age 60 and found that the operative morbidity was less than 2 percent and that over 95 percent of patients were cured of hypercalcemia. Surgery may in fact be technically easier than in many young patients because elderly patients, despite their lack of very high serum calcium levels, more often have larger adenomas than younger adults. The incidence of parathyroid carcinoma does not appear to be increased in the elderly. Although studies have been anecdotal in nature and have not rigorously evaluated mental status, a number of reports suggest that dramatic improvement in mental status may occur after removal of parathyroid adenomas in older persons with modest hypercalcemia [64–69]. Hypercalcemia due to hyperparathyroidism should thus be considered an important treatable cause of memory failure in older individuals.

Some patients are not candidates for parathyroid removal because of medical contraindications to surgery. In addition, many patients have serum calcium levels of less than 11.5 mg per dl and no symptoms or signs of hyperparathyroidism. Scholz et al. [71] followed 140 patients for 10 years who initially had a serum calcium concentration of less than 11 mg per dl and had no symptoms and no evidence of renal involvement or bone disease. Twenty percent of these patients eventually required surgery for hyperparathyroidism. This study indicates that although many patients with minor elevations of calcium will do fine in long-term follow-up, a substantial number will deteriorate and require surgery, and there is no way of predicting initially who these patients will be. If a decision is made not to operate or use medical therapy on these patients, the patient should be followed regularly and carefully every six months to a year to allow early detection of complications should they develop. A controlled trial comparing surgery with observation and various forms of medical therapy in this large group of patients is clearly needed.

Some patients should be considered for medical therapy instead of surgery or observation. These patients have only mild degrees of hypercalcemia, less than 11.5 mg per dl. They have none of the classic symptoms of hyperparathyroidism but may instead complain of a variety of nonspecific symptoms such as fatigue, weakness, and memory failure, which could be due to the hypercalcemia but could also be due to other causes. They may have osteoporosis, which could be caused by hyperparathyroidism but is also very common in the elderly in the absence of an elevated parathyroid hormone level. Although these patients may not be surgical candidates, a trial of medical therapy may be indicated to evaluate whether reduction in the serum calcium level will result in improvement in mental symptoms or reduce bone loss.

Dietary calcium restriction is generally not effective. Diuretics such as furosemide increase urinary calcium excretion and can be effective therapy in some elderly patients. However, they can lead to a worsening of calcium balance in patients who do not have excessive calcium absorption, and if fluid intake is not sufficient, as may occur in many nursing home patients, dehydration could ensue, resulting in decreased renal blood flow, reduced calcium excretion, and worsening hypercalcemia. For this reason, diuretics should be used only in patients who can be followed with careful assessments of volume status and regular measurements of serum and urinary calcium levels.

A number of other therapies are available for the medical management of hyperparathyroidism. Of the drugs available, estrogens appear to be the most effective [72–74]. Ethinyl estradiol in a dose of 30 to 50 mg per day or conjugated estrogens in a dose between 1.25 and 2 mg per day reduces serum calcium an average of 0.8 mg per dl and diminishes urinary calcium excretion and indices of bone turnover such as urinary hydroxyproline. In patients with mild degrees of hypercalcemia, this magnitude of reduction in serum calcium often returns serum calcium to the normal range. Norethindrone, 5 mg per day, has a lesser effect on bone turnover and serum calcium than the other agents. However, it may be preferable for some patients because it has no undesirable effects on the uterus or blood clotting mechanisms.

Oral phosphates have also been used. Neutraphos is the preparation of choice. Each tablet contains 250 mg of elemental phosphorus, and the usual daily dose is somewhere between 1 and 2 gm per day. Broadus et al. [75] studied a number of patients taking oral phosphates for a period of a year and found that serum calcium level decreased an average of 0.3 mg per dl, and calcium excretion decreased as well. However, parathyroid hormone increased, and the long-term effects of this therapy on bone metabolism are uncertain. In addition, many elderly patients [67] do not tolerate oral phosphates because of the gastrointestinal symptoms; thus phosphates are not recommended as the primary therapy for medical management of hyperparathyroidism in the aged. Cimetidine and propranolol were initially reported to suppress parathyroid hormone secretion but have recently been shown in controlled trials not to be effective [76,77]. Dichloromethylene diphosphanate has been shown to inhibit bone turnover in hyperparathyroidism and may be quite effective [78]. This agent is no longer available for clinical use, but other analogues are being developed.

Current data suggest that elderly patients with elevated serum calcium values of less than 11.5 mg per dl and no evidence of complications, patients who are not candidates for surgery, and patients with symptoms that may or may not be due to hypercalcemia should be given a trial of medical therapy. Estrogens are a reasonable choice in elderly females provided there is no obvious contraindication such as breast cancer. Patients treated with estrogens should be carefully monitored for abnormal uterine bleeding. In males, and in females who cannot tolerate or have a contraindication to estrogen therapy, phosphates can be used as initial therapy. Furosemide can be tried in elderly subjects who require diuretic therapy, but volume status, renal function, and serum and urinary calcium levels must be carefully monitored in these patients. If mental function or other symptoms improve after several months of medical therapy, surgical therapy can be considered.

Male Reproductive System
PHYSIOLOGY

The possible existence of a male climacteric analogous to the female menopause has long attracted substantial attention. Early studies suggested a decrease in the levels of testosterone and dihydrotestosterone with age [79]. The re-sults of recent studies on healthy men who were carefully screened to exclude underlying disease are mixed, showing either no effect of age on levels of total testosterone, free testosterone, or the major metabolite, dihydrotestosterone (Fig. 28-3) [80,81], or some decrease in testosterone levels [82]. Even if there is a decrease in average serum testosterone in an aging population, it is clear that this is a variable finding and that many elderly men, even in their nineties, will still have normal testosterone levels. The normal blood levels reported by some authors may still reflect age-related decreases in androgen secretion, since androgen clearance falls with advancing age [79]. Because testosterone is secreted in a pulsatile fashion, it has been suggested that 24-hour integrated testosterone values are of more physiologic relevance than single blood measurements. Studies comparing these two methods in elderly men have also shown disparate results, with some showing a decrease in 24-hour secretion of testosterone with age and others showing an intact diurnal rhythm of testosterone secretion [83,84].

Healthy elderly men have a modest increase in luteinizing hormone (LH) levels [80,81], a marked increase in follicular-stimulating hormone (FSH), and a decrease in LH and FSH response to luteinizing hormone releasing hormone (LHRH), suggesting a decrease in pituitary gonadotropin reserve [85]. Prolactin levels are either unchanged or increase slightly with age [86,87]. In healthy men there appears to be no change in testicular size [85] or in sperm number and morphology [88].

The Duke Longitudinal study has shown that 75 percent of healthy males over age 70 have intercourse at least once a month, and 25 percent of subjects at the age of 78 are still able to engage in regular sexual activity [89]. Martin et al. [90] found that sexual activity in late life correlated with the degree of sexual activity early in life as well as with general health. Sexual response [91] is delayed and greater stimulation is required for a man to attain an erection, which tends to be less firm. The ejaculatory volume is decreased, and men do not appear to have the need to ejaculate with every episode of intercourse. After ejaculation there is a rapid detumescence of the penis, and there is a rather prolonged refractory period before another erection

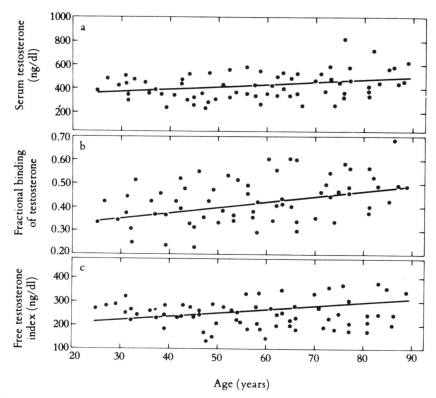

FIGURE 28-3. *Total serum testosterone (a), fractional binding of testosterone (b), and free testosterone index (c) in healthy male participants in the Baltimore Longitudinal Study of Aging. (From S. Harman, et al. Reproductive hormones in aging men. I. Measurement of sex steroids, basal luteinizing hormone, and Leydig cell response to human chorionic gonadotropin. J. Clin. Endocrinol. Metab. 51:35, 1980. © Endocrine Society.)*

is possible. There is no correlation between the levels of serum testosterone and sexual activity in healthy elderly men [92].

IMPOTENCE

Impotence is defined as an inability to obtain or sustain an erection in 25 percent or more of attempts at coitus [93]. Impotence should be differentiated from the occasional erectile failure that occurs in all men as they get older in relation to fatigue, stress, alcohol, and so on and should be pursued only if it persists for a period of at least eight weeks. Impotence is very common in the elderly. Although less than 5 percent of men under the age of 45 are impotent, impotence occurs in over 50 percent of men over the age of 75 [94].

Erection has vascular, neural, and hormonal controls, and erectile dysfunction can result from impairment of any of these factors. Penile blood supply arises from the iliac and pudendal vessels, with neural controls including a local reflex arc in the spinal cord with afferents in the pudendal nerve, a synapse in the S_2 to S_4 spinal segments, and efferents from the parasympathetic nerves. In addition, there is a cortical or psychologic component with efferents in the cranial thoracic sympathetic nerves in the area of T_{12} and L_1. Testosterone is also necessary for the maintenance of sex drive and erectile capacity.

The causes of impotence can be divided into vascular, neurologic, pharmacologic, psychologic, and endocrine causes [95] (Table 28-7). The most common vascular cause is aortoiliac atherosclerosis. Microvascular disease as well as neuropathy probably contributes to the impotence seen in diabetics. Any cause of peripheral neuropathy such as drugs or alcohol and any surgical procedure that disrupts the pelvic nerves such as abdominal perineal resection can lead to impotence. Drugs implicated include antihypertensive agents, psychotropic medica-

TABLE 28-7. *Causes of impotence in elderly males*

Vascular
    Aortoiliac atherosclerosis
    Diabetes
Neurologic
    Peripheral neuropathy
    Surgery affecting perineal nerves
Pharmacologic
    Antihypertensive drugs
    Psychotropic drugs
    Alcohol
Psychiatric
    Depression
Endocrine
    Hypogonadism
    Thyroid disease
    Hyperprolactinemia

tions such as antidepressants, benzodiazepines, and anticholinergic drugs, tranquilizers and other central nervous system depressants, alcohol, and estrogen. Impotence may be the first sign of depression in elderly males.

There are several endocrine causes of impotence in elderly males. Hypogonadism may lead to sexual dysfunction in the elderly. All hypogonadal patients have low testosterone levels. Half of these patients will have peripheral gonadal failure with high levels of LH and FSH, and the other half will have a central form of hypogonadism with a decrease in LH and FSH levels. In patients with low gonadotropin levels, hyperprolactinemia is frequently present. Thyroid disease may also result in impotence, and other systemic diseases affecting gonadal function include hemochromatosis and cirrhosis of the liver.

Few studies have specifically evaluated impotence in the elderly. Recently, Davis et al. [96] reported on 93 men over age 50 who underwent comprehensive evaluation for impotence. Nineteen percent were diabetic. Although 15 percent had psychosocial factors that may have been contributing to their impotence, only 6 percent were depressed or on psychotropic medication. Over 90 percent had abnormal nocturnal penile tumescence, and over 40 percent had evidence of impaired penile blood supply. Nerve conduction disorders were present in 54 percent, most commonly in diabetics. Nine patients had hypogonadism. Four of these had reduced gonadotropin levels, and three of these four had hyperprolactinemia. Two patients were hypo-

thyroid. Over 90 percent had coexisting medical conditions including hypertension or vascular disease, or were taking medications that could have been contributing to their impotence, and 19 percent had previously undergone prostatectomy. This study emphasizes that psychogenic impotence is more common in younger subjects than in the aged. In addition, it illustrates that impotence is frequently multifactorial in this age group.

Wiseman et al. [97] reported that one-third of a group of married, physically and emotionally healthy men between the ages of 60 and 70 suffered from impotence. Increased serum prolactin levels correlated with decreased libido and frequency of sexual activity. Although hyperprolactinemia is an uncommon cause of impotence in younger men, some studies suggest that up to 10 percent of older males may have a pituitary adenoma at autopsy. Based on this information, hyperprolactinemia may be a frequent cause of impotence in elderly men.

Evaluation
Generally, if the impotence has been of gradual onset and associated with a decrease in sexual desire, if there is no evidence of organic pathology, and if the patient and his spouse are not concerned, there is probably no point in investigating further. If the patient desires evaluation, however, the first thing to do is to take a careful history, determining the patient's past and present sexual patterns and his use of prescribed and over-the-counter drugs and alcohol. Impotence of gradual onset suggests an organic cause, whereas a recent and rather abrupt onset suggests a psychiatric cause, particularly if it has been associated with recent life stresses. Patients with psychologic impotence often have selective impotence—i.e., they may be able to have intercourse with certain partners but not others, and they generally also have maintenance of nocturnal tumescence and morning erections. If desire is normal but there is no evidence of erection, a vascular or neurologic cause is more likely. If there is a decrease in both desire and potency, an endocrine cause is probable. The patient should be questioned not only about psychologic symptoms but also about neurologic or vascular symptoms such as claudication and numbness.

The physical examination should concentrate on signs of androgen deficiency or estrogen excess, vascular disease, and neurologic function. Patients should be examined for the presence of a varicocele or testicular atrophy. Reflexes and sensation should be tested in the lower extremities, and perianal sensation and perianal reflexes should be assessed. Pulses should be felt in the lower extremities, and the patient should be examined for bruits.

All patients should have measurements of the serum testosterone level as well as of LH and FSH levels. Because of the pulsatile secretion of these hormones, it is better to take blood samples on three separate mornings or take three samples on the same occasion, 30 to 60 minutes apart. It is also reasonable to perform thyroid function tests and measure prolactin levels in all patients. Patients with hyperprolactinemia should be further evaluated with visual screening, computed tomographic (CT) scanning, and other tests of endocrine function to search for a pituitary tumor. Nocturnal penile tumescence has been the gold standard used to rule out psychogenic impotence. In general, if nocturnal penile tumescence is normal, psychogenic impotence is likely. To formally evaluate this, the patient must be admitted and investigated in a sleep laboratory, which is quite expensive. Recently a snap gauge has become available that may be useful as a screening procedure to determine whether nocturnal penile erections are present.

If the cause of the impotence is not readily apparent after these evaluations, patients can be referred to specialized clinics for more extensive investigations including nerve conduction studies to assess the presence of peripheral neuropathy and Doppler studies or selective angiography to document arterial disease.

Management
Management depends on the underlying cause. In some patients a discussion of the normal aging changes that affect sexual function will allay their anxiety and allow them to resume normal sexual function. Sex counseling may be appropriate for some couples, even in their seventies. Depression should be treated with antidepressants. Surgery to revascularize the arterial supply to the penis should be considered experimental at this time. Any drugs that could be contributing to impotence should be stopped, or alternate medication should be tried, and alcohol consumption should be reduced or discontinued when it may be a contributing factor. In patients with low or borderline testosterone levels, a trial of testosterone may be indicated. Intramuscular preparations are preferred to limit hepatic toxicity. Therapy should be started with 30- to 40-mg injections of testosterone cypionate at three-day intervals, so that the drug can be discontinued if urethral obstruction occurs. The usual maintenance dose is 100 to 200 mg every two to three weeks [95]. In general, the medication must be given for at least two months to determine whether it is beneficial. In patients who respond, it can be withdrawn at six months to see if it is still required. Testosterone is contraindicated in patients with prostate cancer, and it may result in urinary tract obstruction in patients with benign prostatic hypertrophy.

Patients with hyperprolactinemia often show an increase in libido and potency with between 5.0 and 7.5 mg per day of bromocriptine. If all else fails in patients with vascular or neurologic causes, penile prostheses can now be inserted by a number of centers. Although this procedure has not been carefully assessed in older men, studies in younger men suggest that it may be met with patient satisfaction in up to 80 percent of cases.

Adrenal Cortex
The major architectural change with age in the adrenal cortex is an increase in the presence of benign cortical nodular hyperplasia [98]. Autopsy studies indicate the presence of bilateral, multifocal nodules, varying in size from microscopic to macroscopic, in as many as two-thirds of elderly individuals. Even when quite large, these nodules are rarely associated with clinical or chemical evidence of glucocorticoid or mineralocorticoid excess.

CORTISOL
Cortisol, the major glucocorticoid, is produced by the adrenal cortex under the influence of the hypothalamic-hypophyseal axis. Corticotropin-releasing factor (CRF) of hypothalamic origin stimulates the release of adrenocorticotropic

hormone (ACTH) from the anterior pituitary, which in turn stimulates the adrenal cortical production of cortisol. Under normal conditions, there is a nyctohemeral pattern of plasma cortisol, with a peak early in the morning and a stable low value throughout the remainder of the day. In response to stress, this pattern is abolished, and plasma cortisol levels increase abruptly.

Basal cortisol disposal rates decrease by 25 to 35 percent in healthy elderly individuals, presumably secondary to reduced hepatic metabolism of the hormone. This decreased disposal is matched by a 25 to 30 percent reduction in cortisol secretion rates [99]. This balancing of decreased disposal and secretion rates results in the maintenance of normal plasma levels in old age and suggests the presence of an intact negative feedback system by which cortisol is downregulated to compensate for the decreased disposal; thus, excess accumulation of cortisol in plasma is avoided. The 24-hour pattern of cortisol secretion is unchanged with age.

Dynamic studies of glucocorticoid metabolism including stimulation with ACTH and insulin-induced hypoglycemia, suppression with dexamethasone, and testing of the reserve capacity of the hypothalamic-hypophyseal axis (metapyrone) yield similar results in young and old subjects [100,101,102]. In addition, the ACTH and cortisol responses to injection of CRF are unchanged with age in healthy men [103]. Plasma cortisol responses to surgery have also been found to be intact in elderly individuals. Thus, the occasional practice of protecting elderly individuals undergoing surgery with supplemental steroids appears to be without justification in the absence of specific evidence of impaired adrenal reserve.

Contrary to the data on cortisol secretion, there is evidence that adrenal androgen secretion is impaired with age in subjects over 70. Basal levels of dehydroepiandrosterone (DHEA) are one-third the level of that in subjects in their twenties [104]. In addition, DHEA responses to ACTH and CRF are impaired with age.

RENIN AND ALDOSTERONE PHYSIOLOGY

Aldosterone is produced by the zona glomerulosa of the adrenal cortex and is secreted in response to ACTH, elevations of potassium, decreases in plasma sodium, and increases in circulating levels of angiotensin. Aldosterone is an important regulator of sodium reabsorption and potassium excretion in the distal nephron and plays a vital role in the maintenance of volume and composition of the extracellular fluid. As with cortisol, the secretion rate of aldosterone is significantly lower in elderly individuals; however, normal plasma levels are not maintained [105]. Under basal conditions, plasma aldosterone is approximately 30 percent lower in healthy individuals 70 to 80 years of age compared to the level seen in younger adults. In response to a low sodium diet, aldosterone secretion increases threefold in young subjects and doubles in the elderly [106]. The decreased aldosterone levels in old age do not appear to be related to any changes in plasma potassium or extracellular fluid volume; they are most likely related to parallel reductions in renin that are found with advancing age. That the decrease in aldosterone does not represent absolute failure of the adrenal capacity to produce the hormone is suggested by the finding that plasma aldosterone levels after ACTH administration are the same in young and old individuals.

These normal age-related changes in renin and aldosterone are important for several reasons. Since hypertensive individuals are often categorized into different physiologic groups depending on their renin level, an elderly individual with normal renin for his or her age might be incorrectly categorized as a low-renin hypertensive if age-adjusted criteria are not utilized. Lower plasma aldosterone levels in the elderly may predispose them to the development of hyperkalemia. The elderly are particularly vulnerable in this regard because glomerular filtration rate, a prime determinant of potassium disposal, is also impaired with age. This combination of physiologic impairments makes an elderly individual particularly susceptible to the development of hyperkalemia after the administration of potassium-sparing diuretics such as triamterene or spironolactone.

ADRENAL DISEASES

Neither the tests employed in the clinical evaluation of adrenal function nor interpretation of the results are changed by age. Both adrenal hyperfunction (Cushing's disease and Cushing's syndrome) and hypofunction (Addison's disease) are primarily diseases of middle age and occur rarely in the elderly. Cases of hypercorticism in old age are easily overlooked because several of the clinical expressions of glucocorticoid excess including weight gain, osteoporosis, carbohydrate intolerance, and hypertension are commonly seen in elderly individuals with normal adrenal function. Suspicion for Cushing's disease in the elderly must be high to avoid overlooking this treatable entity. The diagnosis can easily be ruled out by giving 1 mg of dexamethasone at midnight and measuring cortisol in the morning. The test is normal if the morning value is less than 5 μg per dl. There are no data to indicate the influence of age on the relative frequency of the causes of glucocorticoid excess (pituitary or adrenal tumors or ectopic production of ACTH). In addition, no studies have been reported to indicate how well the elderly tolerate various forms of therapy for this condition. Neurosurgical procedures for removal of ACTH-producing tumors are well tolerated by all age groups. In patients who are not surgical candidates, a recent case report in an elderly subject suggests that glucocorticoid excess caused by an ACTH-producing pituitary tumor can be managed successfully during the long term with metapyrone, thus avoiding a neurosurgical procedure [107].

Adrenal insufficiency, a rare disease at any age, can easily be misdiagnosed in elderly patients [108]. Addison's disease, idiopathic in about two-thirds of young subjects, is idiopathic in about 40 percent of older subjects; most of the rest of the cases are caused by tuberculosis. Other causes of adrenal insufficiency in the aged include adrenal infarction or hemorrhage associated with sepsis or hypotension and infiltrative diseases including fungal infection, sarcoidosis, or cancer. The presentation of adrenal insufficiency in the elderly is vague and nonspecific. Symptoms include failure to thrive, fatigue and weakness, anorexia and weight loss, gastrointestinal symptoms, confusion, postural dizziness, and arthralgias. Clinical features of adrenal insufficiency include cachexia, orthostatic hypotension or supine hypotension, and

hyperpigmentation. Laboratory findings consist of azotemia, acidosis, hyperkalemia, hyponatremia, anemia, and eosinophilia. Many of the above symptoms, signs, or laboratory findings may be attributed to age or other chronic disease, and the proper etiology may not be appreciated. For example, confusion may be ascribed to dementia, or orthostatic hypotension to age or antihypertensive therapy. The diagnosis of adrenal insufficiency should be suspected in an older individual who has the nonspecific symptoms described above when they are associated with supine hypotension or normotension (if the patient has been previously hypertensive), hyperpigmentation, hypoglycemia, hyponatremia, azotemia, hyperkalemia, and eosinophilia. The diagnostic workup is the same in older as in younger individuals, but particular care must be taken to exclude tuberculosis.

In approaching the treatment of adrenal insufficiency from whatever cause, the decreased disposal of cortisol with age should be taken into account. Frequently, normal plasma cortisol values can be obtained with a total dose of 25 mg of hydrocortisone daily. Doses of 37.5 mg or even 50 mg per day, which are commonly prescribed in the young, may result in development of a mild hypercorticism over long periods of time. As in younger patients with adrenal insufficiency, patients will require larger doses of steroids during times of stress. The prognosis is excellent with treatment in all age groups provided that the underlying pathologic process that led to adrenal insufficiency can be corrected.

AUTONOMIC NERVOUS SYSTEM
The recent development of reliable techniques for the measurement of catecholamines in plasma has stimulated studies of the possible relation between aging and the sympathoadrenal system. The general consensus of opinion at the present time is that basal circulating norepinephrine is not decreased with normal aging, and it is likely that it is increased [109] (Fig. 28-4). The physiologic significance of such an increase might relate to several age-related physiologic changes including decreased end-organ responsiveness because of receptor downregulation or central nervous system changes resulting

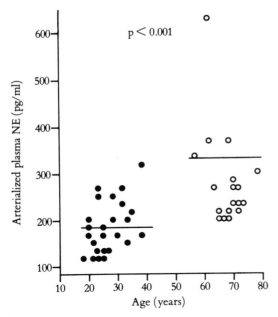

FIGURE 28-4. *Arterialized plasma norepinephrine levels in healthy young (●) and old (○) subjects. (From R. C. Veith, et al. Age differences in plasma norepinephrine kinetics in humans.* J. Gerontol. *41:319, 1986.)*

in less tonic inhibitory input into the brain stem areas regulating sympathetic outflow.

SYMPATHETIC RESPONSIVENESS

The plasma norepinephrine responses to a variety of stimuli including upright posture, exercise, hand grip, and cold pressor tests increase with age [109]. Since increasing fatness is associated with increasing norepinephrine levels and age is associated with increases in total body fat, the relative contributions of age per se and obesity to the results noted above have been questioned. To address this issue, Sowers et al. [110] examined the effects of age on plasma norepinephrine response to upright posture and isometric handgrip exercise in nonobese individuals up to age 75. They found that basal levels of norepinephrine increased significantly with advancing age (slightly more than twofold between the ages of 40 and 70) and that, in the absence of obesity, there persisted statistically significant progressive increases with advancing age in plasma norepinephrine response to upright posture and hand grip. Another question

has been raised about the effects of physical fitness on circulating plasma norepinephrine levels. To address this, Lehmann and Keul [111] determined plasma catecholamine responses to the incremental cycling exercise in young and old competitive cyclists. Norepinephrine levels were higher at each level up to VO_2 max in the older individuals than in their younger counterparts.

The age-related increase in plasma norepinephrine responses in older persons is due in part to increased norepinephrine release and in part to decreased norepinephrine clearance. Employing the tritium-labeled norepinephrine isotope dilution technique, Veith et al. [112] found that basal plasma norepinephrine appearance rate was 32 percent higher, whereas the norepinephrine clearance rate was 19 percent lower in a healthy older group (mean age 68 years) than in their younger counterparts (mean age 27 years). The authors conclude that the principal factor accounting for the 54 percent higher basal plasma norepinephrine levels of older individuals was an increase in the appearance rate.

In another recent study, Hoeldtke and Cimli [113] performed isotope dilution studies on healthy young and old subjects. They found that basal apparent norepinephrine secretion was increased 40 percent in the elderly. Norepinephrine production estimated from urinary excretion of norepinephrine metabolites was similar in young and old subjects, indicating that the increased release of norepinephrine to the circulation did not depend on an increased production of norepinephrine from tyrosine. These authors concluded that in aging there is an alteration in the local disposition of sympathetic norepinephrine.

ADRENAL MEDULLA

Adrenal medullary function, as estimated by circulating epinephrine values, does not appear to be greatly influenced by age. Basal epinephrine values do not change with age, but clearance of epinephrine is enhanced [114], suggesting that the secretion of epinephrine by the adrenal medulla may actually be increased with age. The response of epinephrine to various physiologic stimuli such as mental effort and insulin-induced hypoglycemia is unchanged with age [102].

Parasympathetic Function

Althought there is a need for more studies in this area, there appears to be a decrease in cardiac parasympathetic activity with age [115]. The well-characterized decline in baroreflex sensitivity with age discussed in Chapter 14 could explain both the decrease in parasympathetic activity and the increase in sympathetic nervous system activity. Iris parasympathetic activity is also reduced with age.

Conclusions

The relationship of age-related increases in basal and stimulated norepinephrine to the well-described decrease in response of the aged myocardium to beta-adrenergic stimulation is unclear. Also worthy of study is the relationship between increases in circulating norepinephrine under basal conditions and in response to stress and a number of clinical disorders associated with aging including sleep disorders and hypertension. Since catecholamines can impair glucose tolerance, it was once postulated that the sympathetic overactivity that occurs with aging may play a role in the carbohydrate intolerance of aging. Recent data do not support this hypothesis [116]. Of particular interest is the apparently persistent observation that the capacity to inhibit sympathetic activity after response to a stimulus appears to be blunted in the elderly, resulting in longer peak norepinephrine excursions in older individuals compared to their younger counterparts. Persistent stimulation throughout the day accompanied by a longer peak response might result in development of a gradual hyperadrenergic state in the elderly, a state that might have important physiologic as well as pathologic implications.

It has long been held that an age-related decline in sympathetic nervous system function led to the increased frequency of such disorders as accidental hypothermia and orthostatic hypotension in the elderly. As can be seen from the data already reviewed, current evidence indicates that sympathetic activity probably increases and certainly does not decrease with normal aging. Thus these disorders, although they may be based in part on autonomic nervous system dysfunction with age, should be viewed as pathologic in nature and do not represent extensions of the normal aging process.

Accidental Hypothermia

Accidental hypothermia is the unintentional drop of body temperature below 95°F (35°C). Exposure to freezing air is generally not the provocative cold stress, although exposure to cold air during winter or doing outdoor work, or immersion in cold water can certainly cause hypothermia. Rather, most afflicted aged patients become hypothermic while at home in mildly cold environments, with most episodes initiated by air temperatures near 60°F.

Current prevalence, incidence, and mortality data regarding accidental hypothermia are inadequate. In a large community survey conducted in Great Britain during the winter of 1972, it was found that 10 percent of the elderly population experienced early morning core temperatures of 35.5°C or less [117]. There was no correlation between low body temperature and living alone, being housebound, lack of central heating, or lack of indoor plumbing, all suggesting that increased urbanization does not reduce the risk of hypothermia in the elderly. The only American data were collected in a study in Maine [118]. These authors surveyed 97 elderly subjects (average age 74) from an internal medicine clinic, many of whom were poor or were living in subsidized housing. No subject was found to have a basal body temperature of less than 35.5°C. The mortality from hypothermia is also difficult to determine because there are no definite pathologic findings with this syndrome, most dead bodies are cold when found, and the index of suspicion of physicians for this diagnosis is low. Even if the inadequacy of death certificate data is acknowledged, American data support a substantially increased risk of death from hypothermia in patients over the age of 75 [119]. Hypothermia may also result in significant morbidity. A recent study in Britain showed that among malnourished patients, there was a midwinter peak in hip fracture incidence and a higher mortality after hip fracture [120]. Malnourished patients were frequently hypothermic on admission to the hospital, whereas well-nourished patients had normal body temperatures. It is presumed that malnutrition leads to impaired heat generation, hypothermia, lack of coordination, and subsequent injury. Recent data also suggest that elderly diabetics have a six times greater risk of hypothermia, probably due to vascular disease, which alters thermoregulatory mechanisms [121].

ETIOLOGY

The usual factors implicated in the genesis of hypothermia are environmental cold, age-related physiologic changes in thermoregulation, drugs, and diseases that either decrease heat production, increase heat loss, or impair thermoregulation [122] (Table 28-8). Environmental cold can clearly result in accidental hypothermia even in young individuals, and only minor degrees of cold can cause hypothermia in elderly debilitated individuals. There are a number of physiologic changes with age that predispose the elderly to hypothermia. The elderly appear to have a diminished perception of cold. Changes with age in response to endogenous catecholamines result in a reduced vasoconstrictor response to cold and a decreased shivering response to a cold stimulus. Other factors that predispose old people to hypothermia include reduced physical activity and decreased caloric intake, which reduce the ability of an older person to generate heat. The decrease in lean body mass that occurs with age means that even if shivering occurs, it is less effective in heat production.

TABLE 28-8. *Causes of hypothermia in the elderly*

Environmental cold
Physiologic changes
Diminished perception of cold
Changes in autonomic nervous system function
Decreased physical activity
Decreased caloric intake
Decreased muscle mass
Drugs
Tranquilizers
Sedatives
Antidepressants
Alcohol
Diseases
Decreased heat production
Increased heat loss
Impaired thermoregulation

A number of diseases and drugs may alter thermoregulatory mechanisms. Decreased heat production occurs in hypothyroidism, hypopituitarism, hypoglycemia, starvation, and malnutrition. Forced or involuntary inactivity as in Parkinson's disease, arthritis, paralysis, and dementia decreases heat production and may increase the risk of hypothermia. Increased heat loss can occur secondary to inflammatory skin disease, alcohol-induced vasodilation, cold exposure, and Paget's disease.

Central hypothalamic temperature regulation can be disturbed by a variety of events including stroke, subarachnoid hemorrhage, subdural hematoma, and brain tumor. Uremia and carbon monoxide poisoning may also affect thermal regulation. Many drugs, including phenothiazines, tricyclic antidepressants, benzodiazepines, barbiturates, reserpine, and narcotics, depress central thermoregulation and predispose a person to accidental hypothermia. Chlorpromazine, which also inhibits shivering, is the best known offender.

DIAGNOSIS

The diagnosis of accidental hypothermia depends on the ability to measure body temperature below 95°F. Clinical custom with ill patients is to search for and exclude fever, and body temperature is then recorded as high or normal. The standard clinical thermometer is calibrated from 94 to 108°F. The highest temperature of a hypothermic patient is 94°F. A rectal thermometer reading from 84 to 108°F is available from most hospital suppliers, although it is not in common use. In the absence of a low-reading thermometer, more expensive thermistors or thermocouples have been used. If hypothermia is suspected based on the history or physical examination, core temperature should be recorded using one of the low-reading instruments.

Most clinical laboratory data are not specific for hypothermia. Hemoconcentration, dehydration, leukocytosis, lactic acidosis, bronchopneumonia, ileus, and thrombocytopenia are all common signs of this condition. There are, however, a few distinctive indicators of hypothermia. The electrocardiogram may exhibit a major diagnostic clue. A junctional or J wave

[123] is a small deflection that occurs early in the ST segment, positive in the left and negative in the right ventricular lead. Although it is present in only about one-third of hypothermic patients, when found, it always signifies hypothermia. Another more common electrocardiographic finding frequently found in the nonshivering hypothermic patient is a regular oscillation of the baseline produced by the imperceptible tremor and increased muscle tone.

The blood glucose findings in hypothermic patients have been a point of confusion. Hypothermia produces hyperglycemia by increasing gluconeogenesis through increased steroid and catecholamine secretion. Additionally, although insulin secretion is stimulated, cold interferes with insulin's action, further raising glucose concentration. When hypothermic patients are hypoglycemic, the causality is reversed—that is, hypoglycemia, usually drug-induced, produces hypothermia.

SIGNS AND SYMPTOMS

The symptoms of hypothermia are insidious and transient [122]. Although elderly people with temperatures between 95 and 97°F usually complain of cold, patients with established hypothermia do not. The clinical findings are numerous but nonspecific, and without suspicion of hypothermia they suggest stroke or metabolic disorder. The patient feels cool to the touch and has a history of progressive confusion and sleepiness that may have progressed to coma during the previous two to three days.

Neurologic findings include thick, slow speech, ataxic gait, and depressed reflexes. Pathologic reflexes and plantar responses may be present, and pupils may be dilated and sluggishly reactive. Focal signs, seizures, paralysis, and sensory loss have also been reported.

Although shivering may occur at temperatures higher than 95°F, most reports find that shivering is strikingly absent in hypothermic elderly patients. Instead, marked rigidity with a generalized increase in muscle tone, occasionally accompanied by a fine tremor, may be found.

Although many people have cold extremities in winter, a hypothermic patient has a cold abdomen and back as well. The skin has a cadaveric pallor and chill, and pressure points show erythematous, bullous, or purpuric patches. Subcutaneous tissues are firm, probably from edema. Edema also produces a puffy appearance, especially of the face.

The cardiovascular system is initially stimulated by cold, resulting in peripheral vasoconstriction, tachycardia, and blood pressure elevation, but as hypothermia progresses, the myocardium is depressed, producing hypotension and progressively slow sinus bradycardia. Severe hypothermia can reduce blood pressure and heart beat to barely detectable levels, sometimes leading to an erroneous pronouncement of death. The bradycardia, uninfluenced by atropine or vagotomy, is thought to be a direct result of myocardial depression. In addition to sinus bradycardia, a variety of cardiac arrhythmias have been reported as temperature drop continues, including atrial fibrillation and flutter, premature ventricular beats, and idioventricular rhythm.

Death usually occurs from cardiac failure or ventricular fibrillation. The temperature at which each cardiac event appears is variable, but at temperatures below 85°F, lethal events are a major risk, particularly in patients with an underlying heart disease. Movement or excessive stimulation of hypothermic patients may provoke some of the cardiovascular abnormalities noted above and should be done as gently as possible. It is important to remember that resuscitation should be prolonged and aggressive in patients who are profoundly hypothermic. Remarkable recoveries have been reported in patients when resuscitation has been continued while rewarming occurs. Most authorities agree that these patients should not be pronounced dead until cardiopulmonary resuscitation is shown to be ineffective when body temperature has been raised to at least 96.5°F.

The gastrointestinal response to hypothermia consists of decreased peristalsis, producing abdominal distention and decreased or absent bowel sounds and, less often, acute gastric dilatation with vomiting. Pancreatitis may also occur but is usually not apparent until rewarming has occurred. Hepatic metabolism is depressed, and the metabolism of many drugs may therefore be sharply reduced.

Pulmonary findings include depression of respiration and cough reflex. Atelectasis is universal, and pneumonia is common enough to be expected. Pulmonary edema during recovery may be related to increased vascular permeability as well as to congestive heart failure.

Early in hypothermia, cold suppresses secretion of antidiuretic hormone and diminishes tubular responsiveness to its action, provoking a diabetes insipidus-like diuresis. Later, as glomerular filtration and renal blood flow diminish as a result of volume depletion, oliguria and tubular necrosis will follow.

TREATMENT

Patients with accidental hypothermia need to be carefully managed and should be hospitalized and monitored. If the body temperature is below 90°F, patients should probably be treated in an intensive care unit. Treatment of hypothermia includes a slow, spontaneous rewarming or a rapid, active rewarming. Rapid active rewarming is the standard treatment for otherwise healthy young adults suffering from intense exposure-induced hypothermia, but the dogma has been that rapid active rewarming can contribute to the death of aged hypothermic patients by producing profound and irreversible hypotension. Slow steady rewarming (SSR) allows body temperature to rise slowly to normal by conserving the heat that is still being produced and has been the standard treatment for elderly patients with hypothermia.

The technique commonly used has been to insulate the patient in a warmed room to conserve what heat is being produced and to minimize further loss. Body temperature is monitored and allowed to rise 1°F per hour. Even using slow steady rewarming, a more rapid rise in temperature may produce hypotension. In the patient who is hypothermic because of primary hypoglycemia, restoration of blood glucose level usually results in a rapid return of normal temperature. In one report rapid active rewarming [124] under optimal intensive care unit (ICU) monitoring has been advocated as the preferred treatment for hypothermia in the elderly, especially if slow steady rewarming produces inadequate temperature rise. Such ICU care would include familiarity with and readiness to use tracheal intubation with full ventilatory assistance, temporary cardiac pacing, pharmacologic circulatory support, and intracardiac pressure monitoring.

Several other options exist for rewarming the hypothermic patient. Core temperature can be raised successfully in some patients by having the patient inhale warm, humidified oxygen. Peritoneal or hemodialysis with warmed solutions has also been used to induce core central rewarming. Insertion of a nasogastric tube and gastric lavage with warm isotonic saline has been tried in selected cases as well. In general, patients with core temperatures above 92°F can be managed with slow external rewarming and perhaps humidified oxygen. In patients with body temperatures below 90°F consideration should be given to central rewarming with intubation and ventilation, peritoneal dialysis, or gastric lavage.

Insulin effectiveness declines progressively as body temperature falls, and the hyperglycemia of hypothermia is absolutely unresponsive to insulin when the body temperature is below 85°F. Therefore, insulin should be used cautiously in a hypothermic diabetic who is being rewarmed in order to avoid rebound hypoglycemia as temperature rises and insulin effectiveness increases. If the hyperglycemic hypothermic patient is not known to have diabetes, insulin should not be given unless blood glucose is very high, (greater than 350 mg/dl) because in a nondiabetic person hyperglycemia often disappears spontaneously during warming and rehydration as endogenous insulin becomes more effective. There is no evidence to suggest that the routine use of corticosteroids, antibiotics, anticoagulants, or thyroid hormone in the absence of specific indications for the use of these drugs is beneficial.

CONCLUSION

Prevention of accidental hypothermia is preferable to treatment. Since survival correlates with a milder degree of hypothermia, educating the elderly, particularly those with known risk factors, to seek medical attention earlier should reduce mortality and also prevent some cases. Old people with identifiable predisposing problems should have thermostats set at 65°F or higher and should keep a reliable thermometer separate from the thermostat and check it daily, especially during very cold weather. Additional indoor clothing, particularly covering for exposed areas such as hands, feet, and head should be worn. Frequent periods of exercise can increase heat production, and adequate food intake and caloric intake are of prime importance. Drugs that may alter thermoregulatory mechanisms should be discontinued whenever possible.

References

1. Hurley, J. R. Thyroid disease in the elderly. *Med. Clin. North Am.* 67:497, 1983.
2. Sawin, C. T., et al. The aging thyroid. Thyroid deficiency in the Framingham Study. *Arch. Intern. Med.* 145:1386, 1985.
3. Livingston, E. H., et al. Prevalence of thyroid disease and abnormal thyroid tests in older hospitalized and ambulatory persons. *J. Am. Geriatr. Soc.* 35:109, 1987.
4. Greenspan, S. L., et al. Pulsatile secretion of thyrotropin in man. *J. Clin. Endocrinol. Metab.* 63:661, 1986.
5. Harman, S. M., Wehmann, R. E., and Blackman, M. R. Pituitary-thyroid hormone economy in healthy aging men: Basal indices of thyroid function and thyrotropin responses to constant infusions of thyrotropin-releasing hormone. *J. Clin. Endocrinol. Metab.* 58:320, 1984.
6. Ingbar, S. H. The Effects of Aging on Thyroid Hormone Economy in Man. In R. J. Soto, A. DeNicola, and J. Blaquer (eds.). *Physiology of Endocrine Diseases and Mechanisms of Hormone Action.* New York: Liss, 1981. Pp. 135–145.
7. Inada, M., Nishikawa, M., and Kawa, I. Hypothyroidism associated with positive results of the perchlorate discharge test in elderly patients. *Am. J. Med.* 74:1010, 1983.
8. Sawin, C. T., et al. The aging thyroid. Relationship between elevated serum thyrotropin level and thyroid antibodies in elderly patients. *Am. J. Med.* 79:591, 1985.
9. Davis, P. J., and Davis, F. B. Hyperthyroidism in patients over the age of 60 years. *Medicine* 53:161, 1974.
10. Tibaldi, J. M., et al. Thyrotoxicosis in the very old. *Am. J. Med.* 81:619, 1986.
11. Sawin, C. T., et al. The aging thyroid. *J.A.M.A.* 242:247, 1979.
12. Rosenbaum, R. L., and Barzel, U. S. Levothyroxine replacement dose for primary hypothyroidism decreases with age. *Ann. Intern. Med.* 96:53, 1982.
13. Sawin, C. T., et al. Aging and the thyroid: Decreased requirement for thyroid hormone in older hypothyroid patients. *Am. J. Med.* 75:206, 1983.
14. Greenspan, F. S., and Rapoport, B. Thyroid Nodules and Thyroid Cancer. In F. S. Greenspan, and P. H. Forsham (eds.), *Basic and Clinical Endocrinology.* San Francisco: Lange Medical Publications, 1986. Pp. 192–199.
15. Chopra, I. J. Euthyroid sick syndrome: Abnormalities in circulating thyroid hormone physiology in nonthyroidal illness (NTI). *Med. Grand Rounds* 1:201, 1982.
16. Wartofsky, L., and Burman, K. G. Alterations in thyroid function in patients with systemic illness: The "euthyroid sick syndrome." *Endocrine Rev.* 3:164, 1982.
17. Ragatanavin, R., and Braverman, L. E. Euthyroid hyperthyroxinemia. *J. Endocrinol. Invest.* 6:493, 1983.
18. Kaplan, M. M., et al. Prevalence of abnormal thyroid function test results in patients with acute medical illness. *Am. J. Med.* 72:9, 1982.
19. Slag, M. F., et al. Hypothyroxinemia in critically ill patients as a predictor of high mortality. *J.A.M.A.* 245:43, 1981.
20. Chopra, I. J., et al. Serum thyroid hormone binding inhibitor in nonthyroidal illness. *Metabolism* 35:152, 1986.
21. Brent, G. A., and Hershman, J. M. Thyroxine therapy in patients with severe nonthyroidal illnesses and low serum thyroxine concentration. *J. Clin. Endocrinol. Metab.* 63:1, 1986.
22. Davidson, M. B. The effect of aging on carbohydrate metabolism: A review of the English literature and a practical approach to the diagnosis of diabetes mellitus in the elderly. *Metabolism* 28:688, 1979.
23. Graf, R. J., et al. Glycosylated hemoglobin in normal subjects and subjects with maturity onset diabetes. *Diabetes* 27:834, 1978.
24. Elahi, D., et al. Effect of age and obesity on fasting levels of glucose insulin, growth hormone and glucagon in man. *J. Gerontol.* 37:385, 1982.
25. Chen, M., et al. The role of dietary carbohydrate in the decreased glucose tolerance of the elderly. *J. Am. Geriatr. Soc.* 35:417, 1987.
26. Minaker, K. L., et al. Clearance of insulin: Influence of steady state insulin levels and age. *Diabetes* 31:132, 1982.
27. Meneilly, G. S., et al. Insulin action in aging man: Evidence for tissue-specific differences at low physiologic insulin levels. *J. Gerontol.* 42:196, 1987.
28. Rowe, J. W., et al. Characterization of the insulin resistance of aging. *J. Clin. Invest.* 71:1581, 1983.
29. Fink, R. I., et al. The role of the glucose transport system in the postreceptor defect in insulin

action associated with human aging. *J. Clin. Endocrinol. Metab.* 58:721, 1984.

30. Abbott, R. D. Diabetes and the risk of stroke. The Honolulu heart program. *J.A.M.A.* 257:949, 1987.

31. Pyorala, K. Relationship of glucose tolerance and plasma insulin to the incidence of coronary heart disease; results from two population studies in Finland. *Diabetes Care* 2:131, 1979.

32. Welborn, T. A., et al. Coronary heart disease incidence and cardiovascular mortality in Busselten with reference to glucose and insulin concentrations. *Diabetes Care* 2:154, 1979.

33. Zavaroni, I., et al. Effect of age and environmental factors on glucose tolerance and insulin secretion in a worker population. *J. Am. Geriatr. Soc.* 34:271, 1986.

34. Hollenbeck, C. B., et al. Effect of habitual physical activity on regulation of insulin-stimulated glucose disposal in older males. *J. Am. Geriatr. Soc.* 33:273, 1984.

35. Seals, D. R., et al. Glucose tolerance in young and older athletes and sedentary men. *J. Appl. Physiol.* 56:1521, 1984.

36. Reaven, G. M., et al. Age, glucose tolerance, and non–insulin-dependent diabetes mellitus. *J. Am. Geriatr. Soc.* 3:286, 1985.

37. Leblanc, J., et al. Effects of physical training and adiposity on glucose metabolism and I-125 insulin binding. *J. Appl. Physiol.* 46:235, 1979.

38. Bodgardus, C., et al. Effects of physical training and diet therapy on carbohydrate metabolism in patients with glucose intolerance and non–insulin-dependent diabetes mellitus. *Diabetes* 33:311, 1984.

39. Tonino, R. P., et al. Effect of physical training on the insulin resistance of aging. *Clin. Res.* 34:557A, 1986.

40. Seals, D. R., et al. Effects of endurance training on glucose tolerance and plasma lipid levels in older men and women. *J.A.M.A.* 252:645, 1984.

41. Harris, M. I., et al. Prevalence of diabetes and impaired glucose tolerance and plasma glucose levels in U.S. population aged 20–74 years. *Diabetes* 36:523, 1987.

42. Jaspan, J. Monitoring and controlling the patient with non–insulin-dependent diabetes mellitus. *Metabolism* 36 (Suppl. 1):22, 1987.

43. Jarrett, R. J., et al. The Bedford Survey: Ten year mortality rates in newly diagnosed diabetics, borderline diabetics, and normoglycemic controls and risk indices for coronary artery disease in borderline diabetics. *Diabetologia* 22:79, 1983.

44. Kannel, W. B., and McGee, D. L. Diabetes and glucose tolerance as risk factors for cardiovascular disease: The Framingham Study. *Diabetes Care* 2:120, 1979.

45. Minaker, K. L. Aging and diabetes as risk factors for vascular disease. *Am. J. Med.* 82:47, 1987.

46. Schnider, S. L., and Kohn, R. R. Effects of age and diabetes mellitus on the solubility and non-enzymatic glucosylation of human skin collagen. *J. Clin. Invest.* 67:1630, 1981.

47. Pirart, J. Diabetes mellitus and its degenerative complications. A prospective study of 4,400 patients observed between 1947 and 1973. *Diabetes Care* 1:168, 1978.

48. Coppan, R. Determining the most appropriate treatment for patients with non–insulin-dependent diabetes mellitus. *Metabolism* 36 (Suppl.):17, 1987.

49. Boden, G. Treatment strategies for patients with non–insulin-dependent diabetes mellitus. *Am. J. Med.* 79 (Suppl. 2B):23, 1985.

50. Melander, A. Clinical pharmacology of sulfonylureas. *Metabolism* 36 (Suppl. 1):12, 1987.

51. Asplund, K., et al. Glibenclamide associated hypoglycemia: A report on 57 cases. *Diabetologia* 24:412, 1983.

52. University Group Diabetes Program. A study of the effects of hypoglycemic agents on vascular complications in patients with adult onset diabetes. *Diabetes* 19 (Suppl.):747, 1971.

53. Cahill, G. F. Hyperglycemic hyperosmolar coma: A syndrome almost unique to the elderly. *J. Am. Geriatr. Soc.* 31:103, 1983.

54. Wachtel, T., et al. Predisposing factors for the diabetic hyperosmolar state. *Arch. Intern Med.* 147:499, 1987.

55. Wiske, P. S., et al. Increases in immunoreactive parathyroid hormone with age. *N. Engl. J. Med.* 300:1419, 1979.

56. Gallagher, J. C., et al. The effect of age on serum immunoreactive parathyroid hormone in normal and osteoporotic women. *J. Lab. Clin. Med.* 95:373, 1980.

57. Insogna, K. L., et al. Effect of age on serum immunoreactive parathyroid hormone and its biological effects. *J. Clin. Endocrinol. Metab.* 53:1072, 1981.

58. Bolamore, J. R., et al. Effect of age on calcium absorption. *Lancet* 2:535, 1970.

59. Gallagher, J. L., et al. Intestinal calcium absorption and serum vitamin D metabolites in normal subjects and osteoporotic patients. *J. Clin. Invest.* 64:729, 1979.

60. Tsai, K. S., et al. Impaired vitamin D metabolism with aging in women; Possible role in pathogenesis of senile osteoporosis. *J. Clin. Invest.* 73:1668, 1984.

61. Pearson, M. W. Asymptomatic primary hyperparathyroidism in the elderly—a review. *Age Aging* 13:1, 1984.
62. Heath, H., III, et al. Primary hyperparathyroidism. *N. Engl. J. Med.* 302:189, 1980.
63. Mundy, G. R., et al. Primary hyperparathyroidism: Changes in the pattern of clinical presentation. *Lancet* 1:1317, 1980.
64. Nudelman, I., et al. Surgical treatment of primary hyperparathyroidism in the elderly patient. *Isr. J. Med. Sci.* 19:150, 1983.
65. Alveryd, A., et al. Indications for surgery in the elderly patient with primary hyperparathyroidism. *Acta Chir. Scand.* 142:491, 1976.
66. Mannix, H., Jr., et al. Hyperparathyroidism in the elderly. *Am. J. Surg.* 139:581, 1980.
67. Peskin, G., et al. Expanding indications for early parathyroidectomy in the elderly female. *Am. J. Surg.* 136:45, 1978.
68. Heath, D. A., et al. Surgical treatment of primary hyperparathyroidism in the elderly. *Br. Med. J.* 280:1406, 1980.
69. Tibblin, S., et al. Hyperparathyroidism in the elderly. *Ann. Surg.* 197:135, 1983.
70. Bilezikian, J. P., et al. The medical management of primary hyperparathyroidism. *Ann. Intern. Med.* 96:198, 1982.
71. Scholz, D. A., et al. Asymptomatic primary hyperparathyroidism. *Mayo Clin. Proc.* 56:473, 1981.
72. Selby, P. L., et al. Ethinyl estradiol and norethindrone in the treatment of primary hyperparathyroidism in postmenopausal women. *N. Engl. J. Med.* 314:1481, 1986.
73. Gallagher, J. C., et al. Treatment with oestrogens of primary hyperparathyroidism in postmenopausal women. *Lancet* 1:503, 1972.
74. Marcus, R., et al. Conjugated estrogens in the treatment of post-menopausal women with hyperparathyroidism. *Ann. Intern. Med.* 100:633, 1984.
75. Broadus, A. E., et al. A detailed evaluation of oral phosphate therapy in selected patients with primary hyperparathyroidism. *J. Clin. Endocrinol. Metab.* 56:953, 1983.
76. Glaser, B., et al. Effect of acute cimetidine administration on indices of parathyroid hormone action in healthy subjects and patients with primary and secondary hyperparathyroidism. *J. Clin. Endocrinol. Metab.* 59:993, 1984.
77. Vora, A. M., et al. Parathyroid hormone secretion: Effect of β-adrenergic blockade before and after surgery for primary hyperparathyroidism. *J. Clin. Endocrinol. Metab.* 53:599, 1981.
78. Shane, E., et al. Effects of dichloromethylene diphosphonate on serum and urinary calcium in primary hyperparathyroidism. *Ann. Intern. Med.* 95:23, 1981.
79. Vermeulen, A., et al. Testosterone secretion and metabolism in male senescence. *J. Clin. Endocrinol. Metab.* 34:730, 1972.
80. Sparrow, D., et al. The influence of age, alcohol consumption and body build on gonadal function in man. *J. Clin. Endocrinol. Metab.* 51:508, 1980.
81. Harman, S., et al. Reproductive hormones in aging men I: Measurement of sex steroids, basal luteinizing hormone and Leydig cell response to human chorionic gonadotropin. *J. Clin. Endocrinol. Metab.* 51:35, 1980.
82. Deslypere, J. P., et al. Leydig cell function in normal men: Effect of age, life-style, residence, diet and activity. *J. Clin. Endocrinol. Metab.* 59:955, 1984.
83. Zumoff, B., et al. Age variation of the 24 hour mean plasma concentrations of androgens, estrogens and gonadotropins in normal adult men. *J. Clin. Endocrinol. Metab.* 54:534, 1982.
84. Murono, E. P., et al. The aging Leydig cell VI: Response of testosterone precursors to gonadotropin in men. *Acta Endocrinol. (KOH).* 100:455, 1982.
85. Harman, S. M., et al. Reproductive hormones in aging men, II: Basal pituitary gonadotropins and gonadotropin responses to luteinizing hormone releasing hormone. *J. Clin. Endocrinol. Metab.* 54:537, 1982.
86. Hassdorf, T., et al. Secretion of prolactin in healthy men and women of different ages. *Aktuel Gerontol.* 10:119, 1980.
87. Blackman, M. R., et al. Basal serum prolactin levels and prolactin responses to constant infusions of thyrotropin releasing hormone in healthy aging men. *J. Gerontol.* 41:699, 1986.
88. Nieschlag, E., et al. Reproductive functions in young fathers and grandfathers. *J. Clin. Endocrinol. Metab.* 55:676, 1982.
89. Pfeiffer, E., et al. Sexual behavior in aged men and women. *Arch. Gen. Psychiatr.* 19:753, 1968.
90. Martin, C. E. Factors affecting sexual functioning in 60–79 year old married males. *Arch. Sex. Behav.* 10:399, 1981.
91. Masters, W. H. Sex and aging—Expectations and reality. *Hosp. Pract.* August 15:175, 1986.
92. Tsitouras, P. D., et al. Relationship of serum testosterone to sexual activity in healthy elderly men. *J. Gerontol.* 37:288, 1982.
93. Morley, J. E. Impotence. *Am. J. Med.* 80:897, 1986.
94. Pearlman, C. K. Frequency of intercourse in

males at different ages. *Med. Aspects Human Sexuality* 6:92, 1972.

95. Harman, S. M., et al. Alterations in Reproductive and Sexual Function: Male. In R. Andres, et al. (eds.), *Principles of Geriatric Medicine.* New York: McGraw-Hill, 1985. Pp. 337–353.

96. Davis, S. S., et al. Evaluation of impotence in older men. *West. J. Med.* 142:499, 1985.

97. Weizman, A., et al. The correlation of increased serum prolactin levels with decreased sexual desire and activity in elderly men. *J. Am. Geriatr. Soc.* 31:485, 1983.

98. Dobbie, J. W. Adrenal cortical nodular hyperplasia: The aging adrenal. *J. Pathol.* 9:1, 1969.

99. West, C. D., et al. Adrenal cortical function and cortisone metabolism in old age. *J. Clin. Endocrinol.* 10:1197, 1961.

100. Blichert-Toft, N., et al. Pituitary adrenal corticoid stimulation in the aged as reflected in levels of plasma cortisol and compound S. *Acta Med. Scand.* 136:665, 1970.

101. Blichert-Toft, N. The Adrenal Glands in Old Age. In R. B. Greenblatt (ed.), *Geriatric Endocrinology.* New York: Raven, 1978.

102. Meneilly, G. S., et al. Counterregulatory responses to insulin-induced glucose reduction in the elderly. *J. Clin. Endocrinol. Metab.* 61:178, 1985.

103. Pavlov, E. P., et al. Responses of plasma adrenocorticotropin, cortisol, and dehydroepiandrosterone to ovine corticotropin-releasing hormone in healthy aging men. *J. Clin. Endocrinol. Metab.* 62:767, 1986.

104. Orentreich, N., et al. Age changes and sex differences in serum dehydroepiandrosterone sulfate concentrations throughout adulthood. *J. Clin. Endocrinol. Metab.* 59:551, 1984.

105. Flood, C., et al. The metabolism and secretion of aldosterone in elderly subjects. *J. Clin. Invest.* 46:960, 1967.

106. Weidmann, P., et al. Effect of aging on plasma renin and aldosterone in normal man. *Kidney Int.* 8:325, 1975.

107. Donchier, J., et al. Successful control of Cushing's disease in the elderly with long-term metapyrone. *Postgrad. Med. J.* 62:727, 1986.

108. Moss, C. N., et al. Adrenal insufficiency (Addison's disease) in the elderly. *J. Am. Geriatr. Soc.* 33:63, 1985.

109. Rowe, J. W., et al. Sympathetic nervous system and aging in man. *Endocrine Rev.* 1:167, 1980.

110. Sowers, J. R., et al. Plasma norepinephrine responses to posture and isometric exercise increase with age in the absence of obesity. *J. Gerontol.* 38:315, 1983.

111. Lehmann, M., et al. Age-associated changes of exercise-induced plasma catecholamine responses. *Eur. J. Appl. Physiol.* 55:302, 1986.

112. Veith, R. C., et al. Age differences in plasma norepinephrine kinetics in humans. *J. Gerontol.* 41:319, 1986.

113. Hoeldtke, R. D., et al. Effects of aging on catecholamine metabolism. *J. Clin. Endocrinol. Metab.* 60:479, 1985.

114. Wilkie, F. L., et al. Age-related changes in venous catecholamines basally and during epinephrine infusion in man. *J. Gerontol.* 40:133, 1985.

115. Pfeifer, M. A., et al. Differential changes of autonomic nervous system function with age in man. *Am. J. Med.* 75:249, 1983.

116. Chen, M., et al. Plasma catecholamines, dietary carbohydrate, and glucose intolerance: A comparison between young and old men. *J. Clin. Endocrinol. Metab.* 62:1193, 1986.

117. Fox, R. H., et al. Body temperatures in the elderly: A national study of physiologic, social and environmental conditions. *Br. Med. J.* 1:200, 1973.

118. Keilson, L., et al. Screening for hypothermia in the ambulatory elderly. The Maine experience. *J.A.M.A.* 254:1781, 1985.

119. Rango, N. Hypothermia in the elderly. Testimony before U.S. House Select Committee on Aging, Subcommittee on Health and Long-Term Care, February 3, 1982.

120. Bastow, M. D., et al. Undernutrition, hypothermia and injury in elderly women with fractured femur: An injury response to altered metabolism. *Lancet* 1:143, 1983.

121. Neil, H. A. Risk of hypothermia in elderly patients with diabetes. *Br. Med. J. (Clin. Res.)* 293:416, 1986.

122. Besdine, R. W. Accidental hypothermia in the elderly. *Med. Grand Rounds* 1:36, 1982.

123. Emslie-Smith, D. Accidental hypothermia: A common condition with a pathognomonic electrocardiogram. *Lancet* 2:492, 1958.

124. Nicholas, F., et al. Vingt-quatre observations d'hypothermies accidentelles. *Anesth. Analg.* 31:485, 1974.

29

Osteoporosis

CAROL C. PILBEAM
NEIL M. RESNICK

ALL PEOPLE lose bone with age. If bone becomes so fragile that fracture can occur spontaneously or with minimal trauma, the condition is called *osteoporosis*. Examples of osteoporotic fractures include vertebral crush fractures secondary to compressive stresses generated during normal weight bearing and hip or Colles' fractures resulting from falls from standing height.

Osteoporosis is a common disease, affecting 15 to 20 million adults in the United States and accounting for about 70 percent of all fractures occurring in people over 45 years of age [1]. The total cost of osteoporosis and related fractures in the United States was estimated to be over 6 billion dollars in 1983, with the major morbidity, mortality, and medical costs resulting from the more than 200,000 hip fractures that occur each year [2]. Despite the severity of the problem, we cannot yet predict who will develop osteoporotic fractures, nor do we have reliable treatment for those who do. Moreover, the magnitude of the problem is expected to increase as the elderly population continues to grow.

In this chapter we provide a brief overview of bone anatomy and physiology, review age-related bone losses and fracture patterns, discuss some aspects of the pathogenesis of osteoporosis, and summarize the current status of the diagnosis and treatment of osteoporosis. Although we attempt to separate the physiology

of normal aging from the pathology of osteoporosis, this separation is not always possible, especially among the very old.

Anatomy and Physiology of Bone

The bony skeleton contains about 99 percent of the total body calcium in the form of hydroxyapatite. Approximately 80 percent of the body's bone is cortical (compact) bone and consists largely of lamellae arranged concentrically around longitudinal vascular channels (haversian systems). It is this type of bone that forms the shafts of long bones and the cortices of other bones. The remaining 20 percent of bone is the more porous trabecular (cancellous) bone that is found at the end of long bones and predominates in vertebral bodies. It consists of an open framework of interconnected fragments of lamellar systems, bordered on one side by a shell of cortical bone and interfacing on the other with bone marrow. The proportions of these two types of bone vary in different regions of the body. The proportion of trabecular bone is about 70 percent in vertebral bodies, 50 percent in the femur between the greater and lesser trochanters, 25 percent in the femoral neck, and less than 5 percent at midradius [3].

Throughout life bone is being remodeled at discrete loci through a cyclic process of resorption coupled with formation [4]. The cycle begins with the recruitment and differentiation of cells derived from hematopoietic stem cells [4,5], which eventually become the major bone-resorbing cells, the osteoclasts. A week or two of resorption is followed by a relatively inactive (reversal) phase of several weeks, characterized by the presence of mononuclear phagocytes, which lay down a cementing substance on the resorption surface. Subsequently, preosteoblasts (derived from stromal stem cells [4,5]) appear, followed by osteoblasts, which begin a matrix formation phase lasting two to three months. Mineralization of osteoid begins soon after formation but may continue long after formation is complete. The rate of remodeling is up to eight times higher in trabecular bone (turnover on the order of 20 percent a year) than in cortical bone, and hence metabolic bone diseases frequently affect trabecular bone first. In addition to its importance in the maintenance of mineral homeostasis, remodeling may also play a role in repair of microfractures.

Remodeling is regulated by the complicated and varying interactions of local and systemic factors that act directly and indirectly on bone [6,7]. Two of the main systemic factors are parathyroid hormone (PTH) and calcitriol (1,25-dihydroxyvitamin D), the active metabolite of vitamin D. Because these hormones are the major calcium-regulating hormones, they play a prominent role in integrating bone remodeling with calcium homeostasis. When serum calcium falls, PTH stimulates mobilization of calcium from bone by accelerating resorption and/or by inhibiting formation. PTH also acts on the kidney to stimulate the reabsorption of calcium, the excretion of phosphate, and the synthesis of calcitriol. Calcitriol stimulates intestinal absorption of calcium and phosphorus and also acts directly on bone to stimulate resorption. The combined actions of PTH and calcitriol maintain serum calcium and phosphorus concentrations, which in turn permit normal calcification of osteoid. Calcitonin in pharmacologic doses inhibits bone resorption and decreases renal tubular reabsorption of calcium and phosphate. Because there are no clearly definable clinical syndromes of calcitonin excess or deficiency, its importance in calcium homeostasis is controversial [8].

Interaction of systemic hormones with cells at the bone–bone marrow interface leads to the differentiation and proliferation of bone-resorbing or bone-forming cells, but the specific interactions at the cellular level are only beginning to be understood. For example, although PTH is a major mediator of bone resorption, causing an increase in osteoclast number and activity, PTH receptors are found on osteoblasts or osteoblast precursor cells but not on osteoclasts [5]. Moreover, depending on conditions, PTH can either stimulate or inhibit formation [7]. The complexity of the system is further highlighted when one realizes how many other factors may be involved in the regulation of remodeling—other systemic hormones (glucocorticoids, sex steroids, insulin, thyroxine, growth hormone), growth factors (somatomedin, epidermal growth factor), local factors (prostaglandins, osteoclast-activating factor), calcium and phosphate ions, and mechanical stress [6,7].

Pattern of Bone Loss with Aging

Maximum bone mass is attained in the mid- to late twenties. After a period of stability, bone mineral decreases with aging. Women begin to lose cortical bone mineral in their early fifties, with overall losses of 20 to 40 percent by age 80 [9–12]. The rate of loss is highest immediately after estrogen withdrawal, on the order of 2 to 3 percent per year [13,14], but slows to about 1 percent a year within a few years. In very elderly women loss of cortical bone may cease. Hui and colleagues [15] studied 42 subjects over age 70 (mean age 87), all of whom were followed repeatedly with single photon absorptiometry of the mid-radius for at least six years. Of the 42 individual rate loss estimates, approximately 30 percent were significantly positive, 30 percent were significantly negative, and 40 percent were not significantly different from zero.

Cortical bone in men declines at a rate that is one-half or less the rate found in women [9,16, 17]. Male participants in the Baltimore Longitudinal Study of Aging, followed with x-ray measurements of cortical thickness in the second metacarpal from 1958 to 1981, were found to lose approximately 2 percent of their cortical bone per decade over their adult life span [17].

Average cortical thickness decreased with age from ages 30 to 90, but the peak losses occurred between the ages of 45 and 70. Cross-sectional and longitudinal analyses were similar, indicating that cohort differences and secular changes did not influence the results significantly.

Spinal trabecular bone mineral loss in women begins in the thirties or earlier with average annual losses of 0.7 to 1.2 percent, resulting in overall losses of 40 to 60 percent by age 80 to 90 [9,10,12,18]. Dual photon absorptiometry (DPA) measurements, which give an integral measurement of cortical and trabecular bone mineral density, show no effect of menopause on trabecular bone loss, but quantitative computed tomography (QCT) measurements, which measure trabecular bone separately, show an increase in trabecular bone loss in the immediate postmenopausal or postoophorectomy period [18,19]. Women followed repeatedly with QCT during this period of accelerated loss have shown spinal trabecular bone losses of 8 to 9 percent per year, although there is wide individual variation [19]. The discrepant results probably stem from the difference in the two techniques and from the short duration of accelerated vertebral bone loss, which makes it difficult to detect by studies that do not follow women closely through the perimenopausal period [10].

Rates of spinal bone mineral loss for men vary from about 2 percent per decade by DPA [9] to 8 to 12 percent per decade by QCT [16, 18], with losses beginning in early adulthood. The average loss rate by QCT is similar to that observed for women.

Relation of Fracture to Bone Loss

Traditionally, osteoporosis is defined as proportional loss of bone mineral and matrix, resulting in reduced bone mass per unit volume to such an extent that fractures can occur with minimal or no trauma. In practice, osteoporosis is defined by the occurrence of such fractures. How do these fractures relate to bone loss of aging?

All osteoporotic fractures in women increase in frequency with age (Fig. 29-1). The incidence of vertebral fractures increases after menopause and continues to rise with age. Based on unpublished data from Rochester, Minnesota, it has been estimated that one-third of women over 65 will have vertebral fractures [12]. The incidence of Colles' fractures also rises soon after menopause but reaches a plateau in the sixties [12]. The incidence of hip fracture rises in the early forties and continues to double every five to six years throughout life, with no acceleration around menopause [20]. At any age, white women have twice or more the risk of black women or white men for hip fracture [21]. Riggs and Melton [12] estimate that one-third of white women and one-sixth of white men will have had a hip fracture by age 90.

FIGURE 29-1. *Incidence rates for common osteoporotic fractures as a function of age and sex. Data are from the community population of Rochester, Minnesota. (From B. L. Riggs and L. J. Melton, III. Involutional osteoporosis. Reprinted, by permission of* The New England Journal of Medicine *[314:1676, 1986].)*

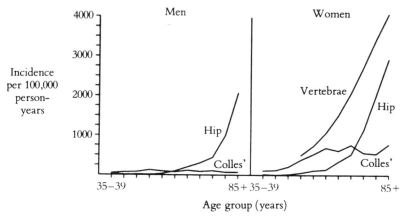

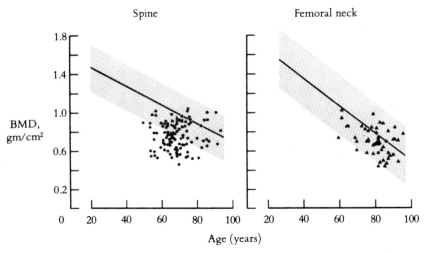

Spine   Femoral neck

FIGURE 29-2. *Bone mineral density (BMD), measured by dual photon absorptiometry, for vertebrae and femoral neck as a function of age. Lines represent the regression on age for women without fractures, and the shaded areas indicate the 90 percent confidence limits. Patients with vertebral fractures and hip fractures are represented by closed circles and triangles, respectively. (From B. L. Riggs and L. J. Melton, III. Involutional osteoporosis. Reprinted, by permission of* The New England Journal of Medicine *[314: 1676, 1986].)*

It is generally agreed that age-related bone loss accounts for much of the increasing incidence of fracture with aging. Multiple studies have shown that the incidence and prevalence of osteoporotic-type fractures increase with decreasing bone mineral density [12,21]. Nevertheless, fracture risk is not easily predictable from bone mineral density measurements because of the considerable overlap of measurements from osteoporotics and normals (Fig. 29-2). The population of women with vertebral fractures can be discriminated from normals by lower average spinal bone mineral measurements [9,18], but the large overlap of the distributions for normals and for women with vertebral fractures limits individual prediction of fracture risk. The problem is worse for the very elderly population. Although hip fracture patients have reduced cortical and trabecular bone mass compared to younger subjects, they do not have significantly lower bone density in the femoral neck or elsewhere than age-matched subjects without fractures [3,23].

Undoubtedly contributing to the increased incidence of hip fractures with age is the age-related increase in frequency of falls from standing height [24]. However, there are a variety of factors, in addition to excessive bone loss, that may diminish bone strength with aging, including reduced microfracture repair, altered physical and structural properties of bone, and impaired mineralization (osteomalacia) [24]. Laboratory testing of bone has shown that cortical and trabecular breaking strengths correlate

with bone density but that strength decreases more rapidly with age than does density [e.g., 25]. In this regard, Parfitt and colleagues [26] have found that loss of spinal trabecular bone immediately after menopause occurs predominantly by a reduction in the *number* of trabecular plates, with trabecular thinning adding significantly to bone loss only later in hip fracture patients. Disruption of the trabecular network in this manner could lead to a disproportionate (and irreversible) loss of strength.

Based on the epidemiology of osteoporotic fractures and their relationship to menopause, Riggs [12] has divided osteoporosis into two types. Type I (postmenopausal osteoporosis) develops within 15 to 20 years after menopause, is associated with accelerated trabecular bone loss, and is characterized mostly by vertebral fractures. Type II (senile osteoporosis) occurs later, is characterized by both hip and vertebral fractures, and is related to the more gradual loss of both cortical and trabecular bone. Hence, type I osteoporotics are distinguished, on average, by lower spinal bone mineral density than normals, whereas type II osteoporotics cannot at present be distinguished from normals on the basis of bone density.

Pathogenesis of Age-Related Bone Loss

Expansion or contraction of the volume of bone undergoing remodeling can give rise to a reversible bone mineral decrease or increase, but a net imbalance between resorption and formation must underlie age-related bone loss. Such an imbalance could occur through a net negative balance at each local remodeling unit as a result of increased resorption relative to formation or of decreased formation relative to resorption. Or resorption might be uncoupled from formation—i.e., formation might be delayed or not occur at all after resorption has been completed [4]. Although such uncoupling might be related to local regulating factors or to impaired osteoblast function, it might also be the result of focal perforation of thin trabeculae by resorption, thereby removing the site for subsequent formation [26]. Once this imbalance is in effect, factors that stimulate or depress cycle activity will result in greater or lesser bone loss.

It is generally agreed that acceleration of bone turnover, with resorption being more accelerated than formation, is important in early postmenopausal bone loss, although an inappropriate formation response may also play a role [6,27]. There is continuing debate about the rate of bone turnover in senile osteoporosis. Serum levels of bone Gla-protein (BGP), a proposed marker for bone formation, increase linearly with age in both men and women, suggesting that bone turnover continues to increase even in the very elderly [28], although the increase could be associated with age-related changes in metabolism and excretion of BGP. On the other hand, data from histologic studies of iliac crest biopsies have consistently suggested an age-related decrease in formation and resorption depth in trabecular bone [29,30].

We discuss below some of the systemic metabolic factors that may influence age-related bone loss and osteoporosis directly or through interactions with local factors. Because it is not possible at present to separate completely age-related bone loss from osteoporosis, it is often impossible to isolate causal factors. Some aspects of therapy are covered, since the ultimate test of a hypothesis proposing that a deficiency of a substance causes bone loss is to prevent the loss with replacement therapy.

ESTROGEN

Fuller Albright first pointed out the association between menopause and osteoporosis in the 1940s when he noted that most subjects with osteoporosis were postmenopausal women. As discussed above, bone loss is accelerated after menopause and oophorectomy. Significant decreases in vertebral mineral density have also been seen in amenorrheic women athletes [31]. Multiple studies have shown that estrogen replacement therapy slows cortical [13,14,32–34] and trabecular [19] bone loss and that loss resumes once therapy is stopped [14,35] (Fig. 29-3). Furthermore, retrospective case-control studies have found a protective effect of postmenopausal estrogen use against vertebral, hip, and distal radius fractures [2]. However, it has not been possible to distinguish between osteoporotic postmenopausal women and normal postmenopausal women based on levels of endogenous estrogen [9,36], although decreased serum estrogen levels have been found in early postmenopausal women with rapid bone loss [36].

Although the relation of estrogen deficiency to age-related bone loss is impressive, it is obviously not the whole story, since men also lose bone with aging. As discussed above, loss of trabecular bone begins well before menopause, as does the rise in hip fracture incidence [20]. Moreover, black women in the United States have hip fractures at one-half or less the rate for white women, their hip fracture rate being similar to that seen in black and white men, although their age at menopause is not different from that of white women [21].

Estrogen is thought to slow bone loss by inhibiting resorption, and it has been suggested that estrogen makes bone less sensitive to the resorptive stimulus of PTH [27]. The main clinical evidence for this hypothesis is the observation that postmenopausal women with primary hyperparathyroidism show a decrease in serum and urine calcium with estrogen therapy [37]. Because no receptors for estrogen have been found in bone and estrogen does not in-

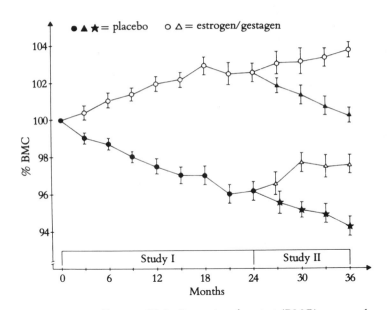

● ▲ ★ = placebo   ○ △ = estrogen/gestagen

FIGURE 29-3. *Bone mineral content (BMC), measured by single photon absorptiometry, for the distal forearm as a function of time and treatment in women within three years of menopause. Subjects were randomized to treatment with hormones or placebo and subsequently switched to the other therapy at 24 months. Initial BMC was taken as 100 percent. (From C. Christensen, M. S. Christensen, and I. Transbol. Bone mass in postmenopausal women after withdrawal of oestrogen/gestagen replacement therapy, Lancet 1:459, 1981.)*

hibit bone resorption in vitro, the mechanism of the estrogen–PTH interaction remains unknown [6].

Withdrawal of estrogen may also influence bone loss by decreasing the production of the calcium-regulating hormones calcitriol and calcitonin. The possible role of these hormones in osteoporosis is discussed further below.

CALCIUM-REGULATING HORMONES
Vitamin D
Vitamin D_3 is made in the skin on exposure to sunlight and, to a lesser degree, derived from the diet, whereas vitamin D_2 is obtained only from the diet. Both vitamins D_3 and D_2, hereafter called vitamin D, are hydroxylated in the liver to calcidiol (25-OH-D) and again in the kidney to the most active metabolite, calcitriol $(1,25\text{-}(OH)_2\text{-}D)$. The activity of the renal hydroxylase is stimulated by PTH. In women estrogen may also regulate the production of calcitriol to some extent because renal production of calcitriol has been found to increase with increases in endogenous estrogen [38]. Although total calcitriol increases with estrogen supplementation [39], free calcitriol concentration is probably unchanged [40].

Levels of calcidiol, the usual measure of vitamin D status, fall with age [11,41–43]. Al-

though the ability to synthesize vitamin D_3 in the skin decreases with age, the decrease in calcidiol levels is mainly the consequence of changes in sunlight exposure and diet [44]. Intestinal absorption of vitamin D is probably unchanged with age [44]. Levels of the active metabolite calcitriol have been found to remain constant with age [43] or to decrease [45]. Women with spinal osteoporosis may have slightly lower levels of calcitriol than normals [40,46]. The ability to hydroxylate calcidiol to calcitriol in the kidney appears to decrease with age and may be further decreased in women with hip fractures [45], suggesting that elevated PTH levels may be required to maintain calcitriol levels.

Changes in vitamin D metabolism have been associated with age-related bone loss and osteoporosis through the effects of vitamin D on calcium absorption. Calcium absorption decreases in women with age [47] and may be more reduced in women with spinal osteoporosis than in normals [39]. Estrogen replacement may increase absorption in postmenopausal women [39]. These observations have led to two hypotheses. The first, which has been used to explain type I or postmenopausal osteoporosis, assumes that the primary abnormality is excessive bone resorption secondary to estrogen deficiency, with the increased calcium mobilization subsequently reducing PTH secretion and thereby decreasing calcitriol production and calcium absorption. In this hypothesis vitamin D metabolism is only indirectly involved in osteoporosis. The second hypothesis, applicable to senile or type II osteoporosis, emphasizes impaired calcium absorption caused by insufficient calcitriol, due either to decreased hydroxylation of calcidiol as a result of an age-related decline in renal mass or to a lack of substrate. The decrease in calcium absorption causes increased PTH secretion, resulting in increased mobilization of calcium from bone.

Results of therapeutic trials with calcitriol have been unimpressive [48]. One study showed a short-term improvement in calcium balance with a waning of improvement after two years [49]. Nevertheless, long-term therapy was associated with an increase in trabecular bone volume. On the other hand, a therapeutic trial of calcitriol in early postmenopausal and 70-year-old women found no effect on cortical bone loss [50]. However, it has been argued that calcitriol therapy has been inadequately tested because of the low doses that were necessarily used to prevent hypercalcemia/hypercalciuria (0.5 μg/day or less) compared to the amount of calcitriol normally produced per day (approximately 1–2 μg) [51].

Parathyroid Hormone
Serum levels of carboxyterminal and midregion PTH increase with age in men and women [52]. Although this rise may be in part due to accumulation of inactive PTH fragments associated with an age-related decrease in renal function, the accompanying increase in urinary cyclic adenosine monophosphate (cAMP) suggests that PTH activity also increases [52]. No consistent difference in PTH levels between women with and without vertebral crush fractures has been detected, but, as noted above, the rise in

PTH has been hypothesized to contribute to senile osteoporosis by stimulating increased bone resorption.

Calcitonin
Calcitonin levels and response to calcium challenge may decrease with age in both men and women, and women may have lower basal and stimulated calcitonin levels than age-matched men [53]. Although, as noted earlier, the physiologic function of calcitonin is unclear, these changes with age have suggested an association with age-related bone loss. Moreover, estrogen administration may raise calcitonin levels [54], and hence it has been postulated that calcitonin mediates the effect of estrogen on bone. However, the involvement of calcitonin in osteoporosis now appears less likely because of a study showing that patients with osteoporosis do not have lower basal or stimulated calcitonin levels than age-matched controls [55]. Calcitonin, when given alone, is generally considered ineffective therapy for osteoporosis [6,8].

CALCIUM AVAILABILITY
Women consume less calcium than men, with more than 75 percent of women over age 35 ingesting less than the RDA of 800 mg [47]. Osteoporotic women may consume less calcium than normals [47]. As noted above, calcium absorption decreases with age and may be more reduced in osteoporotic persons than normals; moreover, the ability to enhance absorption to adapt to a low calcium diet decreases with age [56] (Fig. 29-4). Calcium balance in women is negative before menopause and becomes more negative after menopause: one study has suggested that the negative balance may be reversed by increasing calcium intake to 1,000 mg per day before menopause and 1,500 mg per day after menopause [57]. The major effect on bone of mild calcium nutritional deficiency is thought to be increased PTH-stimulated calcium mobilization from bone.

Calcium deficiency is assumed to play a major role in bone loss with aging, but most epidemiologic studies of calcium intake and bone mass have found little relation between the two [2,47]. As reviewed by Cummings et al. [2], several early studies of calcium supplementa-

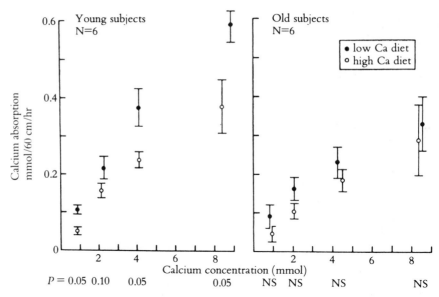

FIGURE 29-4. *Effect on calcium absorption of liberal and restricted calcium intakes in healthy young and old subjects. (From P. Ireland and J. S. Fordtran. Effect of dietary calcium and age on jejunal calcium absorption in humans studied by intestinal perfusion. Reproduced from The Journal of Clinical Investigation, 1973, 52: 2672, by copyright permission of the American Society for Clinical Investigation.)*

tion found some slowing of cortical bone loss, and one study [58] suggested a reduction in vertebral fracture, but the protection provided in all cases was small compared to that provided by estrogen. A study comparing groups of early postmenopausal women on calcium intakes ranging from 1,000 to 2,000 mg per day (including a 500 mg/day supplement) during two years found radial bone mineral losses of 1.6 to 2 percent per year in all groups [59]. In two recent studies, early postmenopausal women were given daily calcium supplements of 1,000 mg (average dietary intake about 500 mg/day) [60] or 2,000 mg (average dietary intake about 1,000 mg/day) [61] for a two-year period. Spinal trabecular mineral loss, measured by both QCT [59] or DPA [61], was unaffected by supplementation and averaged about 5 percent per year in the QCT study [60]. In the DPA study [61], a small but significant slowing of radial cortical bone mineral loss was observed, consistent with the earlier studies noted above. In both studies, women treated with estrogen had no loss of either cortical or trabecular bone during the two years. Preliminary results from another recent study suggest that dietary calcium intakes ranging from about 300 to 2000 mg per day in normal pre- and postmenopausal women are unrelated to cortical or trabecular bone mineral loss [62].

The minimal effect of increased calcium intake on bone loss in early postmenopausal women is consistent with the hypothesis that the primary abnormality in these women is estrogen depletion associated with excessive bone resorption and negative calcium balance. However, the importance of calcium intake for preventing bone loss in the very elderly, who may have elevated levels of PTH, remains relatively unexplored.

OTHER RISK FACTORS

In addition to age, sex, estrogen status, and calcium/vitamin D nutrition, there are multiple other risk factors for osteoporosis, including heredity, race, and geographic area [2]. For example, black women in the United States have greater bone density and fewer osteoporotic fractures than white women. Slender body build, cigarette smoking, and heavy alcohol use are more frequent among osteoporotics [2]. Medical conditions associated with the development of osteoporosis include hypogonadism, hyperthyroidism, hyperparathyroidism, Cushing's disease, rheumatoid arthritis, liver disease, gastrectomy, immobilization, and possibly diabetes. Acceleration of bone loss has also been related to use of drugs such as corticosteroids, anticonvulsants, heparin, and excessive thyroid hormone replacement.

Hip Fracture

For the very elderly, the risk of hip fracture may depend heavily on risk of falling. Physiologic accompaniments of normal aging, particularly increased body sway and postural hypotension, magnify the risk of falling considerably. Postural control mechanisms deteriorate with advancing age, particularly in women, with elderly individuals demonstrating much greater postural instability than younger adults [63]. Postural hypotension also increases markedly with age, as baroreflex sensitivity declines. Thirty percent of community-dwelling elders over age 75 have orthostatic blood pressure drops in excess of 20 mm Hg systolic and 10 mm Hg diastolic; 5 percent have more than a 40-mm Hg systolic decline. The changes are more marked and prevalent with advancing age [64]. Because of these physiologic changes, coupled with normal declines in muscle strength, eyesight, and hearing, falling is common even in healthy independent elderly individuals. About 25 to 30 percent of persons over age 65 fall, and women fall more frequently than men [2]. As many as 6 percent of falls may result in fractures [65].

Given these predisposing factors, it is not surprising to find that psychotropic drug use increases the risk of falling and fractures in elderly persons. A recent study [66] found that a significantly increased dose-related risk for hip fracture was associated with the use of hypnotics-anxiolytics with elimination half-lives of more than 24 hours, tricyclic antidepressants, and antipsychotics. It was estimated that as many as 14 percent of hip fractures could be attributable to the current use of psychotropic drugs [66].

Clinical Features

CLINICAL CONSEQUENCES

Patients with vertebral compression or crush fractures may present with acute or chronic back pain, or they may be asymptomatic with the fracture discovered incidentally on x-ray. Fracture may be associated with an abrupt onset of pain localized over the fracture or radiating toward the abdomen. Maneuvers that increase intraabdominal pressure, such as coughing or defecation, increase the pain, whereas lying flat reduces it. Pain generally dissipates over several weeks, and resolution occurs in most patients by two to three months. However, it is more common for patients to present with dull, chronic back pain, perhaps from muscle spasm, that is relieved by rest. Repeated fractures result in diminished height (by as much as 6–9 inches) and development of a "dowager's hump" (kyphosis). Loss of lumbar lordosis increases hip and knee flexion and the potential for contractures. With progressive fractures, the lower ribs come to rest on the anterior iliac crest causing pain, abdominal distention, and constipation. Although the consequences of multiple vertebral fractures can be devastating, the frequency of these serious consequences is unknown.

Colles' fractures (fractures of the distal radius) are considered to carry little permanent disability, but such a fracture in an elderly woman with multiple medical problems may require hospitalization and subsequent rehabilitation. Hip fractures are usually associated with falls from standing height; the frequency of spontaneous fracture is unknown. The greatest morbidity and mortality of all osteoporotic fractures occur with hip fractures. The mortality rate in the first year after fracture is about 12 to 20 percent higher than expected; the risk of dying increases with advanced age, institutionalization, and disability before fracture [2]. Some 15 to 25 percent of those who were previously functionally independent are institutionalized for at least one year after fracture, and another 25 to 35 percent return home but never recover normal ambulation [2].

DIFFERENTIAL DIAGNOSIS

In clinical practice the diagnosis of postmenopausal or type I osteoporosis is usually made after excluding other causes of vertebral compression fractures and osteopenia. Although osteopenia may be generalized in postmenopausal osteoporosis, it is usually most evident in the axial skeleton. However, 30 percent or more of bone must be lost before osteopenia can be diagnosed reliably on x-ray. In addition to the anterior wedging or complete collapse of the vertebrae that generally define the condition, spine films may also show relative accentuation of cortical surfaces, ballooning of intervertebral disks (Schmorl's nodes), biconcavity of vertebrae ("codfishing"), and prominence of vertical trabeculae secondary to loss of horizontal trabeculae. Vertebral wedging characteristically occurs above T_6; wedging solely above T_4 should suggest malignant disease, trauma, or infection.

Evaluation includes an assessment of risk factors for osteoporosis, including race, sex, body build, and sex steroid status. History of any contributing drugs should be elicited (glucocorticoids, anticonvulsants, chronic heparin therapy, excessive thyroid hormone therapy, and heavy alcohol use). Malignant disease, especially multiple myeloma, may occasionally be associated with fractures, bone pain, and diffuse radiographic osteopenia, and evaluation should include a complete blood count and serum protein electrophoresis. Further laboratory evaluation should include renal and hepatic function tests, thyroid function tests to screen for hyperthyroidism (especially important in the elderly who may have masked or apathetic hyperthyroidism), and, in selected cases, a dexamethasone suppression test. Serum calcium, phosphorus, and alkaline phosphatase are generally normal in postmenopausal osteoporosis but should be obtained to screen for primary hyperparathyroidism and osteomalacia.

In the very elderly it may be important to consider vitamin D status. As noted above, calcidiol levels decrease with age, and some 15 percent of healthy American elderly may be vitamin D-deficient [42]. Hip fracture has been associated with an increased incidence of low-grade osteomalacia in some studies [41]. Although osteomalacia is often accompanied by symptoms of bone pain and proximal muscle weakness and by abnormalities of serum chemistries (mild hypocalcemia, hypophosphatemia, and increased alkaline phosphatase concentration), the low-grade osteomalacia in hip fracture patients is usually asymptomatic and is often associated with normal serum chemistries. Calcidiol levels are the accepted means of screening for vitamin D deficiency. Calcium and calcitriol concentrations may be maintained in the normal range by secondary hyperparathyroidism, an early manifestation of vitamin D deficiency, although urinary calcium level may be decreased. In the absence of abnormal serum chemistries, poor vitamin D nutrition can generally be corrected by one or two multivitamins (with 400–800 IU of vitamin D) daily; high-dose vitamin D therapy is not warranted.

In very selected cases bone biopsies may be useful, since the definitive diagnosis of osteomalacia can be made only by bone biopsy. For unambiguous interpretation, the biopsy sample should be taken after two courses of tetracycline have been given to permit assessment of mineralization rate. However, since the biopsy must be processed in undecalcified form, this test is not widely available and is rarely needed. As therapy for established osteoporosis becomes more specific, bone biopsies may become useful for determining the bone turnover state so that an appropriate therapeutic regimen can be designed.

Preventive Measures
SCREENING FOR OSTEOPOROSIS
A goal of osteoporosis research is to be able to predict those individuals at high risk before they suffer osteoporotic fractures. The risk factors discussed above are useful in assessing patients, but their univariate specificity is low, and their multivariate specificity is unknown. Thus, photon absorptiometry and QCT have been advocated for screening perimenopausal and postmenopausal women.

In single photon absorptiometry (SPA), the bone to be studied is placed in the path of a collimated beam of monoenergetic radiation from a radionuclide source; the bone mineral content is inversely proportional to the transmitted energy. Dual photon absorptiometry (DPA) is similar to SPA but uses two different energies, permitting correction for overlying tissue. SPA is restricted to use at appendicular skeletal sites (proximal and distal radius), whereas DPA can be used at both appendicular (hip, radius) and axial (spine) sites. Both SPA and DPA give a measurement of bone mineral content that is a summation of cortical and trabecular bone. QCT is the only method that permits separate measurement of trabecular bone. Radiation exposure varies with technique but is around 5 mrad for SPA of the radius and 15 mrad for DPA of the spine [67]. Although QCT of the spine can be performed with as little as 150 mrad exposure [67], in practice the exposure can be as high as 1,000 mrad. Costs in 1984 ranged from 35 to 120 dollars for SPA to 95 to 350 dollars for QCT [67]; only SPA is covered by third-party payment at present.

Precision or reproducibility of measurements (the standard deviation of the mean expressed as a percentage of the mean) in controlled research environments is estimated to be 1 to 6 percent for all these techniques, with measurements of spinal bone mineral density being the least precise [18,67–69]. In the clinical setting, precision is expected to be lower because of difficulties in reproducing the area of interest (especially in osteoporotic spines with marked inhomogeneities), because less attention is paid to technique (especially important for DPA), and because calibration procedures are very demanding (especially important for QCT). The accuracy (closeness of the test result to an independent measure of the bone mineral density) of spinal measurements may be decreased in osteoporotic subjects because of spinal deformities and extraosseous calcification. Increased marrow fat with age results in apparent decreased bone density by QCT [18]. Further problems are encountered in attempting to compare test results. In one study, data obtained using the same measurement technique (QCT) and calibration procedures but different instruments varied significantly, and rates of change obtained with different techniques (DPA and QCT) at the same spinal positions on the same subjects correlated poorly [69].

Compared to spinal measurement techniques, measurement of the bone mineral density of the radius is less costly, simpler to perform, and less subject to problems that may reduce precision and accuracy. However, it is generally agreed that even though radial measurements (especially in the distal radius with its high proportion of trabecular bone) correlate moderately well with spinal densities, the correlation is not good enough to predict spinal density [70] and certainly inadequate to predict rates of spinal loss [10].

A single measurement of bone density made with any noninvasive technique has limited usefulness for predicting fracture risk in asymptomatic subjects. As discussed briefly above, spinal measurements with DPA [9] or QCT [18] can differentiate the population of women with vertebral fractures from the population of women without fractures, but there is still significant overlap. In the former study [9], some 50 percent of women with fractures lay within the 90 percent confidence limits for normal women. In the latter study [18], although only 4 percent of women with vertebral fractures were found to be above an arbitrarily selected fracture threshold, some 45 percent of normal women were below it. Distributions of bone mineral density for women with and without hip fractures almost totally overlap [3].

Obtaining multiple measurements of bone density during a period of time to get the rate of bone loss has been advocated as a means of assessing risk in perimenopausal women and of monitoring treatment results. However, with current techniques, even in the most experienced hands, more measurements than are practical in a clinical setting are needed to obtain precise rate estimates [68,69]. Given the relative imprecision of screening techniques and the more acceptable routine use of estrogen replacement after menopause, widespread uncontrolled screening for osteoporosis is not recommended because measurement results can contribute little useful data to therapeutic decisions [68]. For the very elderly, the reduced precision of bone mineral density measurements and the lower rates of bone density change [15] make measurement of bone density changes difficult. Because of these factors, plus the inability of bone mineral density measurements to distinguish women with hip fracture from those without, we do not recommend screening in the very elderly. For the time being, noninvasive measurements of bone density should probably be confined to osteoporosis study centers, where the data can be obtained in a standardized manner and used to increase our understanding of age-related bone loss.

PROPHYLAXIS

Estrogen

As discussed in the earlier section on pathogenesis, estrogen replacement therapy (ERT) prevents the accelerated loss of cortical and trabecular bone following menopause [13,14,19, 32–34] and protects against osteoporotic fractures during use and many years after discontinuation [2]. Inhibition of bone loss has been found in women started on therapy ten years or more after cessation of menses [33] and persists for at least eight to ten years [35]. On stopping ERT, bone mineral loss resumes at approximately the same accelerated rate seen immediately after oophorectomy or menopause [14, 35]. Hence, ERT can only delay bone loss. The minimum effective daily dose of oral estrogen replacement has been determined to be 0.625 mg of conjugated estrogens (Premarin) or 15 µg of ethinyl estradiol [19,71].

Estrogen replacement is associated with some risk. The risk for gallbladder disease may be doubled in estrogen users owing to increasing cholesterol supersaturation of bile and decreasing bile secretion [72]. Case-control studies have generally shown that the risk for endometrial cancer (the baseline detection rate being on the order of 5–10 per 10,000) increases three- to eightfold in estrogen users, with higher risks for longer duration of use and among obese women [73–76]. The increased risk is thought to be related to continuous unopposed stimulation of the endometrium. On the other hand, ERT may provoke endometrial bleeding, which may lead to earlier detection of asymptomatic disease; it has been shown that selection of controls from the population of women presenting for uterine bleeding substantially lowers the calculated risk associated with ERT [77]. Nevertheless, the risk may still be elevated for up to ten years after stopping estrogen in those who have used estrogen for at least one year, and this continuing risk cannot be explained by early detection bias [76]. The addition of progestogen to ERT lowers the risk for endometrial cancer and may even protect users [73]. Most studies have found little or no increased risk of breast cancer with ERT [78].

Although ERT given orally acts on the liver to produce elevated levels of angiotensin and renin activity, there is generally no elevation of blood pressure with ERT [79]. However, because of isolated case reports of hypertension with ERT, blood pressure should be monitored for idiosyncratic elevation. Little is known about the effect of ERT on coagulation, and data from oral contraceptive studies are not applicable because the estrogenic potency of contraceptives is about five times that of low-dose ERT. There is no evidence of increased risk of venous thromboembolic disease in ERT users [80]. The effect of ERT on lipids and lipoproteins is to reduce both total cholesterol and low-density lipoprotein (LDL) cholesterol and to elevate high-density lipoprotein (HDL) cholesterol and triglycerides [80]. These effects, excluding triglycerides, have been considered to be at least partially responsible for the generally favorable effects of ERT on cardiovascular risk. Of 17 diverse studies, eight (including four large prospective studies) showed a statistically significant reduction of cardiovascular risk among ERT users [80–84]. Only one small case-control study and the Framingham Study [84] showed a statistically significant increased risk. Although there was no increased risk for all-cause mortality, the Framingham Study [84] found a significantly elevated relative risk (3.3) for total cardiovascular disease (including asymptomatic myocardial infarction and angina) in smokers and a significantly elevated relative risk (2.3) for cerebrovascular disease in nonsmokers. Because of its discrepant results, this study is being further analyzed. Currently, the weight of the evidence suggests that ERT protects against cardiovascular disease in women.

The effect on cardiovascular risk of the addition of progestogen to ERT is not known. The more androgenic progestogens have been found to reduce or reverse the beneficial effects of estrogens on serum lipoproteins, whereas medroxyprogesterone does not appear to do so [85,86]. To avoid the metabolic side effects that might be secondary to the alteration of hepatic functions, ERT has been given experimentally by absorption through the skin. Percutaneous estradiol has been found to be effective in preventing postmenopausal bone loss [87] and, after a delay of about six months, to produce changes in lipids and lipoproteins similar to those produced by oral estrogen [86].

Although it is generally agreed that women

undergoing bilateral oophorectomy prior to menopause should receive ERT, there is still no consensus regarding prophylactic use of ERT in postmenopausal women. The decision should be made by an informed patient and doctor after considering the risks and benefits for the individual patient. If ERT is to be used, it should be started promptly after estrogen withdrawal to obtain maximum benefit, although positive results have been seen when estrogen was given for the first time to 70-year-old women [50]. Many authorities advocate performing an endometrial biopsy at the start of therapy and as a check on irregular uterine bleeding. If ERT is combined with calcium supplementation, it may be possible in the future to lower the minimum estrogen dose required to prevent bone loss [60].

Addition of progestogen to ERT in the woman with an intact uterus is still controversial. A clinical decision-analysis approach has been used to argue that the beneficial cardiovascular effects of estrogen overshadow the increased risk of endometrial cancer to such an extent that estrogen therapy without progestogen provides a significant gain in quality-adjusted life expectancy [88]. Moreover, many women find the continuation of menstruation on combination therapy to be unacceptable. Nevertheless, to reduce the risk of endometrial cancer, despite the side effects of combination therapy, we recommend that estrogen be given on a cyclic schedule of 1 to 25 days with the addition of a progestogen (e.g., 10 mg of Provera) for the last 10 to 12 days of estrogen therapy.

Calcium and Vitamin D

Results of studies examining the effects of calcium intake on bone mineral loss have been discussed in the section on pathogenesis and suggest that calcium supplementation offers little protective effect against the accelerated trabecular bone loss of early postmenopausal osteoporosis [2,59–62]. The major effect of calcium nutrition may be to determine peak bone mass in the young adult, as suggested by a study of two districts in Yugoslavia with high and low calcium intakes [89]. This study found similar rates of age-related cortical bone loss in both districts, but there was higher bone mass at any age (and lower hip fracture frequency) in the high-calcium district.

However, as discussed above, there is substantial evidence that most adult women have calcium intakes far below the optimal intake suggested by calcium balance studies and that calcium absorption decreases with age [47]. Moreover, the decrease in cortical bone loss that occurs with calcium supplementation in early postmenopausal women [61] may offer some protection later against senile osteoporosis. Hence, we recommend a daily intake of 1,000 mg of calcium in premenopausal women and 1,500 mg in postmenopausal women. Because the elderly have a dietary intake of about 300 to 500 mg per day, supplementation of about 1,000 to 1,200 mg per day is adequate (equivalent to five to six Tums, three to four 8-oz glasses of low-fat milk, two to three Oscal 500-mg tablets, or four to five Oscal 250-mg tablets with vitamin D). In the absence of renal insufficiency, hypercalciuria, or primary hyperparathyroidism, little toxicity is to be expected at this level of calcium intake because the 24-hour excretion of urine calcium is expected to increase on average by less than 70 mg for each 1-gm increase in calcium intake [47]. The 24-hour urinary calcium excretion rate should be kept below 300 mg to prevent renal stones.

The absorption of calcium from calcium carbonate is impaired in the fasting state in achlorhydria, a common condition in the elderly, but normal if given with meals [90]. Alternatively, calcium citrate may be used [90]. Calcium should probably be given in divided doses to increase absorption, but giving most of the dose at night may have the advantage of blunting the evening increase in PTH. Dolomite and bone meal should be avoided because of the relatively high levels of heavy metals in these preparations. Since calcium can cause constipation, patients' diets should contain adequate fiber.

As discussed above, therapy with vitamin D or calcitriol has not proved very effective at decreasing bone loss [48–50], and both calcitriol and high-dose vitamin D (50,000 IU) are commonly associated with hypercalcemia and hypercalciuria [48]. However, given the age-related decrease in calcium absorption and in vitamin D nutritional status, a daily supplement of 400–800 IU of vitamin D (equivalent to one or two multivitamin tablets) is recommended for the elderly, especially the institutionalized elderly.

Physical Activity

Skeletal stresses are important in maintaining skeletal homeostasis. Prolonged immobilization or weightlessness is commonly associated with hypercalcemia, hypercalciuria, and osteoporosis in young to middle-aged persons, probably secondary to increased bone resorption and decreased bone formation [91]. Simple bed rest can result in spinal mineral loss of about 1 percent per week in similar aged subjects, which can be mostly restored on reambulation [92]. It has been proposed that exercise may be able to slow age-related bone loss and stimulate bone formation. As little as two to three hours a week of exercise have resulted in an increase in spinal and radial bone mineral content in early postmenopausal women [93,94]. Both femoral neck and lumbar bone mineral density have been found to be significantly correlated with physical fitness (as defined by predicted maximal oxygen uptake) in healthy women aged 20 to 75 [95]. In a nursing home study, elderly women (mean age 82) who performed 30 minutes of exercises three times a week while sitting showed a significant gain in radial cortical bone compared to controls [96]. Although it is important to emphasize physical activity throughout life to maintain healthy bones, the importance of activity in later life should not be overlooked. An individualized exercise program may be the most effective intervention for age-related bone loss that we have to offer the elderly at present.

Established Disease

FRACTURE THERAPY

Acute pain secondary to vertebral compression fracture may be reduced by bed rest, either strict or with bathroom privileges depending on the patient's discomfort when upright [97]. However, bed rest should be as short as possible because of its adverse side effects. Three weeks of bed rest in young volunteers has been shown to reduce postural tone and stability and cardiovascular fitness; more than four weeks of active retraining was necessary for recovery [98]. It is

expected that these changes in the elderly are more pronounced and will aggravate the increased postural sway, postural hypotension, and impaired cardiovascular fitness already prevalent in this age group. Additionally, bed rest predisposes to thromboembolic events and may increase bone resorption. If pain persists despite bed rest, a back support may be necessary for ambulation [97]. Analgesics should be used judiciously. If opiates are needed, constipation should be treated expectantly with bulk agents. For chronic back pain, measures to improve posture, including back-extension exercises (and avoiding back-flexion maneuvers), may be most helpful [97].

A frequent complication of hip fracture in an elderly patient is an acute confusional state (Chap. 27). There are many potentially contributing factors, including pain, analgesics, anesthetics, new and confusing surroundings, and the many medical problems that can arise during the hospital course (e.g., fecal impaction and urinary retention secondary to bed rest and opiates, hyponatremia secondary to intravenous administration of 5% dextrose in water, plus an age-related decreased ability to excrete free water). Among the most serious complications of hip fractures are deep venous thrombosis and pulmonary embolism. Without anticoagulation, deep venous thrombosis occurs in more than 40 percent of elderly hip fracture patients, with an incidence of fatal pulmonary embolism exceeding 4 percent [99]. Although low-dose (5,000 units subcutaneously every 8 or 12 hours) heparin may be adequate prophylaxis in patients with vertebral fractures, neither low-dose heparin nor aspirin provides adequate protection against deep venous thrombosis and pulmonary embolism in hip fracture patients [99]. Warfarin anticoagulation, dextran, external pneumatic compression, and pressure-gradient stockings have been recommended as prophylaxis by the National Institutes of Health Consensus Conference [99]. Prophylaxis should be continued until the patient is ambulatory.

MEDICAL THERAPY

There is still little to offer in the way of medical therapy that might reverse established disease. A conservative approach is to follow the same recommendations given for prophylaxis. As discussed earlier, calcitonin and calcitriol have not been found very effective in slowing bone loss. Furthermore, calcitonin must be given by injection and costs roughly $2,500 per year. The ideal agent would increase bone formation. Estrogen, calcitonin, and calcium slow bone loss by decreasing bone resorption, and because of coupling they also reduce bone formation. Moreover, the inhibition of turnover by these agents may delay the repair of microfractures and ultimately weaken bone [100]. Anabolic steroids may be able to increase bone formation [101], but they are limited by their cardiovascular and androgenic side effects and are still investigational at present.

The only oral medication that preferentially stimulates bone formation is sodium fluoride, but its role is still controversial [102]. Fluoride is incorporated into bone as fluoroapatite, increasing crystal size. Although histologic studies have shown a large increase in trabecular bone volume with high doses of fluoride, there is also an increase in unmineralized bone (osteoid), which may occur even with supplemental vitamin D and calcium [102]. Furthermore, the increase in trabecular bone may be associated with a decrease in cortical bone mass [101]. One study [59] has shown a dramatic decrease in vertebral fracture with fluoride, but 40 percent of those treated did not respond; there are some criticisms of the study design, including lack of patient randomization [100]. In contrast, a recent three-year study found an increase in incidence of vertebral fracture in the treated group relative to controls during the first year and no difference in fracture incidence thereafter [103]. Side effects of fluoride treatment are common with currently administered doses (affecting up to 50 percent of patients). They include gastrointestinal irritation, painful swollen joints, and new bone excrescences. Because of concerns about the possible side effects of osteomalacia and cortical bone loss, both of which may increase risk of hip fractures, sodium fluoride is not recommended for use in very elderly patients at present. Its current use should probably be confined to treatment of patients with severe progressive vertebral crush fractures at research centers.

Among new therapies that appear promising is a combination of daily subcutaneous injection of PTH and oral calcitriol [104]. Preliminary results showed a marked increase in spinal trabecular bone in a small group of osteoporotic men, and the therapy is currently being evaluated for women. Frost has proposed the approach of manipulating individual loci of bone remodeling (bone remodeling units) so that formation is preferentially increased over resorption [105]. One attempt to implement this approach combined continuous oral phosphate (to induce secondary hyperparathyroidism and stimulate recruitment of remodeling units) and intermittent parenteral calcitonin (to shift the remodeling units into the formation phase) [106]. Preliminary results showed an increase in trabecular bone.

Summary

The difficulties in dealing with osteoporosis begin with our inability to make the diagnosis until fracture has occurred. Attempts to set fracture thresholds based on bone density are of limited usefulness to the individual, not only because of the large overlap of populations with and without fracture, but also because there is still no reliable and convenient therapy for increasing bone mass. The difficulties in defining the disease reflect our lack of understanding of its underlying causes, despite the identification of many factors potentially involved in the process. Efforts to develop effective therapy are limited by the inability to assess bone strength or functional state directly and by the long skeletal turnover time. Prevention of the disease would appear to be the most effective approach at the current time. Estrogen replacement therapy does provide consistent and reproducible protection if started in the early years after estrogen withdrawal, but the side effects and risks associated with ERT make it unacceptable to many women. We are still unable to define precisely the high-risk groups who should receive prophylactic ERT. For the very elderly, a conservative program of adequate calcium and vitamin D nutrition with regular exercise and an emphasis on preventing falls is probably the best we have to offer at present. It is hoped that research on this important problem, which has been centered on early postmenopausal women, will be directed more toward the elderly in the future.

References

1. National Institutes of Health. *Osteoporosis*. NIH Consensus Conference Statement. Washington, D.C.: National Institutes of Health, 1984.
2. Cummings, S. R., et al. Epidemiology of osteoporosis and osteoporotic fractures. *Epidemiol. Rev.* 7:178, 1985.
3. Riggs, B. L., et al. Changes in bone mineral density of the proximal femur and spine with aging. *J. Clin. Invest.* 70:716, 1982.
4. Baron, R., Vignery, A., and Horowitz, M. Lymphocytes, Macrophages and the Regulation of Bone Remodeling. In W. A. Peck (ed.), *Bone and Mineral Research*. New York: Elsevier, 1983. P. 175.
5. Nijweide, P. J., Burger, E. H., and Feyen, H. M. Cells of bone: Proliferation, differentiation, and hormonal regulation. *Physiol. Rev.* 66:855, 1986.
6. Raisz, L. G. Osteoporosis. *J. Am. Geriatr. Soc.* 30:127, 1982.
7. Raisz, L. G., and Kream, B. E. Regulation of bone formation. Parts I and II. *N. Engl. J. Med.* 309:29, 83, 1983.
8. Austin, L. A., and Heath, H. Calcitonin: Physiology and pathology. *N. Engl. J. Med.* 304:269, 1981.
9. Riggs, B. L., et al. Differential changes in bone mineral density of the appendicular and axial skeleton with aging. *J. Clin. Invest.* 67:328, 1981.
10. Riggs, B. L., et al. Rates of bone loss in the appendicular and axial skeletons of women. *J. Clin. Invest.* 77:1487, 1986.
11. Sowers, M. R., et al. Parameter related to 25-OH-D levels in a population-based study on women. *Am. J. Clin. Nutr.* 43:621, 1986.
12. Riggs, B. L., and Melton, L. J. III. Involutional osteoporosis. *N. Engl. J. Med.* 314:1676, 1986.
13. Lindsay, R., et al. Prevention of spinal osteoporosis in oophorectomised women. *Lancet* 2:1151, 1980.
14. Christiansen, C., Christensen, M. S., and Transbol, I. Bone mass in postmenopausal women after withdrawal of oestrogen/testagen replacement therapy. *Lancet* 1:459, 1981.
15. Hui, S. L., et al. A prospective study of change in bone mass with age in postmenopausal women. *J. Chronic Dis.* 35:715, 1982.
16. Meier, D. E., Orwoll, E. S., and Jones, J. M. Marked disparity between trabecular and cortical bone loss with age in healthy men. *Ann. Intern Med.* 101:605, 1984.
17. Fox, K. M., Tobin, J. D., and Plato, C. C. Longitudinal study of bone loss in the second metacarpal. *Calcif. Tissue Int.* 39:218, 1986.
18. Cann, C. E., et al. Quantitative computed tomography for prediction of vertebral fracture risk. *Bone* 6:1, 1985.
19. Genant, H. K., et al. Quantitative computed tomography of vertebral spongiosa: A sensitive method for detecting early bone loss after oophorectomy. *Ann. Intern Med.* 97:699, 1982.
20. Brody, J. A., Farmer, M. E., and White, L. R. Absence of menopausal effect on hip fracture occurrence in white females. *Am. J. Public Health* 74:1397, 1984.
21. Farmer, M. E., et al. Race and sex differences in hip fracture incidence. *Am. J. Public Health* 74:1374, 1984.
22. Jensen, G. F., et al. Relationship between bone mineral content and frequency of postmenopausal fractures. *Acta Med. Scand.* 213:61, 1983.
23. Cummings, S. R. Are patients with hip fractures more osteoporotic? *Am. J. Med.* 78:487, 1985.
24. Melton, L. J. III, and Riggs, B. L. Risk factors for injury after a fall. *Clin. Geriatr. Med.* 1:525, 1985.
25. Leichter, I. O., et al. The relationship between bone density, mineral content, and mechanical strength in the femoral neck. *Clin. Orthop. Rel. Res.* 163:272, 1982.
26. Parfitt, A. M., et al. Relationships between surface, volume, and thickness of iliac trabecular bone in aging and in osteoporosis. *J. Clin. Invest.* 72:1396, 1983.
27. Heaney, R. P., Recker, R. R., and Saville, P. D. Menopausal changes in bone remodeling. *J. Lab. Clin. Med.* 92:964, 1978.
28. Epstein, S., et al. Differences in serum bone GLA protein with age and sex. *Lancet* 1:307, 1984.
29. Eriksen, E. F., Mosekilde, L., and Melsen, F. Trabecular bone resorption depth decreases with age: Differences between normal males and females. *Bone* 6:141, 1985.
30. Lips, P., Courpron, P., and Meunier, P. J. Mean wall thickness of trabecular bone packets in the iliac crest: Changes with age. *Calcif. Tissue Res.* 26:13, 1978.
31. Drinkwater, B. L., et al. Bone mineral content of amenorrheic and eumenorrheic athletes. *N. Engl. J. Med.* 311:277, 1984.
32. Horsman, A., et al. Prospective trial of oestrogen and calcium in postmenopausal women. *Br. J. Med.* 2:789, 1977.
33. Recker, R. R., Saville, P. D., and Heaney, R. P.

Effect of estrogens and calcium carbonate on bone loss in postmenopausal women. *Ann. Intern Med.* 87:649, 1977.

34. Nachtigall, L. E., et al. Estrogen replacement therapy I: A 10-year prospective study in the relationship to osteoporosis. *Obstet. Gynecol.* 53:277, 1979.

35. Lindsay, R., et al. Bone response to termination of oestrogen treatment. *Lancet* 2:1325, 1978.

36. Riis, B. J., Rodbro, P., and Christiansen, C. The role of serum concentrations of sex steroids and bone turnover in the development and occurrence of postmenopausal osteoporosis. *Calcif. Tissue Int.* 38:318, 1986.

37. Selby, P. I., and Peacock, M. Ethinyl estradiol and norethindrone in the treatment of primary hyperparathyroidism in postmenopausal women. *N. Engl. J. Med.* 314:1481, 1986.

38. Buchanan, J. R., et al. The effect of endogenous estrogen fluctuation on metabolism of 25-hydroxyvitamin D. *Calcif. Tissue Int.* 39:139, 1986.

39. Gallagher, J. C., Riggs, B. L., and DeLuca, H. F. Effect of estrogen on calcium absorption and serum vitamin D metabolites in postmenopausal osteoporosis. *J. Clin. Endocrinol. Metab.* 51:1359, 1980.

40. Nordin, B. E. C., et al. Calcium Absorption Studies in Normal and Osteoporotic Women. In A. W. Norman, et al. (eds.), *Vitamin D: A Chemical, Biochemical and Clinical Update.* New York: Walther de Gruyter and Co., 1985. P. 1028.

41. Parfitt, A. M., et al. Vitamin D and bone health in the elderly. *Am. J. Clin. Nutr.* 36:1014, 1982.

42. Omdahl, J. L., et al. Nutritional status in a healthy elderly population: Vitamin D. *Am. J. Clin. Nutr.* 36:1225, 1982.

43. Orwoll, E. S., and Meier, D. E. Alterations in calcium, vitamin D, and parathyroid hormone physiology in normal men with aging: Relationship to the development of senile osteopenia. *J. Clin. Endocrinol. Metab.* 63:1262, 1986.

44. Holick, M. F. Vitamin D requirements for the elderly. *Clin. Nutr.* 5:121, 1986.

45. Tsai, K. S., et al. Impaired vitamin D metabolism with aging in women. *J. Clin. Invest.* 73:1668, 1984.

46. Gallagher, J. C., et al. Intestinal calcium absorption and serum vitamin D metabolites in normal subjects and osteoporotic patients. *J. Clin. Invest.* 64:729, 1979.

47. Heaney, R. P., et al. Calcium nutrition and bone health in the elderly. *Am. J. Clin. Nutr.* 36:986, 1982.

48. Schwartzman, M. S., and Franck, W. A. Vitamin D toxicity complicating the treatment of senile, postmenopausal, and glucocorticoid-induced osteoporosis. *Am. J. Med.* 82:224, 1987.

49. Gallagher, J. C., et al. 1,25-dihydroxyvitamin D_3: Short- and long-term effects on bone and calcium metabolism in patients with postmenopausal osteoporosis. *Proc. Natl. Acad. Sci.* 79:3325, 1982.

50. Christiansen, C. Osteoporosis and Vitamin D Metabolites: A Status Report. In A. W. Norman, et al. (eds.), *Vitamin D: Chemical, Biochemical and Clinical Endocrinology of Calcium Metabolism.* New York: Walther de Gruyter and Co., 1982. P. 915.

51. DeLuca, H. F. Significance of Vitamin D in Age-Related Bone Disease. In M. L. Hutchinson and H. N. Munro (eds.), *Nutrition and Aging.* New York: Academic Press, 1986. P. 217.

52. Marcus, R., Madvig, P., and Young, G. Age-related changes in parathyroid hormone and parathyroid hormone action in normal humans. *J. Clin. Endocrinol. Metab.* 58:223, 1984.

53. Deftos, L. J., et al. Influence of age and sex on plasma calcitonin in human beings. *N. Engl. J. Med.* 302:1351, 1980.

54. Stevenson, J. C., et al. Regulation of calcium-regulating hormones by exogenous sex steroids in early postmenopause. *Eur. J. Clin. Invest.* 13:481, 1983.

55. Tiegs, R. D., et al. Calcitonin secretion in postmenopausal osteoporosis. *N. Engl. J. Med.* 312:1097, 1985.

56. Ireland, P., and Fordtran, J. S. Effect of dietary calcium and age on jejunal calcium absorption in humans studied by intestinal perfusion. *J. Clin. Invest.* 52:2672, 1973.

57. Heaney, R. P., Recker, R. R., and Saville, P. D. Menopausal changes in calcium balance performance. *J. Lab. Clin. Med.* 92:953, 1978.

58. Riggs, B. L., et al. Effect of the fluoride/calcium regimen on vertebral fracture occurrence in postmenopausal osteoporosis. *N. Engl. J. Med.* 306:446, 1982.

59. Nilas, L., Christiansen, C., and Rodbro, P. Calcium supplementation and postmenopausal bone loss. *Br. Med. J.* 289:1103, 1984.

60. Ettinger, B., Genant, H. K., and Cann, C. E. Postmenopausal bone loss is prevented by treatment with low-dosage estrogen with calcium. *Ann. Intern Med.* 106:40, 1987.

61. Riis, B., Thomsen, K., and Christiansen, C. Does calcium supplementation prevent postmenopausal bone loss? *N. Engl. J. Med.* 316:173, 1987.

62. Riggs, B. L., et al. Dietary calcium intake and rates of bone loss in women. *J. Clin. Invest.* 80:979, 1987.

63. Hasselkus, B. R., and Shambes, G. M. Aging and postural sway in women. *J. Gerontol.* 30: 661, 1975.
64. Caird, R. L., Andrews, G. R., and Kennedy, R. D. Effect of posture on blood pressure in the elderly. *Br. Heart J.* 35:527, 1973.
65. Gryfe, C. I., Amies, A., and Ashley, M. J. A longitudinal study of falls in an elderly population: I. Incidence and morbidity. *Age Aging* 6: 201, 1977.
66. Ray, W. A., et al. Psychotropic drug use and the risk of hip fracture. *N. Engl. J. Med.* 316:363, 1987.
67. Health and Public Policy Committee. American College of Physicians. Radiologic methods to evaluate bone mineral content. *Ann. Intern. Med.* 100:908, 1984.
68. Cummings, S. R., and Black, D. Should perimenopausal women be screened for osteoporosis? *Ann. Intern. Med.* 104:817, 1986.
69. Ott, S. M., Kilcoyne, R. F., and Chestnut, C. H. Longitudinal changes in bone mass after one year as measured by different techniques in patients with osteoporosis. *Calcif. Tissue Int.* 39:133, 1986.
70. Mazess, R. B., et al. Does bone measurement on the radius indicate skeletal status? *J. Nucl. Med.* 25:281, 1984.
71. Lindsay, R., Hart, D. M., and Clark, D. M. The minimum effective dose of estrogen for prevention of postmenopausal bone loss. *Obstet. Gynecol.* 63:759, 1984.
72. Boston Collaborative Drug Surveillance Program: Surgically confirmed gallbladder disease, venous thromboembolism, and breast tumors in relation to postmenopausal estrogen therapy. *N. Engl. J. Med.* 290:15, 1974.
73. Gambrell, R. D., Bagnell, C. A., and Greenblatt, R. B. Role of estrogens and progesterone in the etiology and prevention of endometrial cancer: Review. *Am. J. Obstet. Gynecol.* 146:696, 1983.
74. Braunstein, G. D. The benefits of estrogen to the menopausal woman outweigh the risks of developing endometrial cancer (pro). *CA* 34:210, 1984.
75. Morrow, C. P. The benefits of estrogen to the menopausal woman outweigh the risks of developing endometrial cancer (con). *CA* 34:220, 1984.
76. Shapiro, S., et al. Risk of localized and widespread endometrial cancer in relation to recent and discontinued use of conjugated estrogens. *N. Engl. J. Med.* 313:969, 1985.
77. Horowitz, R. I., and Feinstein, A. R. Alternative analytic methods for case control studies of estrogens and endometrial cancer. *N. Engl. J. Med.* 299:1089, 1978.
78. Hiatt, R. A., et al. Exogenous estrogen and breast cancer after bilateral oophorectomy. *Cancer* 54:139, 1984.
79. Mashchak, C. A., and Lobo, R. A. Estrogen replacement therapy and hypertension. *J. Reprod. Med.* 30 (Suppl. 10):805, 1985.
80. Bush, T. L., and Barrett-Connor, E. Noncontraceptive estrogen use and cardiovascular disease. *Epidemiol. Rev.* 7:80, 1985.
81. Henderson, B. E., Ross, R. K., and Paganini-Hill, A. Estrogen use and cardiovascular disease. *J. Reprod. Med.* 30 (Suppl. 10):814, 1985.
82. Criqui, M., et al. Postmenopausal estrogen use and mortality (abstract). *Am. J. Epidemiol.* 120: 466, 1984.
83. Stampfer, M. J., et al. A prospective study of postmenopausal estrogen therapy and coronary heart disease. *N. Engl. J. Med.* 313:1044, 1985.
84. Wilson, P. W. F., Garrison, R. J., and Castelli, W. P. Postmenopausal estrogen use, cigarette smoking, and cardiovascular morbidity in women over 50. The Framingham Study. *N. Engl. J. Med.* 313:1038, 1985.
85. Hirvonen, E., Malkonen, M., and Manninen, V. Effects of different progestogens on lipoproteins during postmenopausal replacement therapy. *N. Engl. J. Med.* 304:560, 1981.
86. Jensen, J., et al. Long-term effects of percutaneous estrogens and oral progesterone on serum lipoproteins in postmenopausal women. *Am. J. Obstet. Gynecol.* 156:66, 1987.
87. Riis, B. J., et al. The effect of percutaneous estradiol and natural progesterone on postmenopausal bone loss. *Am. J. Obstet. Gynecol.* 156:61, 1987.
88. Hillner, B. E., Hollenberg, J. P., and Pauker, S. G. Postmenopausal estrogens in prevention of osteoporosis. *J.A.M.A.* 80:1116, 1986.
89. Matkovic, V., et al. Bone status and fracture rates in two regions of Yugoslavia. *Am. J. Clin. Nutr.* 32:540, 1979.
90. Recker, R. R. Calcium absorption and achlorhydria. *N. Engl. J. Med.* 313:70, 1985.
91. Stewart, A. F., et al. Calcium homeostasis in immobilization: An example of resorptive hypercalciuria. *N. Engl. J. Med.* 306:1136, 1982.
92. Krolner, B., and Toft, B. Vertebral bone loss: An unheeded side effect of therapeutic bed rest. *Clin. Sci.* 64:537, 1983.
93. Krolner, B., et al. Physical exercise as prophylaxis against involutional vertebral bone loss: A controlled trial. *Clin. Sci.* 64:541, 1983.

94. Smith, E. L., et al. Bone involution decrease in exercising middle-aged women. *Calcif. Tissue Int.* 36:S129, 1984.
95. Pocock, N. A., et al. Physical fitness is a major determinant of femoral neck and lumbar spine bone mineral density. *J. Clin. Invest.* 78:618, 1986.
96. Smith, E., Reddan, W., and Smith, P. Physical activity and calcium modalities for bone mineral increase in aged women. *Med. Sci. Sports Exer.* 13:60, 1981.
97. Sinaki, M. Postmenopausal spinal osteoporosis. Physical therapy and rehabilitation principles. *Mayo Clin. Proc.* 57:699, 1982.
98. Taylor, H. L., et al. Effects of bedrest on cardiovascular function and work performance. *J. Appl. Physiol.* 2:223, 1949.
99. NIH Consensus Conference. Prevention of venous thrombosis and pulmonary embolism. *J.A.M.A.* 256:744, 1986.
100. Kanis, J. A. Treatment of osteoporotic fracture. *Lancet* 1:27, 1984.
101. Chesnut, C. H. III, et al. Stanozolol, an Anabolic Steroid, in the Treatment of Postmenopausal Osteoporosis—An Update. In J. Menzel, et al. (eds.), *Osteoporosis.* New York: Wiley, 1982. P. 385.
102. Kanis, J. A., and Meunier, P. J. Should we use fluoride to treat osteoporosis? A review. *Q. J. Med. (New series LIII)* 210:145, 1984.
103. Dambacher, M. A., Ittner, J., and Ruegsegger, P. Long-term fluoride therapy of postmenopausal osteoporosis. *Bone* 7:199, 1986.
104. Slovik, D. M., et al. Restoration of spinal bone in osteoporotic men by treatment with human parathyroid hormone (1-34) and 1,25-dihydroxyvitamin D. *J. Bone Min. Res.* 1:377, 1986.
105. Frost, H. M. Treatment of osteoporosis by manipulation of coherent bone cell populations. *Clin. Orthop.* 143:227, 1979.
106. Marie, P., et al. Treatment of Postmenopausal Osteoporosis with Phosphate and Intermittent Calcitonin. In J. Menczel, et al. (eds.), *Osteoporosis.* New York: Wiley, 1982. P. 407.

30

Fractures in the Elderly

Tobin N. Gerhart

FRACTURES IN THE ELDERLY are a major cause of morbidity and mortality. Compared with those of a younger population, their fractures differ in frequency of occurrence, anatomic location within the bone, and type of fracture pattern. Most result from low-energy injuries and involve bone weakened by osteoporosis or other pathologic processes. The prognosis for uncomplicated healing also differs for elderly patients. They have a greater tendency to develop joint stiffness with immobilization and are at higher risk for medical complications with enforced bed rest. To avoid these complications and because of a shortened anticipated life span, treatment goals in the elderly emphasize rapid return to activities necessary for independent living rather than attempting to achieve a more perfect long-term result by such means as prolonged casting or traction. Most elderly persons are retired. They no longer need to perform manual labor, and high-strength functional capabilities are not a priority. By placing less stress on their musculoskeletal system, the elderly often do well with fracture alignments or prosthetic replacements that would be unsuitable for a younger population.

Epidemiology

The incidence of osteoporotic fractures in the United States has been estimated at a total of 1.2 million per year in 1985. About 247,000 of these were hip fractures occurring in persons over age 45, with the great majority in persons over age 70 [1]. As the population ages, the problem grows. From 1965 to 1981 the number of hip fractures in the United States tripled, and it is expected to triple again in the next two decades. One-third of women and one-sixth of men who live to age 90 will sustain a hip fracture [2]. After hip fracture, an excess mortality rate of 12 to 20 percent occurs during the first year compared with persons of the same age and sex. Of functionally independent patients who live at home before a fracture, 15 to 25 percent will require long-term institutional care for more than a year, and another 25 to 30 percent will become dependent on mechanical aids of assistive personnel. Osteoporotic fractures also afflict other sites, with an estimated 172,000 occurring in the distal radius and 538,000 in the spine in 1985.

Only certain kinds of fractures, however, have an increasing incidence with age. Long bone shaft fractures involve predominantly cortical bone and bear no positive correlation with age. In contrast, vertebral body and hip fractures have a low incidence until the fifth and sixth decades and then increase dramatically [3]. Fractures of the proximal humerus, wrist, tibia, and pubic rami follow a similar pattern. The sites of all these fractures involve predominantly trabecular bone.

450

Etiology

Falls are the most common cause of fractures in the elderly. An estimated 90 percent of geriatric hip, forearm, and pelvic fractures result from a fall. Part of the problem is that the elderly fall more frequently due to a higher incidence of underlying medical conditions: failing vision, neurologic diseases and their sequelae, arthritis impairing lower limb function, and the use of sedatives and other medications. In addition, slowed reflexes, decreased muscle strength, and impaired coordination may reduce their ability to dissipate the impact of a fall and thus increase the likelihood of fracture [4]. Thus, most fractures in the elderly result from the relatively low-energy trauma incurred with a fall on level ground.

Descriptive and Anatomic Terms

A typical long bone is divided into three anatomic regions: the diaphysis, the metaphysis, and the epiphysis. The diaphysis, or shaft, consists of a tube of cortical bone surrounding a medullary cavity of hemopoietic or fatty marrow. The epiphysis lies at the end of the bone between the growth plate, or physis, and the articular surface. The metaphysis is the intermediate flared region, joining the other two. The skeleton is made of two different forms of bone: cortical and trabecular. Trabecular or porous bone composes most of the metaphysis and epiphysis. It varies widely in density and strength depending on its skeletal location, the patient's age, and pathologic conditions such as osteoporosis. Cortical or lamellar bone composes the diaphysis. Its dense histologic architecture of parallel Haversian systems gives it great strength.

Use of standard terminology facilitates the description of fracture patterns. The terms *proximal, midshaft,* and *distal* describe the location of a fracture. The orientation of a fracture line may be *transverse, oblique,* or *spiral. Comminution* refers to the degree of fragmentation. *Open* or *closed* indicates whether the fracture communicates to the outside through a wound in the soft tissue covering. The archaic terms *simple* and *compound* should be avoided. *Alignment* refers to the relative position of the main fracture fragments. Their apex may point *anterior, posterior, lateral* (varus angulation), or *medial* (valgus angulation). The bone ends themselves may be *overriding, distracted,* or *impacted.*

Biomechanics

The force required to break a bone depends on both its material properties and its geometry. Material properties determine the force per unit area required to cause failure of a material and are referred to as ultimate tensile or ultimate compressive strength (expressed in metric units in megapascals [MPa], in which 1 MPa = 145 pounds per square inch). The ultimate tensile strength of cortical bone decreases only slightly with aging from about 140 MPa in the second decade to about 120 MPa in the eighth decade. Remodeling of the diaphysis occurs with aging, causing it to enlarge in cross section. Bone is resorbed from the inner or endosteal surface and is added to the outer or periosteal surface [5]. This redistribution increases the resistance of the diaphysis to bending forces and compensates for the decrease in strength of the cortical bone. Thus fractures of the diaphysis do not increase in frequency with aging.

The ultimate compressive strength of trabecular bone is proportional to the density squared and ranges between 1 and 10 MPa. Fractures of the vertebrae and ends of the femur do not occur until their bone density falls below a threshold of 1.0 gm/cm^2 [6]. Since normal cancellous bone has a density above 1.4 gm/cm^2, a density of 1.0 gm/cm^2 represents a halving of strength. Reduction in density cannot be detected on ordinary radiographs until at least 25 percent of bone mineral is lost. The great majority of fractures in the elderly occur in the metaphyseal region, which does not remodel with age and thus does not compensate for the decreased density of trabecular bone.

Pathologic Fractures
CLINICAL PRESENTATION

The term *pathologic fracture* refers to any fracture involving abnormal bone. Although it may involve an underlying malignancy, the pathologic process may also be a benign bone tumor, metabolic disorder, infection, or osteoporosis. All these conditions can weaken bone so that it will fracture when subjected to relatively low stress.

Thus, any patient who presents with a fracture after minimal trauma must be suspected of having a pathologic fracture. Questioning will usually reveal a prior history of progressively increasing pain in the affected region, especially noticeable at night and with weight-bearing. Recognition is important, for choice of treatment and prognosis for healing can be greatly altered by the pathologic condition [7,8].

Frequently, patients present with an impending pathologic fracture that has not yet broken entirely through the bone. Such patients will have pain in the affected area associated with use of the limb. Rising out of a chair, for instance, can cause thigh pain in a patient with a lesion of the femur. Prophylactic internal fixation of these fractures with metal plates, rods, or prostheses is often indicated to prevent displacement, provide pain relief, and permit the patient to remain functional. Otherwise, if the impending fracture breaks through completely and displaces, treatment would be considerably more difficult, with increased morbidity and a poorer result for the patient.

MALIGNANCY

Metastatic lesions account for the great majority of skeletal malignancies, with metastases from the breast, lung, prostate, gastrointestinal tract, kidney, and thyroid being the most common. The typical radiographic appearance is that of multiple destructive lesions. All can produce lucent lesions on radiographs, and prostatic and breast metastases may also cause sclerosis. Primary bone malignancies occur with much less frequency than metastatic disease. Myeloma and lymphoma are the most common histologic types; osteosarcoma, fibrosarcoma, and chondrosarcoma are rare.

OSTEOPENIA

The radiographic appearance of abnormally decreased bone density is termed *osteopenia*. It is caused by four conditions that are indistinguishable on radiographs but involve completely different pathologic processes: osteoporosis, too little bone; osteomalacia, decreased mineralization; hyperparathyroidism, increased resorption; and myeloma, bone destruction by tumor. Consequently, patients with osteopenia require laboratory tests for evaluation of underlying en-

docrine and renal diseases that may be causing these conditions. A thorough screening series would include a complete blood count with differential, sedimentation rate, serum calcium, phosphorus, and alkaline phosphatase measurements, blood urea nitrogen, blood sugar, serum glutamic-oxaloacetic transaminase (SGOT), T4, serum immunoelectrophoresis, and bone scan. Osteoporosis causes no abnormalities in these tests. It is most accurately detected and measured by specialized scanning techniques including photon absorptiometry and quantitative computed tomography (CT) scanning. Because osteoporosis is so prevalent in the elderly, it is not considered a pathologic process in the usual sense. About 90 percent of women over 75 years of age are estimated to have osteoporosis affecting the lumbar spine [3].

Normal Fracture Healing

Clinical management of fractures is based on an understanding of the physiology of bone repair [9,10]. The process of fracture healing can be divided temporally into three overlapping phases: inflammation, repair, and remodeling. The inflammatory phase includes the body's initial response to injury and lasts for several days. The trauma that fractures the bone also injures the surrounding blood vessels, muscles, and other soft tissues. Hemorrhage at the fracture site forms a hematoma. Traumatic devascularization of the fracture ends and fragments results in nonviable or necrotic bone. All this necrotic material elicits an immediate and intense acute inflammatory reaction. Clinically, the fracture site is characterized by swelling and tenderness. The reparative phase begins within 24 hours after injury and reaches peak activity after one to two weeks. Diaphyseal fractures that are not rigidly stabilized heal by the rapid formation around the fracture site of new bone called the external callus. External callus is not visible radiographically until about three to six weeks postinjury. Until sufficient external callus forms and provides stability, a process that can take several months for long bone fractures, collapse and displacement of the fracture can occur. Metaphyseal fractures heal by direct union of the trabecular bone, a faster process that begins within two to three weeks. During the remodeling phase, the rapidly laid down initial callus is slowly resorbed and replaced by mechanically stronger bone distributed to best resist load-bearing stresses. This process proceeds slowly in the elderly and may account for symptoms of discomfort lasting many months after a fracture.

Specific Fractures

Fractures of the proximal humerus, distal radius, pelvic rami, proximal femur, proximal tibia, and thoracic and lumbar vertebral bodies occur with disproportionate frequency in the elderly. These sites involve predominantly trabecular bone that is often seriously weakened by osteoporosis. Usually these fractures are caused by low-energy trauma such as a fall on level ground. With the exception of hip fractures, the great majority are treated nonoperatively. Nonetheless, rehabilitation is a prolonged and often incomplete process. Usually several months to a year pass before patients regain their preinjury capabilities.

PROXIMAL HUMERUS

Presentation and Classification

The most common mechanism of injury is a fall on the outstretched hand. Patients present with shoulder pain and inability to move the arm. Radiographically, the proximal humerus may show up to four separate fragments: an articular fragment containing the humeral head, greater and lesser tuberosity fragments, and a distal fragment including the humeral shaft. These fragments are prone to displacement owing to the pull of the supraspinatus, subscapularis, and pectoralis muscles. Fortunately, about 80 percent of proximal humeral fractures [11] are minimally displaced, with less than 45 degrees of angulation and less than 1 cm displacement of any fragment. When displaced, the articular fragment may not lie in a satisfactory position above the humeral shaft on anteroposterior and lateral radiographs. Displaced fractures are classified in increasing order of severity into two-, three-, and four-part patterns. Those associated with a glenohumeral dislocation are usually the result of major trauma and constitute the most severe injuries.

Treatment and Prognosis

Treatment and prognosis depend on the number and extent of displacement of the fracture fragments. Patients should be told to expect considerable swelling and discoloration in the lower arm. If the alignment and position of the fragments are satisfactory, the arm may be immobilized with a sling. Otherwise, closed reduction should be attempted. If satisfactory alignment cannot be achieved by manipulation, then open reduction with internal fixation or insertion of a prosthetic replacement may be indicated.

The importance of beginning range of motion exercises as soon as possible cannot be overemphasized. The most common complication following shoulder fractures is adhesive capsulitis resulting from sticking together of the inflamed surfaces of the joint capsule. This can cause chronic pain as well as functional disability due to restricted motion. Physical therapy referral is indicated to instruct and monitor the exercises. For a stable two-part fracture, active motion and use of the hand and wrist should be encouraged immediately. At one week, pendulum exercises in the sling are started. The patient leans forward and, using the noninjured arm to assist, swings the injured arm like a pendulum, making circles with the elbow. The sling may be removed daily to allow bathing and elbow motion. By two weeks, the patient should begin active and passive elevation of the arm. It may take several months to regain the ability to do overhead activities such as combing the hair.

DISTAL RADIUS

Clinical Presentation and Classification

In 1814 Abraham Colles first described the classic silverfork deformity of the wrist that bears his name [12]. The dorsal trabecular bone of the distal radius impacts into itself, resulting in angulation and shortening. Patients present with pain, tenderness, and swelling of the wrist. The mechanism of injury is usually a fall on the outstretched hand.

Treatment and Prognosis

The severity and need for reduction is assessed radiographically [13]. On the anteroposterior view, shortening of the radial styloid compared with the ulna should ideally be less than 0.5 cm. On the lateral view, dorsal tilting of the articular surface of the distal radius should not go beyond neutral. Patients with minimally displaced fractures or low functional demands are treated with a short arm cast or splint. For those fractures requiring closed reduction, some form of anesthesia is necessary. Aspiration of the hematoma and local injection of lidocaine may be sufficient, but intravenous regional or general anesthesia are superior for relaxation and pain relief. Fractures with severe shortening or intra-articular comminution may require application of an external fixator [14]. In the operating room, pins are inserted through the skin into the metacarpals and proximal radius or ulna. Then a metal external frame or plaster cast is applied to the pins, which then maintain the fracture reduction.

Prognosis and Complications
The most frequent complication of distal radius fractures is stiffness of the fingers and shoulder [15]. For this reason, active motion of the fingers, elbow, and shoulder should be strongly encouraged. Elevation of the hand above the heart is also important to combat swelling. Cast immobilization is usually maintained from three to eight weeks depending on the fracture's stability. Patients can expect gradually diminishing pain and weakness in their wrist for up to 6 to 12 months after injury. Physical therapy exercises help to speed recovery. Most patients will eventually regain satisfactory pain-free function.

PELVIC RAMUS
Clinical Presentation and Anatomy
The usual mechanism of injury is a fall on level ground. Patients present with pain and inability to walk. Physical examination reveals local tenderness in the groin and pain with movement of the legs. The clinical appearance mimics fractures of the proximal femur, and the diagnosis is made radiographically. Usually only a single ramus is fractured, with the pubic ramis breaking twice as often as the ischial ramus. Less commonly, two or more rami are fractured, either on the same or opposite sides of the symphysis pubis.

The weight-supporting function of the pelvis is borne mainly through strong bony arches in the ilium with the pubic and ischial rami acting as secondary tie arches. When the pelvis is traumatized, the rami tend to fracture first. If only a single ramus is broken, the pelvic ring remains intact with almost no loss of stability. If both pubic and ischial rami on the same side are broken, the secondary tie arch is weakened, but the main ilial weight-bearing arches remain intact.

Treatment and Prognosis
Hospitalization is required because initially the patient is usually unable to stand or even sit without considerable pain. Analgesics and anti-inflammatory medication help symptomatically. To avoid the complications of bed confinement, patients should be encouraged to begin full weight-bearing ambulation as soon as possible. Most are able to use a walker by one week. Pubic rami fractures typically heal without permanent functional disabilities [16].

HIP FRACTURES, FEMORAL NECK
Clinical Presentation and Classification
Femoral neck fractures can be classified as either occult, impacted, nondisplaced, or displaced. Occult fractures may occur in the elderly after minimal or even no apparent trauma. The patient complains persistently of groin pain with weight bearing, but plain radiographs of the hip reveal no fracture. The initial trauma produces a radiographically undetectable crack that can continue to propagate across the femoral neck with the cyclic stresses of walking. Weight bearing must be avoided, or eventually complete displacement can occur. Bone scans are positive before radiographs show a fracture line.

Patients with impacted and nondisplaced femoral neck fractures also present with groin pain and no deformity on physical examination. Radiographs of impacted, or Garden I, fractures show the femoral head to be slightly tilted into valgus with an incomplete fracture line leaving the medial cortex intact. Nondisplaced, or Garden II, fractures extend completely across both cortices of the femoral neck and are more unstable. Patients with displaced femoral neck fractures, Garden III and IV, present with groin pain and a shortened, externally rotated leg that is too painful to move.

Classification of these fractures reflects the varying amount of disruption of the femoral head blood supply and has crucial implications for treatment and prognosis [17]. Because the femoral head is intraarticular, its sole blood supply comes from vessels traveling through three structures: the bone of the femoral neck, the surrounding hip capsule, and the ligamentum teres. A displaced fracture completely disrupts the femoral neck blood vessels and can also tear those of the hip capsule. The vessels in the ligamentum teres are nonfunctioning in two-thirds of adults. Thus a displaced fracture often completely devascularizes the femoral head [18]. Although a devascularized femoral head can heal if it is securely stabilized, the incidence of complications due to poor healing is considerable. Nonunion occurs in 15 to 20 percent of patients, and osteonecrosis of the femoral head results in another 15 to 30 percent.

Treatment and Prognosis
Occult, impacted, and nondisplaced femoral neck fractures are usually treated with internal fixation with multiple pins in elderly patients. This stabilization permits the patient to begin immediate full weight-bearing ambulation and prevents the occurrence of a displaced fracture. Since the blood supply to the femoral head is not greatly disrupted, these fractures usually heal well.

Two main treatment options, operative stabilization and prosthetic replacement, exist for displaced fractures, and each has advantages and disadvantages. With their much higher incidence of nonunion and osteonecrosis of the femoral head, displaced fractures are often treated by removal of the femoral head fragment, which is then replaced with a prosthesis. Open reduction and internal fixation is usually reserved for vigorous patients under 70 years of age who are able to comply with a postoperative regimen of protected weight-bearing using crutches. The patient's femoral head is preserved, and successful healing gives a nearly normal hip. But if osteonecrosis or nonunion develops, the result is a painful nonfunctional joint that requires a second procedure, total hip

replacement, for correction. For this reason, elderly and less active patients are often treated by prosthetic replacement of the femoral head, which permits immediate full weight-bearing and faster return to independent functioning.

The simplest and historically earliest prosthetic design consists of a smooth metal sphere attached to a stem that is wedged into the medullary canal of the femur. The Moore prosthesis is an example. Drawbacks include a tendency to cause wear of the acetabular articular surface and pain from a loose fit of the stem in the femoral canal. More recent developments include use of acrylic cement and porous ingrowth to stabilize the stem of the prosthesis and an internal metal-polyethylene bearing to reduce acetabular wear [19]. For patients who develop acetabular arthritis, total hip replacement may be performed as a secondary procedure. Primary total hip replacement in acute femoral neck fractures is reserved for those patients with severe preexisting arthritis, since this more extensive operation has a higher associated morbidity than either hemiarthroplasty or internal fixation with pins.

HIP FRACTURES, INTERTROCHANTERIC
Clinical Presentation and Classification
Intertrochanteric hip fractures are usually caused by a fall, often on level ground. On physical examination of displaced fractures, the leg is shortened and externally rotated due to the pull of the leg muscles and gravity. Hemorrhage from multiple bone fragments and associated soft tissue injuries can be extensive and may cause hypovolemic shock in elderly patients.

Intertrochanteric hip fractures are classified according to the number of fracture fragments present and whether the pattern is inherently stable or unstable with respect to weight-bearing forces. Typically, two-part fractures have a single break sloping obliquely between the greater and lesser trochanter on the anteroposterior radiographic view. Three-part fractures have in addition a lesser trochanteric fragment, and four-part fractures include a greater trochanteric fragment. The stability of the fracture pattern depends on whether it is possible to achieve a reduction that maintains continuity of the weight-bearing medial femoral cortex. As a rule, three- and four-part fractures are inherently unstable due to comminution of the medial femoral cortex. Fractures involving the intertrochanteric region of the proximal femur usually allow satisfactory blood supply to be retained by all the fragments, and therefore avascular necrosis and nonunion rarely occur.

Treatment and Prognosis
Intertrochanteric hip fractures are treated by surgical stabilization unless an absolute medical contraindication exists [20]. Healing does occur with traction, but this usually requires four to eight weeks and involves all the hazards of immobilization in bed. Furthermore, traction often cannot adequately control the deforming muscle forces around the hip, which then heals in a shortened and externally rotated position, thereby causing a poor functional result.

The most commonly used fixation device today is the sliding compression hip screw, which provides rigid stabilization yet allows impaction of the fracture fragments, thus ensuring healing. Postoperatively, most patients can begin immediate full weight bearing with a walker for support. Usually 6 to 12 weeks are required before patients are able to switch to a cane.

TIBIAL PLATEAU
Clinical Presentation and Classification
Fractures of the proximal tibia usually result from a lateral bending force such as that occurring when a pedestrian is struck from the side by an automobile. As the leg angulates, the femoral condyle drives the tibial articular surface down into the underlying metaphyseal bone, which gives way easily in the elderly because it is weakened by osteoporosis. Patients present with knee pain and effusion, proximal tibial tenderness, and inability to bear weight. Displaced fractures are readily apparent on standard anteroposterior and lateral radiographs. However, occult fractures can occur that are not well visualized on standard views. In this case, oblique views are often helpful. The presence of fat globules in blood aspirated from the knee joint is also diagnostic of an occult fracture.

Prognosis and Treatment
Patients generally require hospitalization for elevation and observation of the leg to avoid

neurovascular complications due to swelling of the surrounding soft tissues. Traction or continuous passive motion can be used initially to help mold the fragments. Then restricted weight bearing in a long leg brace or cast for 8 to 12 weeks is required. Patients need physical therapy assistance to learn to walk using ambulatory aids such as crutches or walkers. Displacement of the articular surface less than 0.5 to 1.0 cm is usually acceptable for elderly patients [21]. Severely displaced fractures require operative reduction of the articular surface with inclusion of a bone graft to fill the void left by the impacted trabecular bone. Unfortunately, the patient must then refrain from weight bearing on the leg for two to three months postoperatively until healing has occurred.

Young, active patients may in time develop osteoarthritis due to the disruption of the joint surface. The elderly are at less risk for this, and for them total joint replacement is a good option if it does occur.

THORACIC AND LUMBAR VERTEBRAL BODY COMPRESSION FRACTURES
Clinical Presentation
The mechanism of injury in the elderly is usually some activity that increases the compressive load on the spine, such as lifting, forward bending, or a misstep while walking. Patients often present with acute pain that is made worse by sitting or standing. Physical examination reveals well-localized percussive tenderness over a specific region of the spine. Associated neurologic deficits are rare.

Many vertebral body fractures, however, occur silently, because elderly patients often have radiographic evidence of fractures for which no history of symptoms exists. Osteoporosis weakens the trabecular bone of the vertebral bodies and leaves the posterior elements relatively unaffected. Excessive loads then compress the vertebral bodies into a wedge-shaped configuration as the trabecular bone impacts into itself.

Treatment and Prognosis
Vertebral body compression fractures always heal. The trabecular bone is really just impacted into itself, and the blood supply is not impaired. Neurologic deficits due to bony im-

pingement rarely occur. These fractures are relatively stable because the intact posterior elements prevent translational displacement. The clinical problem is progressive kyphotic deformity due to wedging and loss of height of the vertebral bodies.

Initially hospitalization for bed rest may be necessary for pain relief. Analgesics, antiinflammatory medication, and laboratory screening tests for other causes of osteopenia are indicated. Patients should be encouraged to begin sitting up as soon as possible and walking for short periods of time. Patients may require a week to return to independent ambulation and have considerable back pain for 6 to 12 weeks afterward. Sometimes, a month or more later, the pain will shift from the site of the original fracture to a higher or lower location, probably due to altered mechanical stresses caused by the deformity.

Bracing probably does little to prevent deformity but can help in relieving pain and permitting more rapid return to activities. Bracing is only useful for fractures of the lumbar and lower thoracic spine because adequate support cannot be achieved above this level. Hyperextension braces, such as the Jewett brace, are the most effective biomechanically but are not the most comfortable. They apply three-point stabilization of the spine through anterior abdominal and chest pads and a third posterior pad located at the level of the fracture. Corsets or abdominal binders are a better tolerated and effective alternative for patients with midlumbar fractures.

Diagnosis
PHYSICAL EXAMINATION
Most fractures are quite evident due to swelling, deformity, or pain with attempted movement. Minimally displaced, stress, or impending fractures have findings of tenderness with palpation and pain with weight bearing or loading of the involved bone. In noncommunicative patients, refusal to move an extremity may be the only sign of a fracture or dislocation. Careful assessment of sensory, motor, and circulatory status of the injured extremity is important prior to initiation of therapy. After application of a cast, splint, or traction, or after manipula-

tion of a fractured extremity, the neurovascular status of the limb should always be rechecked.

When injuries or lack of patient cooperation make physical examination unreliable, radiographs are required to avoid overlooking a fracture. For instance, the presence of a hip fracture can prevent an adequate examination of the contralateral leg due to pain caused by motion. Because the incidence of coexisting injuries is not negligible, all patients with a femoral or pelvic fracture require radiographs showing both hips and the pelvis to avoid missing a second injury.

Joint aspiration is a useful diagnostic and therapeutic maneuver for patients with suspected hemarthrosis. The possibility of an acute effusion secondary to gout, pseudogout, or infection can be suggested by inspection of the fluid and confirmed by laboratory tests. Aspiration of blood confirms that an intraarticular injury such as a fracture or torn ligament or meniscus has occurred. The presence of fat globules mixed in the blood, which can be easily seen when the aspirate is viewed in an open container, implies the existence of a fracture, which allows fat from the marrow cavity to enter the joint.

X-RAYS
Routine radiographic evaluation of suspected fractures should always include both anteroposterior and lateral views. On a single view the characteristic displacement, discontinuity in contour, or altered alignment of a fracture may be hidden owing to overlapping or projection. When standard views are ambiguous, as sometimes occurs with minimally displaced spiral fractures, oblique views can be helpful. The trap of restricting the initial radiographs to too small an area should be avoided. Musculoskeletal pain is often poorly localized or referred. A patient complaining of thigh and knee pain, for instance, may actually have a hip fracture that would be missed unless radiographs of the entire femur are taken.

Computer tomography (CT) is a useful adjunct to plain radiographs in several circumstances. It helps to visualize occult fractures, particularly in areas where difficulties arise due to overlying bony structures, such as in the cervical spine. It aids the evaluation of joint fractures in determining the extent to which the articular surface has been disrupted. It is also valuable in assessing suspected pathologic fractures for the presence of bone destruction and soft tissue masses.

BONE SCAN

Total body scanning to detect focal injury to bone from any cause is performed using technetium-99-labeled pyrophosphate or similar analogs. These analogs are incorporated in the skeleton anywhere new bone formation occurs such as in response to infection, arthritis, tumor, or fracture. Bone scans can demonstrate occult fractures not yet detectable on plain radiographs. They are useful to differentiate such conditions as osteomyelitis and osteonecrosis, which can mimic a fracture by presenting with acute pain and swelling. Patients suspected of pathologic fractures require bone scans for evaluation of metastatic and metabolic bone disease, which are evident by involvement of other areas besides the fracture site.

BLOOD TESTS

Certain laboratory tests have special relevance in the evaluation of fracture patients. The hematocrit (Hct), which is the volume of packed red cells, is the most widely used clinical test for evaluating blood loss due to fractures or surgery. A 3-point drop in Hct corresponds to the loss of roughly one unit of blood in a normally hydrated patient. Patients with acute bleeding or dehydration may have a falsely elevated Hct that falls when their intravascular volume is repleted with intravenous fluids. Since elderly patients are generally at high risk for development of cardiac ischemia, their red cell volume should not be allowed to drop below a level suitable to maintain sufficient oxygen-carrying capacity. As a clinical guideline, a Hct below 30 indicates the need for blood transfusion, especially preoperatively. In postoperative hip fracture patients, the Hct should be monitored for at least four days following injury or surgery because a 4- to 8-point drop can occur owing to reequilibration or continued bleeding.

A low hematocrit can also be a warning sign of a serious underlying medical condition that has important implications for the fracture patient. For instance, gastrointestinal bleeding can be dangerously exacerbated by the anticoagulants otherwise routinely given to immobilized patients for prophylaxis of deep venous thrombosis. Anemia may be the first indicator of multiple myeloma or other malignancy that has weakened a bone enough to permit a pathologic fracture.

Serum alkaline phosphatase concentration is elevated whenever there is increased bone turnover. This increase occurs during the natural course of fracture healing but may also indicate a malignancy or metabolic abnormality such as Paget's disease. The serum calcium level is elevated with endocrine disturbances such as hyperparathyroidism and with metastatic disease, especially breast carcinoma. When patients with Paget's disease are placed on bed rest, excessively rapid bone resorption may also elevate the serum calcium concentration.

Treatment

INITIAL IMMOBILIZATION OF FRACTURES

Proper initial immobilization of injured extremities is important to prevent further damage from occurring before definitive stabilization can be achieved. Movement of sharp fracture ends can cause serious soft tissue trauma and even puncture the skin, converting a closed injury to an open one. Immobilization also serves to aid patient transport and relieve pain, thus decreasing the need for narcotic medication.

Injuries located about or distal to the knee or elbow can usually be immobilized initially with splints. A wide variety of splints are available including those made of preformed aluminum or plastic, inflatable clear plastic, and easily adjustable splints with Velcro closures. Plaster of Paris splints molded individually for each patient are perhaps the most comfortable for long-term use. All splints are best applied by holding the injured extremity with gentle longitudinal traction while an assistant applies the splint.

Most injuries of the shoulder, upper arm, and elbow can be effectively immobilized by using a sling. If further restraint is required, the arm can be kept close to the body by adding an elastic wrap or swathe. Hip fractures can be treated by careful positioning with pillows or by light skin traction.

AMBULATORY AIDS

Canes, crutches, and walkers can assist elderly patients with ambulation both initially after injuries or operations and subsequently for chronic disability. Walkers provide a moveable stable platform that gives patients security from falling. Although quite useful and popular with the elderly, walkers have limitations. They offer little protection of fractures from weight-bearing forces, cause considerable slowing of gait, and are not suitable for use on stairs. Ordinary crutches are usually inappropriate for the elderly, who lack the upper body strength and motor coordination necessary for their use. Canadian crutches with a forearm support and hand grip require less strength and may be considered for chronic disabilities. Canes are effective for assisting with balance and for reducing the weight-bearing forces across the hip. The cane is of correct length if the patient's elbow is only slightly bent when maximum force is being applied. For proper use, the cane should be held in the contralateral hand for hip injuries and in the hand of preference for knee, ankle, and foot injuries.

CASTS

Casts are used to control the alignment of a fracture while healing occurs. Traditionally, casts are made from rolls of stiff muslin impregnated with Plaster of Paris (calcium sulfate hemihydrate). Inexpensive and easy to mold, plaster is often used for initial casts and those that need frequent changing. Plaster casts are relatively heavy, deteriorate with heavy use, and weaken if they become wet. Casting materials made of polymeric resins and fiberglass have recently been introduced. They are stronger, stiffer, and half as heavy as plaster casts. Water will not weaken the cast itself, but if the underlying padding becomes wet, the cast must be changed to avoid skin breakdown.

To provide effective immobilization, the cast must extend across one joint above and one joint below the fracture site. Thus, for a distal radius fracture, the cast should theoretically extend from above the elbow to just proximal to the metatarsal joint. Because joint stiffness is a major problem in the elderly, this rule is often compromised by ending the cast below the elbow to allow joint motion.

Patients with casts must be given careful instructions to follow. For the first 24 to 48 hours postinjury the casted limb should be elevated constantly to avoid swelling. Rhythmic flexion and extension of the fingers or wiggling of the toes are encouraged to facilitate venous return. Symptoms of progressive or unrelenting pain, pressure, or numbness in the casted extremity should be reported immediately. Swelling of an extremity within the unyielding confines of a circular cast can cause pressures high enough to stop tissue perfusion, thus creating a compartment syndrome.

TRACTION

Traction is used in the elderly only when no satisfactory alternative treatment exists, which may occur if the fracture is too comminuted for a cast or surgical stabilization or if the patient's medical condition will not permit an operation. Associated complications of traction include pressure sores, deep venous thrombosis, depression, disorientation, loss of appetite, atelectasis, and pulmonary infection. Meticulous and aggressive nursing care is required. Specially designed mattresses with alternately inflatable compartments help reduce skin breakdown and increase patient comfort.

Skin traction is particularly hazardous in the elderly. It is only indicated to provide temporary gentle restraint of the limb for patient comfort. More than 5 pounds should never be used. It is applied through foam boots or carefully wrapped moleskin strips. Vigilant monitoring is required. The strong and prolonged traction required to maintain position of a fracture must be applied through skeletal pins. The proximal tibia is the preferred traction pin site for femoral and acetabular fractures.

OPERATIVE STABILIZATION

Operative stabilization of fractures can offer compelling benefits for elderly patients. Especially for lower extremity fractures for which nonoperative treatment would entail a prolonged period of immobility, the risks of surgery are usually outweighed by the likelihood of medical complications resulting from enforced bed rest. Patients with hip fractures, for instance, can usually begin ambulating within days after surgical stabilization.

Despite these advantages, surgical treatment of most fractures should be postponed for correction of acute medical abnormalities. Only fractures associated with such limb-threatening conditions as an impending compartment syndrome, neurovascular compromise, or open wound would require urgent treatment. Furthermore, some conditions are a relative contraindication to surgery. The presence of sepsis that could infect the operative site prohibits the use of metallic implants. Severely osteoporotic bone with poor mechanical properties is also a relative contraindication to internal fixation because the hardware will displace if it cannot obtain secure purchase in the bone.

A deep postoperative wound infection is a serious complication that frequently necessitates removal of all implanted hardware, prolonged daily dressing changes, and weeks of intravenous antibiotics. Studies have shown that with use of prophylactic antibiotics, postoperative infections in hip fracture patients can be reduced to an incidence of about 1 percent [22]. Cephalosporins are currently the agent of choice. An appropriate regimen would be 1 gm cefazolin given intravenously in the hour prior to surgery, followed by 1 gm every eight hours for the next 24 hours.

Complications
COMPARTMENT SYNDROMES
A closed space or compartment syndrome is the most frequent limb-threatening complication associated with trauma to an extremity [23]. Swelling of injured muscle within a confined compartment surrounded by an unyielding envelope such as fascia or a cast can lead to elevated tissue pressures that block normal perfusion of the limb. The resulting tissue ischemia in turn leads to further muscle injury and swelling and higher tissue pressures. The only solution to this ever-intensifying cycle is to remove completely all confining envelopes around the swollen muscular compartment, which means that casts, splints, or dressings should be thoroughly loosened immediately in all patients complaining of increasing pain or distal numbness in an immobilized injured extremity. If the muscle swelling has increased to the point that its surrounding fascia has become a constricting envelope, then an emergency fasciotomy must be performed. Even a few hours of muscle ischemia can lead to irreversible injury and necrosis. The most reliable clinical signs of impending compartment syndrome are progressively increasing pain in an immobilized extremity, pain with passive flexion or extension of the toes or fingers, and numbness in a specific peripheral nerve distribution. The presence of pulses distally in a limb does not ensure that a compartment syndrome has not developed. Muscle necrosis and irreversible nerve damage occur at tissue pressures much lower than those required to obliterate arterial flow.

THROMBOEMBOLISM
Pulmonary emboli are the most frequent fatal complication following lower extremity trauma [24]. About 50 percent of untreated hip fracture patients develop deep venous thrombosis, about 10 percent have pulmonary emboli, and about 2 percent have fatal pulmonary emboli. The major predisposing factors for deep venous thrombosis are advanced age, trauma or surgery involving the lower extremities, prior history of deep venous thrombosis, immobilization, malignancy, and obesity. Sole reliance on clinical findings such as complaints of pain, swelling, tenderness, Homan's sign (pain with forced dorsiflexion of the foot), fever, and leukocytosis leads to marked underdiagnosis of deep venous thrombosis. Only 5 to 30 percent of cases of deep venous thrombosis can be detected by physical examination alone. An autopsy study of patients who died after hip fracture revealed that 38 percent died of pulmonary emboli. Without autopsy fatal pulmonary embolism was recognized clinically in only 2 percent of patients dying after hip fracture.

Thromboembolic disease ideally should be treated prophylactically by anticoagulation begun at time of admission. Studies in elective surgical patients show that 50 percent of thromboses develop by the end of an operation. For orthopedic patients at high risk of deep venous thrombosis, such as those with hip fractures, warfarin and dextran are considered to be the most effective prophylactic agents. Aspirin, low-dose heparin, or external pneumatic boot compression have not been shown to provide as much protection. Anticoagulation should be begun immediately on hospitalization and continued until the patient is fully ambulatory. The initial dose of warfarin is between 2.5 and 10 mg depending on the patient's age and weight. Subsequently, daily doses are given with a goal of maintaining the protime (PT) in a range 1.5 times that of control.

References

1. National Center for Health Statistics. *Advance Data from Vital and Health Statistics: 1985 Summary: National Hospital Discharge Survey.* (U.S. Public Health Service Publication No. (PHS) 86-1250.) Hyattsville, MD: Public Health Service, 1986.
2. Melton, L. J. III, et al. Fifty-year trend in hip fracture incidence. *Clin. Orthop.* 162:144, 1982.
3. Holbrook, T. L., et al. *The Frequency of Occurrence, Impact and Cost of Selected Musculoskeletal Conditions in the United States.* Chicago: American Association of Orthopaedic Surgeons, 1984.
4. Ray, W. A., et al. Psychotropic drug use and the risk of hip fracture. *N. Engl. J. Med.* 316:363, 1987.
5. Ruff, C. B., and Hayes, W. C. Bone-mineral content in the lower limb. Relationship to cross-sectional geometry. *J. Bone. Joint. Surg. [Am.]* 66:1024, 1984.
6. Hayes, W. C., and Gerhart, T. N. Biomechanics of Bone: Applications for Assessment of Bone Strength. In W. A. Peck (ed.), *Bone and Mineral Research.* Vol. 3. Amsterdam: Elsevier, 1985.
7. Harrington, K. D. New trends in the management of lower extremity metastases. *Clin. Orthop.* 169:53, 1982.
8. Behr, J. T., et al. The treatment of pathologic and impending pathologic fractures of the proximal femur in the elderly. *Clin. Orthop.* 198:173, 1985.
9. Brighton, C. T. The biology of fracture repair. *Instr. Course Lect.* 33:60, 1984.
10. Simmons, D. J. Fracture healing perspectives. *Clin. Orthop.* 200:100, 1985.
11. Mills, H. J., et al. Fractures of the proximal humerus in adults. *J. Trauma* 25:801, 1985.
12. Peltier, L. F. Fractures of the distal end of the radius. *Clin. Orthop.* 187:18, 1984.
13. Solgaard, S. Classification of distal radius fractures. *Acta Orthop. Scand.* 56:249, 1985.
14. Cooney, W. P. External fixation of distal radius fractures. *Clin. Orthop.* 180:44, 1983.
15. Stewart, H. D., et al. The hand complications of Colles' fractures. *J. Hand Surg. [Br.]* 10:103, 1985.
16. Spencer, J. D., et al. The mortality of patients with minor fractures of the pelvis. *Injury* 16:321, 1985.
17. Barnes, R., et al. Subcapital fractures of the femur. A prospective review. *J. Bone Joint Surg. [Br.]* 58:22, 1976.
18. Stromqvist, B., et al. Pre-operative and post-operative scintimetry after femoral neck fracture. *J. Bone Joint Surg. [Br.]* 66:49, 1984.
19. Giliberty, R. P. Hemiarthroplasty of the hip using a low-friction bipolar endoprosthesis. *Clin. Orthop.* 175:86, 1983.
20. James, E. T., et al. The treatment of intertrochanteric fractures—a review article. *Injury* 14:421, 1983.
21. Blokker, C. P., et al. Tibial plateau fractures. An analysis of the results of treatment in 60 patients. *Clin. Orthop.* 182:193, 1984.
22. Williams, D. N., et al. The use of preventive antibiotics in orthopaedic surgery. *Clin. Orthop.* 190:83, 1984.
23. Masten, F. A., 3d. A practical approach to compartmental syndromes. Part I. Definition, theory, and pathogenesis. *Instr. Course Lect.* 32:88, 1983.
24. Montrey, J. S., et al. Thromboembolism following hip fracture. *J. Trauma* 25:534, 1985.

31

Rheumatic Disease

Fred G. Kantrowitz
David F. Giansiracusa

Erythrocyte Sedimentation Rate

The erythrocyte sedimentation rate (ESR), an easily performed laboratory test used to evaluate the presence of various diseases and to monitor their activity [1], measures the settling of red blood cells suspended in anticoagulated blood in a vertically positioned tube of specific dimensions for a 60-minute period. Normal values depend on the dimensions of the tube used [2]. Generally quoted normal ESR values in millimeters per hour by the Westergren method are less than 15 for men and less than 25 for women; by the Wintrobe method, they are 0 to 6.5 for men and 0 to 16 for women.

The sedimentation rate is affected predominantly by red blood corpuscle rouleau formation, which, by increasing the size of the particle and weight relative to the surface area, accelerates the rate of red corpuscle fall. Large, asymmetric plasma molecules facilitate rouleau formation. Fibrinogen is the predominant plasma protein responsible for this, while alpha and gamma globulins contribute to lesser degrees. An elevated ESR may reflect the presence of a malignancy, infection, systemic rheumatic disease, paraproteinemia, or renal failure [3].

The effects of aging must be considered when interpreting the ESR. Several studies examining ESRs in healthy individuals of various ages indicate a linear increase with each advancing decade [4]. A study of 1,457 healthy men and 1,021 women with the Westergren method revealed a constant increase in men of 0.85 mm per hour and in women of 0.53 mm per hour every five years until age 50 [5]. After menopause, the ESR increased 2.8 mm per hour every five years [6]. Thus, for individuals older than 65, an ESR up to 40 mm per hour with the Westergren method may be normal for the patient's age.

Possible explanations for the increased ESR seen in elderly individuals include the presence of an occult disease process or an increase in the production or a decrease in the catabolism of asymmetric plasma proteins.

Antinuclear Antibodies

Antinuclear antibodies are immunoglobulins predominantly of the IgG class directed against various nuclear constituents, including deoxyribonucleic acid (DNA), ribonucleic acid (RNA), and nucleoprotein [7]. The homogeneous or diffuse pattern reflects antibody to deoxyribonuclear protein (DNP) and occurs in approximately 98 percent of patients with systemic lupus erythematosus (SLE). The diffuse pattern also occurs in individuals with other systemic rheumatic diseases and chronic active hepatitis.

The peripheral or rim pattern is seen when antibody to double-stranded DNA and occasionally to single-stranded DNA is present. Patients with active SLE frequently have high-titer antinuclear antibodies with a peripheral pattern that may change to a lower-titer homogeneous pattern during remissions. Although antibodies to single-stranded DNA may occur in various diseases, such as rheumatoid arthritis, scleroderma, and chronic active hepatitis, antibodies in significant titers to double-stranded or native DNA are specific for SLE [8].

The speckled pattern of immunofluorescence frequently reflects antibody to an extractable nuclear antigen that is composed of ribonuclear protein (RNP) and the Sm antigen. This pattern is seen in patients with Sjögren's syndrome, rheumatoid arthritis, systemic lupus erythematosus (SLE), progressive systemic sclerosis, and mixed connective tissue disease. Antibody to the Sm antigen component of extractable nuclear antigen occurs with SLE. The nucleolar pattern reflects antibody to nucleolar ribonucleoprotein. It occurs most commonly in patients with progressive systemic sclerosis but is also seen in patients with SLE and Sjögren's syndrome.

In addition to these disease states, antibodies to nuclear constituents occur with relatively high frequency in normal elderly individuals. In one study antinuclear antibodies were found in 3 percent of normal individuals 16 to 59 years of age and in 16 percent of individuals 60 to 91 years of age [9].

Antinuclear antibodies occurring as a "normal" function of age typically have a homogeneous or diffuse immunofluorescent pattern and occur in low titer (less than 1 : 16) [10]. They are directed against nucleic acid-histone; antibodies to purified DNA do not occur simply as a function of aging.

In summary, antinuclear antibodies in low titer may occur in normal elderly individuals and in patients with systemic rheumatic diseases. High-titer antinuclear antibodies with peripheral (or rim), speckled, or nucleolar patterns occur in the setting of various systemic rheumatic diseases and are an extremely unusual finding in a normal elderly person.

Rheumatoid Factor

Rheumatoid factor is an antibody, usually IgM. These antibodies occur (1) in 70 to 80 percent of individuals with rheumatoid arthritis; (2) with lesser frequency in other systemic rheumatic diseases such as SLE; (3) with infectious diseases such as tuberculosis, leprosy, leishmoniasis, syphilis, and subacute bacterial endocarditis; (4) with chronic inflammatory processes of unknown etiology such as sarcoidosis and interstitial pulmonary fibrosis; and (5) with hematologic and oncologic diseases such as multiple myeloma and macro-globulinemic states [11].

Rheumatoid factors occur with increasing frequency with advancing age. Using the latex fixation method, they were found in 1 to 3 percent of individuals less than 65 and in 16 percent of a group of 325 people between the ages of 65 and 103. In over half of these 16 percent, the titer was 1 : 80 or less. In a fifth of those with positive rheumatoid factor, the titer was greater than 1 : 160 [12]. Other studies have found rheumatoid factor activity in approximately 25 percent of healthy individuals older than 70 years of age [13].

Gamma Globulins

Various changes of B- and T-lymphocyte function with advancing age may alter gamma globulin concentrations in elderly individuals. Several studies reveal that after the fourth decade, concentrations of IgA levels remain constant [14,15].

Benign monoclonal gammopathies occur in approximately 3 percent of healthy individuals older than 70 and in as many as 19 percent of healthy individuals over 90 [16]. Monoclonal immunoglobulinemia is the presence in the serum and/or urine of a homogeneous globulin composed of immunoglobulin molecules or fragments produced in excess by a clone of immunocytes. A characteristic M spike in the gamma globulin area noted on protein electrophoresis of the serum and urine can identify the specific immunoglobulin class. Immunoelectrophoresis using monovalent anti-heavy-chain and anti-light-chain sera can then be performed to identify specific fragments [16].

Monoclonal immunoglobulin disorders may be due to a variety of benign and malignant conditions. Malignant immunocytopathies include multiple myeloma, Waldenström's macroglobulinemia, amyloidosis, and heavy-chain diseases. Monoclonal immunoglobulin elevation can also occur in association with various conditions such as carcinomatosis, hepatic cirrhosis, diseases of suspected autoimmune origin, and chronic inflammatory diseases [16].

The clinician may be confronted with the problem of distinguishing a benign from a malignant gammopathy. Several features indicative of a malignant immunocytopathy help to make this distinction [16]. These include (1) a serum M component IgG concentration equal to or greater than 2 gm per dl or a concentration of IgM or IgA M component equal to or greater than 1 g per dl; (2) the presence of Bence Jones proteinuria; (3) a progressive increase in the serum paraprotein concentration over time; (4) a marked decrease in the synthesis of normal immunoglobulins; (5) serum hyperviscosity; (6) marrow plasmacytosis greater than 20 percent, with an increase in the number of immature and atypical cells; (7) a decrease in the number of peripheral blood B-lymphocytes; and (8) the presence of hypoalbuminemia [16].

Recommendations for evaluation and follow-up study of individuals found to have a monoclonal immunoglobulin elevation include (1) evaluation for covert carcinomatosis and malignant immunocytic disease with yearly bone marrow examinations; (2) serum and urine electrophoresis every three months for the first year and then repeated at six-month intervals; and (3) determinations of hemoglobin, white blood count, platelet count, serum iron, and total iron-binding capacity every six months [16].

Amyloid and Amyloid Arthropathy

This section reviews the biochemical and immunologic properties of amyloid fibrils and the circulating plasma precursors, the relationship between amyloid protein precursors and the deposition of amyloid material in tissues, and the characteristics of amyloid arthropathy.

Amyloid tissue is characterized by the deposition of protein fibrils in a beta-pleated sheet conformation [17]. A pentagonal serum protein is bound in a calcium-dependent fashion to all amyloid fibrils except for brain plaques in Alzheimer's disease [18].

Amyloidosis has been classified into six categories: (1) amyloidosis associated with plasma cell dyscrasias; (2) secondary amyloidosis that occurs in the setting of a chronic infectious, inflammatory, or malignant process; (3) primary amyloidosis in which no predisposing illness can be identified; (4) heredofamilial amyloidosis, including familial Mediterranean fever; (5) localized amyloidosis; and (6) amyloid deposition occurring with advancing age [19].

The biochemical composition of the amyloid fibril in primary amyloidosis and that associated with plasma cell dyscrasias, called the AL protein, differs from fibrils occurring in other forms of amyloidosis. The AL protein is composed of kappa or lambda immunoglobulin light chains or fragments. The fibrils found in secondary amyloidosis are composed of AA protein, an alpha globulin with a molecular weight of 8,400 daltons that has no structural relationship to immunoglobulin [20].

A plasma protein called SAA, an alpha globulin, has been identified as a precursor of the AA protein [21]. The SAA protein is found in low concentrations in normal individuals. It is elevated in individuals with secondary amyloidosis and, to a lesser degree, in patients with primary amyloidosis and amyloidosis associated with plasma cell dyscrasias.

The concentration of SAA protein also increases with aging, most strikingly after the age of 70 [22] (Fig. 31-1). The observation that some normal individuals older than 70 have normal levels of SAA suggests that the aging process itself may not be responsible for the elevated concentration of SAA protein but rather that the protein may be a marker of an occult inflammatory or neoplastic disease.

Elevated SAA protein concentrations that are associated with advancing age are paralleled by an increased incidence of amyloid deposition in the brain, heart, and pancreatic islets of Langerhans. Cardiac deposits were found in approximately 40 percent of individuals older than 60. In the brain, localized amyloid deposits were found in small cerebral blood vessels or plaques in 50 to 65 percent of individuals older than 60 years. Aortic amyloid deposits, found most frequently at the base of well-developed atheromatous plaques in the area of degenerated inner media, were found in 40 to 50 percent of individuals older than 60 years [23].

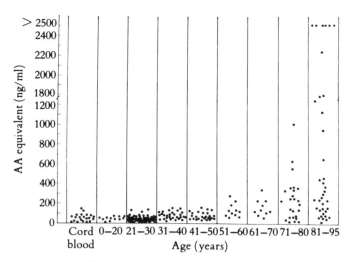

FIGURE 31-1. *Concentration of SAA in a healthy population in relation to age. (From C. J. Rosenthal and E. C. Franklin. Variation with age and disease of amyloid A-related serum component. J. Clin. Invest. 55:746, 1975.)*

Amyloid can also form deposits in the structures of joints, resulting in an arthropathy that may resemble rheumatoid arthritis [24]. Less frequently, amyloid deposits cause joint complaints secondary to bone involvement. Deposits in the marrow space of bones of large joints, most frequently the hip, may form tumefactions, resulting in bone fractures and swelling of the involved joints [25].

Classic multiple myeloma is the underlying disorder found most frequently in amyloid arthropathy, although cases have been reported in association with Waldenström's macroglobulinemia. Although a number of individuals reported in the literature with amyloid arthropathy were thought to have primary amyloidosis, these diagnoses were often made in the absence of bone marrow examination or immunoelectrophoretic evaluation of serum and urine for identification of M spikes. Thus, plasma cell dyscrasias were not definitely ruled out [24].

Amyloid joint involvement occurs most often in the sixth decade of life. The clinical features may be similar to those of rheumatoid arthritis and include morning stiffness, painful joint swelling, and synovial thickening, most commonly in the shoulders, knees, wrists, metacarpophalanges, proximal interphalanges, elbows, and hips [25]. Large as well as small joints are usually involved, including temporo-mandibular and acromioclavicular joints. Flexion contractures are frequent. Subcutaneous nodules, frequently over the olecranon, occur in 70 percent of individuals. Concurrent or antecedent carpal tunnel syndrome occurs in one-third of patients. The prominent shoulder swelling has been described as the "padded shoulder sign." Dorsal synovial thickening of the wrist may have a gritty or nodular feeling on palpation. Although involved joints may be slightly tender, joint inflammation, evidenced by warmth, erythema, and marked tenderness, is conspicuously lacking.

Laboratory studies reveal a monoclonal light-chain or M component in the serum or urine in almost all individuals, with kappa chains occurring eight times more frequently than lambda light chains. Bence Jones proteinuria is found in over two-thirds of those tested.

Radiographic features of amyloid arthropathy include osteolytic lesions, which may be the result of amyloid deposits or myelomatous aggregates. Generalized osteopenia and periarticular soft tissue swelling are common findings. Joint effusions are radiographically apparent in approximately 25 percent of individuals.

Synovial fluid from involved joints tends to be viscous and yellow or xanthochromic. The mean white blood count is 1,000 with a range of several hundred to 10,000. The cells are most commonly mononuclear, but a predominance of neutrophils has also been described. Amyloid deposits in fragments of synovial membrane or as free fibrils are frequently found in aspirated synovial fluid samples when they are stained and viewed under polarized light. Immunoelectrophoresis of the synovial fluid frequently results in identification of immunoglobulin light chains similar to those found in the serum.

Histologic examination of articular tissues frequently reveals amyloid deposits that are located in the synovial layer superficial to or mixed with the synovial lining cells. Articular cartilage and periarticular tissue, including the joint capsule, tendons, ligaments, and bones, may contain amyloid deposits. Cellular reaction to these deposits is minimal.

The natural history of these patients is dependent on the underlying plasma cell dyscrasia. Articular improvement frequently occurs associated with corticosteroid and cytotoxic therapy for the underlying disease.

Changes Associated with Aging of Articular Cartilage

Articular cartilage is formed from mesenchymal cells derived from embryonic mesoderm and is composed of collagen fibers produced by chondrocytes and embedded in a matrix or ground substance. Each collagen macromolecule consists of three tropocollagen fibers or alpha chains, each of approximately 1,000 amino acid sequences wrapped together in an alpha helix structure [26]. Chondrocytes also synthesize the ground substance of articular cartilage, proteoglycans, which are composed of glycosaminoglycans. The highly viscous and strongly hydrophilic properties of proteoglycans provide articular cartilage with resiliency to compression and with lubrication that lessens friction between the articular surfaces [27].

Normal articular cartilage is devoid of blood vessels, lymphatics, and nerves. Chondrocytes derive their nourishment by diffusion through articular cartilage from the synovial fluid and to a lesser extent from subchondral blood vessels. During the developmental stages of articular cartilage (through adolescence), the collagen content increases while the water, hexosamine, chondroitin sulfate, ash, and sialoprotein content decreases [28].

After the age of 30, there are demonstrable changes in articular cartilage. The concentration of keratan sulfate increases, and that of chondroitin sulfate remains constant or decreases [28]. There is no change in total proteoglycan content, but aggregation is abnormal and water content decreases [29].

Osteoarthritis

HISTOLOGIC, BIOCHEMICAL, AND METABOLIC CHANGES OF CARTILAGE

The histologic changes of osteoarthritis are similar to those that occur with aging—that is, loss of superficial, tangential layers of cartilage and an increase in the number of chondrocytes occurring in clones or islands within the cartilage matrix. Other changes occurring specifically in osteoarthritic cartilage include progressive loss of proteoglycan content and extension of vertical clefts into subchondral bone. The defects in the cartilage and subchondral bone formed by these clefts cause scar and reactive bone formation and result in the radiographic appearance of subchondral sclerosis and heterotopic bone formation. The exposed bone becomes sclerotic, and subchondral cysts develop that may be due to small fractures in the trabecular bone or to synovial fluid forced into bone through cartilage defects. The new cartilage that proliferates in the areas of erosions and over marginal osteophytes is mechanically inferior to the normal articular cartilage [28].

Biochemical changes occurring in osteoarthritic cartilage include a decrease in proteoglycan content that is proportional to the severity of the disease and an increase in the content of chondroitin-4-sulfate relative to keratan sulfate [28]. There is also a decrease in proteoglycan chain length in osteoarthritis. Studies of proteoglycan synthesis in osteoarthritic cartilage initially reveal a doubling of synthetic rate compared with normal cartilage. As the osteoarthritis progresses in severity, the rate of proteoglycan synthesis markedly declines [28]. Chondrocyte DNA synthesis as measured by ^{3}H thymidine incorporation is increased, as is collagen synthesis. Chondrocytes in osteoarthritic cartilage produce normal type II $[\alpha_1 (II)]_3$ collagen as well as type I $[\alpha_1 (I)]_2 \alpha_2$, which normally occurs in skin and bone [28].

BIOCHEMICAL AND MECHANICAL PATHOGENESIS

Recognition of the biochemical and histologic features of osteoarthritic joints aids in understanding the pathophysiology of osteoarthritis. Bleeding, which occurs with subchondral bone damage or intrasynovial hemorrhage, is associated with high cytoplasmic quantities of iron pigment in chondrocytes. As chondrocytes phagocytize the iron, lysosomal enzymes are released that degrade cartilage. Repeated articular bleeding decreases metachromatic staining, reflecting loss of proteoglycans, and results in superficial and deep cartilage erosions [28]. Depletion of glycosaminoglycans before fibrillation of the cartilage suggests that degradation of proteoglycans by proteolytic enzymes such as cathepsin may be the initiating process [30]. The levels of cathepsin D are increased in osteoarthritic cartilage [31]. Immunofluorescent studies localize cathepsin D in the chondrocyte lysosomes and in the area of chondrocyte surfaces. Low-molecular-weight proteases, which at a neutral pH digest proteoglycans, may also be present in cartilage. Phagocytosis of particles of abraded cartilage may also cause the release of lysosomal proteases and collagenases.

Normal articular cartilage is resistant to sheer forces due to the low coefficient of friction. With impact, articular cartilage and subchondral bone deform in a manner that maximizes the surface area of contact between the two articular surfaces, thereby distributing the load over the greatest area possible [32]. Repeated impact-loading of joints causes rapid cartilage wear, an increase in the coefficient of friction of the articular surfaces, exposure of subchondral bone, and development of microfractures. With healing, the subchondral bone remodels and loses its ability to absorb stress, which subjects the articular cartilage to increased mechanical stresses and results in progression of cartilage damage. A cycle is thus established of trauma or abnormal physical stresses and proteolytic enzymes damaging articular cartilage and subchondral bone and disrupting the properties of the joint that protect it from physical stresses. The enzymatic damage to cartilage stimulates chondrocyte synthesis of abnormal proteoglycans and articular collagen. The cartilage synthesized in an attempt to repair the damage is inferior to normal articular cartilage with respect to both the collagen and the ground matrix components [30].

CLINICAL FEATURES

Osteoarthritis is a progressive disorder that commonly occurs in later life and is characterized clinically by pain, deformity, and limitation of joint motion. The pathologic features of affected joints include cartilage destruction, subchondral sclerosis, and bone cyst formation as well as osteophytic new bone and cartilage proliferation at joint margins. Degenerative changes at autopsy examination of weight-bearing joints can be demonstrated to occur as early as the second decade and can be found in 90 percent of individuals by age 40. Radiographic changes may be seen in weight-bearing joints in 85 percent of individuals by age 75, only 30 percent of whom are symptomatic. A disparity between the individual's symptoms and the radiographic extent of the disease is common [33]. The cardinal clinical feature of osteoarthritis is pain, which early in the disease occurs with motion, particularly with weight bearing, and is relieved with rest. As the disease progresses, the pain may occur with minimal motion and at rest, may be troublesome at night, may awaken the individual from sleep, and is often of aching quality and poorly localized. Stiffness for several minutes after inactivity and on awakening may occur, but it does not last as long as that seen in patients with rheumatoid arthritis. Progressive loss of range of motion occurs on the basis of joint surface incongruity, muscle spasm, tendon and joint capsule contractures, and the presence of osteophytes [33].

Women tend to be affected with severe osteoarthritis of the knee more commonly than men. Obese women over 50 with varus deformities of the knee are at high risk for developing osteoarthritis of the knee. Patients with osteoarthritis of the knee may complain of a "crunching" sound or sensation with movement and of joint instability. Examination may reveal crepitus on palpation of the joint during motion, limited active and passive ranges of motion, irregular enlargement of the joint due to cartilage and bony proliferation, quadriceps atrophy, instability due to laxity of the collateral ligaments, and knee effusion. Synovial fluid is noninflammatory with less than 2,000 white blood cells and shows a predominance of mononuclear white blood cells and a good mucin clot. Occasionally, cartilage fragments can be seen on synovial fluid analysis. Radiographic studies routinely include anteroposterior (AP) and lateral views. Special studies include the AP view during weight bearing to evaluate the degree of joint space narrowing, which reflects cartilage loss, as well as the degree of genu varus or valgus deformity. Tunnel views with the knee flexed expose the intercondylar notch and are useful in evaluating intraarticular loose bodies and spurs [33].

Osteoarthritis of the hip is more common in men than in women. Although true hip pain is usually appreciated in the groin or inner aspect of the thigh, it may be referred to the buttocks, down the front of the thigh to the knee, or in a sciatic distribution. Low back pain results from an increase in lumbar lordosis that compensates for flexion contractures at the hips. Osteophytes, joint space narrowing, subchondral sclerosis, and cysts occur predominantly on the superior—i.e., the weight-bearing aspect of the hip joint.

The prominent symptom of osteoarthritis of the spine is pain, which may be due to soft tissue reaction of the periosteum, paraspinous ligaments, or joint capsule or to paraspinous muscle spasms. Parasthesias and reflex motor changes may occur secondary to radicular irritation. Changes that may impinge on neural foramina and cause nerve root compression include osteophytes, lateral disk protrusion, and apophyseal joint subluxation. Since the diameter of the spinal canal is smaller in the cervical area than elsewhere in the spine, neurologic abnormalities due to spinal cord compression most commonly occur with osteoarthritis of the cervical spine [33].

Anterior osteophytes are particularly common in the thoracic vertebrae but may extend the entire length of the spine. Radiographic features of osteoarthritis, in addition to anterior osteophytes, include narrowing of the intervertebral disks, which is most severe in the lower cervical and lower lumbar regions, with sclerosis of adjacent vertebral body borders, lateral and posterior vertebral osteophytes, joint space narrowing with vertebral body sclerosis of the posterior apophyseal joints, and subluxation of apophyseal joints. Although osteophytes are generally asymptomatic, severe cases of exostosis with fusion of vertebral body osteophytes has been termed "ankylosing vertebral hyperostosis of the aged," a condition with little pain but marked limitation of motion [33].

Primary osteoarthritis of the hands involves distal and proximal interphalangeal joints of the fingers, the carpometacarpal joint of the thumb, and the first metatarsophalangeal joint of the foot. Women are affected about ten times as frequently as men. Features of this condition include the development of cartilaginous and bony enlargement, usually of multiple distal interphalangeal joints (Heberden's nodes) and proximal interphalangeal joints (Bouchard's nodes). These changes may cause flexion contractures and medial or lateral deviation of the distal phalanx. Involvement of the carpometacarpal joint of the thumb may cause pain. Prominence at the base of the thumb gives it a squared appearance. Involvement of the first metatarsophalangeal joint of the foot usually results in progressive swelling and pain, especially with tight-fitting shoes. Attacks of inflammation of the bursa over the medial aspect of this joint may mimic acute podagra (gout).

Although Heberden's and Bouchard's nodes and arthritis usually develop gradually with little pain, they occasionally develop rapidly and may be associated with erythema, swelling, tenderness, pain, and distal finger paresthesias. The acute onset of Heberden's and Bouchard's nodes associated with inflammatory and degenerative changes of the distal and proximal interphalangeal joints, first metacarpophalangeal and interphalangeal joints is termed *inflammatory osteoarthritis* and occurs almost exclusively in elderly women [34].

Secondary osteoarthritis develops in the setting of joint damage caused by an identifiable condition, including structural abnormalities (congenital hip dysplasia, slipped capital femoral epiphysis) or avascular necrosis of a joint secondary to Legg-Perthes disease, or in association with steroids, SLE, sickle cell anemia, liver disease, Caisson's disease, Gaucher's disease, or trauma. Metabolic diseases associated with cartilage damage, including hemochromatosis, Wilson's disease, ochronosis, Morquio's syndrome, gout, hypophosphatasia, hemophilia with repeated intraarticular hemorrhage, and inflammatory arthritides such as rheumatoid and septic arthritis, also result in osteoarthritis as a final common pathway. Occupational demands and neurologic abnormalities that subject joints to severe mechanical stresses may cause osteoarthritis, including involvement at atypical locations such as the elbows of coal miners and the shoulder of weight lifters.

MANAGEMENT

Treatment of osteoarthritis includes measures to prevent cartilage injury and to delay the progression of joint damage. Once osteoarthritis is established, the major objectives of therapy are relief of pain and preservation of joint motion. Preventive measures include medical treatment of metabolic disorders that predispose to cartilage damage and correction of abnormal mechanical stresses on the joints such as leg length discrepancy, postural abnormalities, meniscal tears, and ligamentous laxity. Maintenance of ideal body weight, appropriate conditioning of the neuromuscular apparatus, avoidance of excessive fatigue during exercise, and use of mechanical assistive devices such as canes or walkers help to minimize mechanical injury to joints.

Medical management of pain associated with osteoarthritis includes the use of appropriate rest, antiinflammatory agents, analgesics, and local steroid injections. Rest as therapy to relieve pain may be divided into two components: rest for the entire body to avoid generalized fatigue, and rest for a particular part of the body in the form of splints or braces. Rest coupled with physical measures such as application of moist heat, massage, and traction may relieve painful muscle spasm.

Medications that provide pain relief include aspirin and other nonsteroidal antiinflammatory drugs (NSAIDs) [35] and a variety of nonnarcotic analgesics, including acetaminophen (Tylenol) and propoxyphene hydrochloride (Darvon). Treatment with NSAIDs, however, remains preferable. Since osteoarthritis requires prolonged therapy, use of narcotic analgesics, which may be associated with addiction and toxicity, should be avoided. A number of NSAIDs

are available. Of these, piroxicam, which is taken once per day, and sulindac and naproxen, which are taken twice per day, appear to be associated with increased compliance. All NSAIDs should be taken with food or an antacid to minimize gastrointestinal side effects. Other potential side effects, such as fluid retention and central nervous system toxicity, must be considered. Indomethacin appears to be associated with increased central nervous system toxicity in the elderly. Phenylbutazone should be avoided.

The nonacetylated salicylate preparations, including salsalate (Disalcid), magnesium choline trisalicylate (Trilisate), and choline salicylate (Arthropan) are poor inhibitors of prostaglandins, are usually well tolerated, and have the advantage, unlike other NSAIDs, of not impairing platelet function and not precipitating a reaction in patients who, when treated with aspirin, develop urticaria and angiodema, often in the face of nasal polyps and a history of bronchial asthma.

Because of the tremendous individual variability of patient response to NSAIDs, failure to achieve benefit and/or development of adverse reactions to one NSAID does not mean that a particular patient will fail to respond to or tolerate another NSAID. A regimen consisting of a NSAID alone, a nonnarcotic analgesic alone, or a combination of a NSAID with a pure analgesic may be tailored to the individual needs of the particular patient.

In the osteoarthritic patient whose problems are localized to a single joint, intraarticular injection of a depot steroid preparation (approximately 40 mg of depot methylprednisolone or its equivalent) mixed with 1 ml of 1% lidocaine may provide relief for weeks to months. Because intraarticular steroids impair the normal synthetic activity of chondrocytes, steroid injections into a given joint should be performed as a rule no more than two to three times and at no shorter intervals than two to three months.

Physical therapy plays an important role in achieving and maintaining joint motion and muscle strength. Flexion contractures at the hips and knees and quadriceps weakness and atrophy are particularly disabling. A program of physical therapy designed specifically to treat these musculoskeletal problems is an essential component of management of the patient with osteoarthritis.

Surgical intervention may be useful, particularly for the correction of deformities such as flexion contractures and for relief of pain [27, 36]. Surgical procedures such as removal of intraarticular loose bodies and repair of a torn meniscus may improve joint function dramatically. The patient with severe pain, particularly at night, or severe impairment of joint function of the hip or knee is a candidate for total joint replacement.

Pseudogout-Calcium Pyrophosphate Dihydrate Crystal Deposition Disease

Deposition of calcium pyrophosphate dihydrate (CPPD) in articular cartilage increases with advancing age and is associated with various clinical presentations of arthritis. Articular chondrocalcinosis, the radiographic finding of abnormal deposition of calcium salts in hyaline and fibrocartilage, increases in incidence with advancing age and by the ninth decade is found in 25 to 30 percent of individuals [37].

A definite diagnosis of CPPD deposition requires either identification of calcium pyrophosphate dihydrate crystals, $Ca_2P_2O_7 \cdot 2H_2O$, in synovial fluid or biopsy specimens or arthritic cartilage, or the presence of typical polyarticular chondrocalcinosis together with identification of weakly positive birefringent crystals on compensated polarized microscopic examination of synovial fluid [38].

The arthritis associated with articular chondrocalcinosis is variable, and six categories—types A through F—have been defined [39]. Type A is an acute monoarticular or oligoarticular arthritis that is termed *pseudogout* because it resembles an acute attack of gout. This type occurs in approximately 25 percent of patients with CPPD deposition disease and is characterized by acute or subacute attacks of inflammation, usually in one appendicular joint, that last from one to four days. The attack may spread to surrounding joints and involve multiple contiguous joints at a given time, resulting in a "cluster" attack. The knee is the most frequently involved joint, being affected in 50 percent of attacks; the ankles, wrists, elbows, and small joints of the hands and feet are involved

less frequently. Between attacks the individual is asymptomatic. Identification of crystals is necessary to establish the diagnosis of an acute pseudogout attack. Various physiologic stresses such as medical illnesses, surgery, and trauma may precipitate an attack.

Type B, or *pseudorheumatoid arthritis,* occurs in approximately 5 percent of individuals with CPPD deposition disease. Attacks last several weeks to months, and multiple joint involvement with synovial thickening, pitting edema, and limited range of motion secondary to flexion contractures and pain may mimic rheumatoid arthritis.

Type C and D presentations have been termed *pseudoosteoarthritis.* These occur in approximately 50 percent of individuals with CPPD crystal deposition disease. Progressive degeneration of multiple joints, commonly in a bilateral and symmetric pattern, is seen clinically and radiographically. Women are affected more commonly than men. The knee is the most common joint involved, but other affected joints include the wrist, metacarpophalangeal, hip, shoulder, elbow, and ankle joints, all of which are seldom involved in classic osteoarthritis. Individuals with superimposed acute attacks of pseudogout are said to have type C; those without the acute episodes have type D.

Type E, the *lanthanic* or asymptomatic form, and type F, the *pseudoneuropathic* form, comprise the final two clinical presentations. In type E, individuals have radiographic articular cartilage calcification without symptoms. Individuals with type F have severe destructive changes characteristic of a neuropathic or Charcot's joint in the presence of articular chondrocalcinosis, but there are no identifiable sensory abnormalities [40].

The radiologic features of CPPD crystal deposition disease are varied. CPPD crystal deposition in fibrocartilage of the menisci, radioulnar joint, triangular cartilage of the wrists, symphysis pubis, and annulus fibrosus of the intervertebral disks appears as dense punctate calcifications. Crystal deposition in hyaline cartilage appears as fine, linear calcifications that parallel the subchondral bone of the femoral condyles and head of the humerus. Crystal deposition in the synovial lining may create an irregular appearance of radiodense focuses similar to calcifications seen in synovial chondroma-tosis. Joint capsule calcifications may occur in the hips, shoulders, elbows, and small joints of the hands. Occasionally, CPPD crystal deposi-tion occurs in the Achilles, triceps, quadriceps, and supraspinatus tendons and in connective tissue of the hip abductors [41]. Hook-like or tear-drop osteophytes at the distal metacarpal heads are characteristic of patients with CPPD crystal deposition disease. Patients with appen-dicular chondrocalcinosis have been demon-strated to have an increased incidence of an-kylosing hyperostosis of the spine [41].

Biopsies performed during acute attacks of pseudogout reveal proliferation of the lining cells of the synovial membrane, vascular con-gestion, fibrinous exudate overlying the syno-vial membrane, and rhomboid-shaped, weakly positive birefringent crystals in the synovial membrane, connective tissue, fibrin exudate, and synovial and tissue-based leukocytes. In the chronic forms of CPPD arthropathy, the syno-vium and underlying connective tissue appear fibrotic, with infiltration of mononuclear cells and the presence of foreign body granulomas. Giant cells are seen in areas of CPPD crystal de-posits. In severe cases the cartilage is replaced by granulation tissue [42]. These fibrotic changes most likely contribute to the flexion contractures seen in the subacute and chronic forms of CPPD-associated arthropathy.

Familial CPPD disease has been described in populations in Chile, Holland, and Czechoslo-vakia. In the last group, the absence of male-to-male transmission suggests X-linked genetics, and the finding of more severe phenotypic expression at a younger age in the homozygote suggests that an enzymatic defect is a possible etiology. In the Chilean and Dutch populations, male-to-male transmission is consistent with autosomal genetics [43].

Various metabolic diseases have been asso-ciated with CPPD disease, including hyper-parathyroidism, hemochromatosis, hypothy-roidism, gout, hypophosphatasia, and Wilson's disease [44]. Patients with CPPD arthropathy should be evaluated for evidence of hyperpara-thyroidism and hypothyroidism, and a family history of pseudogout or other forms of CPPD arthropathy should be obtained. Laboratory investigation should include determination

serum calcium and phosphorus and tests of thyroid function. Serum iron and total iron-binding capacity (TIBC) are a simple screen for hemochromatosis.

An understanding of the pathophysiology of CPPD disease clarifies its association with vari-ous metabolic disorders. An acute attack is ini-tiated when CPPD crystals residing in articular cartilage or joint tissues are shed into the syno-vial fluid. There they are coated with IgG and phagocytized by polymorphonuclear leuko-cytes and monocytes, which then release a low-molecular-weight chemotactic factor that re-cruits additional inflammatory cells. As the leukocytes attempt to phagocytize the CPPD crystals, they release destructive lysosomal en-zymes, including collagenases and elastases [39]. The result of these processes is joint in-flammation and articular cartilage damage.

Calcium ions, Ca^{++}, and pyrophosphonate, P_2O_7-4, are in equilibrium with the crystal-line form of calcium pyrophosphate dihydrate, $Ca_2P_2O_7 \cdot 2H_2O$. Patients with hypophospha-tasia have a deficiency of alkaline phosphatase, a pyrophosphatase. As a result, high concentra-tions of pyrophosphate accumulate, which fa-cilitates formation of the CPPD crystal. Indi-viduals with hyperparathyroidism have elevated Ca^{++} levels, which also facilitate the formation of CPPD crystals. A fall in serum calcium in a patient with hyperparathyroidism, either as a result of medical management or resection of parathyroid tissue, may precipitate an acute at-tack of pseudogout by disturbing the equi-librium between the crystalline and ionic forms of calcium pyrophosphate. Crystals may then be shed into the synovial fluid. The precipita-tion of pseudogout attacks by surgery is also consistent with this pathophysiologic mecha-nism, since a significant (approximately 10 per-cent) fall in serum Ca^{++} occurs after abdominal and thoracic surgical procedures. An additional precipitating factor in patients with hyperpara-thyroidism is the collapse of subchondral bone, which causes "shedding" of crystals into the synovial fluid. Degenerated cartilage may elabo-rate inorganic pyrophosphate, which may ex-plain the increased incidence of chondrocalcino-sis and CPPD arthropathies in the elderly, a population in which osteoarthritis is prevalent, and is consistent with the experimental observation of elevated concentrations of synovial fluid inorganic pyrophosphate, which is elaborated by osteoarthritic articular cartilage but not by normal adult cartilage [39].

The finding of inflammatory synovial fluid with intraleukocytic calcium pyrophosphate dihydrate crystals does not necessarily indicate that the crystals initiated and are the only cause of the joint inflammation. Any inflammatory arthritis, including pyogenic arthritis and acute gout, is associated with a leukocytic response. If calcium pyrophosphate is present in the articular cartilage, the lysosomal enzymes released by the leukocytes may leach the crystals out of the cartilage. Because of this mechanism of lysosomal "enzymatic strip mining," patients with CPPD arthritis must be evaluated for septic arthritis with Gram's stain and culture of the synovial fluid [39].

TREATMENT

Treatment of pseudogout and other forms of CPPD crystal arthropathies includes management of any associated underlying disorder and administration of antiinflammatory medications. An attack of pseudogout treated with an oral NSAID (e.g., ibuprofen, 1,600 to 2,400 mg in three or four divided doses a day; naproxen, 250 to 500 mg twice a day; or sulindac, 150 to 200 mg twice a day) will generally respond within three to four days. Joint aspiration and intraarticular injection of 40 mg of a depot prednisone preparation or its equivalent usually provide relief of signs and symptoms within one to two days [45]. Patients with the more subacute and chronic forms of CPPD arthropathy such as pseudorheumatoid arthritis and the pseudoosteoarthritic forms are generally treated in the same manner as patients with osteoarthritis (see the section on management of osteoarthritis).

Gout

The presence of atypical tophaceous deposits in the soft tissue pads of the terminal digits, the periungual soft tissue crescent, and overlying Heberden's nodes has recently been described. All patients were females with varying degrees of renal insufficiency. None had a prior history of acute gout [46].

Rheumatoid Arthritis

Rheumatoid arthritis (RA) is a chronic, systemic disease of unknown etiology that affects the diarthrodial joints and is associated with multiple extraarticular manifestations. The arthritis tends to be symmetric in distribution and frequently involves the wrist, metacarpophalangeal, proximal interphalangeal, metatarsophalangeal, knee, elbow, ankle, shoulder, and hip joints. Morning stiffness is a common complaint. Objective signs of synovitis are frequently found on examination, and joint destruction may be demonstrated radiographically with joint space narrowing and marginal erosions. Synovial fluids are characteristically inflammatory.

Extraarticular manifestations tend to occur in rheumatoid factor-positive patients who have severe arthritis. Subcutaneous nodules, pericarditis, pleuritis, interstitial lung disease, peripheral neuropathies, anemia, Sjögren's syndrome, and vasculitis may accompany the articular disease [47,48]. The natural history varies from a several-month period of arthritis followed by complete remission, to chronic, active multisystem disease.

Although rheumatoid arthritis occurs most commonly in individuals between the ages of 20 and 60, approximately 10 percent of patients experience the onset of disease after age 60. In one group of elderly patients the arthritis affected men more often than women and was characterized by an acute onset with a predilection for the large joints. These patients had a high frequency of remission within the first year [49]. In a group of 110 patients with onset of rheumatoid arthritis between the ages of 60 and 86, 74 percent had disease identical to rheumatoid arthritis occurring in younger patients [50]. However, the remaining 26 percent (29 patients) experienced remission within 12 to 18 months of onset compared to the usual remission rate of 5 to 10 percent in published series.

The characteristics of this group of 29 patients included the sudden onset of polyarticular arthritis, usually over a one- or two-day period, and severe constitutional symptoms, including anorexia, weight loss, malaise, depression, and severe morning stiffness that lasted as long as four to five hours. All had elevated erythrocyte sedimentation rates with a mean of 95 mm per hour for men and 75 mm per hour for women. Men comprised over half of the 29 individuals. Proximal joint involvement, including shoulders and neck, occurred in about half. In 6 of the 29, manifestations of pain and stiffness of the neck, shoulders, and buttock area suggested a diagnosis of polymyalgia rheumatica until more distal synovitis developed.

All 29 patients had positive rheumatoid factors that varied in titer from 1/32 to 1/5,120. All had radiographic periarticular osteopenia, and 7 of 26 developed erosions. The association of acute onset with good prognosis in this group is similar to the pattern seen in younger populations. This group of elderly individuals is of particular interest because all experienced complete remissions, even those who had disease activity for longer than 12 months. This study of RA in the elderly also revealed that gold therapy was well tolerated and may be prescribed as it is in a younger patient population. Steroids were used in 12 of the 29 patients for severe systemic symptoms. Prednisone in a dose of 5 to 10 mg per day was prescribed for 10 and was never administered in excess of 20 mg on a daily basis. In all patients it was possible to discontinue the steroids eventually [50].

MANAGEMENT

Although the basic therapeutic principles and modalities used to treat rheumatoid arthritis in younger patients apply to the patient in whom rheumatoid arthritis develops in the later years of life, several aspects of treatment of the elderly rheumatoid patient deserve particular attention. First, due to coexisting medical problems such as renal impairment, congestive heart failure, subclinical gastritis, and/or osteopenia, the elderly patient may be more susceptible to the toxicities and side effects of aspirin, other nonsteroidal antiinflammatory agents, and steroids than are younger patients. Differences in drug metabolism and, in the case of aspirin, the decreased ability to perceive tinnitus in the elderly may also predispose them to adverse drug reactions. The elderly patient may also have a greater tendency toward the development of muscle weakness and atrophy, flexion contractures, and progressive bone loss than the younger patient, who may have a stronger musculoskeletal system at the onset of arthritis.

For these reasons, particular attention must be paid to physical therapy, including range of motion and strengthening exercises, and to the appropriate use of joint splints and supplemental dietary calcium and vitamin D, as well as to avoidance of immobilization whenever possible. In the elderly patient whose rheumatoid arthritis is characterized by severe stiffness, constitutional symptoms, and particularly proliferative synovitis, treatment with low-dose steroids (5–10 mg of prednisone per day) used in addition to NSAIDs may be particularly beneficial.

Systemic Lupus Erythematosus

Systemic lupus erythematosus (SLE) is a chronic, multisystem, inflammatory disease characterized by abnormalities in the immune system. Evidence of disordered humoral immunity includes circulating autoantibodies to nuclear and cytoplasmic antigens, lymphocytes, platelets, red blood cells, and various clotting factors as well as identification of nuclear antigen, immunoglobulin, and complement deposition in small blood vessels [48]. Clinical manifestations include polyarthralgias/polyarthritis, alopecia, mucosal ulcerations, Raynaud's phenomenon, skin rashes, fevers, glomerulonephritis, pleuritis, parenchymal lung disease, pericarditis, myocarditis, myositis, peritonitis, cerebritis, meningitis, peripheral neuritis, leukopenia, hemolytic anemia, and thrombocytopenia [52,53].

Although SLE occurs most commonly during adolescence and young adulthood and decreases in incidence and prevalence after age 45, idiopathic SLE may occur at any age. Between 4 and 10 percent of patients with SLE develop the disease after the age of 50 [54]. The percentage of men in whom SLE develops after the age of 50 is higher than in the younger group. In those with onset of disease after age 60, 12.5 percent are men, whereas in younger populations of SLE patients males comprise approximately 5 percent [55]. The onset of SLE in the elderly does not differ significantly from that in younger patients. In the older age group, however, initial symptoms can be confused with those seen in other rheumatic diseases. Myalgias, weight loss, and fatigue may suggest polymyalgia rheumatica. The presentation of arthritis without associated symptoms may suggest rheumatoid arthritis.

The incidence of various manifestations of SLE varies with age of onset [56]. Individuals in whom SLE develops after age 50 have a higher incidence of pneumonitis, pulmonary fibrosis, discoid lupus, and photosensitivity than do younger individuals. Skin rash, alopecia, arthralgias, myalgias, serositis, renal disease, and renal biopsy findings are similar in both groups. Manifestations that occur less frequently in individuals with onset after age 50 include oral ulcers, Raynaud's phenomenon, cutaneous vasculitis, thrombocytopenia, hemolytic anemia, leukopenia, neuropsychiatric manifestations, and hypocomplementemia [56,57].

SLE in elderly individuals in general requires less steroids and azathioprine to suppress the disease [57], which implies that SLE that begins between the ages of 50 and 60 is a milder disease and is more responsive to therapy than is SLE in younger individuals [58]. However, the authors of one study concluded that, like the mode of onset, the prognosis for those developing SLE after age 50 is the same as that for patients developing SLE at a younger age [55].

DRUG-INDUCED LUPUS

A number of medications associated with the development of lupus-like syndromes are administered to elderly individuals. These include procainamide, hydralazine, isoniazid, diphenylhydantoin, propylthiouracil, chlorpromazine, and, less frequently, practolol, methylthiouracil, methimazole, and penicillamine [59]. Positive antinuclear antibodies occur most frequently with administration of procainamide [60], hydralazine, and anticonvulsant therapy and less frequently with chlorpromazine, isoniazid, and alpha-methyldopa. As many as 50 percent of individuals in a prospective study treated for six months with procainamide developed antinuclear antibodies without symptoms of SLE. Positive SLE tests and antibodies to denatured DNA and to deoxyribonucleoprotein (anti-DNP) but not to native DNA occur in one-third to one-half of individuals treated with procainamide for longer than six weeks [60].

The diagnosis of drug-induced lupus is based

on the same clinical features as those characterizing idiopathic SLE. Clinical signs and symptoms may disappear within days to weeks, whereas antinuclear antibodies may remain positive for months to years after the offending drug has been stopped. Rechallenge with the drug results in prompt reappearance of the signs and symptoms [56].

The relationship between drug use and development of lupus-like features may take three forms. Antinuclear antibodies without clinical symptoms of lupus erythematosus may develop. This type of reaction is not associated with production of lymphocytotoxins, Coombs' positivity, or antibodies to native or double-stranded DNA. A second type of reaction is characterized by the development of antinuclear antibodies and symptoms of lupus erythematosus. Exacerbation of preexisting SLE with drug administration is the third type of reaction [61], in which sulfonamides are a frequent offender.

The incidence of clinical features of lupus differs in drug-induced lupus compared with idiopathic SLE. In the former, pleuropulmonic manifestations such as pleuritic pain, pleural effusions, and pneumonitis occur with greater frequency and severity and may be more recalcitrant to therapy [59]. Constrictive pericarditis and cardiac tamponade have both been reported with procainamide-induced lupus [62]. Renal and central nervous system involvement, febrile episodes, dermal manifestations, and hematologic manifestations are much less common in drug-induced SLE than in idiopathic SLE. Antibodies to native or double-stranded DNA do not occur in high titer in drug-induced lupus except when hydralazine is the drug administered [63]. Although hypocomplementemia is a feature of idiopathic SLE, it rarely occurs in drug-induced lupus.

TREATMENT OF SYSTEMIC AND DRUG-INDUCED LUPUS

Other than discontinuing the offending drug, if possible, in cases of documented drug-induced lupus syndromes, the management of idiopathic and drug-induced lupus in the elderly patient does not differ appreciably from the management of idiopathic SLE in younger patients

[53]. Aspirin and other nonsteroidal antiinflammatory agents are helpful in controlling arthralgias, arthritis, myalgias, serositis, fevers, and malaises. Topical steroid preparations are efficacious for skin rashes and mucosal ulcerations. Sun screens should be used in patients with sun sensitivity. Hydroxychloroquine (Plaquenil) may be helpful, particularly for the management of skin and articular manifestations. The occurrence of hemolytic anemia, thrombocytopenia, severe renal disease, pericarditis, pleuritis, peritonitis, fevers, and neurologic manifestations may be an indication for the use of steroids alone or in combination with cytotoxic agents in both elderly and younger patients with lupus erythematosus.

Sjögren's Syndrome

Histologic changes of the salivary glands with aging include fatty degeneration and fibrosis of the parenchyma and lymphocytic infiltration, occasionally causing glandular enlargement [64]. Salivary secretions diminish with advancing age and are associated with loss of filiform papillae on the dorsum of the tongue, resulting in a smooth, glazed appearance. Lacrimal secretions also decrease, causing complaints of dry eyes. Vaginal dryness and dyspareunia may occur in elderly postmenopausal women as the vaginal epithelium becomes thin and dry in the absence of significant levels of circulating estrogens. These various complaints may suggest the presence of Sjögren's syndrome, a specific entity with characteristic clinical and pathologic features.

Sjögren's syndrome is composed of keratoconjunctivitis sicca (dry eyes) and xerostomia (dry mouth) and is often associated with rheumatoid arthritis or another systemic rheumatic disease [65]. Ocular complaints related to lacrimal gland dysfunction are common in patients with Sjögren's syndrome, occurring in over 90 percent. A burning sensation of the eyes or an inability to produce tears results from inadequate lacrimal secretion of the aqueous portion of tears. A sensation of a foreign body or dust in the eyes and of a film covering the eyes and obscuring vision may result from production of an abnormal lacrimal mucus component [66].

Oral manifestations are related to inadequate salivary gland secretions and mechanical problems secondary to salivary gland infiltration. Dryness of the mouth and lips with development of fissures and ulcers on the lips, tongue, and buccal mucosa and loss of sense of taste may occur. Difficulty with mastication and swallowing result from inability to produce adequate saliva to form a bolus of food. Rampant dental caries may also occur due to inadequate salivary gland secretions.

Swelling of the salivary glands, particularly the parotid glands, occurs as a result of lymphocytic infiltration. Discrete episodes of swelling occur in approximately two-thirds of patients, whereas chronic progressive swelling, which is usually symmetric, is seen in about one-third of patients [65]. Although salivary gland swelling may be painful, this finding, especially when accompanied by fever, raises the concern of a complication of Sjögren's syndrome such as suppurative parotitis or development of a lymphoreticular malignancy. The differential diagnosis of parotid swelling is large and includes viral, fungal, and bacterial infections; tuberculosis; sarcoidosis; deficiency of vitamins C, B_6, or A; iodide ingestion, hyperlipidemia types III, IV, and/or V; diabetes mellitus; cirrhosis; and primary or metastatic neoplasms [65].

Since the symptoms of Sjögren's syndrome may be found in many healthy elderly individuals, definite criteria have been developed to establish the diagnosis. These include objective evidence of keratoconjunctivitis sicca or xerostomia and characteristic histopathologic findings on biopsy of the minor salivary glands [66]. Various tests to document keratoconjunctivitis sicca include Schirmer's test, which measures tear production with filter paper placed at the intercanthus of the lower eyelid, measurement of tear lysozyme, and conjunctival and corneal staining. Clinically, Schirmer's test is performed as a screening examination, but since tear production decreases with age, the test lacks specificity [67]. Conjunctival and corneal staining with rose bengal or fluorescein and viewed with a slit lamp can be performed as a more specific examination. The stain collects in areas of devitalized and epithelialized corneal and conjunctival tissue and reflects damage occurring as a result of lacrimal dysfunction. Evaluation of salivary gland function includes determination of salivary flow rates, technetium salivary gland radionuclide scans, and sialography [68].

Biopsy of the minor salivary glands of the lower lip is done for histopathologic documentation. This procedure has evolved owing to complications from parotid gland biopsies such as fistula formation and facial nerve damage and from the recognition that the minor salivary glands are involved in Sjögren's syndrome [68]. Major changes include parenchymal acinar atrophy, fibrous and adipose tissue replacement, lymphocytic infiltration, hyperplasia and proliferation of intraglandular ductal lining cells, and epimyoepithelial islands, the most specific of the histologic findings for Sjögren's syndrome. The severity of the histologic changes correlates well with the severity of sicca symptoms [66].

Even though the clinical and diagnostic features emphasize lacrimal and salivary gland involvement, Sjögren's syndrome is a systemic disease [65]. In addition to eye and oral involvement, the skin, respiratory tract, genitourinary tract, and gastrointestinal systems may be affected. Clinically, manifestations include dryness of the skin with lack of sweating, non-thrombocytopenic hyperglobulinemic purpura, nasal dryness, chronic nonproductive cough, pleurisy and pleural effusions, atelectasis, pulmonary fibrosis, dyspareunia, hyposthenuria, and proximal renal tubular acidosis with its sequelae (osteomalacia secondary to urinary phosphate wasting, hypokalemia, and nephrocalcinosis), dysphagia and abnormal esophageal motility, liver function abnormalities, pancreatitis, and peripheral neuropathies. Histologic studies reveal lymphocytic infiltration in the affected organs. Raynaud's phenomenon is also associated with Sjögren's syndrome, as is the presence of multiple circulating antibodies to tissue constituents, including antibodies to thyroglobulin, gastric parietal cells, and salivary ductal cells. Hypergammaglobulinemia, especially IgG, is common. Antinuclear antibodies occur in one-third to two-thirds of patients, and IgM rheumatoid factor occurs in about two-thirds of patients with documented Sjögren's syndrome. B_2-microglobulin, be-

lieved to be a product of lymphocytes and consisting of polypeptide chains homologous to immunoglobulin, is found in serum, salivary gland secretions, and urine [65] and reflects the degree of lymphocytic infiltration in these organs and the general activity of the disease. Elevated concentrations of immunoglobulin G and of IgM rheumatoid factors are also found in salivary gland secretions. Erythrocyte sedimentation rates are frequently elevated. An increased incidence of anergy associated with impaired lymphocyte transformation to phyto-hemagglutinin in vitro is another immunologic abnormality seen in patients with Sjögren's syndrome. In the peripheral blood, B-lymphocytes are increased, whereas T-lymphocytes are decreased [66].

The immunologic features and the animal model of Sjögren's syndrome, the F_1 hybrid population of New Zealand black/white (NZB/NZW) mice, provide evidence that Sjögren's syndrome results from a deficiency of suppressor T-cell lymphocytes, leading to excessive B-lymphocyte activity [69,70].

The natural history of patients with Sjögren's syndrome is now appreciated as a spectrum, ranging from benign lymphocytic infiltration of various exocrine glands to lymphocyte infiltration of viscera described as pseudolymphoma to frank lymphoproliferative malignancies or hyperviscosity syndromes [71] (Fig. 31-2). In a given patient, however, the disease usually does not evolve through all three stages. Striking elevation in the concentration of B_2 microglobulin may reflect lymphocytic proliferation and signal the development of a lymphoproliferative malignancy [72]. A progressive increase in IgM levels may signal the development of a macroglobulinemic hyperviscosity syndrome. Several features of Sjögren's syndrome are risk factors for development of lymphoproliferative malignancies. These include parotid enlargement, lymphadenopathy, and splenomegaly, as well as an increased frequency of the HLA-Dw3 antigen that appears to serve as a marker of patients with Sjögren's syndrome without rheumatoid arthritis [73].

TREATMENT

Treatment of patients with Sjögren's syndrome includes supplementation of the inadequate ex-

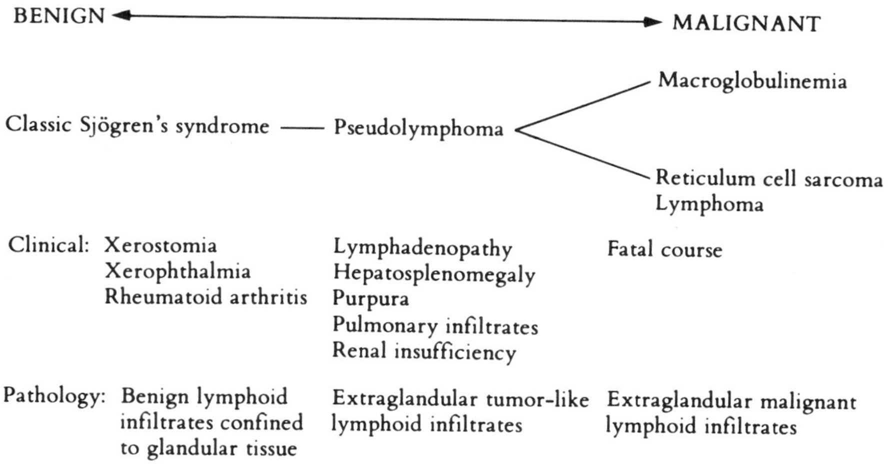

BENIGN ◄──────────────────────────────────► MALIGNANT

```
                                              ╱─ Macroglobulinemia
Classic Sjögren's syndrome ──── Pseudolymphoma ◄
                                              ╲─ Reticulum cell sarcoma
                                                 Lymphoma
```

Clinical: Xerostomia   Lymphadenopathy   Fatal course
           Xerophthalmia   Hepatosplenomegaly
           Rheumatoid arthritis Purpura
                               Pulmonary infiltrates
                               Renal insufficiency

Pathology: Benign lymphoid   Extraglandular tumor-like Extraglandular malignant
           infiltrates confined lymphoid infiltrates   lymphoid infiltrates
           to glandular tissue

FIGURE 31-2. *The spectrum of benign to malignant lymphoproliferation in Sjögren's syndrome, with pertinent clinical and histologic features noted. (From N. A. Cummings, et al. Sjögren's syndrome—newer aspects of research, diagnosis, and therapy. Ann. Intern. Med. 75:937, 1971.)*

ocrine gland secretions and management of complications. The treatment of lacrimal gland insufficiency includes the use of methylcellulose or polyvinylpyrol-based tears. Various maneuvers to retard loss of tears, such as the use of shielding eyeglasses and humidification of the environment, are useful. Infectious conjunctivitis should be treated aggressively. Oral symptoms can be treated with secretagogues including sugarless chewing gum and Slippery Elm lozenges. Meticulous dental care must be observed, including brushing and flossing after meals and frequent visits to a dentist and dental hygienist. Patients treated with cyclophosphamide for lymphoproliferative complications have noted improvement in sicca symptoms, but cytotoxic therapy is not indicated for uncomplicated Sjögren's syndrome.

Polymyalgia Rheumatica

Polymyalgia rheumatica is a specific clinical entity consisting of proximal muscle aching and stiffness that occurs in individuals over the age of 50, with peak incidence in the midsixties. It occurs twice as frequently in women as in men and infrequently in nonwhite populations, and is associated with an elevated erythrocyte sedimentation rate [74].

The onset of myalgias often starts with the posterior neck muscles and spreads to the shoulder and pelvic girdles. Initially, the distribution may be unilateral, but most frequently it becomes symmetric and affects muscles of both the shoulders and hips. The onset of myalgias may be either insidious or abrupt. Exercise may aggravate the discomfort. Morning stiffness may last about an hour, sometimes suggesting rheumatoid arthritis in the differential diagnosis. The stiffness may be so severe that getting out of a bed or chair becomes very difficult. Myalgias at night may interfere with sleeping. Fatigue, lethargy, anorexia, weight loss, malaise, apathy, and depression are commonly associated symptoms.

Objective abnormalities may include limited range of motion of the shoulders and hips secondary to muscle discomfort. Muscles of the shoulder and pelvic girdles and posterior neck may be tender to palpation. Although the individual may make a poor effort on strength testing due to discomfort, true muscle weakness is not part of the clinical picture of polymyalgia rheumatica. Peripheral arthritis with synovial fluid white counts up to 20,000 have been described, especially in the knees [75].

Laboratory studies reveal an elevated erythrocyte sedimentation rate, usually greater than 50. A normochromic anemia, elevated α_2 globulins, and hypoalbuminemia are associated findings. Muscle enzyme measurements, electromyograms, and muscle biopsies are normal in contrast to those seen in polymyositis and dermatomyositis [76]. Joint scans may be positive in the areas of the shoulders and hips in some individuals with polymyalgia rheumatica [77]. Abnormal liver function tests occur as reflected by increased bromsulphalein (BSP) retention and elevation of alkaline phosphatase [78].

The differential diagnosis of polymyalgia rheumatica includes virus-induced myalgias, rheumatoid arthritis, polymyositis, and hypothyroidism. Viral infections are characteristically of less than one month's duration and are associated with fever and normal sedimentation rates. In polymyalgia rheumatica the ESR is elevated and fever is unusual unless giant cell arteritis is present. In rheumatoid arthritis initial symptoms may include upper arm myalgias and morning stiffness that may be indistinguishable from that seen in polymyalgia rheumatica [74]. Knee effusions described in polymyalgia rheumatica makes this "differential" even more difficult, as can the finding of a positive rheumatoid factor in the elderly patient with polymyalgia rheumatica. With time, the development of a peripheral synovitis, nodules, and radiographic changes such as periarticular osteopenia and marginal erosions help establish the diagnosis of rheumatoid arthritis. Polymyositis can be distinguished from polymyalgia rheumatica on the basis of weakness, abnormal muscle enzymes, electromyograms, and muscle biopsies.

The myalgias of polymyalgia rheumatica characteristically improve dramatically when the patient is given low-dose steroids (10 mg per day of prednisone), usually within 12 hours to four days. Decrease in the sedimentation rate occurs within days, while the associated anemia improves over a few weeks. Most commonly, polymyalgia rheumatica runs approximately a two-year course, although disease activity may persist for several years.

TREATMENT

The goal of therapy for polymyalgia rheumatica in the absence of giant cell arteritis is to relieve symptoms until the disease has run its natural course. Nonsteroidal antiinflammatory drugs may significantly relieve muscle stiffness and pain, but steroids are usually necessary. Prednisone, in a dose of 5 to 15 mg a day, usually provides rapid improvement, often within 12 to 24 hours, of the musculoskeletal symptoms. After approximately one month of steroid therapy, the dose may be reduced as the symptoms permit. The erythrocyte sedimentation rate usually decreases to normal while the patient is treated with even low doses of steroids. If, however, the sedimentation rate remains markedly elevated—i.e., greater than 60 to 70 mm per hour by the Westergren method—after four to six weeks of steroid therapy, the possibility that the patient may also have occult giant cell arteritis must be considered.

Giant Cell Arteritis

Giant cell arteritis is a form of vasculitis of unknown etiology that occurs most frequently in individuals in the seventh decade. The clinical symptoms in any given patient may include those of polymyalgia rheumatica as well as symptoms secondary to vascular inflammation [79]. Onset occurs most frequently between 65 and 73 years of age, with a range of 48 to over 90 years of age [76]. Although giant cell arteritis occurs almost exclusively in white individuals and has a 2 : 1 predominance of women to men, nonwhite patients have been reported with biopsy-documented giant cell arteritis. The onset and character of the myalgias associated with giant cell arteritis may be indistinguishable from the symptoms that occur with only polymyalgia rheumatica. Symptoms of polymyalgia rheumatica have been noted in 40 to 60 percent of individuals with giant cell arteritis. Of patients presenting with polymyalgia rheumatica symptoms alone, 40 percent have characteristic histologic features of giant cell arteritis on temporal artery biopsies [79]. Low-grade fevers are present in about half of the individuals with giant cell arteritis and may be the initial manifestation of this disease. For this reason, temporal artery biopsy is recommended as part of the evaluation of fever of unexplained origin in an elderly individual [80].

In addition to polymyalgia rheumatica symptoms, patients with giant cell arteritis may have constitutional symptoms, including fever, malaise, weight loss, fatigue, and apathy, as well as symptoms due to vasculitic lesions. The most commonly involved vessels are the branches of arteries originating from the aortic arch, although almost any artery may be involved. Pathologic examinations at postmortem from patients dying of giant cell arteritis reveal frequent involvement of superficial temporal, vertebral, ophthalmic, and posterior ciliary arteries, with the internal carotid, external carotid, and central retinal arteries being involved less frequently [81]. Classic symptoms include headache, claudication of muscles of mastication, scalp pain and tenderness and visual disturbances.

Headache occurs in 44 to 98 percent of individuals with giant cell arteritis and is the initial symptom in 30 to 45 percent [82]. Headaches may be localized over the arteries of the scalp, but the type and location are variable. A significant feature of the history is either a change in the pattern or severity of old headaches or the onset of new headaches. Visual disturbances include ptosis, diplopia, transient or permanent visual impairment, and complete blindness. Visual impairment and blindness are most commonly due to involvement of the posterior ciliary arteries and branches of the ophthalmic artery and less commonly to central retinal artery involvement. Visual symptoms usually occur several weeks or months after other symptoms such as myalgias or headaches have developed. Transient visual disturbances frequently precede the development of blindness, but the sudden onset of blindness may be the first visual symptom. Although complete blindness usually does not improve with corticosteroid therapy, lesser degrees of visual impairment improve in about 15 percent of patients. Visual impairment due to involvement of the posterior circulation has been reported but is a much less frequent cause than ciliary and ophthalmic artery vasculitis. Other symptoms of vasculitis include the aortic arch syndrome, with claudication of the upper extremities, renal artery vasculitis, brain stem strokes due to vasculitis of the posterior circulation, and aortic aneurysm dissections and ruptures [83].

Physical findings in patients with giant cell arteritis include impairment of visual acuity. Funduscopic examination may reveal fundic hemorrhages, cotton wool patches, and pallor and edema of the optic disk. Arterial examination may reveal tenderness, dilation of the involved arteries, diminished pulses, and bruits distal to the vasculitic lesions. Although palpa-

tion of the superficial temporal arteries may reveal tenderness, warmth, firm nodules, or diminished pulses, in approximately half of patients the temporal arteries are normal on examination [79]. Palpation of occipital arteries may elicit tenderness. Other findings include evidence of synovitis, primarily of the knee.

Lesions occur in arteries with elastic fibers in the vessel walls. The pathologic features of giant cell arteritis include inflammation of the internal elastic lamina, thrombosis at the site of vessel inflammation, necrosis of the arterial wall, granuloma formation, and infiltration of histiocytic giant cells, lymphocytes, plasma cells, and fibroblasts. Polymorphonucleocyte (PMN) infiltration is minimal [79,81].

Vascular involvement tends to be segmental. Skip lesions are found in 28 percent of patients with some focuses of vasculitis as short as 330 μ in length [84]. The need to examine temporal artery specimens of several centimeters in length with multiple sections thus becomes clear. For this reason angiography has been performed to localize involved segments of the temporal artery for biopsy. Although angiography is a sensitive method for localizing arterial narrowing, the angiographic patterns demonstrated are not specific for giant cell arteritis and may be caused by other processes such as atherosclerosis [85].

The major laboratory abnormality is elevation of the erythrocyte sedimentation rate. An ESR of greater than 100 mm per hour is common in patients with untreated giant cell arteritis. Rare cases of biopsy-proven giant cell arteritis have been reported, however, with normal or near-normal sedimentation rates. Mild normochromic or hypochromic anemias are common. White blood cell counts may be normal or moderately elevated. Platelet counts are normal or elevated. Antinuclear antibody and rheumatoid factors are negative. Fibrinogen and α_2 globulins are elevated, and albumin is depressed. Immunoglobulin levels are occasionally elevated. Liver function abnormalities occur in approximately one-third of patients. Alkaline phosphatase elevations are most frequently found, but serum glutamic-oxaloacetic transaminase (SGOT) and prothrombin elevations may also occur. Joint imaging may reveal increased uptake of radionuclide in the hips and shoulders [77]. Synovial fluids may be mildly inflammatory, with white blood cells ranging from 1,000 to 8,000 with a differential of 50 percent PMN and poor mucin clots. Synovial biopsies may reveal nonspecific synovial proliferation and lymphocytic infiltration. Muscle biopsies of individuals with giant cell arteritis and polymyalgia are normal.

Treatment

The goal of treatment of giant cell arteritis is to suppress the vasculitis, thereby preventing sequelae. Once a diagnosis is suspected clinically, prednisone should be started immediately at a dose of 40 to 60 mg per day. A several-centimeter temporal artery biopsy should be obtained and examined with multiple sections. The histology of the vasculitic lesions is not altered significantly by several days of high-dose steroid therapy, which should be maintained until the sedimentation rate plateaus or returns to normal and all reversible symptoms disappear. This process generally takes two to four weeks. At that time, the dose of prednisone may be tapered off gradually by approximately 10 percent every two to three weeks while the ESR and symptoms are followed closely. If the ESR rises or arteritic symptoms recur with steroid tapering, the dose must be increased. Patients are at risk of developing arteritic sequelae as long as the ESR is elevated.

Although giant cell arteritis has been considered a self-limited disease, the authors of a study of giant cell arteritis over a seven-year period found that, due to either symptomatic relapses or elevation in the sedimentation rate, many of the 34 patients with biopsy-proven cases required steroids for longer than two years [86]. These authors saw a typical patient with giant cell arteritis whose disease recurred 10 years after the original diagnosis was made clinically and confirmed by a positive temporal artery biopsy. The patient's initial episode of giant cell arteritis had responded to a year of prednisone therapy, and she had been asymptomatic with a normal ESR for the subsequent nine years before her recurrence, which was also documented by temporal artery biopsy. Giant cell arteritis is therefore now often thought of as a chronic or relapsing disease.

References

1. Marquis, D. The Blood. In J. B. Miale (ed.), *Laboratory Medicine* (5th ed.). St. Louis: Mosby, 1977.
2. Fischel, E. E. The Erythrocyte Sedimentation Rate. In A. S. Cohen (ed.), *Laboratory Diagnostic Procedures in Rheumatic Disease* (2nd ed.). Boston: Little, Brown, 1975.
3. Zacharski, L. R., and Kyle, R. A. Significance of extreme elevations of erythrocyte sedimentation rate. *J.A.M.A.* 202:264, 1967.
4. Hayes, G. S., and Stinson, I. N. Erythrocyte sedimentation rate and age. *Arch. Ophthalmol.* 94:939, 1976.
5. Boyd, R. V., and Hoffbrand, B. I. Erythrocyte sedimentation rate in elderly hospital inpatients. *Br. Med. J.* 1:901, 1966.
6. Bottiger, L. E., and Svedberg, C. A. Normal erythrocyte sedimentation rate and age. *Br. Med. J.* 2:85, 1967.
7. Notmann, D. D., Kurata, N., and Tan, E. M. Profiles of antinuclear antibodies in systemic rheumatic diseases. *Ann. Intern. Med.* 83:464, 1975.
8. Kredich, N. M., Skyler, J. S., and Foote, L. J. Antibodies to native DNA in systemic lupus erythematosus. *Arch. Intern. Med.* 131:639, 1973.
9. Svec, K. H., and Viet, B. C. Age-related antinuclear factors: Immunologic characteristics and associated clinical aspects. *Arthritis Rheum.* 10:509, 1967.
10. Ritchie, R. F. The clinical significance of titered antinuclear antibodies. *Arthritis Rheum.* 10:544, 1967.
11. Christian, C. L. Rheumatoid Factors, In A. S. Cohen (ed.), *Laboratory Diagnostic Procedures in Rheumatic Disease* (2nd ed.). Boston: Little, Brown, 1975.
12. Cammarata, R. J., Rodnan, G. P., and Fennell, R. H. Serum anti-gamma-globulin and antinuclear factors in the aged. *J.A.M.A.* 199:115, 1967.
13. Litwin, S. D., and Singer, J. M. Studies of the incidence and significance of anti-gamma globulin factors in the aging. *Arthritis Rheum.* 8:538, 1965.
14. Rowe, D. S. Standardization of Quantitative Measurements of Human Immunoglobulins G, A, M. In E. Merler (ed.), *Immunoglobulins: Biologic Aspects and Clinical Uses*. Washington, D.C.: National Academy of Sciences, 1970.
15. Buckley, C. E., and Dorsey, F. C. The effect of aging on human serum immunoglobulin concentration. *J. Immunol.* 105:964, 1970.
16. Zawadski, Z. A., and Edwards, G. A. Clinical

significance of monoclonal immunoglobulin-emia. *Bull. Rheum. Dis.* 25:810, 1974–1975.

17. Glenner, G. G. Amyloid deposits and amyloidosis: The B-fibrilloses. *N. Engl. J. Med.* 302:1283, 1980.

18. Skinner, M., et al. P Component of amyloid: Isolation, characterization and sequence analysis. *J. Lab. Clin. Med.* 84:604, 1974.

19. Cohen, A. S. Studies of amyloidosis. *Arthritis Rheum.* 20:S76, 1977.

20. Natvig, J. B., and Anders, R. F. Characterization of four different immunochemical classes of amyloid fibril proteins. *Clin. Rheum. Dis.* 3:589, 1977.

21. Benson, M. D., and Cohen, A. S. Serum amyloid A protein in amyloidosis, rheumatic, and neoplastic diseases. *Arthritis Rheum.* 22:36, 1979.

22. Rosenthal, C. J., and Franklin, E. C. Variation with age and disease of amyloid A-related serum component. *J. Clin. Invest.* 55:746, 1975.

23. Kyle, R. A., and Bayrd, E. D. Amyloidosis: Review of 236 cases. *Medicine* 54:271, 1975.

24. Cohen, A. S., and Canoso, J. Rheumatological aspects of amyloid disease. *Clin. Rheum. Dis.* 1:149, 1975.

25. Wiernik, P. H. Amyloid joint disease. *Medicine* 51:465, 1972.

26. McDevitt, C. A. Biochemistry of articular cartilage: Nature of proteoglycans and collagen of articular cartilage and their role in aging and in osteoarthritis. *Ann. Rheum Dis.* 32:364, 1973.

27. Pearson, C. M., et al. Diagnosis and treatment of erosive rheumatoid arthritis and other forms of joint destruction. *Ann. Intern. Med.* 82:241, 1975.

28. Mankin, H. J. The reaction of articular cartilage to injury and osteoarthritis. *N. Engl. J. Med.* 291:1285, 1974.

29. Venn, M. F. Variation of chemical composition with age in human femoral head cartilage. *Ann. Rheum. Dis.* 37:168, 1978.

30. Mankin, H. J., et al. Biochemical and metabolic abnormalities in articular cartilage from osteoarthritic human hips: II. Correlation of morphology with biochemical and metabolic data. *J. Bone Joint Surg.* 53A:523, 1971.

31. Howell, D. S. Degradative enzymes in osteoarthritic human articular cartilage. *Arthritis Rheum.* 18:167, 1975.

32. Radin, E. L. Mechanical aspects of osteoarthritis. *Bull. Rheum. Dis.* 26:862, 1975–1976.

33. Moskowitz, R. W. Clinical and Laboratory Findings in Osteoarthritis. In D. J. McCarthy (ed.), *Arthritis and Allied Conditions* (9th ed.). Philadelphia: Lea & Febiger, 1979.

34. Ehrlich, G. E. Inflammatory osteoarthritis: I.

The clinical syndrome. *J. Chronic Dis.* 25:317, 1972.

35. Hasloch, I. Medical treatment of osteoarthritis. *Clin. Rheum. Dis.* 2:615, 1976.

36. Moskowitz, R. W. Treatment of Osteoarthritis. In D. J. McCarty (ed.), *Arthritis and Allied Conditions* (9th ed.). Philadelphia: Lea & Febiger, 1979.

37. Ellman, M. H., and Levin, B. Chondrocalcinosis in elderly persons. *Arthritis Rheum.* 18:43, 1975.

38. McCarty, D. J. Calcium pyrophosphate dihydrate crystal deposition disease: Nomenclature and diagnostic criteria. *Ann. Intern. Med.* 87:240, 1977.

39. McCarty, D. J. CPPD crystal deposition disease—1975. *Arthritis Rheum.* 19:275, 1976.

40. Jacobelli, S., et al. Calcium pyrophosphate dihydrate crystal deposition in neuropathic joints. Four cases of polyarticular involvement. *Ann. Intern. Med.* 79:340, 1973.

41. Genant, H. K. Roentgenographic aspects of calcium pyrophosphate dihydrate crystal deposition disease (pseudogout). *Arthritis Rheum.* 19:307, 1976.

42. Reginato, A. M., et al. Polyarticular and familial chondrocalcinosis. *Arthritis Rheum.* 13:197, 1970.

43. Van der Korst, J. K., Geerards, J., and Driessens, F. C. M. A hereditary type of idiopathic articular chondrocalcinosis: Survey of a pedigree. *Am. J. Med.* 56:307, 1974.

44. Hamilton, E. B. D. Diseases associated with CPPD deposition disease. *Arthritis Rheum.* 19:353, 1976.

45. O'Duffy, J. D. Clinical studies of acute pseudogout attacks. *Arthritis Rheum.* 19:349, 1976.

46. Stern, S. H., et al. Atypical tophaceous deposition in elderly females. *Arthritis. Rheum.* 30:D100, 1987.

47. Williams, R. C. The Clinical Picture of Rheumatoid Arthritis. In D. J. McCarty (ed.), *Arthritis and Allied Conditions* (9th ed.). Philadelphia: Lea & Febiger, 1979.

48. Decker, J. L., and Plotz, P. H. Extra-Articular Rheumatoid Disease. In D. J. McCarty (ed.), *Arthritis and Allied Conditions* (9th ed.). Philadelphia: Lea & Febiger, 1979.

49. Ehrlich, G. E., Katz, W. A., and Cohen, S. H. Rheumatoid arthritis in the elderly. *Geriatrics* 25:103, 1970.

50. Corrigan, A. B., et al. Benign rheumatoid arthritis of the aged. *Br. Med. J.* 1:444, 1974.

51. Brunner, C. N., and Davis, J. S. Immune mechanisms in the pathogenesis of systemic lupus erythematosus. *Bull. Rheum Dis.* 26:854, 1975–1976.

52. Decker, J. L., et al. Systemic lupus erythema-

tosus, contrasts and comparisons. *Ann. Intern. Med.* 82:391, 1975.

53. Fries, J. F., and Holman, H. R. *Systemic Lupus Erythematosus*. Philadelphia: Saunders, 1975.

54. Estes, D., and Christian, C. L. Natural history of systemic lupus erythematosus. *Medicine* 50:85, 1971.

55. Dimant, J., et al. Systemic lupus erythematosus in the older age group: Computer analysis. *J. Am. Geriatr. Soc.* 27:58, 1979.

56. Baker, S. B., et al. Late onset systemic lupus erythematosus. *Am. J. Med.* 66:727, 1979.

57. Foad, B. S. I., Sheon, R. P., and Kirsner, A. B. Systemic lupus erythematosus in the elderly. *Arch. Intern. Med.* 130:743, 1972.

58. Urowitz, M. B. SLE subsets: Divide and conquer. *J. Rheum.* 4:332, 1977.

59. Lee, S. L., and Chase, P. H. Drug-induced systemic lupus erythematosus: A critical review. *Semin. Arthritis Rheum.* 5:83, 1975.

60. Molina, J., et al. Procainamide-induced serologic changes in asymptomatic patients. *Arthritis Rheum.* 12:608, 1969.

61. Stahl, N. I., and Klippel, J. H. Recognizing drug-induced lupus syndromes. *Drug Ther.* September 1978, pp. 80–88.

62. Sunder, S. K., and Shah, A. Constrictive pericarditis in procainamide-induced lupus erythematosus syndrome. *Am. J. Cardiol.* 36:960, 1975.

63. Hahn, B. H., et al. Immune responses to hydralazine and nuclear antigens in hydralazine induced lupus erythematosus. *Ann. Intern. Med.* 76:365, 1972.

64. Bauer, W. H. Old age in human parotid glands with special reference to peculiar cells in uncommon salivary gland tumors. *J. Dent. Res.* 29:686, 1950.

65. Shearn, M. A. *Sjögren's Syndrome, Problems in Internal Medicine*. Vol. II. Philadelphia: Saunders, 1971.

66. Bloch, K. J., et al. Sjögren's syndrome. *Medicine* 44:187, 1965.

67. Van Bijsterveld, O. P. Diagnostic tests in the sicca syndrome. *Arch. Ophthalmol.* 82:10, 1969.

68. Greenspan, J. S., et al. The histopathology of Sjögren's syndrome in labial salivary gland biopsies. *Oral Surg. Oral Med. Oral Pathol.* 37:217, 1974.

69. Medical Staff Conference, University of California, San Francisco. Recent clinical and experimental developments in Sjögren's syndrome. *West J. Med.* 122:50, 1975.

70. Berry, H., Bacon, P. A., and Davis, J. D. Cell-mediated immunity in Sjögren's syndrome. *Ann. Rheum. Dis.* 31:298, 1972.

71. Cummings, N. A., et al. Sjögren's syndrome—newer aspects of research, diagnosis, and therapy. *Ann. Intern. Med.* 75:937, 1971.

72. Michalski, J. P., et al. Beta$_2$ microglobulin and lymphocytic infiltration in Sjögren's syndrome. *N. Engl. J. Med.* 293:1228, 1975.

73. Moutsopoulos, H. M., et al. Sjögren's syndrome (sicca syndrome): Current issues. *Ann. Intern. Med.* 92(Part I): 212, 1980.

74. Anderson, L. G., and Bayles, T. B. Polymyalgia rheumatica and giant cell arteritis. *DM* January 1974.

75. Healey, L. A. Long term follow-up of polymyalgia rheumatica: Evidence for synovitis. *Semin. Arthritis Rheum.* 13:322, 1984.

76. Hunder, G. G., and Allen, G. L. Giant cell arteritis: A review. *Bull. Rheum. Dis.* 29:980, 1978–1979.

77. O'Duffy, J. D., Wahner, H. W., and Hunder, G. G. Joint imagining in polymyalgia rheumatica. *Mayo Clin. Proc.* 51:519, 1976.

78. Long, R., and James O. Polymyalgia rheumatica and liver disease. *Lancet* 1:77, 1974.

79. Fauchald, P., Rygvold, O., and Oystese, B. Temporal arteritis and polymyalgia rheumatica: Clinical and biopsy findings. *Ann. Intern. Med.* 77:845, 1972.

80. Ghose, M. K., Shensa, S., and Lerner, P. I. Arteritis of the aged (giant cell arteritis) and fever of unexplained origin. *Am. J. Med.* 60:429, 1976.

81. Wilkinson, I. M. S., and Russel, R. W. R. Arteritis of the head and neck in giant cell arteritis: A pathologic study to show the pattern of arterial involvement. *Arch. Neurol.* 27:378, 1972.

82. Hamilton, C. R., Shelley, W. M., and Tumulty, P. A. Giant cell arteritis: Including temporal arteritis and polymyalgia rheumatica. *Medicine* 50:1, 1971.

83. Klein, R. G., et al. Large artery involvement in giant cell (temporal) arteritis. *Ann. Intern. Med.* 83:806, 1975.

84. Klein, R. G., et al. Skip lesions in temporal arteritis. *Mayo Clin. Proc.* 51:504, 1976.

85. Layfer, L. F., et al. Temporal arteriography: Analysis of 21 cases and a review of the literature. *Arthritis Rheum.* 21:780, 1978.

86. Beevers, D. G., Harpur, J. E., and Turk, K. A. D. Giant cell arteritis—the need for prolonged treatment. *J. Chronic Dis.* 26:571, 1973.

32

Paget's Disease of Bone

Jonathan Kay
Fred G. Kantrowitz

PAGET'S DISEASE OF BONE has probably existed since prehistoric times [1]. Samuel Wilks reported a case of this disease in 1869 [2], and Sir James Paget first described the condition before the Royal Medico-Chirurgical Society of London on November 14, 1876 [3]. In 1882 he reported seven additional cases of the disorder that he called "osteitis deformans" [4].

Osteitis deformans is a slowly progressive, focal bone disease of uncertain etiology, occurring primarily in geriatric patients, that is initiated by excessive bone resorption and followed by the accelerated formation of disorganized new bone [5].

Epidemiology

The onset of Paget's disease rarely occurs before age 30 [6]. Its incidence increases progressively with age, reaching 5 to 11 percent in the ninth decade [7]. Men are affected more frequently than women. In a series of 4,614 autopsies of patients older than 40 years of age, the prevalence of Paget's disease was 3.0 percent [8]. The prevalence is highest in Britain, New Zealand, Australia, and the northern United States. Paget's disease is rare in Africa, Asia, Scandinavia, and Ireland [9]. Although the disease aggregates in families, there is no definitive genetic transmission [10]. The prevalence of Paget's disease among American blacks is similar to that

among whites despite its rarity among African blacks, suggesting a role for environmental influences [11].

Etiology

Although the etiology of Paget's disease is unknown, evidence is accumulating to support the idea of a slow viral infection. Nuclear and cytoplasmic microcylindric inclusions, resembling viral nucleocapsids, have been demonstrated by electron microscopy in pagetic osteoclasts but not in normal osteoclasts [12,13]. These inclusions have also been demonstrated in the nuclei of cells from a giant cell tumor arising adjacent to pagetic bone in a patient with Paget's disease [14]. Using polyclonal and monoclonal sera, antigens of measles virus and of respiratory syncytial virus have been demonstrated in osteoclasts of patients with Paget's disease but not in osteoclasts from controls. By in situ hybridization, measles virus RNA sequences encoding for the measles virus nucleocapsid protein have been found in osteoclasts, osteoblasts, fibroblasts, and lymphocytes from patients with Paget's disease [15]. Thus, Paget's disease might occur when osteoclasts, in a patient harboring one or more latent paramyxoviruses, express antigens encoded for by previously dormant viral RNA. Although a slow virus infection is suggested by epidemiologic and histologic data, a causative virus has not yet been isolated, and Paget's disease has not been reproduced by passage of involved tissue into a normal host.

Natural History

The natural history of active Paget's disease can theoretically be divided into three phases. However, in an individual patient these phases frequently overlap. The osteolytic phase is brief and consists of excessive bone resorption due to enhanced osteoclastic activity. This increased osteoclastic activity is not due to parathyroid hormone excess [16]. In an active lesion there may be as many as 14 osteoclasts per square millimeter [17]. These osteoclasts are multinucleated; as many as 100 nuclei have been observed within a single cell [18]. Patients are usually in negative calcium balance [7], and urinary hydroxyproline levels increase, reflecting bone resorption [19]. Although radiographs may show focal areas of osteopenia during this phase [20], bone scanning will demonstrate areas of increased vascularity adjacent to diseased bone [21].

The mixed phase of Paget's disease is characterized by an increase in new bone formation to compensate for the ongoing excessive bone resorption. Osteoblasts deposit the newly formed bone in a chaotic manner, resulting in a "mosaic" pattern of lamellar bone. Each individual section of lamellar bone is normal; however, the bone lamellae are oriented toward one another in a haphazard fashion [22]. The serum alkaline phosphatase level is elevated, reflecting the increase in osteoblastic activity. If osteoblastic activity exceeds osteoclastic activity during this phase, positive calcium balance results [7].

The final phase is primarily osteoblastic. There is relatively little cellular activity in the bone. The pagetic bone neither forms osteones nor orients around blood vessels, so it is relatively avascular, heavy, and hard to cut. The marrow space contains mostly fibrous tissue [22]. As osteoblastic activity subsides, the pagetic lesion becomes "quiescent" [23].

Clinical Manifestations

The majority of patients with Paget's disease of bone are asymptomatic, their disease having been detected inadvertently by finding an elevated alkaline phosphatase concentration or characteristic changes on radiographs obtained for other reasons [24]. Although Paget's disease usually presents as pain, the presenting manifestation may be a neurologic deficit or a pathologic fracture [25]. Pain, when it occurs, is usually "dull and boring." However, it may be "sharp and radiating." The pain of pagetic lesions in the vertebrae, pelvis, and lower extremities may be exacerbated by weight bearing [22]. Joint involvement is the commonest cause of pain in Paget's disease [26], especially when both sides of the joint space are involved [27]. Nerve impingement may also be painful. An abrupt increase in pain suggests the development of a fracture or malignant degeneration.

The nature of focal manifestations depends on the site of skeletal involvement. About 25 percent of patients have disease in only one bone ("monostotic involvement"), and the remainder have disease in several bones ("polyostotic involvement"). The bones most commonly involved, in decreasing order of frequency, are the pelvis, the spine, the femur and tibia, and the skull [28].

SKULL

The calvarium is the most frequent site of skull involvement. "Osteoporosis circumscripta," a focal irregular area of osteopenia, is the earliest radiographic manifestation of Paget's disease of the skull [29]. It usually begins in the frontal or occipital region and may spread to involve the entire calvarium. This manifestation of the osteolytic phase is usually asymptomatic [30]. The deposition of pagetic bone on the outer table of the skull, which is greatest in the frontal and occipital bones, causes enlargement of the cranium during the mixed phase [22]. The increased weight of the skull may lead to spasm of the posterior neck muscles, causing headaches [31]. Pagetic remodeling may result in platybasia (basilar impression). Among 64 patients with Paget's disease of the skull, 31 percent had platybasia, whereas only 6 percent had neurologic complications resulting from compression of the structures adjacent to the foramen magnum, the contents of the posterior fossa, and the upper cervical spinal cord [32]. Bilateral trigeminal neuralgia and bilateral hemifacial spasm have each been described in a patient with basilar impression secondary to Paget's disease of the skull [33].

Impairment of hearing is present in 30 to 50 percent of patients with pagetic skull involvement. Pagetic involvement of the temporal bone may lead to atrophy of neural tissue in the cochlea and in the vestibular labyrinth, causing a sensorineural hearing loss and vestibular dysfunction [34]. Ankylosis of the stapes, ossification of the stapedius tendon, and stenosis of the external auditory canal may cause a conductive hearing loss superimposed on the sensorineural hearing loss [35].

With extensive involvement of the skull, blood is shunted into the external carotid arterial system, and there is enlargement of the superficial temporal artery. This "pagetic steal syndrome" leads to diminished cerebral blood flow, which may cause fatigue, confusion, agitation, and cerebrovascular accidents [36].

Of 138 patients with Paget's disease, 20 (15 percent) had involvement of the maxilla, whereas only 3 (2 percent) had involvement of the mandible [37]. Disease in the facial bones may cause localized pain [38]. The teeth develop "hypercementosis" of the roots, and the lamina dura is replaced by pagetic bone, making dental extraction difficult. Progression of the disease may cause the jaws to enlarge, teeth to migrate, and malocclusion to develop [39]. In the rare patient in whom all of the facial bones enlarge, "leontiasis ossea" (a lion-like facial appearance usually associated with fibrous dysplasia of bone) may develop [40].

SPINE

Paget's disease of the spine occurs most frequently in the lumbosacral region, with about one-third of patients having involvement of that area [41]. Most commonly, one vertebra is affected [42]. Back pain, with progressive leg weakness and sensory changes, may result from spinal cord or nerve root compression due to vertebral body enlargement. Spinal cord compression occurs most frequently in the upper thoracic spine; it is rare in the cervical spine [43]. A spinal cord "vascular steal syndrome," which improves with calcitonin and/or diphosphonate (bisphosphonate) therapy, has been postulated as the cause of motor, sensory,

and reflex deficits in patients with active Paget's disease [44,45].

Radiologic features of vertebral involvement include an increase in the size, density, and trabeculation of the body; squaring of the body; and thickening of the margins. An increase in the size of an affected vertebral body without disruption of the cortices helps to differentiate Paget's disease from metastatic tumor to the spine [46].

PELVIS

Osteoblastic pagetic lesions of the pelvis may resemble those due to a malignancy metastatic to bone, especially those of prostatic carcinoma. The "brim sign" is useful in distinguishing Paget's disease from carcinoma metastatic to the pelvis. Thickening of the pelvic brim or arcuate line (iliopectineal line) was seen in 85 percent of 225 patients with Paget's disease involving the pelvis, whereas it was seen in only 1 of 225 patients with carcinoma metastatic to the pelvis. Widening of the ischium and os pubis also occurs in Paget's disease [47].

EXTREMITIES

In long bones, bone resorption may give the radiographic appearance of a "flame shaped or inverted V-shaped advancing edge" (or "wedge") of osteopenia. This advancing edge is the border between the osteopenic pagetic bone and normal bone [20].

Involvement of the femur and tibia causes pain, deformity, and an increase in the temperature of the overlying skin. The femur bows laterally with weight bearing, which, combined with a coxa vara deformity, leads to external rotation of the lower leg. The tibia bows anteriorly and laterally [22]. Knee pain occurs most frequently when Paget's disease involves the distal femur or the proximal tibia. The small bones of the hands and feet are involved in Paget's disease of bone but less frequently than are the large bones [6].

Complications
FRACTURE
Pathologic fractures are the most common complication of Paget's disease of bone [6]. The

true incidence of fractures is virtually impossible to determine; however, it has been estimated that from 8.8 percent [48] to 24.6 percent [49] of patients suffer from pathologic fractures in pagetic bone. Often a pathologic fracture is the presenting manifestation of Paget's disease. There is frequently a history of pain in the affected limb for weeks or months preceding the fracture. Most pathologic fractures in pagetic bone occur spontaneously or following minor trauma [50]. Fractures occur most commonly during the osteolytic and mixed phases of Paget's disease and less frequently during the osteoblastic phase, when the bone becomes sclerotic [6].

In one series of patients, compression fractures of the thoracic and lumbar vertebral bodies were the most frequent pathologic fractures seen in Paget's disease [6]. In other studies the femur was the most frequently involved bone and the tibia was the next most commonly fractured bone [48,50]. The shaft or the subtrochanteric region is involved in 78 percent of pathologic femoral fractures in Paget's disease [48]. In elderly osteoporotic individuals without Paget's disease, however, the majority of femoral fractures occur in the femoral neck [51].

Transverse fractures, descriptively called "chalk-stick fractures," are the type most often seen in Paget's disease of bone [6,51]. Incomplete fissure fractures are also seen frequently in Paget's disease. They occur perpendicular to the surface of the cortex on the convex side of bowed weight-bearing bones and are usually multiple. They present with sudden pain and localized tenderness. Fissure fractures usually heal but may progress to complete transverse fractures [52].

Neoplasia

The development of a malignancy in pagetic bone may present as an abrupt increase in pain, as progressive soft tissue swelling, or as a mass [53]. Malignant transformation occurred in 38 (0.95 percent) of 3,964 patients with Paget's disease of bone seen at the Mayo Clinic between 1927 and 1977 [54]. Osteogenic sarcoma is the most frequent type of "Paget's sarcoma." Fibrosarcomas occur less frequently, whereas chondrosarcomas are rare [55].

"Paget's sarcomas" occur most commonly in the femur, pelvis, and humerus. Men are affected twice as frequently as women. The predominant radiographic appearance of osteosarcomas arising in Paget's disease of bone is a mixed blastic and lytic lesion. However, purely blastic and purely lytic tumors are also seen. Radiographic features include bone destruction, cortical thickening, bone expansion, soft tissue masses, periosteal reaction, and pathologic fractures. Osteogenic sarcoma in patients older than 50 years almost always occurs in the presence of Paget's disease of bone [55]. The prognosis of osteogenic sarcoma arising in Paget's disease is poor, with only 4 percent of patients surviving longer than five years, and is worse than that of primary osteogenic sarcoma in patients 39 years of age or older, in which 25 percent of patients survive longer than five years [53].

Benign neoplasms, such as giant cell tumors, arise very rarely in pagetic bone. Unlike the osteogenic sarcoma, the giant cell tumor usually presents as a nontender mass in the skull or facial bones. It infrequently involves the remaining axial or the appendicular skeleton. This tumor responds well to local excision. Its incidence is increased among patients with Paget's disease of bone who trace their ancestors to the Italian town of Avellino, suggesting a role for genetic and possibly for environmental factors in the development of this tumor [56].

Metabolic Complications

Even with extensive bone involvement, hypercalcemia is rarely seen in Paget's disease. When it occurs, it can usually be attributed to a coexisting condition known to cause hypercalcemia. Hypercalcemia most frequently presents when patients with active disease are immobilized for the treatment of fractures [57].

Hypercalciuria occurs when the rate of bone resorption exceeds that of bone formation. Thus it is a dynamic phenomenon in Paget's disease of bone. The mean incidence of all types of renal calculi among 1,382 patients with Paget's disease is 5 percent. Although this incidence is slightly higher than the incidence of renal stones in a normal population, it may not be higher than that in a population matched for age and sex. The incidence may be further increased by the discovery of asymptomatic Paget's disease on radiographs taken to investigate urinary calculi [7].

RHEUMATIC DISEASE

Osteoarthritis is the most common rheumatic manifestation of Paget's disease [58]. Involvement of the acetabulum and femoral head may lead to the development of osteoarthritis of the hip. The medial joint space is narrowed in pagetic coxopathy, while the superior joint space is narrowed from the stress of weight-bearing in osteoarthritis. Projection of the femoral head into the pelvis ("protrusio acetabuli") may occur either with medial joint space narrowing alone, when advanced Paget's disease involves the hip, or with both superior and medial joint space narrowing, when osteoarthritis is superimposed on Paget's disease of the hip [59]. Deformities of the femur or tibia can lead to osteoarthritis of the knee joint. In symptomatic patients, radiographs of the knee reveal severe joint space narrowing with prominent osteophytes [27].

Osteoarthritis develops in joints adjacent to pagetic bone because of accelerated endochondral ossification. The increased blood flow to pagetic bone increases the number of small blood vessels at the junction of the subchondral bone and the calcified layer of the articular cartilage. This hypervascularity accelerates endochondral ossification. The newly formed pagetic bone erodes the overlying articular cartilage from below. The remaining cartilage is irregular and narrowed, resulting in secondary osteoarthritis. Structural changes of bones involved by Paget's disease lead to mechanical abnormalities that also accelerate the development of secondary osteoarthritis [60].

In his first description of osteitis deformans, Paget commented on its coexistence with gouty arthritis [3]. In one series of severe pagetic patients, 40.4 percent of the 47 patients in whom serum uric acid levels were determined had hyperuricemia that was not attributable to drug use or to renal disease. The incidence of hyperuricemia in patients of both sexes was greater than in normal individuals. The level of serum uric acid correlated positively with the percent-

age of bone involved. The incidence of gouty arthritis among pagetic patients in this series was "that expected for the general hyperuricemic population" [27]. In another series of 290 patients with "moderately severe" Paget's disease, 11 (4 percent) gave a history of gouty arthritis, whereas in only one was there documentation of monosodium urate crystals in the synovial fluid. Of the 149 patients in whom serum uric acid was measured, only 20 percent were hyperuricemic [58]. Of 26 patients with gout proved by demonstration of monosodium urate crystals in the synovial fluid, six (23 percent) also had Paget's disease in contrast to seven (2.1 percent) of 333 nongouty patients. The six patients with both gout and Paget's disease had significantly higher serum alkaline phosphatase levels than did the 20 patients with gout alone [61]. The degradation of nucleic acids from the actively dividing cells of pagetic bone might add to the body pool of urate and might account in part for the increased incidence of hyperuricemia among patients with Paget's disease [27].

Calcific periarthritis is also prevalent. Of 55 patients with severe Paget's disease, 36.4 percent had radiographic evidence of calcific periarthritis. The shoulder was most commonly involved, but areas of calcification were also seen about the elbow, wrist, hip, knee, metacarpophalangeal, and interphalangeal joints. Only half of the periarticular calcifications seen were adjacent to pagetic bone. An acute inflammatory process occurred in 44 percent of involved sites and responded to therapy with oral nonsteroidal antiinflammatory drugs or with intralesional corticosteroid injections [27].

In contrast to the increased incidence of gouty arthritis and calcific periarthritis, articular chondrocalcinosis and pseudogout occur less frequently than would be expected in the age group affected by Paget's disease [27,58]. A possible explanation for this is that patients with Paget's disease have elevated levels of alkaline phosphatase, a pyrophosphatase. Pyrophosphatases, by preventing the accumulation of pyrophosphate, may retard the formation of calcium pyrophosphate dihydrate crystals, which deposit in articular chondrocalcinosis and may result in pseudogout.

CARDIOVASCULAR COMPLICATIONS

High-output cardiac failure can occur when there is active Paget's disease involving at least 35 percent of the skeleton [62]. Most of the increased blood flow to involved extremities in Paget's disease of bone is due to cutaneous vasodilatation [63], which is manifested by warmth and erythema of the skin overlying involved bone and by enlarged draining veins. Increased blood flow through the capillary bed of pagetic bone, not anatomic arteriovenous shunting, also contributes to the increased cardiac output seen in some patients with Paget's disease [64].

In a retrospective autopsy study, individuals with Paget's disease were found to have a four-fold higher incidence of anatomic calcific aortic valve disease than a matched control population. The frequency of aortic valve disease correlated with the severity of the bone disease. There was no association of Paget's disease with a greater frequency of mitral valve disease [65].

OPHTHALMIC MANIFESTATIONS

Disciform macular degeneration is the most commonly seen ophthalmic complication of Paget's disease of bone [66]. Pagetic involvement of the orbit, with compression of the orbital contents, can lead to papilledema, optic atrophy, exophthalmos, and extraocular muscle paresis. Angioid streaks, due to linear cracks in a calcified, degenerated Bruch's membrane, are seen on funduscopic examination in 8 percent of patients with Paget's disease [67,68].

GASTROINTESTINAL SIGNS

Two patients with Paget's disease and diarrhea have been reported, one of whom had a low serum folate level. Both patients' abdominal symptoms improved significantly within one week after beginning oral folic acid supplementation. Folate deficiency, due to the increased demand for this vitamin associated with increased cellular proliferation, together with the relative ischemia of the bowel have been postulated to cause this reversible malabsorption syndrome [69].

Evaluation
LABORATORY TESTS

Laboratory tests useful in evaluating Paget's disease include the 24-hour urinary hydroxypro-line excretion test and serum alkaline phosphatase measurement. The former, when measured in an individual with normal renal function, reflects the turnover of collagen [70]. Thus it reflects osteoclastic activity. In a group of patients with severe Paget's disease, the 24-hour urinary hydroxyproline excretion test correlated both with the serum alkaline phosphatase level and the extent of skeletal involvement [27].

The serum level of bone alkaline phosphatase reflects osteoblastic activity. It usually correlates with the extent of pagetic bone disease except in two situations. Isolated involvement of the skull is associated with levels of alkaline phosphatase that are much higher than would be expected for the extent of bone disease. Paget's disease limited to the pelvis, lumbosacral spine, and femoral heads is associated with relatively low levels of alkaline phosphatase for the extent of bone involved [27]. Patients with limited anatomic spread of disease may have normal serum alkaline phosphatase levels [25].

IMAGING

Bone scans provide information about both the state and the activity of Paget's disease. Radionuclide (technetium-99m diphosphonate) is taken up by areas of bone where active remodeling is occurring [71]. Bone scintigraphy is more sensitive than radiography in Paget's disease, with about 20 percent of lesions being detected on bone scans but not on radiographs. Thus bone scanning is useful in detecting early Paget's disease [28]. Skeletal scintigraphy can be used to evaluate the extent of Paget's disease [71]. Serial bone scans may be useful in monitoring response to therapy [72].

Although bone scanning is more sensitive than radiography in detecting Paget's disease, radiography is more specific. When an area of increased radionuclide uptake appears on a bone scan, radiographs can be used to differentiate Paget's disease from bone tumors, fibrous dysplasia, healing fractures, and osteomyelitis. Certain radiographic findings are pathognomonic for Paget's disease of bone: coarsening and thickening of the trabecular pattern, "osteoporosis circumscripta" in the skull [29], an increase in the size of a sclerotic vertebral body without disruption of the cortex [46], the pelvic "brim sign" [47], and a "flame-shaped or inverted V-shaped advancing edge" of osteopenia in a long bone [20]. Radiographs can detect pathologic fractures and bone tumors, which may present as increased pain in a pagetic bone. Radiographs can also be used to determine the cause of joint pain and to evaluate the extent of joint damage in Paget's disease. Radiography, computed tomography, and myelography may be indicated when a patient with Paget's disease presents with neurologic deficits [43]. Computed tomography of the spine is especially useful in diagnosing spinal stenosis caused by Paget's disease [73]. Radiographs can be used to follow a patient's response to calcitonin therapy because calcitonin may induce the remineralization of osteolytic pagetic bone [74].

Therapy

The goals of therapy for Paget's disease are to relieve pain, to maintain skeletal function, and to minimize local and systemic complications. Asymptomatic disease requires no treatment. Minimal pain may improve with analgesic therapy. Symptoms due to rheumatologic complications may respond to nonsteroidal antiinflammatory drug therapy [27]. Definite indications for therapy with specific antipagetic medications are severe bone pain, high-output cardiac failure, hypercalcemia due to Paget's disease, and recurrent renal calculi due to hypercalciuria. Possible indications for such therapy include multiple fractures in pagetic bone, anticipated orthopedic surgery involving pagetic bone or prolonged immobilization, skeletal compression of nerve tissue, and the early onset of Paget's disease that may result in disabling deformities [22]. The three medical forms of therapy—calcitonin, disodium etidronate, and mithramycin—all decrease bone resorption.

CALCITONIN

Calcitonin is a peptide hormone that is predominantly synthesized by the C-cells of the mammalian thyroid gland [75]. Porcine, salmon, and human calcitonin have all been used to treat Paget's disease. Calcitonin specifically decreases bone collagen resorption [76]. Within 30 minutes, calcitonin decreases the number of osteoclasts in pagetic bone and causes their ruffled borders to retract from sites of previously active bone resorption [77]. Following a single subcutaneous injection, the plasma calcium level and urinary hydroxyproline excretion decrease acutely but return to baseline within 24 hours [78]. With chronic administration, after several weeks of therapy, urinary hydroxyproline excretion remains lowered and the serum alkaline phosphatase level gradually falls [79]. Bone formed following the institution of calcitonin therapy has a normal lamellar structure [80].

Calcitonin significantly reduces bone pain in up to 80 percent of patients with Paget's disease. Pain relief usually begins during the first two months of therapy and reaches a maximum after 6 to 12 months of treatment. Skin temperature, if increased over involved bones, can fall and high-output congestive heart failure may disappear with calcitonin therapy. Neurologic deficits may improve during calcitonin treatment [81]; however, deafness rarely improves [82]. Calcitonin therapy reduces hemorrhage associated with orthopedic surgery of pagetic bone [83]. In the osteolytic phase, calcitonin therapy arrests progression of the lytic front and produces radiologic evidence of healing [74]. However, disease relapses after calcitonin has been discontinued [83].

Up to 40 percent of patients on salmon calcitonin therapy for longer than four months acquire resistance to the drug [84]. Although all patients who form antibodies to this foreign protein develop resistance, not all of those who become resistant have circulating antibodies to calcitonin [85].

Highly purified synthetic human calcitonin (Cibacalcin) is now available for use in patients with Paget's disease. Antibodies to synthetic human calcitonin have been found in only one patient who was treated with this drug for 16 months [86]. Thus synthetic human calcitonin is useful in patients with antibodies to heterologous calcitonins [87].

Calcitonin is usually given as a subcutaneous injection. Salmon calcitonin (Calcimar) is administered in a dose of 50 to 100 MRC (Medical Research Council) units daily. The dosage can be reduced to three times weekly with maintenance of a clinical response [79]. Salmon calcitonin also suppresses bone turnover in Paget's disease of bone when given as an intranasal spray or as a suppository [88]. The initial recommended dose of synthetic human calcitonin is 0.5 mg given subcutaneously daily for six months.

The most common side effect of subcutaneously administered calcitonin is nausea, which occurs in up to 50 percent of patients. Facial flushing, lasting for one to two hours after the drug has been administered, also occurs frequently. Local skin reactions and urticaria, palmar and plantar erythema, abdominal cramps and diarrhea, and pruritus also occur [75]. Systemic side effects have not occurred in a small number of normal volunteers and patients receiving salmon calcitonin by nasal spray or by rectal suppository [88].

DIPHOSPHONATES

Diphosphonates are compounds, not found in untreated humans or animals, that have similar physiochemical activity to pyrophosphate but resist enzymatic hydrolysis. They contain a P–C–P group that resembles the P–O–P group found in pyrophosphate [89]. Diphosphonates inhibit bone resorption by reducing the number of osteoclasts that are attached to the mineralized matrix [90]. They also uncouple bone formation from bone resorption, thus reducing bone turnover. Three diphosphonates have been studied in patients with Paget's disease of bone: 1-hydroxyethylidene-1, 1-bisphosphonic acid (EHDP), dichloromethylidenebisphosphonic acid (Cl_2MDP), and 3-amino-1-hydroxypropylidene-1, 1-bisphosphonic acid (APD).

EHDP (Didronel) is the only diphosphonate that is commercially available to treat Paget's disease. The initial course of therapy for most patients is 5 to 10 mg per kg per day orally for six months. Because diphosphonates are excreted in the urine, the dose must be reduced in patients with renal impairment. Retreatment for another six months is indicated if symptoms recur with an increase in serum alkaline phosphatase or in urinary hydroxyproline excretion. Of 93 patients with symptomatic Paget's disease and with alkaline phosphatase levels and/or hydroxyproline excretion rates more than two times the upper limit of normal, 40 percent did not require retreatment during an average follow-up period of 6.2 years. Disease associated with higher initial alkaline phosphatase levels and/or hydroxyproline excretion tended to relapse earlier [91]. With therapy, urinary hydroxyproline excretion decreases over several weeks, followed by a fall in the serum alkaline phosphatase level. Radionuclide bone scanning may show decreased uptake [92]. In patients with severe Paget's disease, a paradoxical increase in bone pain may occur four to six weeks after the initiation of therapy. Pathologic fractures of long bones develop in patients taking high doses of EHDP (10 to 20 mg per kg per day) [93]. Patients treated with as little as 5 mg per kg per day of disodium etidronate may develop focal osteomalacia [90]. Thus EHDP may be contraindicated in patients with predominantly osteolytic lesions [94].

EHDP (7.5 mg per kg per day by mouth) has been given in combination with synthetic human calcitonin (0.5 mg subcutaneously daily) to nine patients with Paget's disease and bone pain. Bone pain improved during the second month of therapy. The reduction in serum alkaline phosphatase level and in urinary hydroxyproline excretion was greater than that achieved with double the dose of calcitonin alone, and osteomalacia did not occur [95].

Three patients treated with Cl_2MDP developed leukemia [17]. Although a causal relationship has not been proved, this drug is not commercially available in the United States.

APD is 10 to 20 times more potent than EHDP. Unlike EHDP, which increases osteoid by causing osteomalacia, APD reduces osteoid surface by reducing bone formation. Of 170 patients with Paget's disease who were treated with either oral or intravenous APD, 90 percent had normal serum alkaline phosphatase levels and urine hydroxyproline excretion rates within one year. APD arrests the radiographic progression of Paget's disease. Recommended therapy consists of 20 mg of intravenous APD daily for 10 days, followed by 300 mg of APD by mouth twice daily until urinary hydroxyproline excretion has normalized. Oral APD causes nausea and gastric mucosal irritation in 30 percent of patients at a dose of 600 mg per day, but lower doses are better tolerated. Fever and transient lymphopenia can occur on initiation of oral APD therapy. Intravenous APD causes no known side effects [17]. APD is not commercially available in the United States.

MITHRAMYCIN

Mithramycin is a cytotoxic antibiotic that binds to DNA, thus blocking RNA synthesis. It seems to be more toxic to osteoclasts than to osteoblasts [96]. Bone pain may disappear within four to five days after treatment [97]. Intravenous therapy with 15 μg per kg per day of mithramycin for three days followed by 10 μg per kg per day for seven additional days provided relief of pain for up to five years after treatment despite the return of the serum alkaline phosphatase to pretreatment levels [98]. Nausea and vomiting may begin about four hours after the infusion of mithramycin; it lasts for several hours and responds to antiemetic therapy [99]. A transient hepatitis can occur with mithramycin therapy. Fewer than 5 percent of patients treated develop prerenal azotemia. In the rare patient, the blood urea nitrogen (BUN) level may remain slightly elevated even after therapy has been discontinued. Transient severe thrombocytopenia occurs very infrequently during treatment of Paget's disease with mithramycin. No hemorrhagic episodes have been reported in association with mithramycin used to treat Paget's disease of bone [96]. Because it is more toxic than calcitonin and the diphosphonates and because it requires ten days of hospitalization for intravenous infusion, mithramycin should not be used as an initial drug in the management of Paget's disease.

SURGERY

As an adjunct to medical therapy, surgery is occasionally necessary to treat several of the complications of Paget's disease. Total hip arthroplasty is performed to treat severe pagetic coxarthrosis and protrusio acetabuli [100]. Pathologic fractures are often treated with internal fixation [50]. Suboccipital decompression and high cervical laminectomy are performed to treat the neurologic manifestations of basilar impression of the skull [101]. Insertion of a ventriculoatrial shunt can result in improvement of the progressive dementia, impaired gait, and urinary incontinence caused by hydrocephalus due to basilar impression [102]. Decompressive laminectomy may be useful to relieve spinal cord or nerve root compression [103]. To reduce the risk of hemorrhage associated with elective surgery on pagetic bone, calcitonin should be given for three months prior to surgery and for six to twelve months postoperatively [83].

Prevention

There is currently no method available to prevent the development of Paget's disease of bone. Because it is most likely caused by infection with one or more slow viruses, perhaps in a genetically susceptible host, efforts at prevention should be directed toward immunizing individuals against the causative virus or viruses. First, the virus or viruses must be isolated and shown to reproduce Paget's disease in a previously uninfected host. Then, a vaccine should be developed to immunize uninfected individuals. The major problem, once a vaccine has been developed, will be to determine which group should receive the vaccine. Because Paget's disease is found primarily in people over the age of 40 and because measles virus and respiratory syncytial virus, the most likely etiologic agents, predominantly infect children, it will be important to determine what other factors predispose to developing Paget's disease so that not all children would have to be subjected to the risks of vaccination.

References

1. Singer, F. R. *Paget's Disease of Bone.* New York: Plenum, 1977. P. 17.
2. Wilks, S. Case of osteoporosis, or spongy hypertrophy of the bones (calvaria, clavicle, os femoris, and rib, exhibited at the Society). *Trans. Pathol. Soc. Lond.* 20:273, 1869.
3. Paget, J. On a form of chronic inflammation of bones (osteitis deformans). *Med. Chir. Trans.* 60:37, 1877.
4. Paget, J. Additional cases of osteitis deformans. *Med. Chir. Trans.* 65:225, 1882.
5. Hamdy, R. C. *Paget's Disease of Bone.* New York: Praeger, 1981. P. 22.
6. Dickson, D. D., Camp, J. D., and Ghormley, R. K. Osteitis deformans: Paget's disease of the bone. *Radiology* 44:449, 1945.
7. Nagant de Deuxchaisnes, C. N., and Krane, S. Paget's disease of bone: Clinical and metabolic observations. *Medicine* 43:233, 266, 1964.
8. Schmorl, G. Über Osteitis deformans Paget. *Virchows Arch. Pathol. Anat.* 283:694, 1932.

9. Barker, D. J. P. The epidemiology of Paget's disease of bone. *Br. Med. Bull.* 40:396, 1984.
10. Sofaer, J. A., Holloway, S. M., and Emery, A. E. H. A family study of Paget's disease of bone. *J. Epidemiol. Commun. Health* 37:226, 1983.
11. Guyer, P. B., and Chamberlain, A. T. Paget's disease of bone in two American cities. *Br. Med. J.* 280:985, 1980.
12. Rebel, A., et al. Osteoclast ultrastructure in Paget's disease. *Calcif. Tissue Res.* 20:187, 1976.
13. Mills, B. G., and Singer, F. R. Nuclear inclusions in Paget's disease of bone. *Science* 194:201, 1976.
14. Mirra, J. M., Bauer, F. C. H., and Grant, T. T. Giant cell tumor with viral-like intranuclear inclusions associated with Paget's disease. *Clin. Orthop.* 158:243, 1981.
15. Baslé, M., et al. On the trail of paramyxoviruses in Paget's disease of bone. *Clin. Orthop.* 217:9, 1987.
16. Burckhardt, P. M., Singer, F. R., and Potts, J. T., Jr. Parathyroid function in patients with Paget's disease treated with salmon calcitonin. *Clin. Endocrinol.* 2:15, 1973.
17. Harinck, H. I. J., et al. Efficacious management with aminobisphosphonate (APD) in Paget's disease of bone. *Clin. Orthop.* 217:79, 1987.
18. Rasmussen, H., and Bordier, P. *The Physiological and Cellular Basis of Metabolic Bone Disease.* Baltimore: Williams & Wilkins, 1974. P. 243.
19. Dull, T. A., and Henneman, P. H. Urinary hydroxyproline as an index of collagen turnover in bone. *N. Engl. J. Med.* 268:132, 1963.
20. Jacobs, P. Osteolytic Paget's disease. *Clin. Radiol.* 25:137, 1974.
21. Rausch, J. M., et al. Bone scanning in osteolytic Paget's disease: Case report. *J. Nucl. Med.* 18:699, 1977.
22. Singer, F. R., et al. Paget's disease of bone. In L. V. Avioli, and S. M. Krane (eds.), *Metabolic Bone Disease.* Vol. II. New York: Academic, 1978. Pp. 490–575.
23. Hamdy, R. C. *Paget's Disease of Bone.* New York: Praeger, 1981. P. 36.
24. Guyer, P. B. The clinical relevance of radiologically revealed Paget's disease of bone (osteitis deformans). *Br. J. Surg.* 66:438, 1979.
25. Harinck, H. I. J., et al. Relation between signs and symptoms in Paget's disease of bone. *Q. J. Med.* 58:133, 1986.
26. Khairi, M. R. A., et al. Paget's disease of bone (osteitis deformans): Symptomatic lesions and bone scan. *Ann. Intern. Med.* 79:348, 1973.
27. Franck, W. A., et al. Rheumatic manifestations of Paget's disease of bone. *Am. J. Med.* 56:592, 1974.
28. Vellenga, C. J. L. R., et al. Untreated Paget disease of bone studied by scintigraphy. *Radiology* 153:799, 1984.
29. Sosman, M. C. Radiology as an aid in the diagnosis of skull and intracranial lesions. *Radiology* 9:396, 1927.
30. Singer, F. R. *Paget's Disease of Bone.* New York: Plenum, 1977. P. 56.
31. Singer, F. R. *Paget's Disease of Bone.* New York: Plenum, 1977. P. 57.
32. Bull, J. W. D., et al. Paget's disease of the skull and secondary basilar impression. *Brain* 82:10, 1959.
33. Gardner, W. J., and Dohn, D. F. Trigeminal neuralgia—Hemifacial spasm—Paget's disease: Significance of this association. *Brain* 89:555, 1966.
34. Nager, G. T. Paget's disease of the temporal bone. *Ann. Otol. Rhinol. Laryngol.* 84(Suppl. 22):1, 1975.
35. Lindsay, J. R., and Suga, F. Paget's disease and sensori-neural deafness: Temporal bone histopathology of Paget's disease. *Laryngoscope* 86:1029, 1976.
36. Singer, F. R. *Paget's Disease of Bone.* New York: Plenum, 1977. P. 116.
37. Stafne, E. C., and Austin, L. T. A study of dental roentgenograms in cases of Paget's disease (osteitis deformans), osteitis fibrosa cystica, and osteoma. *J. Am. Dental Assoc.* 25:1202, 1938.
38. Spilka, C. J., and Callahan, K. R. A review of the differential diagnosis of oral manifestations in early osteitis deformans. *Oral Surg.* 8:809, 1958.
39. Tillman, H. H. Paget's disease of bone: A clinical, radiographic, and histopathologic study of twenty-four cases involving the jaws. *Oral Surg.* 15:1225, 1962.
40. Singer, F. R. *Paget's Disease of Bone.* New York: Plenum, 1977. P. 62.
41. Guyer, P. B., and Clough, P. W. L. Paget's disease of bone: Some observations on the relation of the skeletal distribution to pathogenesis. *Clin. Radiol.* 29:421, 1978.
42. Guyer, P. B., and Shepherd, D. F. C. Paget's disease of the lumbar spine. *Br. J. Radiol.* 53:286, 1980.
43. Schmidek, H. H. Neurologic and neurosurgical sequelae of Paget's disease of bone. *Clin. Orthop.* 127:70, 1977.
44. Herzberg, L., and Bayliss, E. Spinal-cord syndrome due to non-compressive Paget's disease of bone: A spinal-artery steal phenomenon reversible with calcitonin. *Lancet* 2:13, 1980.
45. Douglas, D. L., et al. Spinal cord dysfunction in Paget's disease of bone: Has medical treatment a vascular basis? *J. Bone Joint Surg.* 63B:495, 1981.
46. Schreiber, M. H., and Richardson, G. A. Paget's

disease confined to one lumbar vertebra. *Am. J. Roentgenol.* 90:1271, 1963.

47. Marshall, T. R., and Ling, J. T. The brim sign: A new sign found in Paget's disease (osteitis deformans) of the pelvis. *Am. J. Roentgenol.* 90:1267, 1963.

48. Galbraith, H.-J. B., Evans, E. C., and Lacey, J. Paget's disease of bone—a clinical and genetic study. *Postgrad. Med. J.* 53:33, 1977.

49. Traver, C. A. The association of fractures and Paget's disease (osteitis deformans). *N.Y. State J. Med.* 36:242, 1936.

50. Verinder, D. G. R., and Burke, J. The management of fractures in Paget's disease of bone. *Injury* 10:276, 1979.

51. Singer, F. R. *Paget's Disease of Bone.* New York: Plenum, 1977. P. 92.

52. Allen, M. L., and John, R. L. Osteitis deformans (Paget's disease): Fissure fractures—their etiology and clinical significance. *Am. J. Roentgenol.* 38:109, 1937.

53. Huvos, A. G., Butler, A., and Bretsky, S. S. Osteogenic sarcoma associated with Paget's disease of bone: A clinicopathologic study of 65 patients. *Cancer* 52:1489, 1983.

54. Wick, M. R., et al. Sarcomas of bone complicating osteitis deformans (Paget's disease): Fifty years' experience. *Am. J. Surg. Pathol.* 5:47, 1981.

55. Haibach, H., Farrell, C., and Dittrich, F. J. Neoplasms arising in Paget's disease of bone: A study of 82 cases. *Am. J. Clin. Pathol.* 83:594, 1985.

56. Jacobs, T. P., et al. Giant cell tumor in Paget's disease of bone: Familial and geographic clustering. *Cancer* 44:742, 1979.

57. Nathan, A. W., et al. Hypercalcaemia due to immobilization of a patient with Paget's disease of bone. *Postgrad. Med. J.* 58:714, 1982.

58. Altman, R. D., and Collins, B. Musculoskeletal manifestations of Paget's disease of bone. *Arthritis Rheum.* 23:1121, 1980.

59. Roper, B. A. Paget's disease involving the hip joint: A classification. *Clin. Orthop.* 80:33, 1971.

60. Goldman, A. B., et al. Osteitis deformans of the hip joint. *Am. J. Roentgenol.* 128:601, 1977.

61. Lluberas-Acosta, G., Hansell, J. R., and Schumacher, H. R., Jr. Paget's disease of bone in patients with gout. *Arch. Intern. Med.* 146:2389, 1986.

62. Howarth, S. Cardiac output in osteitis deformans. *Clin. Sci.* 12:271, 1953.

63. Heistad, D. D., et al. Regulation of blood flow in Paget's disease of bone. *J. Clin. Invest.* 55:69, 1975.

64. Rhodes, B. A., et al. Absence of anatomic arteriovenous shunts in Paget's disease of bone. *N. Engl. J. Med.* 287:686, 1972.

65. Strickberger, S. A., Schulman, S. P., and Hutchins, G. M. Association of Paget's disease of bone with calcific aortic valve disease. *Am. J. Med.* 82:953, 1987.

66. Mackie, E. G. Paget's disease and the eye. *Trans. Ophthalmol. Soc. U.K.* 76:267, 1956.

67. Gass, J. D. M., and Clarkson, J. G. Angioid streaks and disciform macular detachment in Paget's disease (osteitis deformans). *Am. J. Ophthalmol.* 75:576, 1973.

68. Scholz, R. O. Angioid streaks. *Arch. Ophthalmol.* 26:677, 1941.

69. Somayaji, B. N. Malabsorption syndrome in Paget's disease of bone. *Br. Med. J.* 4:278, 1968.

70. Kivirikko, K. I. Urinary excretion of hydroxyproline in health and disease. *Int. Rev. Connect. Tiss. Res.* 5:93, 1970.

71. Miller, S. W., et al. Technetium 99m labeled diphosphonate bone scanning in Paget's disease. *An:. J. Roentgenol.* 121:177, 1974.

72. Vellenga, C. J. L. R., et al. Bone scintigraphy in Paget's disease treated with combined calcitonin and diphosphonate (EHDP). *Metab. Bone Dis. Rel. Res.* 4:103, 1982.

73. Zlatkin, M. B., et al. Paget disease of the spine: CT with clinical correlation. *Radiology* 160:155, 1986.

74. Murphy, W. A., Whyte, M. P., and Haddad, J. G., Jr. Paget bone disease: Radiologic documentation of healing with human calcitonin therapy. *Radiology* 136:1, 1980.

75. Deftos, L. J., and First, B. P. Calcitonin as a drug. *Ann. Intern. Med.* 95:192, 1981.

76. Krane, S. M., et al. Urinary excretion of hydroxylysine and its glycosides as an index of collagen degradation. *J. Clin. Invest.* 59:819, 1977.

77. Singer, F. R., Melvin, K. E. W., and Mills, B. G. Acute effects of calcitonin on osteoclasts in man. *Clin. Endocrinol.* 5(Suppl.): 333s, 1976.

78. Krane, S. M., et al. Acute effects of calcitonin on bone formation in man. *Metabolism* 22:51, 1973.

79. DeRose, J., et al. Response of Paget's disease to porcine and salmon calcitonins: Effects of long-term treatment. *Am. J. Med.* 56:858, 1974.

80. Woodhouse, N. J. Y., et al. Human calcitonin in the treatment of Paget's bone disease. *Lancet* 1:1139, 1971.

81. Chen, J.-R., et al. Neurologic disturbances in Paget disease of bone: Response to calcitonin. *Neurology* 29:448, 1979.

82. Walker, G. S. Effect of calcitonin on deafness due to Paget's disease of skull. *Br. Med. J.* 2:364, 1979.

83. MacIntyre, I., et al. Chemistry, physiology, and therapeutic applications of calcitonin. *Arthritis Rheum.* 23:1139, 1980.

84. Haddad, J. G. Jr., and Caldwell, J. G. Calcitonin resistance: Clinical and immunologic studies in subjects with Paget's disease of bone treated with porcine and salmon calcitonins. *J. Clin. Invest.* 51:3133, 1972.

85. Singer, F. G., Fredericks, R. S., and Minkin, C. Salmon calcitonin therapy for Paget's disease of bone: The problem of acquired clinical resistance. *Arthritis Rheum.* 23:1148, 1980.

86. Dietrich, F. M., Fischer, J. A., and Bijvoet, O. L. M. Formation of antibodies to synthetic human calcitonin during treatment of Paget's disease. *Acta Endocrinol.* 92:468, 1979.

87. Rojanasathit, S., Rosenberg, E., and Haddad, J. G., Jr. Paget's bone disease: Response to human calcitonin in patients resistant to salmon calcitonin. *Lancet* 2:1412, 1974.

88. Nagant de Deuxchaisnes, C., et al. New modes of administration of salmon calcitonin in Paget's disease: Nasal spray and suppository. *Clin. Orthop.* 217:56, 1987.

89. Fleisch, H. Experimental basis for the use of bisphosphonates in Paget's disease of bone. *Clin. Orthop.* 217:72, 1987.

90. Boyce, B. F., et al. Focal osteomalacia due to low-dose diphosphonate therapy in Paget's disease. *Lancet* 1:821, 1984.

91. Altman, R. D. Long-term follow-up therapy with intermittent etidronate disodium in Paget's disease of bone. *Am. J. Med.* 79:583, 1985.

92. Altman, R. D., et al. Influence of disodium etidronate on clinical and laboratory manifestations of Paget's disease of bone (osteitis deformans). *N. Engl. J. Med.* 289:1379, 1973.

93. Kantrowitz, F. G., et al. Clinical and biochemical effects of diphosphonate in Paget's disease of bone. *Arthritis Rheum.* 18:407, 1975.

94. Khairi, M. R. A., et al. Sodium etidronate in the treatment of Paget's disease of bone: A study of long-term results. *Ann. Intern. Med.* 87:656, 1977.

95. Hosking, D. J., et al. Paget's bone disease treated with diphosphonate and calcitonin. *Lancet* 1:615, 1976.

96. Ryan, W. G., and Schwartz, T. B. Mithramycin treatment of Paget's disease of bone: Exploration of combined mithramycin-EHDP therapy. *Arthritis Rheum.* 23:1155, 1980.

97. Russell, A. S. Calcitonin or mithramycin for Paget's disease. *Lancet* 1:884, 1980.

98. Russell, A. S., et al. Long term effectiveness of low dose mithramycin for Paget's disease of bone. *Arthritis Rheum.* 22:215, 1979.

99. Lebbin, D., Ryan, W. G., and Schwartz, T. B. Outpatient treatment of Paget's disease of bone with mithramycin. *Ann. Intern. Med.* 81:635, 1974.

100. Stauffer, R. N., and Sim, F. H. Total hip arthroplasty in Paget's disease of the hip. *J. Bone Joint Surg.* 58A:476, 1976.

101. Taylor, A. R., and Chakravorty, B. C. Clinical syndromes associated with basilar impression. *Arch. Neurol.* 10:475, 1964.

102. Goldhammer, Y., Braham, J., and Kosary, I. Z. Hydrocephalic dementia in Paget disease of the skull: Treatment by ventriculoatrial shunt. *Neurology* 29:513, 1979.

103. Hartman, J. T., and Dohn, D. F. Paget's disease of the spine with cord or nerve-root compression. *J. Bone Joint Surg.* 48A:1079, 1966.

33

Gastrointestinal System

KENNETH L. MINAKER
PETER BONIS
JOHN W. ROWE

FUNCTIONAL AND PATHOLOGIC gastrointestinal abnormalities are common in the elderly; 20 percent of geriatric deaths are caused by gastrointestinal illnesses [1]. Studies of community-dwelling elderly show that even when nutritional supplements and vitamins are excluded, 42 percent of nonprescription drugs are gastrointestinal medications. Nearly 27 percent of geriatric medical admissions are due to gastrointestinal disease [2]. The incidence of gastrointestinal malignancy is second only to skin cancer, and its mortality is second only to cancer of the lung.

Diagnostic difficulties are particularly common in geriatric gastroenterology. One-half of patients referred for gastroenterologic consultation who are examined carefully and followed for one year have no identifiable pathologic explanation for their complaints [3]. The long "silent period" of many gastrointestinal diseases compounds the notorious underreporting and late presentation of illness characteristic of the geriatric population.

Invasive and noninvasive techniques requiring patient cooperation are more difficult and uncomfortable for the less mobile elderly patient. However, since the prevalence of gastrointestinal malignancy increases progressively with age and comprises 30 to 40 percent of all malignancies of very old patients, accurate diagnosis of any significant symptom is clearly crucial in the elderly population. The aged patient is thus often in the unfavorable position of being overinvestigated with uncomfortable techniques for fear of missing a malignant lesion. The proper approach to diagnosis and therapy of gastrointestinal disease must be pursued on an individual basis. In general, each case should receive the least investigation leading to specific diagnosis. Therapy should be based on awareness of the good potential life expectancy of otherwise healthy old individuals.

Oral Cavity
PHYSIOLOGY
Normal aging affects oral function minimally. Since our Western diet is soft and refined, tooth wear generally does not cause significant dental loss. The finding that caries and periodontal disease are virtually nonexistent in some elderly populations outside Western countries suggests that dental loss is likely to be disease-related. The normal changes with age, including reduction in dentine production, shrinkage and fibrosis of root pulp, gingival retraction, and loss of bone density in the alveolar ridge, all contribute to the increased vulnerability of the elderly to dental disease.

The normal reductions in taste and smell with age interfere little with nutrition but certainly minimize enjoyment of food. The number of tongue papillae and taste buds decreases with normal aging. Clinical studies have shown increased taste thresholds for individual amino acids, salt, and sugars. Older people clearly have more difficulty recognizing common smells and flavors, and food odor is apparently the main gustatory factor that decreases [4]. The net effect is that bitter tastes predominate and more concentrated sugar is required to experience a sweet taste.

Mucous and parotid gland secretions show no age-related declines and cannot be considered a contributor to xerostomia in the elderly. Oral mucosal changes with advancing age are mainly due to loss of submucosal elastic tissue. The tongue may develop a lobular appearance and papillary loss may be marginal or diffusely distributed. The most frequent change is appearance of sublingual varicosities on the ventral surface of the tongue in 50 percent of the over-60 population.

Masticatory muscle function and masticatory coordination decline significantly with age, resulting in significant lengthening of the time required for individuals to chew their food adequately and create a bolus that can subsequently be swallowed.

Cosmetically important is a progressive loss in the tone of circumoral muscles, which accounts for the tendency of older persons not to close their mouths tightly and predisposes to development of drooling. Patients may complain of increased amounts of saliva, whereas the actual problem relates to circumoral muscle laxity.

PATHOLOGY

In our Western civilization dental caries affect 99 percent of our population. Dental caries are largely a dietary problem, in which sticky carbohydrate-containing foods provoke proliferation of acid-producing bacteria in plaque, periodontal pockets, and dental crevices. With advancing age the bacteriology of the accumulated plaque and calculus changes; the usual mixture of fusospirochetal organisms remains stable, but the gram-negative anaerobic rods are increasingly replaced by gram-positive facultative cocci. The two processes contribute to the startling loss of secondary dentition in our community. Changes in the dental status of older individuals represent one of the more striking secular changes that have occurred during the past several decades. Cross-sectional studies in 1957 showed that 55 percent of individuals over the age of 65 had no teeth, but this figure has steadily declined to 46 percent in 1973 and 34 percent in 1980.

With progressive improvements in medical and dental care, as well as public health measures such as fluoridation, this trend is likely to continue. Perhaps even more important, the average dentulous individual over the age of 65 now has 19 teeth, clearly an adequate number for very significant dental function. The presence of more teeth implies a greater need for expertise in identifying and managing the special dental problems of the elderly. The clearest example is root caries, which are much more common in older individuals because the gums recede with age. The more familiar caries that occur earlier in life occur on the tooth crown.

The elderly are seen more frequently by their physicians than by dentists, emphasizing the need for physician competence in the oral screening examination, which involves intraoral and extraoral examinations as well as obtainment of a history of unusual signs or symptoms [5]. The most critical component of routine oral examinations is screening for oral cancer, which accounts for 5 percent of all malignancies in men and 2 percent in women in the United States [6]. For the edentulous patient [7] evaluation for denture-related pathologic conditions is important. Fully 50 percent of the elderly population experience painful traumatic lesions of the oral cavity due to dental fractures and maladjusted or malfitting plates. These changes may be ulcerative, atrophic, such as occurs in lichen planus, or hyperplastic, such as the changes occurring in leukoplakia.

Once teeth are lost, the alveolar ridge loses height rapidly (50 percent over three years), which makes denture-fitting and refitting an ongoing necessity. Denture comfort becomes a decreasing reality as there is less purchase for plates. Mandibular bony integrity is impaired in the edentulous jaw. Fully 20 percent of edentulous mandibular fractures result in nonunion, probably due to a combination of osteoporosis and structural weakness. The facial collapse consequent to alveolar bony loss causes muscular incompetence and predisposes to angular cheilitis, which is commonly complicated by monilial infection. This mechanical cause of angular cheilitis is more prevalent than iron or riboflavin deficiency.

Monilial infections are now being recognized, along with iron deficiency, as common causes of red, beefy tongues. The classic flat surface of the tongue in pernicious anemia remains a clue to that specific geriatric disease. Enlargement of the tongue is commonly seen in the aged and may be compensatory for or related to loss of teeth in several ways. The tongue may have increased masticatory function and hypertrophy, or it may have enlarged passively because of the increased space afforded it by dental loss [8].

Dry mouth is a complaint of 20 percent of elders. The major contributors are obstructing nasal disease that causes mouth breathing and anticholinergic drugs or drugs that cause volume depletion. Middle-aged and elderly women may develop Sjögren's syndrome, which in full form consists of keratoconjunctivitis sicca, salivary gland enlargement, xerostomia, and seronegative peripheral polyarthritis. Awareness of the frequent partial expression of this syndrome will lead to its inclusion in the differential diagnosis of dry mouth. The consequences of xerostomia are disturbed taste sensation, increased vulnerability of the oral mucosa, and decreased clearance of bacteria prominent in causing caries. Severely dehydrated elderly patients may develop acute bacterial parotitis, often due to *Staphylococcus aureus*.

Malignancies of the oral cavity are 90 percent squamous cell carcinomas and are statistically associated with smoking and alcohol use. The peak incidence of these lesions occurs in the seventh decade. Inspection of the lower lip, back of the tongue, gingiva, and floor of the mouth will cover the major sites of occurrence. Lesions may present as ulcers in high-wear areas and hypertrophic masses in sheltered areas.

Esophagus

PHYSIOLOGY

Esophageal function is essentially preserved during normal aging. The major change consists of smooth muscle weakness with normal vagal enervation [9]. On esophageal manometry the only change with age is a decreased amplitude of peristalsis, with no increased prevalence of clinically important abnormalities of motility. No clear physiologic changes can be identified as being responsible for the increased prevalence of hiatus hernia with age.

PATHOLOGY

Esophageal dysfunction is common in the elderly and is usually secondary to diseases of the nervous system that cause neuromuscular incoordination. Parkinson's disease, amyotrophic lateral sclerosis, pseudobulbar palsy, peripheral neuropathy, diabetes mellitus, and stroke are the most prevalent disorders. The common radiologic picture on cinesophagoscopy reveals absent or reduced peristalsis, tertiary contractions, delay in esophageal emptying, and esophageal dilation. The motility pattern is similar to that seen in diffuse esophageal spasm. In contrast to that disorder, however, patients with esophageal dysfunction are usually asymptomatic. Symptoms, when present, include aspiration, painless dysphagia, which often occurs more with solids than with liquids, and progressive protein-calorie malnutrition.

The differential diagnosis of dysphagia does not change dramatically with advanced age, but there are some variations in the underlying diseases. Increasing numbers of patients report angina-like chest pain and are subsequently found to have normal or near normal coronary arteriograms. In these patients subsequent studies for esophageal disease are common. In some series 30 percent of patients with recurring chest pain resembling angina pectoris have normal coronary arteries. If 500,000 coronary angiograms are performed each year in this country, it can be hypothesized that as many as 150,000 patients per year have unexplained—and therefore possibly esophageal—chest pain. Potentially 60 percent of patients with noncardiac chest pain may have an identifiable esophageal abnormality. The major esophageal motility disorder patterns include

1. Achalasia, 5 to 10 percent
2. Diffuse esophageal spasm, 0 to 24 percent
3. "Nutcracker esophagus," 28 to 45 percent
4. Hypertensive lower esophageal sphincter, 0 to 23 percent

5. Nonspecific esophageal motility disorder, 23 to 55 percent

Esophageal spasm, esophageal webs, and classic achalasia are relatively unusual in the elderly; Zenker's diverticulum and neuromuscular disease are given priority in the differential diagnosis of upper esophageal dysphagia in elderly men. Vascular dysphagia due to dilatation or aneurysm of the aorta and osteophytic disease of the cervical spine causing dysphagia are uniquely geriatric.

Cancer of the esophagus is the most common cause of progressive dysphagia in the elderly. Fifty percent of the lumen must be stenotic before symptoms appear. Squamous cell carcinoma occurs above the diaphragm, whereas adenocarcinoma predominates at and below the esophagogastric junction. Eight percent of all cancers of the esophagus are found in the cervical region, 25 percent occur in the upper thorax, 17 percent are lower thoracic, and 50 percent are found at the esophagogastric junction.

Hiatus hernia, common in the elderly, is demonstrable in 60 percent of patients over the age of 60. Fortunately, it is rarely symptomatic, and symptoms, when present, can usually be controlled.

MANAGEMENT

In the geriatric patient, who has often accumulated several illnesses that may affect the esophagus, adequate diagnosis requires several types of relatively complex studies. Barium swallow studies should be supplemented by cinesophagograms and fiberoptic esophagoscopy when symptoms are progressive or are associated with weight loss or bleeding. Concurrent with these studies, a Bernstein or Tensilon (edrophonian chloride) study to provoke pain may reveal the diagnosis in fully one-third of patients. Hiatus hernia symptoms are responsive to weight reduction, reduction in the size of meals, particularly before lying down, and elevation of the head of the bed. Foaming agents taken after meals create a bubble of antacid in the less dependent areas of the stomach and esophagus, which is helpful in reducing peptic symptoms. Antacid regimens are otherwise similar to those for duodenal ulceration.

Esophageal malignancy yields a dismal 10 percent five-year survival with any mode of therapy, and the debate over the best mode of therapy continues. Treatment that aggressively attempts to control the spread of disease tends to lead to a poorer quality of survival. The best survival rates are reported when combined staged surgical and radiotherapeutic approaches are used. For individuals who are unsuitable surgical risks (up to 75 percent of this largely geriatric population), fluoroscopically guided dilatation and placement of a fashioned tube through the lesion can provide excellent palliation with a minimum of discomfort or hospitalization time. Palliative radiation can be added. Individualization of therapy is crucial here and depends on the patient's preferences, the site and pathologic type of tumor, and the locally available surgical and radiotherapeutic expertise [10].

Stomach and Duodenum
PHYSIOLOGY

The impaired secretory capacity of the aged stomach is well documented. With advancing age, maximal stimulated gastric acid decreases 5 mEq per hour per decade in men and slightly less in women. Enough acid is present, however, to facilitate recurrence and progression of established acid-peptic disease. In asymptomatic patients, serum gastrin levels increase with advancing age and are associated with the presence of antiparietal cell antibodies. Hyposecretion of intrinsic factor may lead to vitamin B_{12} malabsorption. The increasing prevalence of atrophic gastritis, between 28 and 96 percent in the elderly, strongly suggests that aging increases susceptibility to the disease.

Long-term studies show that atrophic gastritis tends to persist, and superficial gastritis progresses slowly to atrophic gastritis. No age differences are observed in the pathologic appearance [11]. Gastric motility may be somewhat impaired in the elderly, but the influence of age on gastric emptying has not been well defined. Gastritis certainly causes delayed gastric emptying.

An indirect index of gastric acid secretion may be found in the ratio of circulatory pepsinogen I (PI), which is secreted by mucous and chief cells in the gastric fundus, to pepsinogen II (PII), which is secreted by cells in the gastric fundus, cardia, and antrum. Employing a PI/

PII ratio of less than 2.9 as indicative of gastric atrophy, the prevalence of this disorder increases from 24 percent between ages 60 and 69 years to 37 percent over age 80 years [29]. Impaired gastric acid production has several clinically relevant consequences including decreased gastric emptying, lowered intrinsic factor levels, enhanced propensity for bacterial overgrowth, and elevated proximal intestinal pH, which influences nutrient and drug absorption.

PATHOLOGY

Peptic disease of the stomach and duodenum will be considered together because they have a similar pathophysiology. Peptic gastric ulcer is more likely to occur at an advanced age and carries a graver prognosis than duodenal ulcer disease, with more than two-thirds of ulcer deaths being caused by gastric ulcers. The 10 : 1 ratio of duodenal to gastric ulcer in the young becomes a 2 : 1 ratio in the elderly. The sex incidence ratio remains unchanged in old age, with a male predominance of 2 : 1. Atypical presentation is likely, and unusual pain or unphysiologic but disturbing symptomatology is common. In contrast, catastrophic complications such as hemorrhage or perforation occur with little forewarning. Fully one-half of gastric ulcer fatalities occur in patients with symptoms of less than one month's duration. Giant benign gastric ulcerations (ulcers with a diameter larger than 3 cm) have a peak incidence in the seventh decade, later than that of the common smaller ulcers.

Anatomically, gastric ulcers in the elderly occur more proximally, 40 percent occurring in a juxtacardia or posterior wall location; in younger patients 85 percent are found within 9 cm of the pylorus. In the long term more than 50 percent of individuals will have recurrent disease. Etiologic factors such as salicylate ingestion may be more common in the elderly because of the high prevalence of arthritic disease.

Although the prevalence of duodenal ulcer does not increase with age, the morbidity and mortality associated with complications are increased. As many as 20 percent of patients hospitalized with peptic ulcer disease are elderly. Peptic ulcer usually begins during middle age. Because current views on the natural history of peptic ulcer suggest a varying course extending 15 to 20 years from the initial symptoms, the risk period for complications or recurrent symptomatology clearly extends into the geriatric age range. Although estimates vary, as many as half of peptic ulcer patients come to physicians with the first symptoms after age 60. Clinical features vary with advancing age. The elderly patient more commonly presents late in the course of the disease or with a complication but with surprisingly little prior symptomatology. Although pain is often present, it is poorly localized with an unusual radiating pattern, and response to food is atypical. Other organs or organ systems may be involved and may provoke the presenting complaint. For example, a patient may present with angina due to anemia caused by chronic low-grade blood loss.

Among the rarer causes of peptic ulceration, 20 percent of cases of Zollinger-Ellison syndrome occur in patients older than 60, and 2 percent occur in those older than 70. The presentation and course of this illness are not strongly influenced by age.

Bleeding is the most common complication of peptic ulcer of any type and is more common in the elderly [12]. In addition, if bleeding is the first symptom, recurrence increases with age, reaching a rate of 7 percent yearly over the age of 70 years. Emergency surgery for bleeding carries a 20 percent mortality in the elderly (much higher than in the younger age group) because of a combination of factors, including delayed presentation and diagnosis and physiologically and pathologically limited reserves to surgical stress. Prognostic factors for the likelihood of recurrent bleeding and indications for surgery do not change with age.

Perforation as a complication of peptic ulcer disease occurs three times as commonly (in 10 to 20 percent of cases) in the elderly as it does in the younger age group. It represents the second major complication. The mortality from perforation is clearly higher. One factor contributing to this excess morbidity and mortality is the delay in diagnosis fostered by the unusual presentation of the "acute abdomen" in the elderly. There may be a minimal past history, poorly localized symptoms, and few signs of peritonitis.

Persistingly painful ulcer disease is uncommon in the elderly and a rare indication for hospitalization or surgery. Finally, gastric outlet obstruction may present in an unusual way in the elderly, with the secondary metabolic or catabolic disturbances leading to atypical presentation. The surgical approach to the latter two conditions is unchanged with advancing age.

CANCER OF THE STOMACH

Cancer of the stomach has a peak incidence in the eighth and ninth decades. Vague symptomatology and delay in diagnosis lead to advanced illness at presentation. The five-year survival of 15 percent has not increased significantly in 40 years. Atrophic gastritis, which is prevalent with advancing age, increases the risk of stomach cancer 20-fold. Pernicious anemia is likewise associated with an increased risk. Poor prognostic indicators at laparotomy include lymph node involvement and more aggressive pathologic classification. Complications are similar to those seen with peptic ulceration.

GASTRITIS

Erosive gastritis causes as much upper gastrointestinal bleeding in the elderly as duodenal ulceration and is second only to gastric ulcer as a source of bleeding. The use of multiple medicines, known to provoke gastritis, is common because of the accumulation of illnesses with advancing age. Salicylates, phenylbutazone, indomethacin, steroids, and nonsteroidal antiinflammatory agents are commonly used for geriatric medical illnesses. The awareness of the prevalence of alcoholism in the elderly makes it important to include alcohol-related gastric disease in the differential diagnosis of this condition.

MANAGEMENT OF DISEASES OF THE STOMACH AND DUODENUM

Once a clear diagnosis is established, treatment for peptic ulcer disease must be modified for the elderly patient. Medical therapy in the elderly has several caveats. Anticholinergic agents in the elderly are prone to cause complications outside of the gastrointestinal tract and should be discouraged. The use of carbenoxolone may cause symptoms related to sodium retention and hypokalemia. Gastric irradiation has been reported to be 50 percent efficacious and noninvasive, but this therapy is rarely employed to-

day because of advances in surgical care and new medical and pharmacologic approaches.

Cimetidine and ranitidine are enjoying popularity in the treatment of peptic ulcer disease. Of the short-term side effects of these agents, confusion and depression are almost completely geriatric syndromes [37, 38]. One factor clearly demonstrated as a cause of confusion is the reduced plasma clearance of these agents with advancing age. Dosage modification is indicated in the elderly, but at present clear, safe guidelines do not exist.

It is of interest that 42 percent of all nonprescription drugs used by the elderly are gastrointestinal medications [13], and a careful drug history is required before any therapy is begun. A standard regimen for the elderly with peptic ulcer disease includes a regular diet and avoidance of foods known to reproduce symptoms. Use of frequent around-the-clock antacids (30-ml doses) or cimetidine in reduced doses four times a day promotes ulcer healing. Known irritant medications, smoking, and alcohol are best avoided. Surgical management of the elderly patient follows the same general principles as those used for patients of any age, but risk-benefit analysis requires closer scrutiny. Since more catastrophic complications are the rule in the elderly, nonemergency surgery is commonly contemplated. Gastric malignancy in the elderly may be cured by gastrectomy if it is discovered early, but most surgical procedures for this illness are deemed palliative. Chemotherapy in the form of 5-fluorouracil with or without a nitrosourea compound seems most useful at the present time. The elderly are more sensitive to the bone marrow suppression of these agents, thus further limiting their marginal effectiveness.

Small Intestine
PHYSIOLOGY

The weight of the small intestine decreases with advancing age. Jejunal biopsies in healthy elderly patients with normal fat, xylose, iron, and folate absorption reveal significant reductions in mucosal surface area. Other structural abnormalities include a reduction in the number of Peyer's patches and in lymphatic follicles within individual patches.

With gastric acid decreasing, the sterility of the upper gastrointestinal tract is threatened, and the elderly harbor fewer anaerobic lactobacilli and larger numbers of coliform bacteria than younger patients [14]. Blood supply to the gut does not alter with aging, dispelling the notion that chronic ischemia influences aging-related gut function.

Absorption of nutrients in the small intestine of elderly individuals is in general preserved. Deficits do exist and when complicated by poor intake predispose the patient to deficiency syndromes. With advancing age D-xylose (a sugar absorbed from the proximal jejunum and duodenum) ingestion results in lower peak blood levels. The gut absorption of this agent appears to be definitely diminished after the age of 80 [15]. Fat absorption is moderately decreased in the elderly, although there is no evidence to suggest that this decrease is clinically important.

Iron transport, and the increased iron transport noted across the intestinal lumen in iron deficiency, is preserved in normal aging [16]. Calcium absorption decreases steadily with aging and is related directly to decreasing values of 1,25-dihydroxyvitamin D_3 [17]. Serum levels of vitamin C decrease gradually with aging. There is a slight decline in the circulating levels of vitamin B_{12} with age, which may be related to B_{12} malabsorption secondary to bacterial overgrowth. These declines are generally not significant enough to result in clinical evidence of vitamin B_{12} deficiency. Absorption of folic acid is adequate in most elderly, which may be due to the fact that the tendency toward decreased absorption induced by higher intestinal pH is compensated by folate production from increased bacterial flora. Vitamin A absorption increases with age, most likely secondary to age-related declines in the unstirred water layer barrier and increases in pH, thus placing the elderly who ingest large doses of vitamin A supplements at risk for vitamin toxicity.

PATHOLOGY
Malabsorption
Malabsorption presents either as steatorrhea or with chronic diarrhea, anemia, and bone pain. Several diagnoses predominate in the differential diagnosis of this condition in the elderly.

Celiac disease may present at an advanced age even though it is often a lifelong illness. Slow or incomplete recovery characterizes the elderly individual's response. However, consideration should be given to the existence of a complicating lymphoma in such slow-to-respond cases. Pancreatic insufficiency from benign or malignant disease should be considered next, with abdominal pain a major clue to the presence of the malignancy [18].

A distinctive geriatric syndrome of malabsorption caused by bacterial overgrowth in solitary or multiple duodenal or jejunal diverticula seems clearly defined. Small bowel biopsy is normal, and radiographic examination fails to show a malabsorption pattern. The clinical presentation is one of general debility rather than diarrhea or steatorrhea specifically. Also known in the elderly is malabsorption secondary to bacterial overgrowth in the absence of an anatomic blind pouch. Diagnosis is supported by ^{14}C-glycocholate breath testing; the therapeutic response to a broad-spectrum antibiotic is excellent [19].

The final major cause of malabsorption in the elderly is the postgastrectomy syndrome. Gastrectomy is associated with mild fat and protein malabsorption and iron malabsorption, and vitamin B_{12} deficiency may develop after many years.

MANAGEMENT
In spite of the vast array of illnesses potentially responsible for small bowel dysfunction, there are a limited number of major causes for malabsorption in the elderly as outlined. The approach to diagnosis is identical at all ages, with perhaps an earlier trial of tetracycline therapy to assess the possibility of the presence of bacterial overgrowth in the elderly patient.

Crohn's Disease
Five percent of Crohn's disease patients may present initially after age 60 years. Ileal disease is the predominant lesion, presenting in more than 50 percent of cases as an isolated lesion. Although previous reports have indicated a second peak in the incidence of left-sided segmental colonic disease in women in their eighties, this peak was not observed in a recent report.

Symptoms and diagnostic approach were unchanged with advancing age, and thus the main barrier is physician awareness of the possibility of the presence of this condition. The increased prevalence of diverticular disease and ischemic colitis may, however, make the diagnosis more problematic. The necessity for surgical intervention appears to be unchanged with age, and when disease is limited to the ileal region, recurrence rates are relatively lower (30 to 40 percent) [43].

Liver and Biliary Tract

PHYSIOLOGY

In individuals who die of unrelated illnesses, the liver decreases modestly with age in absolute and relative weight, from 4 percent of body weight in the neonate to 2 percent in the elderly, changes that parallel the general reduction in lean body mass [20]. Light microscopy shows a mild increase in hepatic fibrous tissue. Hepatic blood flow shows a 1.5 percent fall per year, resulting in a 50 percent reduction in blood flow from maturity to advanced old age. Giant parenchymal cells with multiple nucleoli appear. The intracellular organelles also show changes. The Golgi apparatus size decreases with age. Mitochondria decrease in number but morphologically increase in size and have an increased density of cristae. There appear to be more lysosomes. There are a large number of reports

in the literature concerning the hepatic enzyme systems of numerous intrahepatic enzymes in mammals, the majority showing no change with aging, some an increase, and some a decrease [21]. The overall pattern is a decrease in the inducible microsomal enzymes involved in redox mechanisms and an increase in hydrolytic enzymes. This finding is compatible with the electron microscopy findings already discussed relating to numbers and morphology of intracellular organelles. Drugs that are altered in metabolism secondary to these changes are shown in the following table (Table 33-1).

Standard liver function studies including bromsulphalein (BSP) retention do not change with age [22]. Serum albumin falls slightly with age, influencing some hormone and drug-binding characteristics.

PATHOLOGY

Hepatitis and Jaundice

Jaundice in the elderly patient is an ominous sign (Table 33-2); the most common cause of progressive jaundice in the elderly is cancer, with pancreatic neoplasms accounting for half of all cases. Jaundice caused by viral hepatitis carries a mortality rate approaching 25 percent and is now most commonly due to non-A, non-B hepatitis. Other diagnostic considerations include choledocholithiasis or drug-related jaundice (which is equal in rate of occurrence to viral hepatitis in the elderly) [23].

TABLE 33-1. *Changes in drug metabolism with age*

DRUG	CHANGE IN HEPATIC DRUG METABOLISM WITH AGE	REFERENCE
Phenytoin	Increase in clearance	Hayes, et al. (1975b)
Aminopyrine	Decreased plasma disappearance	Jori, et al. (1972)
Acetanilide	Increased half-life	Farah, et al. (1977)
Isoniazid	No change	Farah, et al. (1977)
Ethanol	No change	Vestal, et al. (1977)
Nitrazepam	No change in half-life	Castleden, et al. (1977)
Diazepam	Increased half-life	Klotz, et al. (1975)
Phenazone (antipyrine)	Increased half-life	Vestal, et al. (1975)
Phenylbutazone	Increased half-life	O'Malley, et al. (1971)
Amylobarbitone	Increased half-life	Irvine, et al. (1974)
Propranolol	Increased half-life	Castleden, et al. (1975)
Paracetamol (acetaminophen)	Increased half-life	Triggs and Nation (1975)
Chlordiazepoxide	Increased half-life	Roberts, et al. 1978

SOURCE: From H. Mooney, et al. Alterations in the liver with aging. *Clin. Gastroenterol.* 14:757, 1985.

TABLE 33-2. *Causes of jaundice in the elderly**

REFERENCE	MALIGNANT	STONES	DRUGS	HEPATIC	HAEMOLYSIS
Eastwood (1971)	35	16	20	24	5
Huete-Armijo and Exton-Smith (1962)	44	29	7	16	4
O'Brien and Tan (1970)	32	12	6	48	2
Malchow-Moller, et al. (1981)	31	28		41	
Naso and Thompson (1967)	30	29		51	
Parbhoo (1978)	62	27		11	
Vowles (1979)	50	50			

*Figures given are percentages.
SOURCE: From J. R. Croker. Biliary tract disease in the elderly. *Clin. Gastroenterol.* 14:773, 1985.

Toxic and Drug-Related Hepatitis

For numerous reasons the elderly are susceptible to chemical hepatotoxicity. They are frequent recipients of hepatotoxic drugs, commonly receive multiple drugs, and often have reduced clearance of them. Common patterns of toxicity seen in the elderly include a hepatitis-like reaction, intrahepatic cholestasis, and a mixed pattern. Examples of drugs causing a hepatitis-like reaction are antidepressants (monoamino-oxidase inhibitors), anticonvulsants (carbamazepine, phenytoin), antituberculosis drugs (rifampin, isoniazid), and antirheumatic drugs (gold, allopurinol, acetaminophen). The incidence and severity of isoniazid hepatitis increases with age. Age influences the choice and use of this drug for antituberculosis prophylaxis. Currently, reports suggest that this agent is safe in the elderly.

The intrahepatic cholestasis pattern of liver injury may be caused by chlorpromazine, antidepressants, oral hypoglycemic agents (sulfonylureas), benzodiazepines, thiazides, phenylbutazone, antithyroid drugs (propylthiouracil), and sulfonamides. The mixed pathology is seen with antituberculosis drugs, sulfonamides, oral antidiabetic drugs, methyldopa, and erythromycin estolate [24].

Although alcoholic hepatitis is usually a disease of early middle age, it is certainly reported in the elderly. Cirrhosis of the liver may be the major predisposing factor in the United States for the development of hepatoma. Of individuals with biopsy-proven hepatoma, 66 percent have preexisting cirrhosis of the liver associated with alcohol intake [25]. Although the incidence of alcoholic hepatitis and cirrhosis of the liver peaks in early middle age, between 30 and 60 percent of hepatoma patients are over the age of 60, making it a geriatric illness. Males outnumber females with this disease by a 3 : 1 ratio. Symptoms of abdominal discomfort (62 percent), weight loss (34 percent), and abdominal swelling (30 percent) are the common presenting symptoms. The majority have hepatomegaly (75 percent) and ascites (30 percent) at the time of diagnosis. Most will have abnormal liver function studies (serum glutamic oxaloacetic-transaminase is increased in 88 percent; alkaline phosphatase in 78 percent). Alpha-fetoprotein levels are elevated in 74 percent, and in most series hepatitis-associated antigen is rarely found to be positive. Various paraneoplastic syndromes such as polycythemia, thrombocytosis, hypoglycemia, hypercalcemia, and fever may cloud the presentation and delay diagnosis. Median survival with this illness is about six months from diagnosis.

Viral Hepatitis

Although other causes of jaundice predominate in the elderly, the possibility of acute viral hepatitis must not be overlooked. The clinical setting is usually a patient with an unrelated disease receiving multiple drugs and often with a history of recent surgery and anesthesia or blood transfusion. In the most common type of viral hepatitis (non-A, non-B) the serum bilirubin and aminotransferase concentrations are often lower than in other types, and the serologic markers are absent. Because the elderly are more likely to have had hepatitis in the past, the presence of antibodies (IgG type) to hepatitis A and B may create a diagnostic problem.

Diagnosis is based on clinical and laboratory factors and the exclusion of other causes. Although the histopathologic changes of viral hepatitis are characteristic, they do not enable one to differentiate between hepatitis A, hepatitis B, and non-A, non-B hepatitis, which are best distinguished with serologic testing. Liver biopsy is indicated when the diagnosis remains uncertain and when the clinical course is atypical, particularly if it is prolonged or severe.

The sophistication of serologic testing has led to a clearer understanding of the documented higher morbidity of the elderly from hepatitis. Severe hepatitis in elderly patients is essentially all secondary to blood product transfusion, with non-A, non-B hepatitic agents being implicated in 95 percent of cases. Type A hepatitis is rare and is clinically benign in the elderly. The increased severity and decreased survival in the aged due to hepatitis thus result from the greater frequency of non-A, non-B hepatitis than type A hepatitis, associated poor nutrition, the high prevalence of associated medical illnesses, and impaired immune response. Elderly patients with posttransfusional non-A, non-B hepatitis either recover spontaneously or progress to a chronic phase with intermittent mildly elevated liver function tests.

The higher frequency of progression to chronic hepatitis in the elderly, now better understood as chronicity (approximately 50 percent of cases), is consistent with non-A, non-B hepatitis. The main histologic types of chronic hepatitis are chronic persistent hepatitis, which is usually considered a nonprogressive form in which the architecture of the liver is maintained, and chronic active hepatitis, which is associated with more necrosis. Because chronic persistent hepatitis is a benign disease its therapy is expectant. Corticosteroids are contraindicated in chronic active hepatitis B, and no controlled studies in chronic non-A, non-B hepatitis have been reported. Even in the autoimmune type of chronic active hepatitis, judgment must be exercised before embarking on corticosteroid therapy. The use of corticosteroids in elderly patients should be considered only in those who have chronic disease in the presence of marked symptoms because of the high incidence of complications including osteoporosis and fractures, sodium retention, hypertension, and diabetes mellitus. If at the end of a therapeutic trial period of 30-mg prednisolone daily, unequivocal laboratory and histologic evidence of decreased disease activity is not apparent, corticosteroids should be withdrawn [41].

Type A hepatitis is endemic throughout the world, the prevalence of specific antibodies in serum being closely related to age and socioeconomic factors. Individuals older than 50 years of age are two to four times more likely to have specific antibodies than those less than 20 years. Prior exposure to hepatitis A, as determined by serologic testing, rises to approximately 75 percent in the elderly.

Cholelithiasis and Biliary Tract Surgery

Recent studies of age-related factors that contribute to the supersaturation of bile with cholesterol may help to explain the increased prevalence of cholelithiasis from 10 to 20 percent at age 55 to 65 years to 35 to 40 percent after age 80 years. Most stones are "silent" and are unpredictably present with severe complications. The natural history of gallstones in patients undergoing cholecystography not operated on and free from complications for the following year is as follows: During the next decade nearly 20 percent will develop severe complications (jaundice, pancreatitis, acute cholecystitis, carcinoma), and a further 20 percent will require elective surgery for pain. Should one advise routine cholecystectomy for patients with gallstones? Some surgeons advocate this policy in younger patients. Complications increase with age, but so do the risks of surgery. Present opinion suggests that silent stones are innocent and that routine prophylactic surgery is unnecessary. A further argument advanced for prophylactic cholecystectomy is related to the prevention of gallbladder cancer. However, the risk of developing carcinoma of the gallbladder in patients with asymptomatic stones is less than the fatalities associated with elective cholecystectomy, making surgery impractical and unsafe in the elderly. Unfortunately, gallstone dissolution is unsuitable and ineffective in the elderly. At present we do not know which silent stones are likely to cause problems for elderly patients in the future. Choledochal stones are more common in the elderly, with some series

TABLE 33-3. *Age-related mortality rates for cholecystectomy performed electively and as an emergency*

	ELECTIVE		EMERGENCY		
AGE	N	MORTAL-ITY (%)	N	MOR-TALITY	REFERENCE
50	3803	0.1	765	0.4	
50	3610	0.9	878	2.2	McSherry and Glenn (1980)
65		2.5		3.4	Lygidakis (1983)[a]
65–74	55	1.8	15	26.0	
74	33	0	15	26.0	Houghton and Donaldson (1983)
80		0		12.5	Sullivan, et al. (1982)[b]
70	50	2.0	43	14.0	Huber, et al. (1983)
60		2.3		16.7	Ibach, et al. (1968)

[a]Total N for elective + emergency = 789.
[b]Total N for elective + emergency = 42.
SOURCE: From J. R. Croker. Biliary tract disease in the elderly. *Clin. Gastroenterol.* 14:773, 1985.

reporting a fourfold greater incidence in older patients. These stones are generally believed to be more dangerous than stones in the gallbladder. In a few patients stones may cause sudden severe illness. In most, however, symptoms such as pain, infection, or abnormal liver function tests are present. The approach to the elderly is to investigate accurately and quickly patients presenting with these clues.

The morbidity and mortality of complicated biliary tract disease increases with aging. Again, delayed diagnosis and intercurrent disease are largely responsible (Table 33-3).

One form of acute cholecystitis is uniquely geriatric—acute emphysematous cholecystitis in which gas-producing organisms such as *Clostridium welchii*, anaerobic streptococci, *Escherichia coli, S. aureus, Pseudomonas,* and *Klebsiella* have been implicated. The course is more toxic and is associated with more severe pain than uncomplicated cholecystitis.

Carcinoma of the gallbladder is three times more common in patients over the age of 70 and is a disease of elderly women. It is usually associated with chronic calculous cholecystitis. Its rarity precludes its use as an indication for prophylactic cholecystectomy except when gallbladder calcification is present. In patients in this situation there is a 25 percent incidence of carcinoma.

Endoscopic papillotomy is promising and is well tolerated by the elderly [26]. It is now increasingly accepted that an elderly patient with stones in the common bile duct should be managed by endoscopic sphincterotomy and gallstone removal. Mortality is less than 2 percent.

Preoperatively, vitamin K is given to bring the prothrombin time within three seconds of control values. Antibiotics are given to patients in whom the gallbladder is still in situ, to those who have suffered a recent episode of cholangitis, and when adequate drainage is not achieved. Care must be exercised in titrating sedation during duodenoscopy in the elderly, particularly in very frail and debilitated patients. Full radiologic screening must be available, and x-rays are taken. The technique of endoscopic sphincterotomy is well established. Following sphincterotomy, many stones will pass spontaneously, and most of the remainder can be removed with a basket. The success rate for duct clearance is now around 85 percent. Stones less than 1 cm in diameter can almost always be removed, but there is progressive difficulty with stones over 15 to 20 mm. Crushing baskets may extend the success of the endoscopist. Results are unpredictable because some stones are soft and break up. There may be narrowing of the bile duct below the stone, and stones above real strictures cannot be removed.

Pancreas
PHYSIOLOGY
Pancreatic size increases or remains unchanged with aging. Structurally, duct ectasia is common and follows hyperplastic change in ductules. Various microscopic changes occur, including islet cell atrophy and amyloid and adipose infiltration. There is no reduction in volume of pancreatic fluid or its content of trypsin, amylase, or bicarbonate with aging.

Since 90 percent of pancreatic function must be impaired before significant fat malabsorption occurs, clinically important maldigestion of fat does not occur as a consequence of normal aging.

PATHOLOGY

The incidence of pancreatitis increases with advancing age. Biliary tract disease, hypothermia, carbon monoxide poisoning, and steroid and thiazide therapy are all more common in the elderly and may be contributory causes of pancreatitis. Atypical location of pain, frequently altered mental function, and higher morbidity characterize elderly patients with pancreatitis. The differential diagnosis of abdominal pain and hyperamylasemia is more difficult with advancing age because of the increased prevalence of illnesses well known to cause hyperamylasemia, such as dissecting abdominal aortic aneurysm and acute arterial and venous obstruction. Assessment of amylase clearance helps to differentiate the condition from macroamylasemia but not the other conditions. Pancreatitis in the very elderly is often painless, further confusing the clinical picture.

The incidence of pancreatic carcinoma is increasing steadily and has become the fourth most common death-causing cancer in the United States for males. Peak incidence occurs in the sixth decade with a 3 : 1 male-to-female ratio. Diagnosis is notoriously difficult, leading in all age groups to late advanced presentation. Recently developed diagnostic modalities such as retrograde pancreatography and computed tomography may permit earlier diagnosis of this cancer. The paraneoplastic syndrome of psychosis or depression as the initial presentation of pancreatic malignancy may be a diagnostic clue in a previously stable geriatric patient.

MANAGEMENT

The management of pancreatitis, aside from pain management, is unchanged with advancing age. Analgesic effectiveness increases with advancing age, necessitating a reduction in doses of major analgesics. A careful search for common bile duct stones is indicated.

Pancreatic malignancy carries a less than 5 percent five-year survival, but when operation is possible survival increases modestly to 15 percent at five years.

Large Bowel
PHYSIOLOGY

The large bowel has active resorptive (water, chloride, sodium) and secretory (mucus, potassium, bicarbonate) functions. In addition, food residues and bacteria are compacted and stored temporarily before evacuation. Alterations in gastrointestinal flora occur in the elderly, as discussed previously. Analysis of transit time of radiopaque markers in healthy elderly subjects reveals that the first marker is always excreted in three days, and 80 percent have passed by five days [28]. The transit time from cecum to rectum is short, with most of the delay in evacuation occurring below the sigmoid colon. These transit times are no different than those seen in healthy, young, normal individuals. Normal stool frequency is between 3 and 20 stools per week. The reflex action in defecation involves a voluntary response to anal canal relaxation that occurs when the rectum is distended by fecal material. Study has shown that elderly individuals have normal sensibility to balloon distention of the rectum.

PATHOLOGY
Ischemic Colitis

Narrowings of major intestinal arteries by atheroma become significant in the geriatric age group. Once two vessels are blocked or severely compromised, the large bowel mucosa is vulnerable to any further insult, which may include digoxin overdose (intestinal vasospasm and increased oxygen demands), heart failure (compromised perfusion), or polycythemia (stasis). Three distinct clinical pictures may result, depending on the acuteness of the obstruction. They include transient abdominal ischemia, slow development of ischemic stricture, and gangrenous colitis. The first two appear clinically as food avoidance, postprandial abdominal pain, and rectal bleeding with normal rectal mucosa. If a segment is totally infarcted, an intraabdominal catastrophe results. More often, spontaneous resolution occurs, with subsequent development of a long, smooth stricture in the watershed area of the arterial blood supply at the splenic flexure.

Ulcerative Colitis

The demonstration of a second peak in the incidence of ulcerative colitis at age 60 establishes a bimodal age distribution for this disease [29]. Retrospective studies suggest that the disease produces a more rapid appearance of significant symptoms, less systemic involvement, and lower relapse rates in the elderly. Therapeutic principles are unchanged with advancing age.

Angiodysplasia

When conventional methodology short of angiography has failed to disclose the source of colonic bleeding, the most likely cause is venous ectasia. These lesions are felt at present to be degenerative immature venules and capillaries [30]. Similar lesions occur in association with aortic stenosis. These lesions occur almost exclusively in the elderly, are usually in the right colon, and are best identified by angiography during acute hemorrhage. Venous ectasia usually presents with recurrent bright red or maroon-colored rectal bleeding, but massive or occult bleeding may also occur. Colonoscopy may visualize the lesion, but the most specific diagnostic test is angiography. Therapy consists of surgical removal of the involved colonic segment.

Diverticular Disease

Several surveys of asymptomatic healthy volunteers indicate a progressive development of colonic diverticula with advancing age, with prevalence rates of 18 percent at ages 40 to 59, 29 percent at ages 60 to 79, and 42 percent above age 80. There is a female preponderance in a ratio of approximately 1.5 : 1. Most patients with radiologically confirmed diverticula are asymptomatic. The risk of hemorrhagic complications appears to be increased in the elderly (particularly those who are hypertensive). Management both at the time and prophylactically is the same as that in the younger age groups—high-residue diets (bran) or Metamucil. Peridiverticular abscess requires close in-hospital observation, bowel rest, and antibiotics (since the elderly seem to have less capacity to avoid free peritonitis). Pneumaturia should lead to suspicion of diverticular disease in the otherwise healthy geriatric patient.

Appendicitis

With advancing age there is a decreased amount of lymphoid tissue in the appendix. Obliteration of the lumen is common. Appendicitis is more complicated in the elderly and has a higher incidence of perforation; less than 20 percent of these patients are able to leave the hospital in the usual five postoperative days. The classic principles of atypical pain, delay in presentation, and intercurrent disease in the geriatric patient are of major importance in the diagnosis of appendicitis in the elderly. There is a strong relation between delay in presentation and perforation, with a 60 percent rate of perforation after a less than 48-hour delay and a 90 percent perforation rate for those delaying more than 48 hours [31]. Nonoperative management of appendicitis, which may be necessary in some compromised elderly patients, requires bowel rest, antibiotics for aerobic gram-negative rods and anaerobic bacteria, and carefully planned interval appendectomy.

A rare variant of appendicitis, appendicitis occurring in a femoral hernia, occurs almost exclusively in postmenopausal women and should be included in the differential diagnosis of inflammatory right groin masses in such patients. Appendiceal abscesses complicate 3 percent of cases of acute appendicitis. Although death is unusual, 28 percent have significant complications perioperatively and extended hospital stays. Interval appendectomy after medical treatment of abscess is associated with a 19 percent complication rate; if the appendectomy is not performed (usually because of serious associated illness), less than 10 percent are likely to have recurrent symptoms.

Incidental appendectomy should be avoided in the elderly. In individuals over the age of 65, 100 incidental appendectomies need to be done to avoid a single case of appendicitis in the remaining lifetime of the individual. The common confounding differential diagnoses in younger individuals, such as ectopic pregnancy, salpingitis, and ruptured ovarian cysts, are less relevant in the elderly. Because of the relative rarity of death from appendicitis (3.5 percent), it would take 3,000 incidental appendectomies to save a single elderly person's life [32].

Overall, the mortality from appendicitis in the elderly has fallen gradually and progressively from 54.0 percent in 1928 to 3.5 percent in 1978, which is a more dramatic improvement than improvement in anesthetic risk alone would allow. These figures suggest an improvement in the natural history of the disorder.

Constipation

Constipation and laxative use become more prevalent with age. Between 40 and 60 percent of elders use laxatives regularly, largely on a self-administered basis. Many individuals who take laxatives regularly do not consider themselves constipated but wish to maintain a preconceived idea of regular bowel function. Of those who claim to be constipated, 25 percent have normal bowel transit times [28]. Clearly, physiologic bowel function is perceived as abnormal and is manipulated by self-prescribed agents. The cost of this routine in the United States has been estimated at 130 million dollars per year. Bills for cathartics in chronic-care hospitals often approach 15 percent of their drug budget.

The elderly become constipated for the same reasons that younger people do. The main reason for the increased prevalence in the elderly is the role played by multiple etiologies in overcoming normal physiologic habit. Some of the factors provoking constipation include the following:

1. Insufficient dietary fiber
2. Inactivity
3. Anxiety or depression
4. Drugs
5. Inadequate fluid intake
6. Laxative abuse
7. Poor muscle power
8. Dementia
9. Anal disease
10. Neurologic disease
11. Others: carcinoma, hypothyroidism, diverticulitis, strictures, hypercalcemia, hypokalemia

Some of the drugs causing constipation are narcotic analgesics, anticholinergics, narcotic-containing cough medicines, iron, phenothia-zines, tricyclic antidepressants, antiparkinsonian agents, and any drug leading to oversedation and thus neglect of the call to stool [33]. In long-term care facilities as many as two-thirds of the patients consume one or more drugs on this list.

One cause of constipation that demands consideration is carcinoma of the colon. This concern prompts investigation of any change in bowel habits, particularly constipation. A primary care physician caring for 3,000 people with a typical age range is likely to encounter one case of colorectal carcinoma every 16 months in his or her geriatric patients. Aggressive investigation is indicated in high-risk cases, especially in the presence of weight loss or bleeding. Additional risk factors include previous colon, endometrial, or bladder cancer; immunodeficiency states; inflammatory bowel disease; previous sporadic polyps; and Gardner's or familial polyposis syndrome. The minimum relevant investigation in a newly identified constipated patient includes a hematocrit, rectal examination, sigmoidoscopic examination, and three stools for occult blood testing.

Therapy for constipation has not received much physician interest. Many agents are available, and it is evident from institutional surveys that no clear prescribing practices exist. The regimen popularly suggested now includes a two-level therapeutic prescription of bulk laxative followed by an irritative cathartic should this first agent not be satisfactory. Bulk laxatives such as bran are easily introduced into the daily diet at doses of 5 gm twice a day. Metamucil can be considered an equivalently efficacious agent. One of the senna derivatives can be an effective second agent should bulk laxatives fail.

The institution and continued administration of these agents must be considered carefully and reviewed in the context of encouraging a general plan of management. This plan should include educating the patient in normal bowel habits, making modifications in diet, recommending an increase in activity, encouraging him or her to heed the call to stool, and minimizing or eliminating painful local conditions or contributing drugs.

Complicated constipation may present as spurious diarrhea and usually requires more aggressive acute and chronic therapy. The atonic megacolon of the neglected, chronically consti-pated patient requires vigorous local therapy in the form of enemas to clear the colon of residue and a comprehensive plan of therapy. No clear guidelines exist regarding types and frequencies of enemas or strong cathartics. Perforation of the rectum with enema nipples may not be im-mediately reported and will obviously worsen the presenting difficulty.

Fecal Incontinence

Fecal incontinence, a socially isolating disease of predominantly institutionalized demented geri-atric patients, may be caused by local anal dis-ease, fecal impaction, or neurologic disorder perhaps secondary to diabetes mellitus. Occa-sional cases may result from diarrheal illnesses or laxative abuse. Clearly, senile dementia of the Alzheimer's type or obvious neurologic dis-order is almost always present. Studies have shown that neurologically intact, fecally incon-tinent patients often demonstrate intense rectal contractions that are not observed in continent subjects and that are reminiscent of the findings in patients with detrusor hyperreflexia and uri-nary incontinence [34].

Evaluation of fecal incontinence has recently been described by Wold and consists of careful history, physical examination, and several spe-cific tests, especially an incontinence calendar (Table 33-4) [40]. The abnormalities causing fecal incontinence yield reasonably characteris-tic clinical findings (Table 33-5).

Biofeedback therapy has proved beneficial for patients with prior anal surgery, for idio-pathic cases, and with modifications in diabetic patients. Elderly patients commonly have fecal impaction due to impaired mobility and cogni-tion. Treatment begins with hypertonic enemas twice a day until there is no fecal return. Sub-sequently, planned period evaluations with a phosphate enema followed by a mildly irritant suppository once or twice a week will provide effective management.

Therapy for this disturbing problem is diffi-cult. Once fecal impaction and proximal or local pathology have been excluded by specific studies, the best form of therapy is a low-residue diet, pharmacologic induction of con-stipation, and periodic planned evacuation. Other modalities such as operant conditioning or rigorous bowel habit training may be useful in patients with more resistant cases.

TABLE 33-4. *Evaluation of fecal incontinence*

History
    Frequency, duration, severity
    Pattern (diurnal, nocturnal, both)
    Associated symptoms (e.g., urgency, lack of warning, diarrhea, constipation, straining at defecation)
    Other relevant factors (e.g., anorectal trauma or sur-gery, diabetes, laminectomy, urinary incontinence, immobility, dementia, neurologic disease, multiple childbirths, inflammatory bowel disease)
Physical examination
    Rectal examination (prolapse, fecal impaction or rectal mass, anal deformity or disease, anal "gaping," atro-phy of gluteal muscles)
    Neurologic examination (mental status, sacral reflexes, perineal sensation, basic neurologic evaluation)
Initial investigation
    Sigmoidoscopy (proctitis, tumor, melanosis coli)
    Biochemical survey (hematologic study, glucose and electrolyte evaluation)
    Incontinence calendar
    Presence of diarrhea (stool for culture, ova, and para-sites; 72-hour stool collection for weight, fat, reduc-ing substances; barium enema; small bowel series; medication and diet histories)

TABLE 33-5. *Abnormalities causing fecal incontinence*

	MOTIVATION	RESERVOIR CAPACITY	RECTAL SENSATION	ANAL SPHINCTER
Dementia	A	N	N	N
Anal sphincter surgery	N	N	N	A
Idiopathic	N	N	N	A
Diabetes mellitus	N	N	N/A	A
Inflammatory bowel disease	N	A	N	N
Ileoanal anastomosis	N	A	N/A	N
Neurogenic problems	N	N	N/A	A
Encopresis	N/A	N	N/A	N

Key: N = normal most or all of the time; A = abnormal most or all of the time; N/A = may be normal or abnormal.

Carcinoma of the Colon

Of all digestive malignancies, 50 percent are adenocarcinomas of the colon. Pathologic studies have indicated less distant disease in the elderly, thus usually allowing local symptoms and prolonged course to dominate the clinical picture.

Symptoms provoked by the primary tumor are unchanged across the age spectrum. In the elderly, confounding factors are introduced by the presence of concomitant benign disease that could also explain the same symptomatology, leading to both patient delay in reporting and physician delay in appropriate investigation.

Metabolic or nonmetastatic manifestations of cancer may dominate the clinical picture in the elderly and lead to the oft-quoted "altered presentation." Nonspecific vague symptomatology often includes loss of drive and interest, anorexia, weight loss, weakness, malaise, failing mobility, and a tendency to fall. The more typical presentations are rectal bleeding, alteration in stool habit from a previously stable routine, and intraabdominal catastrophes resulting from obstruction and perforation.

Screening and surveillance of patients with or at risk for colonic cancer are becoming clearer but still require an individualized approach in older patients. Because 98 percent of colorectal cancers occur after age 40 and 95 percent occur after age 50, asymptomatic patients who have no other special risk factors should undergo digital examination of the rectum annually. Twelve percent of colorectal cancers and cancer of the prostate will be detected by this method.

If one or more fecal blood test slides show a positive reaction, the patient should be carefully evaluated. About 25 percent of patients perform the test incorrectly despite the best efforts at instruction. Patients with an improperly performed positive test should repeat fecal blood testing.

There is an increasing shift away from the previously recommended investigative pattern, which included rectal examination, sigmoidoscopy, and air contrast barium enema followed if necessary by a barium meal with small bowel radiography and finally colonoscopy. More and more clinicians are now recommending colonoscopy as the first step, followed by barium enema if the entire colon has not been visualized.

The American Cancer Society recommends that asymptomatic patients have a sigmoidoscopic examination at age 50 and every three to five years thereafter as long as findings are normal and the patient remains asymptomatic.

The 65-cm fiberoptic (flexible) sigmoidoscope detects about twice as many cancers and six times as many adenomas as does the rigid sigmoidoscope and is much better tolerated by patients. Fiberoptic sigmoidoscopes are used for screening examinations. In addition to detecting adenomatous polyps, this tool can also be used to remove them. Removal of adenomas in the more proximal colon may result in secondary prevention of cancer.

If a polyp smaller than 1 cm in diameter is discovered, the lesion is subjected to biopsy because about half of such polyps are not neoplastic and require no treatment, evaluation, or special follow-up. If the biopsy shows adenoma or if polyps are larger than 1 cm in diameter, the patient is advised to have colonoscopy with treatment of all polyps. Barium contrast examination of the colon is not advised unless the entire colon cannot be examined with the colonoscope.

Individuals with a family history of colorectal cancer, especially familial cancer syndrome or hereditory site-specific colon cancer, inflammatory bowel disease, past history of colorectal cancer, familial polyposis or Gardner's syndrome, or a history of breast or genital cancer represent higher risk groups for colorectal cancer. Only patients with ulcerative colitis, a past history of carcinoma, or breast or genital malignancy are significant in the geriatric population. A variety of strategies have been suggested for these groups, suggesting insufficient data for specific recommendations. Ulcerative colitis requires progressive concern because significant risk begins eight years after the initial diagnosis if disease is present in the entire colon and 18 years after diagnosis with left-sided disease. For the first four to five years after excision of a colonic malignancy colonoscopy has been recommended by many clinicians, with decreasing intensity of reassessment subsequently.

The general trend toward conservative care for senescent patients with malignancy is based in part on their shorter life expectancy. In some cases it is more desirable to preserve function and quality of life with disease than to invoke disturbing or disfiguring radical therapy. Although it leads to increased cure rates, radical surgery or radiotherapy also involves significant morbidity. Concomitant illness may preclude investigation and therapy and or indeed may hasten or be totally responsible for the elderly patient's demise. Each case must be weighed carefully. Such care is crucially important when one considers the extended life expectancy of otherwise healthy elders.

Principles of palliative care apply equally to young and old patients, but it must be realized that the older patient may have less family support, more complex social isolation, and increased nursing care needs.

Acute Abdominal Pain

A particularly frustrating picture is presented to the clinician assessing acute abdominal pain in the elderly. A history is often lacking because of organic brain disease, confusion, or the absence of family to provide a history. The coexistence of several diseases (multiple pathology) further complicates the picture.

The expected abdominal signs may be minimal or absent. Retroperitoneal and intrathoracic disease may present with abdominal pain. The most common cause of surgical abdominal pain in the elderly is cholecystitis. Intestinal obstruction is the second most common cause of acute abdominal pain requiring surgical investigation. Half of these obstructions are caused by hernias, followed by adhesions and malignancy. In the large bowel, malignancy and colonic volvulus are most likely to cause acute pain. The third most common cause of acute abdominal pain is appendicitis, and the increased difficulties in elderly patients with this diagnosis have been discussed [35].

Gallstone ileus is another unique female geriatric illness. Acute pancreatitis is the most common nonsurgical cause of abdominal pain in the elderly.

Acute mesenteric infarction is almost limited to the geriatric population. Its presentation is variable, and it is often quickly associated with altered mental function and vascular instability,

leading to disastrous results. In addition to abdominal pain, hyperperistalsis, bloody stool, and a pseudoobstructive pattern on x-ray are part of the clinical presentation. This illness may be the most common cause of fatal acute abdominal crisis in the geriatric population.

References

1. McKeown, F. *Pathology of the Aged*. London: Butterworth, 1965.
2. Geboes, K., and Bossaert, H. Gastrointestinal disorders in old age. *Age Ageing* 6:197, 1977.
3. Sklar, M., Kirsner, J. B., and Palmer, W. L. Symposium on medical problems of the aged: Gastrointestinal disease in the aged. *Med. Clin. North Am.* 40:223, 1956.
4. U.S. Department of Health, Education and Welfare. *Special Report on Aging, 1979*. NIH Publication No. 79-1907. Washington, D.C.: U.S. Government Printing Office, 1979. P. 16.
5. Gordon, S. R., and Jahnigen, D. W. Oral assessment of the dentulous elderly patient. *J. Am. Geriatr. Soc.* 34:276, 1986.
6. Bhaskan, S. N. *Synopsis of Oral Pathology (5th ed.)*. St. Louis: Mosby, 1977.
7. Gordon, S. R., and Jahnigen, D. W. Oral assessment of the dentulous elderly patient. *J. Am. Geriatr. Soc.* 31:797, 1983.
8. Klein, D. R. Oral soft tissue changes in geriatric patients. *Bull. N.Y. Acad. Med.* 56:724, 1980.
9. Hollis, J. B., and Castell, D. O. Esophageal function in elderly men. *Ann. Intern. Med.* 80:371, 1974.
10. Cancer of the esophagus: Three different views. *Hosp. Pract.* October 1976. P. 63.
11. Siurala, M., et al. Prevalence of gastritis in a rural population. *Scand. J. Gastroenterology* 3:211, 1968.
12. Narayanan, M., and Steinheber, F. V. The changing face of peptic ulcer in the elderly. *Med. Clin. North Am.* 60:1159, 1976.
13. Law, R., and Chalmers, C. Medicines and elderly people: A general practice survey. *Br. Med. J.* 1:565, 1976.
14. Gorbach, S. L., et al. Studies of intestinal microflora. *Gastroenterology* 53:845, 1967.
15. Guth, P. H. Physiologic alterations in small bowel function with age: The absorption of D-xylose. *Am. J. Dig. Dis.* 13:567, 1968.
16. Marx, J. J. Normal iron absorption and decreased red cell iron uptake in the aged. *Blood* 53:204, 1979.
17. Gallagher, J. C., et al. Intestinal calcium absorp-

tion and serum vitamin D metabolites in normal subjects and osteoporotic patients. *J. Clin. Invest.* 64:129, 1979.

18. Price, H. L., Gazzard, B. G., and Dawson, A. M. Steatorrhoea in the elderly. *Br. Med. J.* 1:1582, 1977.

19. Bayless, T. M. Malabsorption in the elderly. *Hosp. Pract.* August 1979. P. 57.

20. Morgan, Z., and Feldman, M. The liver, biliary tract and pancreas in the aged: An anatomic and laboratory evaluation. *J. Am. Geriatr. Assoc.* 5:59, 1967.

21. Hyams, D. E. The Liver and Biliary system. In J. C. Brocklehurst (ed.), *Textbook of Geriatric Medicine and Gerontology* (2nd ed.). New York: Churchill Livingstone, 1978.

22. Koff, R. S., et al. Absence of an age effect on sulfobromophthalein retention in healthy men. *Gastroenterology* 65:300, 1973.

23. Huete-Armyo, A., and Exton-Smith, A. N. Causes and diagnosis of jaundice in the elderly. *Br. Med. J.* 1:1113, 1962.

24. Hyams, D. E. Gastrointestinal problems in the old. II. *Br. Med. J.* 1:150, 1974.

25. Al-Sarraf, M., et al. Primary liver cancer. *Cancer* 33:574, 1974.

26. Seigel, J. Endoscopic management of choledocholithiasis and papillary stenosis. *Surg. Gynecol. Obstet.* 148:747, 1979.

27. Cancer statistics, 1979. *CA* January/February 1979. P. 811.

28. Eastwood, H. D. H. Bowel transit studies in the elderly. Radiopaque markers in the investigation of constipation. *Gerontol. Clin.* 14:154, 1972.

29. Evans, J. G., and Acheson, E. D. An epidemiologic study of ulcerative colitis and regional enteritis in the Oxford area. *Gut* 6:311, 1965.

30. Stewart, W. B., Gathright, J. B., and Ray, J. E. Vascular ectasias of the colon. *Surg. Gynecol. Obstet.* 148:670, 1979.

31. Owens, B. J., and Hamit, H. F. Appendicitis in the elderly. *Ann. Surg.* 187:392, 1978.

32. Nockerts, S. R., Detmer, D. E., and Fryback, D. G. Incidental appendectomy in the elderly? No. *Surgery* 88:301, 1980.

33. Hutchinson, B. Constipation in the elderly. *Can. Fam. Physician* 24:1018, 1978.

34. Brocklehurst, J. C. Bowel management in the neurologically disabled. The problems of old age. *Proc. R. Soc. Med.* 65:66, 1972.

35. Steinheber, F. V. Interpretation of gastrointestinal symptoms in the elderly. *Med. Clin. North Am.* 60:1141, 1976.

36. Shapiro, P. A., et al. Crohn's disease in the elderly. *Am. J. Gastroenterol.* 76:132, 1981.

37. Greene, D. S., et al. The effect of age on ranitidine pharmacokinetics. *Clin. Pharm. Ther.* 39:300, 1986.

38. Billings, R. F., et al. Depression associated with ranitidine. *Am. J. Psychiatry* 143:915, 1986.

39. Norfleet, R. G. Early detection of colorectal neoplasms. *Postgrad. Med.* 79:121, 1986.

40. Wold, A. Fecal incontinence. *Postgrad. Med.* 3:123, 1986.

41. Mooney, H., et al. Alterations in the liver with ageing. *Clin. Gastroenterol.* 14:757, 1985.

42. Croker, J. R. Biliary tract disease in the elderly. *Clin. Gastroenterol.* 14:773, 1985.

43. Shapiro, P. A., et al. Crohn's disease in the elderly. *Am. J. Gastroenterol.* 76:132, 1981.

34

Research in Gerontology

JOHN W. ROWE

ADVANCES IN THE CARE of the elderly ultimately depend on the development of increased understanding of the aging process. As interest in and support for gerontologic research increase, there is enhanced need for clear recognition of the methodologic obstacles inherent with this type of research. Experience has identified several perils and pitfalls that are characteristic of research in aging [1]. This chapter reviews some of these special considerations with particular emphasis on clinical investigation.

Subject Selection

Several important considerations govern the conduct and evaluation of clinical gerontologic studies. The most important factor is subject selection. In the past, geriatric literature was often tainted by a lack of attention to the medical status of the subjects being studied. Not infrequently, medical students or hospital employees constituted the young group, while the old group comprised residents of long-term care facilities or, in some cases, patients in acute-care hospitals. Although these individuals were generally screened to exclude those with an abnormality of the particular organ system under study, they were often disabled or multiply impaired and were suboptimal for a study of the physiologic concomitants of normal aging. In such studies, differences between young and old

individuals were a complex mixture of disease-related and age-related effects and failed to provide insight into the normal aging process.

During the past several years a new phase in gerontologic research has emerged in which investigators carefully scrutinize study subjects in an effort to avoid, as much as possible, contamination from disease processes. Careful attention to exclusion of diseased individuals and those taking medications, although it may be viewed as "cleaning up" the physiologic data, also entails risk. One must be aware that intensive screening of the population may result in a select group of elderly superperformers whose data do not reflect the influence of age-related changes. For instance, in attempting to exclude diabetics, one might adopt criteria by which individuals with a two-hour postprandial blood glucose level greater than 140 mg per dl would be excluded. Since carbohydrate tolerance is well known to decline with age in nondiabetics, the application of this uniform criterion to all age groups would result in an increasingly stringent selection procedure with advancing age. The marked changes in carbohydrate tolerance with age would result in only a small fraction of individuals in the eighth or ninth decade of life qualifying for the study. Since systolic blood pressure increases with age, a similar selection effect would be introduced in studies excluding all individuals with systolic pressure over 130 mm Hg. In these examples, generally accepted age-adjusted criteria for normality are available and might be applied as a screening technique. However, such guidelines are lacking for most variables.

Investigators embarking on gerontologic studies should also be aware that differences in habits, such as alcohol or caffeine consumption or tobacco use, may introduce apparent age effects. A reasonable approach seems to be that of (1) avoiding the presence of overt clinical diseases or administration of medications, and (2) carefully describing the study population and the selection criteria applied to all age groups.

An additional approach involves including individuals, from across the adult age range rather than just young and old adults. Such a strategy provides insight not only into the status of old individuals but also some view of the change in the variable during the life cycle. Since most age-related changes in physiologic variables have been found to be linear, the finding of a marked change in middle age or late middle age suggests the presence of an underlying disease process.

Clinical Relevance of Aging Changes

Once we define a normal change with age, it is important to understand that normality does not imply harmlessness. If healthy old individuals perform less well on glucose tolerance tests than young individuals, that does not imply that the carbohydrate intolerance of the elderly, which is "normal" for their age, is harmless. That conclusion would require a study of another dependent variable—for example, cardiovascular complications or death—because it may be that among normal 80-year-olds, those with the worst carbohydrate tolerance are actually at greater risk for these complications. Although systolic blood pressure increases "normally" with age, that does not mean that this increase is harmless. Advancing age is a risk factor for disease and death. Just because we define some age-related changes as normative, their potential adverse effects should not be overlooked.

On the other hand, it is important clinically to know which changes occur as a function of normal aging and which do not. Perhaps the

most important change that occurs with age is no change. Too frequently, physicians, because they lack a concept of normative aging, will ascribe a diagnosis to an individual with a normal age-related finding. Hematocrit, for instance, does not change with normal aging [2], and thus "anemia of old age" is not a meaningful diagnosis.

Cross-Sectional and Longitudinal Studies

Two general study designs are available to clinical gerontologists. In cross-sectional studies, groups of various ages are observed, and age-related differences are sought. In longitudinal studies, serial prospective measurements are obtained in one group of subjects at specified intervals, and the slopes for these variables or the age-related changes are determined. Since the human life span is so long, most longitudinal studies follow subjects in several age cohorts throughout the adult age range concurrently; thus, slopes for different ages can be compared.

Cross-sectional studies must be interpreted with caution because there are several ways in which they may not reflect true age-related changes. One error in design is based on a common misconception of the human life cycle. It is often assumed that the growth and development phase ends before the age of 20 and is followed by a prolonged "plateau phase", during which the biologic or physiologic variable under study is stable, and then, at about the age of 60 years, by the onset of a fairly rapid decline. However, in terms of most of the variables that have been found to change with age, the growth and development phase ends near the age of 20 to 30 years and is followed by a gradual, often linear, decline. Misconceptions of the life cycle have also introduced error into animal studies in which the animals (particularly rats) used as the young adult group were still undergoing rapid growth and development and had not yet reached maturity.

SELECTIVE MORTALITY

In the interpretation of cross-sectional studies it is important to remember that subjects over the age of 75 represent a sample of biologically superior survivors from a cohort that has experi-

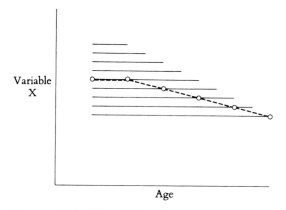

FIGURE 34-1. *Effect of selective mortality in a cross-sectional study. Horizontal lines indicate use of a prospective longitudinal study design. See text for further explanation.*

enced at least a 75 percent mortality. If the variable under study is related to survival, either because it is a risk factor or because it has a protective effect, a cross-sectional study will seem to show age-related differences that do not exist. This effect, called selective mortality, is shown in Figure 34-1. The figure concerns an imaginary study of the influence of age on the plasma concentration of "factor X," a risk factor that is found at widely varying levels in the population but does not change with age. Since X is related to survival, a group with a very high level will have a shortened life span, and, on the basis of this variable, a group with a low level will have a normal life span. In a cross-sectional study, values for the subjects 30 and 40 years old are similar in both means and variance. The 50-year-old cohort, however, has lost its members with the highest values, and the mean value is less, with a lower variance. This trend continues with advancing age, and the cross-sectional results wrongly suggest that factor X declines with age. This serious methodologic obstacle can be avoided with use of a prospective longitudinal study design, in which each subject is followed over time and the rate of change of each variable is calculated for each age group followed. As shown by the horizontal lines in Figure 34-1, no age effect is indicated if this method is applied to the study of factor X. An effect similar to that of selective mortality may be introduced in cross-sectional studies by any cause of variation in follow-up—including death, illness, or change in geographic location—that is related to the level of the variable under study.

CHANGES IN POPULATIONS

Non-age-dependent differences between age groups of a population may introduce error into age trends based on cross-sectional observations. The origin of the differences between age groups may be quite diverse, including educational, nutritional, environmental, and other influences that would result in misleading data regarding the possible effects of age. This type of effect is shown in Figure 34-2, which contains cross-sectional and longitudinal data from the Framingham Study on the impact of age on weight [2]. Whereas the cross-sectional data, based on a single examination, indicate a decline in weight with age, the longitudinal data, based on five examinations over a period of 18 years, suggest a different trend. The 35-year-old subjects are increasing weight rapidly and approaching a weight, eight years after their initial examination, that is clearly higher than that initially recorded for the 43-year-old subjects. Since the analysis includes only subjects who survived for at least 18 years after the first examination, neither selective mortality nor another cause of variation in follow-up study is responsible for this effect. The longitudinal data, shown by the lines in Figure 34-2, indicate

FIGURE 34-2. *Comparison of cross-sectional and longitudinal data on the impact of age on weight. See text for further explanation.*

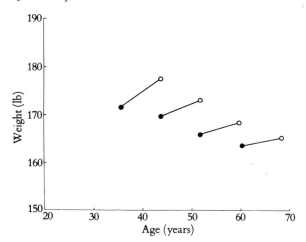

that weight is changing in the entire population and that the general tendency to gain weight decreases with age.

Drawbacks of Longitudinal Studies

Despite their advantages over cross-sectional studies, longitudinal studies may also have major drawbacks, including the need to observe a stable population over a long period and a particular sensitivity to alterations in methods. Subtle changes in laboratory techniques over several years may introduce "laboratory drifts" that are difficult to separate from age-related changes. An example is the "aging" of a sphygmomanometer. In addition, when subjects return at regular intervals and become increasingly familiar with the testing environment, a "learning" or "stress" effect may introduce error into serial measurements.

An example of such an effect is depicted in Table 34-1 in which systolic and diastolic blood pressures at the first seven biannual examinations of the Framingham Study are depicted. The data were selected from a population who had completed all seven examinations, thus removing the possibility of selective mortality or differential follow-up. The researchers set out to determine the influence of age on blood pressure and the impact of high blood pressure on morbidity from heart disease. At the first visit,

TABLE 34-1. *Stress effect in longitudinal studies**

| EXAMINATION NO. | BLOOD PRESSURE (MM HG) | |
	SYSTOLIC	DIASTOLIC
1	133.2	84.6
2	129.6	82.4
3	128.2	81.5
4	130.1	82.6
5	131.9	83.2
6	133.9	84.3
7	135.2	85.1

*Data are for entire study population of the Framingham Study. Examinations are at two-year intervals. To exclude the impact of differential follow-up, analysis includes only subjects present for all examinations.
SOURCE: Data from J. Gordon and D. Shurtleff. In W. B. Kannel and T. Gordon (eds.), *The Framingham Study: An Epidemiologic Investigation of Cardiovascular Disease.* DHEW Publication No. (NIH) 74-478. Washington, D.C.: U.S. Goverment Printing Office, 1973.

the averages were 133 systolic and 85 diastolic. Surprisingly, the second visit produced 129 systolic and 82 diastolic. At the third visit, blood pressure was 128 over 81 and still going down! Six years and many, many dollars later, the investigators had found out that blood pressure declines with age—which was very unlikely! On subsequent visits blood pressure rose, and the initial decrease is attributed to the "stress effect." Familiarity with the testing environment has a measureable effect. Four years passed before the first useful data for calculating slopes were collected. Perhaps one can make more frequent measures in the beginning to accustom participants to the testing environment rather than spending four years doing it. If one ignored the effect and calculated slopes using all the data, the slopes would be much less steep than those reflecting the actual effect of age.

Planning a Longitudinal Study

The major elements in a longitudinal study are the size of the samples, the frequency of measurements, and the duration of the study. Clearly, a variable that changes dramatically with age and is easily measured accurately need only be tested a few times before age-related changes are well defined. On the other hand, variables that change slowly with age and are difficult to measure accurately require frequent observations over a long period. Quantitation of the factors involved in the design of longitudinal studies has been made possible by the work of Schlesselman [3]. Appropriate strategies for each variable can now be estimated once reliable cross-sectional data or limited longitudinal data are available.

Recognition of these special considerations will improve the utility of the data for gerontologic studies and contribute to the necessary expansion of our understanding of the aging process as well as the interaction of aging-related and disease-related changes.

References

1. Rowe, J. W. Clinical research in aging: Strategies and directions. *N. Engl. J. Med.* 297:1332, 1977.
2. Gordon, J., and Shurtleff, D. In W. B. Kannel and

T. Gordon (eds.), *The Framingham Study: An Epidemiologic Investigation of Cardiovascular Disease*. DHEW Publication No. (NIH) 74-478. Washington, D.C.: U.S. Government Printing Office, 1973.

3. Schlesselman, J. J. Planning a longitudinal study: I. Sample size determination. II. Frequency of measurement and study duration. *J. Chronic Dis.* 26:553, 1973.

Index